# The Forensic Pharmacology of Drugs of Abuse

**OLAF H. DRUMMER PhD**

Victorian Institute of Forensic Medicine,
Victoria, Australia

With a contribution by

**Morris Odell**

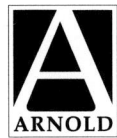

A member of the Hodder Headline Group
LONDON  NEW YORK  NEW DELHI

First published in Great Britain in 2001 by
Arnold, a member of the Hodder Headline Group,
338 Euston Road, London NW1 3BH

http://www.arnoldpublishers.com

Distributed in the United States of America by
Oxford University Press, Inc.,
198 Madison Avenue, New York NY10016
Oxford is a registered trademark of Oxford University Press

© 2001 Olaf H. Drummer and Morris Odell

All rights reserved. No part of this publication may be reproduced or transmitted in any form or by any means, electronically or mechanically, including photocopying, recording or any information storage or retrieval system, without either prior permission in writing from the publisher or a licence permitting restricted copying. In the United Kingdom such licences are issued by the Copyright Licensing Agency: 90 Tottenham Court Road, London W1P OLP.

Whilst the advice and information in this book are believed to be true and accurate at the date of going to press, neither the authors nor the publisher can accept any legal responsibility or liability for any errors or omissions that may be made. In particular (but without limiting the generality of the preceding disclaimer) every effort has been made to check drug dosages; however it is still possible that errors have been missed. Furthermore, dosage schedules are constantly being revised and new side effects recognized. For these reasons the reader is strongly urged to consult the drug companies' printed instructions before administering any of the drugs recommended in this book.

*British Library Cataloguing in Publication Data*
A catalogue record for this book is available from the British Library

*Library of Congress Cataloging-in-Publication Data*
A catalog record for this book is available from the Library of Congress

ISBN 0 340 76257 8 (hb)

1 2 3 4 5 6 7 8 9 10

Commissioning Editor: Georgina Bentliff
Editorial Assistant: Zoë Elliott
Production Editor: Lauren McAllister
Production Controller: Iain McWilliams

Typeset in 9.5/14 pt Sabon and 9/14 pt Gill Sans by Charon Tec Pvt. Ltd, Chennai, India
Printed and bound in Italy by Giunti

# Contents

| | |
|---|---|
| Foreword | xii |
| Preface | xiii |
| Acknowledgements | xiv |
| Abbreviations | xv |
| Definitions and glossary | xvi |

## 1 INTRODUCTORY ASPECTS OF DRUG ACTIONS — 1

### 1.1 General introduction — 2
- Use of drugs in the general community — 2
- Prevalence of drugs in sudden death — 2
- Manufacture and production of psychoactive drugs — 3
- Psychoactive substances — 4
- Alcohol — 5
- Opioids — 6
- Cannabis — 6
- The sedatives and hypnotics — 6
- Amphetamines, cocaine and other abused stimulants — 7
- Other drugs of abuse — 7
- Focus of this book — 7

### 1.2 Specimens and specimen collection procedures — 9
- Specimens and their relative merits — 9

### 1.3 Analysis and measurement — 17
- Cut-off levels and approved assays — 17
- Validation and uncertainty — 18
- Quality assurance — 21

### 1.4 Pharmacokinetics and duration of action — 22
- Absorption and bioavailability — 22
- Volume of distribution — 23
- Clearance — 25
- Half-life — 25
- Metabolism — 27
- Excretion — 28
- Duration of action — 29
- Metabolic interactions — 31

# Contents

|  |  |  |
|---|---|---|
|  | Pharmacokinetics in the elderly | 32 |
|  | Pharmacokinetics in disease states | 33 |
|  | Pharmacokinetics in obesity | 33 |
|  | Pharmacokinetics in children | 34 |
|  | Effect of blood loss and blood replacements | 34 |
| 1.5 | Tolerance and dependence | 36 |
|  | Defining drug dependency | 36 |
|  | Tolerance | 37 |
|  | Side effects and adverse reactions | 37 |
| 1.6 | Toxicology | 38 |
|  | Chemical instability | 38 |
|  | Metabolic changes | 38 |
|  | Postmortem redistribution | 39 |
|  | Other processes | 41 |
|  | Interpretation of toxicological information | 41 |
|  | References for Section 1 | 43 |

## 2 STIMULANTS — 49

|  |  |  |
|---|---|---|
|  | Foreword | 50 |
| 2.1 | Classification and sources of stimulants | 52 |
|  | Historical aspects | 52 |
|  | Structures and sources of amphetamine-like stimulants | 54 |
|  | Synopsis | 59 |
| 2.2 | Pharmacokinetics and duration of action | 60 |
|  | Metabolism | 60 |
|  | Absorption and half-life | 62 |
|  | Half-life | 67 |
|  | Excretion and urine detection times | 68 |
|  | Synopsis | 69 |
| 2.3 | Mechanisms of action | 71 |
|  | Amphetamines | 71 |
|  | Cocaine | 72 |
|  | Synopsis | 72 |
| 2.4 | Pharmacological actions and therapeutics | 74 |
|  | Amphetamines and related stimulants | 74 |
|  | Cocaine | 76 |
|  | Medical uses of stimulants | 77 |
|  | Synopsis | 77 |
| 2.5 | Adverse reactions, tolerance and dependence | 79 |
|  | Abuse potential | 79 |
|  | Adverse reactions | 79 |

| | | Tolerance | 80 |
|---|---|---|---|
| | | Dependence and abstinence | 81 |
| | | Synopsis | 82 |
| | 2.6 | Toxicology | 83 |
| | | Prevalence in forensic cases | 83 |
| | | Toxicology and pathology of stimulants | 84 |
| | | Toxicology and pathology of cocaine | 89 |
| | | Redistribution | 91 |
| | | Tissue concentrations | 91 |
| | | Synopsis | 91 |
| | 2.7 | Case reports | 93 |
| | | Case Report 2.1 Amphetamine- and cocaine-induced self-defence | 93 |
| | | Case Report 2.2 Speed and violence | 93 |
| | | Case Report 2.3 Rave to the grave | 94 |
| | | Case Report 2.4 Amphetamine-induced fatigue | 94 |
| | | Case Report 2.5 Cocaine intoxication leading to death | 94 |
| | | Case Report 2.6 Detection of amphetamine use at the workplace | 95 |
| | | References for Section 2 | 96 |
| 3 | | **BENZODIAZEPINES AND RELATED DRUGS** | **103** |
| | | Foreword | 104 |
| | 3.1 | Source and structures | 105 |
| | | Structural features of benzodiazepines | 105 |
| | | Classification of benzodiazepines | 110 |
| | | Other related anxiolytics and hypnotics | 111 |
| | | Synopsis | 114 |
| | 3.2 | Pharmacokinetics and duration of action | 116 |
| | | Absorption and bioavailability | 116 |
| | | Routes of metabolism | 119 |
| | | Enzyme systems involved in metabolism | 121 |
| | | Excretion | 121 |
| | | Duration of action | 123 |
| | | Metabolic interactions | 124 |
| | | Pharmacokinetics in various physiological states | 126 |
| | | Synopsis | 129 |
| | 3.3 | Mechanisms of action | 130 |
| | | Benzodiazepines | 130 |
| | | Barbiturates | 132 |
| | | Zolpidem and the imidazopyridines | 132 |
| | | Zopiclone and the cyclopyrrolones | 132 |

## Contents

|  |  |  |
|---|---|---|
| | Buspirone and the azapirones | 132 |
| | Synopsis | 133 |
| 3.4 | Pharmacological actions and therapeutics | 134 |
| | Indications for benzodiazepines | 134 |
| | Other hypnotics and sedatives | 136 |
| | Benzodiazepines in the elderly | 137 |
| | Non-medical uses of sedatives | 138 |
| | Therapeutics | 138 |
| | Synopsis | 140 |
| 3.5 | Adverse reactions and tolerance | 141 |
| | Benzodiazepines | 141 |
| | Effect on memory and cognitive functions | 142 |
| | Other anxiolytics | 146 |
| | Effect on driving | 146 |
| | Drug interactions | 147 |
| | Tolerance and dependence | 147 |
| | Barbiturates | 149 |
| | Buspirone, zolpidem and zopiclone | 149 |
| | Synopsis | 149 |
| 3.6 | Toxicology | 151 |
| | Use of benzodiazepines by drug users | 151 |
| | Toxic reactions to benzodiazepines | 151 |
| | Toxic reactions to barbiturates | 157 |
| | Toxic reactions to zolpidem | 157 |
| | Toxic reactions to zopiclone | 159 |
| | Tissue distribution of sedatives | 159 |
| | Synopsis | 161 |
| 3.7 | Case reports | 163 |
| | Case Report 3.1 Negative drug result | 163 |
| | Case Report 3.2 Paradoxical reaction to benzodiazepines | 163 |
| | Case Report 3.3 Behavioural aggression | 164 |
| | Case Report 3.4 Sexual and aggressive fantasies | 164 |
| | Case Report 3.5 Sexual disinhibition due to benzodiazepines | 165 |
| | Case Report 3.6 Death due to flunitrazepam | 165 |
| References for Section 3 | | 166 |

## 4  CANNABIS — 177

| | Foreword | 178 |
|---|---|---|
| 4.1 | Source and structures of cannabinoids | 179 |
| | Historical aspects and synonyms | 179 |

| | | | |
|---|---|---|---|
| | Cannabis species | | 179 |
| | Active constituents of *Cannabis sativa* | | 180 |
| | Cannabis products | | 181 |
| | Other substances with THC-like activity | | 181 |
| | Synopsis | | 182 |
| 4.2 | Pharmacokinetics and duration of action | | 183 |
| | Absorption and bioavailability | | 183 |
| | Prediction of time of administration | | 186 |
| | Metabolism and biological activity of metabolites | | 186 |
| | Excretion | | 188 |
| | Duration of action | | 189 |
| | Alternative sources of cannabinoids | | 194 |
| | Nabilone: a synthetic cannabinoid | | 195 |
| | Synopsis | | 195 |
| 4.3 | Mechanisms of action | | 197 |
| 4.4 | Pharmacological actions and therapeutics | | 198 |
| | Acute physiological effects | | 198 |
| | Acute behavioural changes | | 198 |
| | Chronic and adverse health effects | | 200 |
| | Medical uses | | 201 |
| | Synopsis | | 202 |
| 4.5 | Tolerance and dependence | | 203 |
| | Tolerance | | 203 |
| | Dependence | | 203 |
| | Synopsis | | 204 |
| 4.6 | Toxicology | | 205 |
| | Prevalence of THC in forensic cases | | 205 |
| | Contribution of cannabis use to death | | 205 |
| | Contribution to motor vehicle accidents | | 206 |
| | Impairing blood concentrations of THC | | 207 |
| | Synopsis | | 207 |
| 4.7 | Case reports | | 209 |
| | Case Report 4.1 Proof of cannabis use | | 209 |
| | Case Report 4.2 THC back calculation | | 209 |
| | Case Report 4.3 Cannabis intoxication while driving – 1 | | 210 |
| | Case Report 4.4 Cannabis intoxication while driving – 2 | | 211 |
| | References for Section 4 | | 212 |
| 5 | **OPIOIDS** | | **219** |
| | Foreword | | 220 |

## Contents

| | | | |
|---|---|---|---|
| 5.1 | Source and structures | | 221 |
| | Sources of opioids | | 221 |
| | Structural features | | 222 |
| | Synopsis | | 224 |
| 5.2 | Pharmacokinetics and duration of action | | 225 |
| | Absorption and bioavailability | | 225 |
| | Pharmacokinetics in various physiological states | | 230 |
| | Pharmacokinetic profiles of selected opioids | | 231 |
| | Synopsis | | 237 |
| 5.3 | Mechanisms of action | | 238 |
| | Mu-opioid receptor | | 238 |
| | Delta-opioid receptor | | 238 |
| | Kappa-opioid receptor | | 239 |
| | Other actions | | 239 |
| | Synopsis | | 239 |
| 5.4 | Pharmacological actions and therapeutics | | 241 |
| | Uses of opioids | | 241 |
| | Side effects of opioids | | 242 |
| | Non-medical uses of opioids | | 244 |
| | Therapeutics | | 244 |
| | Synopsis | | 245 |
| 5.5 | Adverse reactions and dependence | | 246 |
| | Dependence and tolerance | | 246 |
| | Withdrawal symptoms | | 246 |
| | Important drug interactions | | 247 |
| | Synopsis | | 248 |
| 5.6 | Toxicology | | 249 |
| | Heroin and morphine | | 249 |
| | Other opioids | | 253 |
| | Toxic concentrations of opioids | | 258 |
| | Distinguishing source of opioid from urine profile | | 258 |
| | Ingestion of poppy seeds and morphine excretion | | 259 |
| | Synopsis | | 260 |
| 5.7 | Case reports | | 261 |
| | Case Report 5.1 Occupational drug testing | | 261 |
| | Case Report 5.2 Acute heroin death | | 261 |
| | Case Report 5.3 Delayed heroin death | | 262 |
| | Case Report 5.4 Methadone death | | 263 |
| | References for Section 5 | | 265 |

# 6 ETHANOL — 273

Foreword — 274

## 6.1 Types and sources of alcohol — 275
- Structures of alcohols — 275
- Physical properties of alcohols — 275
- Historical aspects and source — 276
- Alcoholic content of beverages — 276
- Alcoholic content of commercial products — 277
- Synopsis — 277

## 6.2 Pharmacokinetics, metabolism and duration of action — 278
- Absorption — 278
- Metabolism — 281
- Excretion and detection times — 284
- Drugs affecting absorption and elimination — 285
- Markers of alcohol consumption — 286
- Duration of action — 287
- Effects of alcohol on drug pharmacokinetics — 287
- Synopsis — 289

## 6.3 Mechanisms of action — 290
- CNS mechanisms — 290
- Peripheral mechanisms — 291
- Synopsis — 291

## 6.4 Pharmacological actions and therapeutics — 292
- CNS effects — 292
- Cardiovascular system — 293
- Liver and gastrointestinal system — 293
- Other effects — 294
- Therapeutic uses of ethanol — 295
- Synopsis — 296

## 6.5 Adverse reactions, tolerance and dependence — 297
- Abuse potential — 297
- Adverse reactions — 297
- Tolerance — 298
- Dependence and abstinence — 298
- Synopsis — 299

## 6.6 Toxicology — 300
- Prevalence in forensic cases — 300
- Fermentation — 301
- Collection artefacts — 301

## Contents

|  |  |
|---|---|
| Redistribution and diffusion | 301 |
| Tissue concentrations | 302 |
| Toxicology and pathology of ethanol | 305 |
| Adverse drug interactions | 307 |
| Synopsis | 307 |

### 6.7 Case reports — 309
| Case Report 6.1 Alcohol read-back 1 | 309 |
|---|---|
| Case Report 6.2 Alcohol read-back 2 | 310 |
| Case Report 6.3 Alcohol and homicide | 311 |
| Case Report 6.4 Alcohol and putrefaction | 311 |

References for Section 6 — 313

## 7 OTHER DRUGS OF ABUSE — 321

Foreword — 322

### 7.1 LSD — 323
| Source and structures | 323 |
|---|---|
| Tissue concentrations, metabolism and excretion | 323 |
| Mechanism of action | 324 |
| Pharmacological actions and adverse reactions | 324 |
| Toxicity | 324 |

### 7.2 Phencyclidine and related hallucinogens — 326
| Mechanism of action | 326 |
|---|---|
| Pharmacological actions and adverse reactions | 327 |
| Tissue concentrations, metabolism and excretion | 327 |
| Toxicity | 328 |

### 7.3 Gamma-hydroxy butyrate — 329
| Tissue concentrations, metabolism and excretion | 329 |
|---|---|
| Pharmacological actions and adverse reactions | 329 |
| Mechanism of action | 330 |
| Toxicity | 330 |

### 7.4 Volatile substances — 331
| Types of volatile substances | 331 |
|---|---|
| Tissue concentration, metabolism and excretion | 332 |
| Mechanism and frequency of use | 332 |
| Pharmacological actions and adverse effects | 332 |

### 7.5 Case reports — 334
| Case Report 7.1 PCP and violent behaviour leading to death | 334 |
|---|---|

| | | |
|---|---|---|
| | Case Report 7.2 Driving while intoxicated with GHB | 334 |
| | Case Report 7.3 GHB withdrawal | 334 |
| | Case Report 7.4 GHB intoxication | 335 |
| | References for Section 7 | 336 |

# 8 CLINICAL FORENSIC ASPECTS OF DRUG USE 339

| | | |
|---|---|---|
| | Foreword | 340 |
| 8.1 | Reasons for a forensic medical examination | 341 |
| 8.2 | Health status of drug users | 344 |
| 8.3 | Principles of an examination scheme for drug-affected persons | 345 |
| | Obtaining a history | 345 |
| | The examination | 345 |
| 8.4 | Clinical forensic opinions | 348 |
| 8.5 | Common drug effects seen in clinical medicine | 349 |
| | Stimulants | 349 |
| | Benzodiazepines | 351 |
| | Cannabis | 353 |
| | Opioids | 354 |
| | Alcohol | 357 |
| 8.6 | Case reports | 360 |
| | Case Report 8.1 Fitness for interview | 360 |
| | Case Report 8.2 Drug-affected driving and doctor shopping | 360 |
| | Case Report 8.3 Benzodiazepine overdose | 362 |
| | Case Report 8.4 Methadone toxicity | 363 |
| | Case Report 8.5 Alcohol intoxication | 364 |
| | References for Section 8 | 365 |

## APPENDIX – MONOGRAPHS OF SELECTED DRUGS 367

| | |
|---|---|
| Explanations to monographs | 368 |
| Stimulants | 369 |
| Benzodiazepines | 382 |
| Other sedatives and anxiolytics | 406 |
| Opioids and related drugs | 413 |
| Other monographs | 435 |
| References for Appendix | 442 |

Index 451

# Foreword

Associate Professor Olaf Drummer is a toxicologist and forensic pharmacologist of outstanding repute both in Australia and internationally. It has been my privilege to observe his work at first hand in his position as head of the scientific and research laboratories at the Victorian Institute of Forensic Medicine. And so, it is a pleasure and an honour to write the foreword to this important and informative book. Professor Drummer is also a member of several professional organisations, including the Australian Academy of Forensic Sciences, the Australasian Society for Clinical and Experimental Pharmacology and Toxicology, and the Royal Australian Chemical Institute. He has published over 200 scientific articles related to forensic toxicology and pharmacology.

The scholarship underpinning this book is impeccable. So is the author's attention to detail. He has drawn on his rich knowledge and experience in its compilation.

Drug abuse is a major problem in our society, and many cases that come before our courts are linked to the misuse of drugs. Practitioners working in the field of criminal law, both legal and medical, need to understand patterns of drug usage in the community, the effect that certain drugs have on the human body, and then interpret and apply this information in court proceedings. Forensic pharmacology and toxicology are overlapping fields of science that have become important tools in the law and provide valuable information about the properties of drugs, and the effects that these drugs have on the people using them. In this book the author has categorised the major drugs of abuse in our society today, compiled a comprehensive account of their pharmacological and toxicological properties, and provided case reports to demonstrate their application in court. This book will be, I am sure, a most helpful and authoritative resource for practitioners.

It constitutes a valuable addition to the medico/legal literature.

John Harber Phillips
Chief Justice of Victoria and Chairman of the Council
Victorian Institute of Forensic Medicine
Melbourne, Australia

# Preface

The scope of this book is to provide a comprehensive account of the pharmacological, pharmacokinetic and toxicological properties of the most common drugs of abuse that require expert evidence in courts – the stimulants, the opioids, the benzodiazepines, cannabis, alcohol and others, including the hallucinogens and GHB.

Opioids include heroin and morphine, and other members used in therapeutic practice for analgesia, as well as those used illicitly as drugs-of-abuse.

The amphetamines include 'speed' as well as the designer amphetamines such as 'ecstasy', Adam and Eve, and those drugs used as weak stimulants or as weight-reducing tablets, which can exhibit amphetamine-like properties in high doses. Cocaine is included in this group since it shares many pharmacological similarities with the amphetamines.

Benzodiazepines are a family of drugs known as minor tranquillizers, which include Valium, Normison, Rohypnol, etc. and a series of related sedatives and hypnotics. They are important from a medical point of view since they act on the brain centres involved in thought processes and memory and control of hand–eye–foot movements involved in driving motor vehicles. Benzodiazepines can produce profound changes in behaviour, particularly if abused, and are often a factor in court proceedings.

The pharmacology and pharmacokinetics of the single drugs alcohol and cannabis are covered in separate sections including the effects of their combination.

A section is included to cover the effect of other drugs-of-abuse less commonly encountered in forensic medicine. These include the hallucinogens LSD, PCP, ketamine, GHB, and volatile substances.

An appendix containing monographs for the common drugs-of-abuse discussed in the book is included to provide a quick guide to the most important chemical, toxicological and pharmacokinetic properties of each drug.

The book also contains accounts of actual case examples of how these disciplines can and have been used in court cases and illustrates deficiencies in what conclusions can be drawn from toxicological data.

The aim is to provide a sufficiently authoritative book on the forensic application of pharmacology and toxicology of these drugs to the needs of the law and is directed to legal and medical practitioners and to other experts in the field of pharmacology and toxicology who are involved in interpreting toxicological data for court proceedings.

Olaf H. Drummer<br>Melbourne, Australia

# Acknowledgements

A number of people contributed to the production of this book whose comments and helpful advice are sincerely appreciated. These include Dr Barry Logan from the Washington State Patrol, Dr Michael Robertson formerly of National Medical Services and now the San Diego Medical Examiner facilities, Dr John Caplehorn, epidemiologist and physician, Westmead Hospital and the University of Sydney, Dr David Wells, clinical forensic physician at the Victorian Institute of Forensic Medicine, Dr Jim Gerostamoulos, toxicologist at the Institute, Barrister Francine McNiff, Victorian Director of Public Prosecutions Mr Geoff Flatman, supreme court judges Justice John Coldrey and Frank Vincent, and county court judge John Barnett.

I thank Dr Morris Odell, clinical forensic physician at the Victorian Institute of Forensic Medicine, for writing the section on clinical forensic medicine and assisting with the remainder of the book.

I would also like to particularly thank Kerry Johannes, librarian at the Victorian Institute of Forensic Medicine, who provided so much of my material and references, Professor Stephen Cordner, director of the Institute and the Council members who graciously provided the support to conduct this project. Gratitude goes to Ceril Pereira, my secretarial assistant who provided significant help through the various stages of the book. The assistance of various other members of the Institute is also acknowledged.

Finally, an enormous gratitude goes to my family, particularly my wife Christine who patiently endured months of my solitary confinement and messy papers scattered throughout the house, and to my parents, without whose help my education would not have been possible.

# Abbreviations

| | |
|---|---|
| 5-HT | 5-Hydroxy-tryptophan, or serotonin |
| 6-AM | 6-Acetylmorphine (heroin metabolite) |
| AUC | Area under curve (of blood or plasma drug concentrations over a given period of time) |
| Cl | Clearance (of drugs) |
| $C_{max}$ | Maximum blood concentration |
| $C_{ss}$ | Steady-state blood concentration (during chronic dosing) |
| CV | Coefficient of variation |
| DUID | Driving under the influence of drugs |
| EMIT | Enzyme-multiplied immunoassay |
| GC | Gas chromatography |
| HPLC | High-performance liquid chromatography |
| $K_P$ | Octanol-buffer partition coefficient (often as logarithm) |
| LOQ | Limit of quantitation |
| LSD | Lysergic acid diethylamide |
| MDA | Methylenedioxyamphetamine |
| MDEA | Methylenedioxyethylamphetamine |
| MDMA | Methylenedioxymethamphetamine |
| mg/L | Milligram per litre |
| ng/mL | Nanogram per millilitre |
| PCP | Phencyclidine |
| SD | Standard deviation of the mean |
| $T_{1/2}$ | Half-life |
| THC | $\Delta^9$-Tetrahydrocannabinol |
| $T_{max}$ | Time to maximum concentration |
| $V_D$ | Volume of distribution |
| % | Gram per 100 mL (by weight) |

# Definitions and glossary

| | |
|---|---|
| Abuse potential | The relative potential for a drug to be abused for its pleasurable drug effects. |
| Acetylcholine | Neurotransmitter, involved in transmission of nerve impulses in cholinergic nerves. |
| Acidosis | Low pH of blood. |
| Addiction | A fully-fledged state of drug dependence in which drug withdrawal leads to profound drug-seeking behaviour. See also Dependence. |
| Adrenergic | Nerves utilizing noradrenaline (norepinephrine) as transmitter, e.g. sympathetic nerves. |
| Agonist | A chemical which has the capacity to excite specific receptors and elicit a pharmacological response. |
| Agoraphobia | A feeling of fear at the thought of being alone in an open space. |
| Amnesia | Lack or loss of memory. |
| Analgesic | Pain-relieving medication. |
| Anergia | Decreased physical and psychological energy. |
| Anhedonia | Inability to experience pleasure. |
| Angina (pectoris) | Spasmodic choking or suffocative pain due to anoxia of the myocardium. |
| Antagonist | A chemical which opposes the action of an agonist. |
| Antitussive | Cough suppressant. |
| Apnoea | Transient cessation of the breathing impulse that follows breathing; asphyxia. |
| Aspiration | Breathing or drawing in of gastric material into lungs. |
| Ataxia | Poor co-ordination. |
| Automatism | Performance of non-reflex acts without conscious volition. |
| Autonomic nervous system | The part of the nervous system under involuntary control. |
| Bioavailability | The fraction of drug that is available to the systemic circulation after absorption. Usually refers to the difference in availability between intravenously administered drug and when the same dose is applied through the route in question, e.g. oral. |
| Bradycardia | Low heart rate. |
| Central nervous system | The brain and spinal cord. |

# Definitions and glossary

| | |
|---|---|
| Cholinergic | Nerves utilizing acetylcholine as transmitter, e.g. parasympathetic nerves. |
| Clinical pharmacology | The study of drugs in subjects with particular reference to the study of the pharmacodynamics and pharmacokinetics of drugs. |
| Confirmation test | Test that unequivocally establishes presence of a chemical substance. |
| Cut-off levels | Analytical term referring to an arbitrary concentration below which immunoassay responses or confirmatory results are deemed to be negative. |
| Dependence (drug) | A state in which a person has either a psychological or physiological desire to continue using a drug. |
| Detection limit | Effective lowest concentration limit when a true response is detected. |
| Drug | A chemical, or collection of chemicals such as in herbal remedies, used to alter the physiological or psychological state of a living being, often for the prevention or treatment of disease states. |
| Dysphoria | Disquiet, restlessness, malaise. |
| Enkephalin | Endogenous peptide responsible for opioid-like activity. |
| Entero-hepatic recirculation | The process of re-absorption of drugs from the bowel after being excreted into bile from the liver. |
| Euphoria | Bodily comfort, well-being, absence of pain or distress; an exaggerated sense of well-being. |
| First-pass effect | The degree to which orally administered drugs are metabolized in their first pass through the liver prior to reaching the systemic circulation. |
| First-pass metabolism | The metabolism of drugs during their first-passes through the liver, after oral absorption. |
| Forensic pharmacology | The application of pharmacology to the needs of the law. |
| Forensic toxicology | Deals generally with the toxicological issues in court proceedings and more particularly is concerned with the science of measuring biological specimens for the presence of poisons. |
| Haematocrit | Proportion of red blood cells in whole blood. |
| Haemolysis | Loss of haemoglobin from red blood cells into plasma caused by rupture of cells. |
| Half-life | A pharmacokinetic term to describe the approximate time taken to halve blood concentration of the drug during the terminal phase of drug elimination. |
| Hyperdipsia | Increased intake of water. |
| Hyperphagia | Ingestion of greater than optimal quantity of food. |
| Insomnia | A pathological inability to sleep. Drugs that are used to treat insomnia, and other disorders leading to sleep deprivation, are termed hypnotics. This should not be confused with hypnosis conducted by psychiatrists and other health professionals, although hypnotic drugs can be used to assist in producing a hypnotic state. |

# Definitions and glossary

| | |
|---|---|
| Limit of quantitation (LOQ) | Lowest concentration at which a substance can be accurately measured – best defined as lowest concentration with a CV of 20%. |
| Neuroadaptation | The development of tolerance, either physiological or psychological. |
| Nystagmus | The jerking movement of eyes when moved to their furthest sideways (horizontal) or vertical movement (vertical gaze). |
| Opioids | Substances which act like morphine; opiates. |
| Pharmacodynamics | The study of the relationship between pharmacological effect of a drug with time. |
| Pharmacokinetics | The study and characterization of the time course of drug absorption, distribution, metabolism and excretion. |
| Pharmacology | The science of drugs; deals with understanding their actions and their uses. When knowledge of drug actions are applied to court proceedings, the term 'forensic pharmacology' is used. |
| Poison | Any drug can be a poison in the right circumstance, as can any other chemical substance, and inflict serious harm or even death on a living being. |
| Pro-drug | A substance that is converted metabolically to an active drug after administration. |
| Psychoses | Behavioural disorders. |
| Receptor | Specific recognition site in tissues that is usually functionally connected to a physiological response. |
| Respiration | Process of breathing. |
| Rhabdomyolysis | Disintegration or dissolution of muscle. |
| Screening test | An initial test to show the possible presence of a chemical substance. |
| Sedative | A drug which has calming or tranquillizing action. |
| Serotonin (5-HT) | Neurotransmitter in the brain often involved in affective conditions. |
| Somnolence | Sleepiness or unnatural drowsiness. |
| Terminal elimination phase | The stage of elimination of drug well beyond the time taken to absorb and distribute drug to tissues, usually reflected by the last stage of drug removal from the blood stream. |
| Tolerance | This refers to the physiological state in which drug use has led to a diminution of drug effects resulting in an increase in dose to achieve the original pharmacological effects. |
| Toxicology | The science concerned with the understanding of the toxic effects of drugs and other chemicals. |
| Validation (of testing methods) | The process of establishing that an analytical method is fit for purpose and meets established performance criteria. |
| Volume of distribution | Artificial volume that a drug distributes to the body, defined by the total amount of drug in the body (absorbed dose) by the plasma concentration time at zero. |

# 1 Introductory aspects of drug actions

| | | |
|---|---|---|
| 1.1 | General introduction | 2 |
| 1.2 | Specimens and specimen collection procedures | 9 |
| 1.3 | Analysis and measurement | 17 |
| 1.4 | Pharmacokinetics and duration of action | 22 |
| 1.5 | Tolerance and dependence | 36 |
| 1.6 | Toxicology | 38 |
| **References for Section 1** | | 43 |

# 1.1 General introduction

One of the biggest problems facing society today is the abuse and misuse of drugs. There are numerous drugs available to the community at large. However, the drugs of greatest concern are the psychoactive on the central nervous system (CNS) and are therefore subject to abuse. Many offenders charged with violent crimes, or victims of violent crime, may have been under the influence of psychoactive drugs at the time a crime was committed. Drugs-of-abuse are not only associated with violent crimes. The use of such mind-altering drugs in places of employment, by drivers of motor vehicles, or even to enhance performance in athletic events and sports place other members of the community at risk. Therefore, it is important to understand the possible pharmacological effects associated with the use of these drugs.

## USE OF DRUGS IN THE GENERAL COMMUNITY

The use of drugs for recreational reasons is widespread. Surveys in Australia show that ~30% of the population have used a psychoactive drug for pleasure at some stage in their life, with ~15% using such a drug regularly. The younger population is more likely to use a psychoactive drug, rates being estimated to be as high as 50% in some groups. The most common illegal drugs are cannabis (marijuana), amphetamines, cocaine and heroin.[i]

Surveys in the USA show 34% of full-time college students have used illicit drugs in the last year, of which 28.7% used cannabis, 7.9% used inhalants, 6.8% used LSD, 4.4% used tranquillizers, 4.5% used cocaine, and 4.7% used heroin and other opioids. The use of these drugs in the previous 30 days was collectively 1.8%.[ii] Alcohol was used by 62% in the last month and 81% in the last year.[1]

Household surveys have been conducted in Australia and the USA. These show valuable data on the frequency of use of illicit and other drugs (Table 1.1). Illicit drug use in the last 12 months (1998) consists mainly of cannabis followed by cocaine, heroin, amphetamines, and hallucinogens such as ecstasy and LSD. Similar use of drugs probably exists in other developed countries, and increasingly in other parts of the world.

## PREVALENCE OF DRUGS IN SUDDEN DEATH

The prevalence of drugs in various categories of sudden and unexpected death is shown in Table 1.2. These results show that alcohol is a frequent association with car accidents, homicides, drug deaths and suicides. Other drugs of abuse show significant differences in their prevalence in different types of sudden death. The benzodiazepines show an incidence of

---

[i] *Victorian Drug Strategy Statistics Handbook*, October 1993.
[ii] National Institute on Drug Abuse, http://www.nida.org.

# General introduction

**Table 1.1** Prevalence of drug use in Australia and the USA – surveys of use in the last 12 months – 1998

|  | Australia[a] (%) | USA[b] (%) |
|---|---|---|
| Tobacco | 26 | 31 |
| Alcohol | 81 | 64 |
| Cannabis products | 18 | 8.6 |
| Amphetamines/stimulants | 3.6 | 0.7 |
| Tranquillizers | 3.0 | 0.9 |
| Hallucinogens | 3.0 | 1.6 |
| Cocaine | 1.4 | 1.7 |
| Inhalants | 0.8 | 0.9 |
| Heroin | 0.7 | 0.1 |
| Barbiturates | 0.2 | – |
| Any illicit drug | 22 | 6.2 |

[a] 1998 National Household Survey, aged 14 years and over (Ref. 2); [b] USA 1998 National Household Survey, aged 12 years and older, see www.samsha.gov/NHSDA.htm.

**Table 1.2** Incidence of drugs of abuse in various types of death (%)

| Type of death | Ethanol | Opioids[a] | Benzodiazepines | Stimulants[b] | Cannabis |
|---|---|---|---|---|---|
| Natural death | 15 | 13 | 9.4 | 1.4 | 2.3 |
| Homicide | 38 | 11 | 11 | 4.0 | 16 |
| Drivers of motor vehicles | 27 | 6.2 | 4.3 | 4.3 | 16 |
| Non-drug-related suicide | 33 | 10 | 21 | 2.9 | 13 |
| Licit drug death | 40 | 41 | 59 | 3.2 | 8.0 |
| Illicit drug death | 35 | 96 | 61 | 7.1 | 38 |
| All cases | 27 | 20 | 20 | 3.1 | 12 |

Data obtained from 2000 coroners' cases for deaths occurring in 1997. [a] Includes codeine and propoxyphene; [b] includes legal stimulants, amphetamines and cocaine.

almost 60% in drug deaths, but only ~4% in drivers killed in car accidents. As expected, the opioids dominate the illicit drug deaths, and the amphetamine-like stimulants, including cocaine, show a relatively small prevalence in all types of death, with the highest being in the illicit drug deaths. Cannabis is found in all types of cases.

## MANUFACTURE AND PRODUCTION OF PSYCHOACTIVE DRUGS

The activities of the International Narcotics Control Board (INCB),[iii] a division of the United Nations (UN), collate information on the manufacture, production and seizures of drugs

---

[iii] Available at http://www.undcp.org.

from member countries who are signatories to the Convention on Narcotic Drugs of 1961 and its amended 1972 protocol.

In 1995 production of morphine from opium poppy in legal plantations is estimated to be 236.7 tonnes. This is the equivalent of over 20 billion 10-mg morphine tablets. Much of this morphine goes to codeine production (76%), while other narcotics produced from morphine are dihydrocodeine (12%), pholcodine (3%) and ethylmorphine (1%). These figures do not account for the illegal production of morphine in certain countries, nor do they account for the synthetic manufacture of opioids such as fentanyl and methadone.[3]

Worldwide estimates of the use of benzodiazepines vary. Statistics produced by the UN over the 10 years to 1996 show over 22 billion daily doses of benzodiazepines were used each year throughout the world. This estimate is conservative since some major manufacturers of benzodiazepines do not report their production statistics. On the basis of the figures provided, anxiolytics accounted for ~15 billion doses, and hypnotics ~7 billion doses. The most common anxiolytic benzodiazepines manufactured were diazepam (34% of total manufacture), lorazepam (29%), alprazolam (11%), chlordiazepoxide (6%), and others (20%). The most common hypnotic benzodiazepine was temazepam (23%), nitrazepam (23%), lormetazepam (20%), estazolam (11%), triazolam (9%), and others (14%).

As expected, there are wide variations in types of benzodiazepine available in each country, and their relative prescription frequency. For example, in 1994 haloxazolam and nimetazepam were only available in Japan, whereas diazepam was imported into 89 countries and territories.

Amphetamine production is largely for illicit purposes through clandestine laboratories. The most common are amphetamine, methamphetamine and methylenedioxymethamphetamine (MDMA). Amphetamines are mainly produced in the UK, the Netherlands and Belgium, although significant production exists elsewhere including Asia.[4] Depending on local clandestine activities and ease of importation, local differences exist in the availability of the amphetamine class of drugs.

LSD is one of the oldest illicit drugs and is still widely available throughout the world. In Australia and New Zealand, some 3% of the population have used the drug in the last 12 months. Production is still believed to occur largely in California.[4]

Other hallucinogens such as mescaline, PCP, psilocybin and hyoscine are used by relatively few people in localized areas where such drugs or plant products are available.

Cannabis is widely available in almost all countries of the world, and is arguably the most widely used illicit drug. Its ready growth as a plant in most climates, including its adaptation to hydroponic culture, makes it a cheap and convenient drug for recreational use.

GHB is becoming increasingly available throughout the world, as are other drugs-of-abuse such as khat.

## PSYCHOACTIVE SUBSTANCES

The principal drugs of concern can be divided into the categories shown in Table 1.3.

**General introduction**

Table 1.3  Principal classes of psychoactive substances

| | | |
|---|---|---|
| **CNS depressants** | | |
| 1 | Ethanol[a] | All alcoholic beverages (alcohol) |
| 2 | Benzodiazepines[b] | Alprazolam, diazepam, flunitrazepam, oxazepam, temazepam, triazolam, etc. |
| 3 | Opioids[c] | Codeine, heroin, methadone, morphine, oxycodone, pethidine (meperidine), etc. |
| 4 | Antipsychotics[d] | Chlorpromazine, clozapine, fluphenazine, haloperidol, olanzapine thioridazine, trifluoperazine, etc. |
| 5 | Antidepressants[e] | Amitriptyline, doxepin, dothiepin, fluoxetine, moclobemide, sertraline, venlafaxine, paroxetine, etc. |
| 6 | Marijuana[f] | Various forms of *Cannabis sativa* containing tetrahydrocannabinol |
| 7 | Barbiturates | Amylobarbital, butobarbital, secobarbital, phenobarbital, thiopental, etc. |
| **CNS stimulants**[g] | | |
| 8 | Amphetamines | 'Speed' (methamphetamine), 'ecstasy' (methylenedioxymethamphetamine) and others |
| 9 | Cocaine | Free base 'crack' and hydrochloride |
| 10 | Other stimulants | Ephedrine, pseudoephedrine, phentermine, fenfluramine, diethylpropion, etc. |
| **Other substances** | | |
| 11 | Inhalants[h] | Petrol, solvents, propane (LPG), paint, butane lighter fluid, etc. |
| 12 | Hallucinogens[i] | LSD, ecstasy, plant-derived substances such as mescaline, psilocybin, scopolamine, etc. |
| 13 | Phencyclidine | Usually abbreviated as PCP, and ketamine |
| 14 | Anabolic steroids | Testosterone, stanozolol, etc. |

[a] Common alcohol available in numerous forms from light beer (1–2.5%), to full-strength beer (~5%), wine (8–12%) and spirits (20–40%). [b] These drugs are prescribed as hypnotics (sleeping pills), minor tranquillizers to reduce anxiety, as muscle relaxants and as anti-epileptic drugs, and include some 13 different drugs within the group. [c] These drugs include the drugs of addiction, as well as weaker analgesics such as codeine which are available in numerous over-the-counter and prescription medications. [d] These major tranquillizers are usually prescribed to people with psychoses, schizophrenia and other mental disorders. [e] Antidepressants include both the older tricyclic and tetracyclic groups, and the newer monoamine oxidase inhibitors (type A) and the serotonin re-uptake inhibitors. [f] The active chemical in this plant is $\Delta^9$-tetrahydrocannabinol (THC) and a number of other 'cannabinoids'. [g] This group includes the amphetamines and designer variations as well as the ephedrine-type stimulants used in common cold preparations and slimming tablets. [h] While inhalants are not drugs, they are used recreationally and are recognized as mind-altering substances. Approximately 4% of the population have used inhalants. [i] There are a number of potential hallucinogens including certain species of mushrooms (psilocybin) and from a number of members of the Solanacea family including 'angel's trumpets' (scopolamine).

# ALCOHOL

Ethanol, better known as alcohol, is a simple chemical produced by the fermentation of fruits and other food products. It is widely available as a legal drug packaged in a vast variety of beverages and food products. Unfortunately, it is the most common drug encountered in forensic medicine, and despite its structural simplicity has a complex pharmacology. Alcohol is almost always taken orally, although it is often used by people consuming other drugs.

Other alcohols are only occasionally of interest in forensic cases, and include methanol and some higher alcohols.

## OPIOIDS

Drugs related to morphine comprise a large number of naturally occurring, semi-synthetic and synthetic drugs, all of which share a common property: they act as narcotic drugs and regular users can expect to exhibit major tolerance and dependence phenomena. Opioids have a widespread general medical and specialist use in the treatment of people with pain and undergoing surgical procedures.

The main licit members of this family of drugs are morphine, oxycodone, pethidine (meperidine), methadone, fentanyl, and many others. Heroin is another opioid that has plagued society for decades. This (largely) illicit drug derives from acetylating morphine and is rapidly converted to morphine following administration.

Other members such as codeine, dextromethorphan, dihydrocodeine, ethylmorphine, pholcodine, etc. are relatively weak opioids and used as mild pain relievers and/or as antitussives and show relatively little abuse potential.

The abuse of opioids can lead to serious medical and social harm that often presents in court hearings.

## CANNABIS

Cannabis in its various forms is arguably the second most commonly abused drug after alcohol. While cannabis contains many active substances, $\Delta^9$-tetrahydrocannabinol (THC) is the most important. For many years THC was regarded as a plant-derived chemical producing an unnatural psychic high. However, THC is now regarded as interacting specifically with receptors (recognition sites) in the brain (and elsewhere) modifying the activity of endogenous chemical mediators. Importantly, it is now recognized that THC enhances the activity of other drugs of abuse, notably opioids, and possibly many other drugs. The ability of THC to modify behaviour and psychomotor activity places this drug into an increasingly important role in forensic medicine.

## THE SEDATIVES AND HYPNOTICS

The benzodiazepines are arguably one of the most common class of drug used throughout Australia and the Western world. They are a large family of structurally related drugs, all of which possess an ability to act as sedatives and hypnotics. The benzodiazepines have a relatively wide therapeutic index (wide margin between medical benefit and toxicity), minimal serious adverse reactions, and the absence of undesirable central nervous system side effects when compared with the barbiturates and other older sedative and hypnotic drugs.

They have a widespread general medical and specialist psychiatric use in the treatment of people with sleep disorders, in a variety of anxiety-related conditions including panic and phobic disorders, and in many other conditions.

Other anxiolytics and hypnotics in current use include zopiclone, belonging to the cyclopyrrolone class of drugs, zolipdem, zaleplon and buspirone. The grandfathers of sedatives, chloral hydrate, meprobamate and the barbiturates, while still used in some parts of the world, have largely been replaced by the newer generation drugs. Users of chloral hydrate, meprobamate and barbiturates were liable to become severely dependent on long-term use and these drugs had a narrow margin between therapeutic response and toxicity. Consequently, these drugs are now uncommonly prescribed in developed countries especially when benzodiazepines and the newer generation of sedatives are available for prescription.

Drugs such as the sedating anti-histamines, e.g. doxylamine and diphenhydramine, also possess sedating activity but find little use as sedatives. Clearly, their primary pharmacological properties for the treatment of a variety of allergic conditions determine the medical indications for their use. A number of other drugs including many of the older antidepressant drugs (the tricyclic antidepressants), many of the major tranquillizer drugs used to treat a variety of mental disorders, and propranolol, a drug used to treat angina, high blood pressure and migraines, also possess sedative actions.

## AMPHETAMINES, COCAINE AND OTHER ABUSED STIMULANTS

Amphetamines such as speed or ecstasy are well-known illegal drugs and are members of another large family of drugs that behave as CNS stimulants. They are all subject to clandestine manufacture from a variety of cheap and readily available raw materials, most of which are now controlled by many countries. Abuse of these drugs can lead to disturbing behavioural changes and are often associated with violent crimes.

Many of the legal stimulants prescribed as nasal decongestants or used as slimming tablets are either abused or are converted chemically to stronger stimulants. These include ephedrine, diethylpropion, pseudoephedrine, phentermine and fenfluramine.

Cocaine, the naturally occurring alkaloid from a South American plant (*Coca erythroxylon*), is also widely abused, and together with the amphetamines, can produce disturbing psychological and physiological changes in personality. Violent crimes are also often associated with this drug.

## OTHER DRUGS OF ABUSE

A number of other drugs of abuse are covered, including the hallucinogenic drugs LSD, PCP and ketamine, as well as the emerging drug GHB. A chapter on volatile substances is also included since these are widely abused in some communities.

## FOCUS OF THIS BOOK

This book focuses on the uses and subsequent effects of hypnotics, sedatives and the hallucinogens in humans, with emphasis on alcohol, cannabis, the benzodiazepines, the opioids and the family of stimulants related to amphetamine and cocaine. A summary of the expected blood concentrations, metabolism and excretion of these drugs is described. This book also provides an review of the pharmacological and toxicological consequences of their use and abuse. Case examples from both medical and forensic literature are presented to illustrate their significance and involvement in cases.

# 1.2 Specimens and specimen collection procedures

The collection of the most appropriate specimens in forensic cases is essential in order to maximize the range and accuracy of any analytical tests conducted, and thereby maximize the evidentiary nature of the case history. The specimens collected assume even greater importance in forensic cases since there is rarely an opportunity to re-collect specimens. Bodies have usually been sent out of the mortuary, and in clinical cases the presence of drug at the time of original collection is usually desired, hence any later collection is worthless. Consequently, practitioners must ensure an appropriate collection takes place when the opportunity presents. Specimens can always be stored if analysis is not immediately required.

This chapter reviews the types of specimen that can and should be collected in forensic medicine and discusses their relative advantages.

## SPECIMENS AND THEIR RELATIVE MERITS

The choice of specimens will depend on the type of analysis to be conducted, the instrumentation and methodology available, and, naturally, the specimens that can be collected. In situations involving live persons, the specimens recommended are blood (for plasma or serum) and urine if it can be collected. Other specimens, such as saliva, hair and sweat, are being increasingly used as alternatives to plasma and urine, and can provide important additional information. In deceased persons, the range of specimens can of course extend to those collected during life including solid tissues and gastric contents.

Each of these specimens has its own relative advantages depending on the reason for the test being conducted.[5,6] These are summarized below.

### Blood

Blood is useful to establish whether recent ingestion has taken place and can assist in determining whether the drug affected the person at the time of an offence. While this is one of the most asked questions in court proceedings, blood concentrations are also used to establish compliance or to establish a possible dose of prescribed medication. This latter use is often termed therapeutic drug monitoring.

In clinical cases, blood is usually taken from the veins in the arms (antecubital vein) using a hypodermic needle and syringe. In postmortem cases, blood is preferentially taken from the femoral (upper leg) region to avoid contamination from abdominal fluids and contents, and to reduce artefactual rises in blood concentration due to redistribution (see Chapter 1.5 for details).

If femoral blood cannot be obtained, then other peripheral blood is preferred over heart or cavity blood. Pathologists and assisting technicians should avoid 'milking' the vein since this may contaminate the blood with abdominal blood or other fluids. If no blood can be drawn it is preferable to either try another peripheral site or dissect out the vein. Blood from the heart, abdominal and thoracic cavities should be avoided, unless it is used for screening purposes.

Blood specimens taken from hospitalized persons may pose unforeseen contamination problems. Sampling from an indwelling catheter used to administer drugs will produce completely erroneous and misleading results. When results are unphysiological, contamination may be questioned; however, when results are physiological, they are often not questioned. For this reason, it is advisable to exclude this form of contamination when toxicological results are of importance in a case.

To reduce bacterial degradation of drugs (particularly alcohol and the benzodiazepines), blood should be collected into tubes containing potassium fluoride. Laboratories should aim to use fluoride concentrations of 2% (concentration assuming a full blood tube). There is no clear preference for type of container for most drugs, i.e. glass or plastic, provided it can be properly sealed for forensic purposes and should be frozen to at least $-20°C$.

When blood is collected analytical tests will need to be directed to this specimen. Since blood concentrations of drugs are often quite low, the analytical difficulty is quite high compared with urine, especially if a specific drug is not targeted. Volumes of blood of at least 10 mL, and preferably 20 mL, are recommended to ensure optimal sensitivity and to provide the analyst an opportunity to repeat any analysis.

## Urine

Urine provides a much more convenient specimen over blood for analysts since concentrations of metabolites and/or parent drugs are usually much higher than in blood, and the volume collected can easily exceed 20 mL. Depending on the half-life of the drug, the excretion pattern, and the sensitivity of the analytical test, many drugs may be detected in urine for a few days to a week following last use of the drug.

The disadvantage of this specimen is that the presence of drug in urine does not mean the drug was present in blood, and therefore actively exerting a pharmacological effect. The collection of both blood and urine specimens is therefore recommended in cases since the laboratory can use urine for drug-screening purposes and, if a drug is detected, use the blood for quantitative analyses.

Reliance on urine screening alone is dangerous in clinical and forensic medicine since a recently ingested drug may not yet have been excreted into urine, and the concentration of drug in urine provides little information on the amount present in the blood stream. The absence of morphine in the urine of deaths occurring from heroin use is relatively common when death occurs within minutes of an injection. Reliance on urine testing in the absence of information to suggest a heroin death may result in incorrect death certification.

Drugs-of-abuse testing for the purposes of pre-employment, employment, or sports testing is usually only conducted in urine, since only proof of past use of a drug is required. In this situation, collection of urine must be supervised to preclude tampering or substitution of urine.

## Gastric contents

Gastric contents can provide a very useful indicator of drug exposure, whether it be in a clinical setting following a drug overdose (aspirates), or in a deceased person. The presence of drug in amounts much greater than normal therapeutic use can provide good evidence of recent drug ingestion.

When gastric contents are analysed in postmortem cases, pathologists and forensic technical staff should make sure that all, or essentially all, the contents are provided to the laboratory such that the total drug content in milligrams (mg) or grams (g) can be calculated.

For most drugs, the weight or volume of contents should be recorded and an approximate equivalent volume of water (or other solvent, e.g. methanol, ethanol) added to dissolve any tablet residues. Additional amounts of solvent can be added if required. An alcohol is useful because they are good solvents for most drugs and will precipitate out much of the food material present in the stomach and any inactive excipients present in tablets. The total weight or volume is recorded and the supernatant, or an aliquot of the supernatant, can then be briefly centrifuged to settle any particulate matter. The supernatant at this stage should be quite clear. In cases of suspected overdose serial dilutions in solvent can be performed and assayed separately. These are assayed directly without further extraction for drugs using a validated chromatographic procedure.

In cases where no liquid gastric contents are present the whole stomach should be submitted to the laboratory. Analysts should thoroughly rinse the stomach with alcohol (or another solvent). Analysis can then be conducted directly on the solvent rinse.

Results should be expressed as 'mg' or 'g' drug per contents provided. Results expressed as mg/kg stomach cannot be usefully interpreted without the actual mass of contents collected.

The issue of timing of drug ingestion is not straightforward as is sometimes assumed. The presence of drug, equivalent to several dosage forms (i.e. several multiples of known tablet strengths), is usually indicative of recent ingestion, and may even suggest suicide. However, delayed emptying of stomach contents can occur in persons in a coma such that a few days may be required to completely empty stomach contents.

Gastric lavage or the administration of charcoal (to remove drugs from bowel) will usually prevent the successful use of gastric drug analysis.

The presence of small amounts of drug in stomach contents (i.e. part of a dosage form) may either be evidence of relatively recent ingestion, e.g. a few hours ago, or evidence of contamination from bile. Many drugs are found in bile, particularly the opioids and PCP. Reflux or vomiting can lead to contamination of drug in the gastric contents, leading to a false conclusion of relatively recent drug ingestion.

For example, morphine concentrations in bile in persons using heroin or morphine can exceed 100 mg/L. At 100 mg/L, 10 mL of bile in the stomach contains 1 mg! Clearly much larger amounts of morphine are required in the stomach before a conclusion of oral ingestion is opined.

## Liver and other solid specimens

Liver has traditionally been used by forensic toxicologists (in deceased cases) to measure the concentrations of drugs. Liver is not only the primary metabolic organ, but also it is easily collected and can be readily homogenized. Consequently, liver is used in forensic toxicology to supplement blood concentration data, or often becomes the primary specimen in decomposed cases when blood is not available.

Liver (and other solid tissues) should be finely diced and homogenized in water or a dilute buffer until homogeneous. The use of an ultrasonicating blender is most effective, particularly for fibrous tissues such as muscle (heart). A minimum volume ratio of buffer to tissue is 1 : 1. Higher volume ratios are easier to handle, but will dilute out any drugs present.

Because of the matrix effects of this solid tissue, and many other non-blood tissues, more sophisticated analytical methods are required to reliably detect these drugs. Unfortunately, the absence of data in the toxicological literature from controlled studies reduces the ability to interpret liver concentration data. This limitation applies not only to drugs of abuse, but to all drugs and other solid tissues. Consequently, many cases reported in the literature do not have liver concentration data.

Table 1.4  Recommended specimens for toxicology testing and their principal uses

| Specimen | Advantages and usefulness | Volume sampled |
| --- | --- | --- |
| Blood | Peripheral blood (femoral) most useful to confirm recent use of drug and to infer likely toxicological response | 2 × 10 mL |
| Urine | Most useful for conducting broad-class drug screens and can provide little useful information on timing of drug ingestion | ≥10 mL |
| Liver | Useful solid tissue to supplement blood data in postmortem settings – right lobe preferred | ≥100 g |
| Bile | Useful fluid if urine unavailable, particularly for most opiates in postmortem cases, benzodiazepines, cocaine, cardiovascular and psychiatric drugs | Minimum 5 mL |
| Vitreous humour | Very useful fluid in cases of long postmortem interval, particularly ethanol, digoxin, biochemistry (urea, glucose, creatinine), lithium and many psychotropic drugs | 1–2 mL |
| Hair | Should only be used to supplement other information on drug use; can provide exposure information to drugs for months; very liable to contamination | >50 mg |
| Sweat | Potentially useful specimen clinically to assess recent use of drugs; sweat will contaminate hair | Volume not measurable |
| Saliva | Has been a useful specimen clinically for therapeutic drug monitoring; also useful to establish recent use of illicit drugs | Volume not readily measurable, >100 µL |

Nevertheless, if liver is collected it is advisable to take at least 100 g to ensure the specimen is representative of the drug content in the tissue. Data are available which show that liver concentrations can vary depending on the anatomical site of the liver sample.[7] The right lobe has been advocated to reduce redistribution artefacts from the stomach and gall bladder.

Other solid specimens can be analysed for content of drugs. However, there are few data on the significance of these results. The measurement of drug content in a number of key organs and non-parenchymal tissues (skin, fat, muscle and bone) can be useful when a more accurate estimate of total body load of drug is required.[7,8]

## Bile

Bile is a thick green fluid found in the gall bladder and produced by the liver. Drugs are invariably excreted into this fluid after passing through the liver. Drug concentrations can exceed those in all other specimens, can appear before drug is excreted into urine, and can persist for longer times than blood concentrations.[9-13]

The opioids, PCP and the benzodiazepines are readily detected in bile, often predominantly as glucuronide conjugates. The use of a prior hydrolysis procedure, such as for urine, is strongly recommended.

Bile (~10 mL) can be collected from the gall bladder and stored in 'plain' or potassium fluoride-treated plastic or glass tubes. Storage temperature should be at −20°C or lower. Alcohol is readily produced in bile by fermentation processes.

## Vitreous humour

Vitreous humour is the main fluid component of the eye and can be best considered an isotonic salt solution with little protein content. This specimen has been quite useful for the estimation of alcohol, digoxin and other drugs, particularly when some putrefaction in the body has occurred.[9,14-16] Since it is largely free of protein and other complex substances, analysis of this tissue is relatively straightforward.

Volumes collected are small; however, 1–2 mL can be taken if both eyes are used. Storage needs to be only in normal 2–5 mL plastic 'plain' or potassium fluoride-preserved containers. Storage temperature should be at −20°C or lower.

## Hair

Hair has proven to be a useful specimen for the analysis of drugs of abuse. Studies have shown that most, if not all, drugs and poisons are excreted into hair following exposure. Hair is particularly useful to establish drug use many weeks to months prior to collection, since specimens such as blood and urine will only provide evidence of use from hours to at most a few days. This provides hair a distinct advantage over urinalysis for workplace, pre-employment and custodial situations where proof of abstinence from drugs of abuse is required and may avoid regular urinalysis.

This is true for people exposed to poisonous metals such as arsenic, mercury and lead.[17-19] Human scalp hair has also been shown to be useful for the detection of drugs of abuse,[20,21] as well as therapeutic drugs.[22] A number of review articles on hair analysis are available.[20,23-27]

**Table 1.5** Factors affecting retention and concentration of substances in hair

- Physiochemical properties of substances (basic > neutral > acidic)
- Dose of substance and frequency of administration
- Mechanism of incorporation (blood, sweat, sebaceous secretions, etc.)
- Hair colour and type (African and Asian hair show greatest retention)[29,32,33]
- Bleaching of hair (e.g. cocaine)[34]
- Other hair treatments, including shampoo (e.g. cocaine)[31,34–36]
- Decontamination method used to prepare hair for analysis[22,37–39]
- Extraction method[22]

Unfortunately, contamination of hair can occur because substances enter hair by a number of processes. Incorporation by entrapment from the blood bathing the growing follicle is likely to be one of the mechanisms, although incorporation through direct contact of mature hair with sweat and/or sebaceous secretions is a likely major source of drug entry.[28,29]

Because of the ability of hair to directly absorb drug, contamination of hair by direct environmental exposure should also be reasonably excluded if hair results are to be used. For example, nicotine is found in the hair of non-smokers[30] and cocaine is found in the hair of children of cocaine users.[29]

Experiments on drug-free hair dipped into a solution containing drugs have shown that the hair takes up cocaine,[29,31] and 6-acetylmorphine and morphine.[31] Benzodiazepines are also taken up by this mechanism.

For these reasons, metabolite patterns for drugs to distinguish internal exposure from environmental exposure are rarely useful for drugs of abuse. Heroin, cocaine and the amphetamines and benzodiazepines are present largely as the parent compound. Although 6-acetylmorphine and morphine are also present in the hair of heroin users, both are readily formed spontaneously from heroin. Similarly, cocaine is spontaneously hydrolysed to benzoylecgonine, the major metabolite of cocaine.

There are a number of factors that affect retention of drugs into hair, hence quantitative values are rarely useful. These are summarized in Table 1.5.

Hair is normally collected from the back of the head (nape) and can be stored at room temperature in a sealed plastic bag. The amount of hair collected will depend on the type of analysis required; however, at least 50 mg should be collected. A pencil thickness is often a convenient amount that will allow repeat testing if required.

## Sweat

Sweat is a natural secretion in all humans particularly at higher ambient temperatures. Sweat is produced by eccrine glands located in the transdermal layer of most skin surfaces. Apocrine glands located in axillary and pubic regions also produce sweat. Sweat glands are often associated with hair follicles and therefore the presence of drugs in hair and sweat are difficult to disassociate.

Approximately 50% of all the sweat is produced by the trunk, 25% by the legs, and 35% by the head and upper extremities. Sweat is approximately 99% water, the remainder being sodium chloride. The rate of sweating can be as high as >1 L/min for short periods, although rates of ~20 mL/h are more common.[40]

Sweat patches have been used to absorb sweat. These are typically in contact with skin for 1–5 days. This time allows sufficient sweat to accumulate to enable adequate detection of drugs. Drug-wipe devices have been developed to allow spot tests for on-site detection of drugs in the sweat of persons suspected of using drugs of abuse.

Drugs detected in sweat include the benzodiazepines and barbiturates, as well as alcohol (ethanol), amphetamines, cocaine, heroin, morphine, methadone and PCP. A number of reviews have been published.[41,42]

## Saliva

Saliva is excreted primarily by three glands – the parotid, submaxillary and sublingual – and by other small glands such as labial, buccal and palatal glands.[43] The fluids secreted by these glands differ considerably from each other. Their composition is affected by time of day, food, age, gender, state of health, and drugs. Saliva is made up of the usual electrolytes as well as mucus and amylase. Protein content is less than 5% of plasma.

The flow of saliva is dependent on neurotransmitter stimulation and can vary from zero to several mL/min, although flow rates for the parotid and submaxillary are usually <1 mL/min. Craving for food is clearly an important factor. Flow rates are also dependent on age of person and seasonal influences. The pH ranges from 5.5 to 7.9.[44]

Stimulation of saliva flow can lead to a change in pH. Reviews on the physiology and other analytical aspects of saliva are available.[45,46]

Drugs may enter saliva by passive diffusion from blood, ultrafiltration and active secretion. Passive diffusion is apparently the dominant mechanism.[44,45]

Devices used to stimulate saliva formation and facilitate the collection provide less opportunity for contamination than other means of collecting saliva. The use of devices to stimulate saliva flow will also change the level of drug due to osmotic and possibly pH changes.

Specimens can be stored frozen at −20°C, unless analysis will be conducted shortly after collection. Samples should be centrifuged to ensure particulate and other material does not interfere with sampling.

Saliva can be extracted and analysed as other biological fluids such as blood. In general, there will be less interference with saliva from endogenous compounds than blood or urine. Saliva volumes will usually be small, hence there will be limited ability to repeat analyses. Additionally, not all subjects will be able to provide saliva on demand.

Immunoassays are also directed to metabolites of drugs. This could limit its applicability since profiles of drug metabolites may be different in saliva. Laboratories should validate immunoassay kits properly before use.

Interpretation of saliva drug concentrations is more difficult than blood since saliva concentrations are subject to more variables than blood, such as degree of protein binding, pKa of drug and pH of saliva. Alcohol, the amphetamines and opioids are present in saliva in useful concentrations, while benzodiazepines are present in much lower concentrations than in blood.

Contamination of saliva by recently ingested drug is a real problem, although this may be useful if evidence of recent exposure to a drug (through inhalation or oral use) is required. Cannabis is the best example: its presence in saliva is almost exclusively a result of oral contamination.

# 1.3 Analysis and measurement

The identification of drugs in a biological specimen can be one of the most significant pieces of evidence linking drug use to a crime in a criminal matter or the death of a person in a death investigation. Drug presence may provide important evidence relating to behavioural changes, such as in homicides, suicides, and motor vehicle and industrial accidents, and in some situations may even provide a cause of death. Of course, drug testing in prisons and workplace testing is aimed at reducing drug use. Consequently, the identification process and the estimation of drug content in the specimens provided must stand up to scientific rigour and meet the principles of good laboratory practice.[iv]

The process of identifying a drug in a biological matrix such as urine or blood or another biological specimen is complex and is best left for a specialist analytical chemist or a forensic toxicologist trained in this field. There is, however, a need to provide some information to readers on the range of techniques available for the analysis of specimens for drugs of abuse in forensic laboratories. This chapter provides this information and discusses the limitations and strengths of the principal techniques.

The analytical process of measurement can be split into two distinct steps: the initial screening test, and the confirmation step. The screening step provides a relatively quick process to establish whether a drug, or drug class, is likely to present in a given specimen, while the second step ensures that the drug is present and may also provide an estimate of the amount present. Both screen and confirmatory tests are usually necessary in cases where drugs are detected.

## CUT-OFF LEVELS AND APPROVED ASSAYS

Internationally a convention has existed for some years to set cut-off limits for immunoassay screening methods and confirmation methods. For example, some initial screening tests for morphine-like immunoreactivity have been set at 300 ng/mL. A positive result (i.e. >300 ng/mL response) will require confirmation by GC/MS for morphine at a cut-off level of 300 ng/mL.

Cannabinoids can be screened in urine at 50 ng/mL, but the carboxy-THC metabolite is normally confirmed in urine with a cut-off of 15 ng/mL. Other drugs have different cut-off limits depending on their relative concentrations in urine and sensitivities of the immunoassays (see Table 1.6). The USA has various standards for such testing. An Australian Standard recommends a similar protocol (AS4308) for urine drugs-of-abuse testing. The European Union has also considered recommendations for the reliable detection of illicit drugs in urine.[47]

---

[iv] A term used to define the highest international standards of laboratory procedures including peer review such as through recognized accreditation or certification programmes.

# Introductory aspects

**Table 1.6** Recommended screening cut-off levels in urine

| Drug | SAMSHA[a] | Australia[b] | European Union[d] |
|---|---|---|---|
| Amphetamines | 1000 | 300[c] | 300 |
| Benzodiazepines | – | 200 | – |
| Cannabinoids | 50 | 50 | 50 |
| Opiates | 2000 | 300 | 300 |
| Cocaine metabolite | 300 | 300 | 300 |
| PCP | 25 | – | 25 |
| Barbiturates | – | – | 200 |

[a] Substance abuse and mental health services administration. [b] Australian Standard AS4308 for urine drugs-of-abuse testing using immunoassay; [c] includes amphetamine, methamphetamine and MDMA. Phentermine, ephedrine, and pseudoephedrine also included with cut-off at 500 ng/mL using non-immunoassay screening; [d] Ref. 47 and proposed UK guidelines for workplace testing.

Occasionally other screening and confirmation cut-off values are used depending on the needs of the client. Whatever the cut-off value chosen in a screen, it is imperative that the values used are clearly indicated in the report. Confirmation cut-off values are shown in Table 1.7.

If cut-off values are used it is important to note that a 'not detected' result only implies that no drug was detected at or above the cut-off value chosen. The choice of a lower cut-off value or the use of a more sensitive assay may detect the presence of drug.

For drugs such as the benzodiazepines, the sensitivities of the screening assay will be different. The use of a common cut-off value for benzodiazepines will not indicate to the client what drugs in that group were reasonably excluded, and what drugs could not be detected because of lack of sensitivity.

In forensic cases it is often important to determine whether a drug is present at all. For example, the presence of a trace amount of amphetamine (or other drugs) may be critical in establishing the likelihood of previous drug use and confirm claims made by an accused. This fact could be important if psychosis or other behavioural problems associated with amphetamines is claimed, or if rebound fatigue occurs because of previous (but relatively recent) use of stimulants has occurred. Using cut-offs as a convenient method to exclude positive cases without thought of the consequence of this action can be harmful to the administration of justice. See Case Report 2.6 (p. 95).

Whether these drugs are ultimately confirmed by the laboratory or not, it is strongly recommended to report these (presumptive) results with appropriate comments as to the reasons for not confirming the result. This approach will at least provide clients with the appropriate information and not arbitrarily decide what is useful evidence.

## VALIDATION AND UNCERTAINTY

All analytical methods used to detect drugs in biological specimens and in other specimens, e.g. powders and liquids, must be fit for the purpose intended. This means that the method

**Table 1.7** Recommended confirmation cut-off levels in urine

| Drug | SAMSHA[a] | Australia[b] | European Union[c] |
| --- | --- | --- | --- |
| Amphetamine | 500 | 300 | 200 |
| Methamphetamine | 500 | 300 | 200 |
| MDA | | – | 200 |
| MDMA | | 300 | 200 |
| MDEA | | – | 200 |
| 7-Aminoflunitrazepam | | 200 | 10 |
| Flunitrazepam | | – | 10 |
| Temazepam | | 200 | 100 |
| Oxazepam | – | 200 | 100 |
| Nordiazepam | | 200 | 100 |
| 7-Aminonitrazepam | | 200 | 100 |
| 7-Aminoclonazepam | | 200 | – |
| THC-COOH | 15 | 15 | 15 |
| Morphine | 2000 | 300 | 300 |
| Codeine | 2000 | 300 | 300 |
| 6-AM | 10 | | 10 |
| Dihydrocodeine | – | | 300 |
| Benzoylecgonine | 150 | 150 | 150 |
| Ecgonine methyl ester | – | 150 | – |
| PCP | 25 | – | 25 |
| Barbiturates | – | – | 200 |

[a] Substance abuse and mental health services administration; includes for opiates test 6-AM if morphine >2000 ng/mL at cut-off of 10 ng/mL; and for confirmation of methamphetamine, amphetamine must be >200 ng/mL; [b] Australian Standard AS4308 for urine drugs-of-abuse testing, administration; [c] proposed UK guidelines for workplace testing.

used must be validated against a minimum number of criteria in that specimen type before it can be accepted in actual casework.

Validation criteria for screening methods, confirmatory methods and quantifications are summarized in Table 1.8.

While there is considerable variability in the types of techniques and specimens used in forensic laboratories to provide a drug detection, the criteria listed in Table 1.8 should be met before any confidence can be obtained in results produced by a laboratory. It would not be unreasonable to question the caseworker to ensure the tests used are fit for the purpose intended. Peer review of methods is a useful way to ensure fitness for purpose. Publication in an international peer-reviewed journal is one of the best ways to achieve this aim. Criteria for validation of analytical methods have been published.[47,48]

Uncertainty of analytical measurement is becoming an increasingly important aspect of any quantitative result.[49] The ability to provide a client, including courts, a reasonably reliable

**Table 1.8** Validation criteria for analytical methods

| | |
|---|---|
| Initial tests (screens) | Analytical sensitivity acceptable to determine use of drug or drug class from therapeutic or common doses |
| | Sufficient selectivity to target drug or drug class to ensure a minimum degree of false positives in intended specimen |
| | Sufficient cross-reactivity to most members of particular drug class to provide adequate sensitivity (immunoassays only) |
| | Sufficiently stable and robust to ensure adequate repeatability |
| Chromatographic confirmations and quantifications[a] | Specificity defined by lack of interference from known common drugs and relevant metabolites, and from matrix |
| | Analytical proof of presence strictly defined and includes adequate match of retention time and response by detector |
| | Sufficient accuracy to enable confidence in results |
| | Analytical sensitivity acceptable to determine use of drug or drug class from therapeutic or common doses, defined by limit of detection, limit of quantitation and recovery from matrix |
| | Sufficiently stable and robust to ensure adequate precision and reproducibility, defined by both intra- and inter-assay variability |

[a] Note immunoassays are not regarded as capable of confirmation.

estimate of the uncertainty attached to a quantitative result assists in establishing a possible range attached to the evidence. For example, if a trafficking charge is attracted to a limit of 1 g of substance, then a certificate reporting 1.1 g of the prohibited substance should indicate a possible uncertainty. This allows the court to understand whether it is reasonably likely that the amount detected could be below the statutory limit of 1 g.

Uncertainty of measurement derives from all steps in the processes leading to analytical result, i.e. weighing the substances and analytical standard, purity of the standard, dilutions and pipette errors, calculations of the response and the variation of the extraction and detection. In practice, the greater error derives from the analytical extraction and detection steps.[50] For this reason it may be convenient to assess the coefficient of variation (CV) for replicate measurements over several assays of the same batch. This is often known as the reproducibility. For example, replicate analyses over 10 assays give a CV of 4.1%. The uncertainty of result is $\pm 2 \times 4.1\% = 8.2\%$ if a 95% confidence range is calculated.

Hence a result may be reported as $1.00 \pm 0.08$ mg/L, or as a range 0.92–1.08 mg/L. Alternatively, a laboratory may take off the uncertainty and report 'no less than 0.92 mg/L'. This latter form is usually only useful when a statutory limit applies, e.g. a blood alcohol limit or a drug trafficking limit, i.e. no less than 0.16 g/100 mL alcohol, or no less than 1.1 g of amphetamine.

## QUALITY ASSURANCE

An important step to ensure analytical methods used in a particular laboratory are fit for purpose, and that the staff have adequate skills to act as forensic toxicologists, is to take part in proficiency testing programmes. Such programmes usually involve the submission of an unknown case to a number of laboratories. The results of the investigation are made known to an independent organization that evaluates each laboratory's results and compares results between laboratories. Each laboratory is then compared with other similar laboratories. This provides an independent test for the ability of the laboratory to detect substances, and also to quantify their presence. Laboratories that produce false positive results, i.e. detections of drugs that are not present in the specimen, or that cannot detect substances that other laboratories can, require improvement.

Proficiency programmes can either be submitted externally or if this is not possible then an internal programme can be run, providing the laboratory is not aware of the result before completion of the investigation. Samples blind to the laboratory are clearly preferable, but this can rarely be managed given the nature of case receipt by external clients. Analysts should ensure that proficiency cases are treated no differently to real cases.

The inclusion of quality controls in quantitative assays is strongly recommended. These controls can either be purchased from a commercial source or prepared in the laboratory by an independent process. These controls contain a declared target concentration, and unless shown otherwise, provide a means to establish the accuracy and reliability of an assay. For example, if an amphetamine quality control has a target concentration of 1.0 mg/L, then an assay quantifying unknown samples must return a value for this control of 1.0 mg/L before any result can be accepted as reliable. In practice, there is an inherent uncertainty of any quantitative result (see previous section on uncertainty). This uncertainty is initially defined by the validation process and is typically 5–10% when expressed as a standard deviation from the mean. Acceptance ranges for controls may be set as $\pm 2$ SD or $\pm 20\%$, depending on the local laboratory policy. Any deviation from this range for this example, i.e. $1.0 \pm 0.2$ mg/L, will lead to rejection of the assay on quantitative grounds.

If two or more quality controls are run in an assay, then acceptance rules become more complex. It is recommended to include at least two quality controls in analytical runs (duplicates or two different concentrations) to avoid random errors. In long runs, i.e. >10 samples, more controls are recommended. Laboratories will need to establish their own appropriate acceptance criteria.

The underlying ability of a laboratory to adapt to changing drug use trends and to embrace new and emerging technologies is clearly a desirable feature and should be encouraged, as it forms a process of continuous improvement in a quality systems management environment.

# 1.4 Pharmacokinetics and duration of action

Pharmacokinetics refers to the time course of absorption, distribution into tissues, metabolism and excretion (see also definitions in Chapter 1.1). Pharmacokinetics is a most important concept in pharmacology and provides a useful way to define the time course of drug action, and the rate of removal and inactivation of drugs.

This chapter details some of the more important aspects of the fundamental principles of pharmacokinetics and its applications to cases.

Readers are directed to Gibaldi's *Biopharmaceutics and Clinical Pharmacokinetics*,[51] Avery's *Drug Treatments* (latest edition) and *Goodman and Gilman's The Pharmacological Basis of Therapeutics*,[52] and to a number of review articles and other papers listed in the monographs for each drug (see Appendix).

## ABSORPTION AND BIOAVAILABILITY

For drugs to exert any biological activity, they must be delivered to the biological organism. Intravenous administration results in immediate and complete availability to the body, whereas oral administration results in a relatively slow and often incomplete availability (bioavailability) to the body. Since the amount of drug absorbed often relates to the intensity of the pharmacological response, it is important therefore that the bioavailability of a drug is known for a given route of administration.

### Oral absorption and bioavailability

Absolute bioavailabilities are calculated by comparing the blood concentration of drug for both oral and intravenous administration. Absolute bioavailabilities of less than 100% are caused by a combination of incomplete gastrointestinal absorption and first-pass metabolism in the liver. This first-pass metabolism essentially inactivates the drug before it has a chance to produce a biological response, unless the drug is activated in the liver to an active metabolite. For those drugs that rely on metabolism to an active drug, peak effects will correlate better with the active metabolite, rather than the precursor, or pro-drug form.

For oral administration, food can often affect the absorption process in terms of both rate and extent, leading to an enhanced, reduced or unchanged bioavailability. For example, the absorption of ethanol can be markedly affected by food. Where food is known to affect bioavailability mention is made in the individual drug sections.

### Other routes of administration

Other routes of administration are used for drugs. These include intravenous, intramuscular, dermal, nasal insufflation, intravaginal, ocular, inhalation, rectal and sublingual.

All of these routes have their own special pharmacokinetic properties that vary between drugs. Pharmaceutical preparations are especially designed for each route of administration to optimize the absorption process. Casual non-medical use of drugs given by routes not designed for the preparation will not usually give optimal absorption characteristics.

For example, heroin and the amphetamines are often injected intravenously, while cocaine is inhaled through the nose (nasal insufflation). The vapours of heroin and cocaine can also be inhaled leading to absorption through the lungs. Drugs such as many asthma medications and anaesthetics are delivered by inhalation of aerosols.

Intramuscular administration is a relatively common alternative site for medical use of benzodiazepines and other drugs. The rate and extent of absorption from this site would be expected to be somewhere between that of intravenous and oral administrations. For example, the benzodiazepine midazolam is rapidly absorbed intramuscularly with drug detectable after 5 min, and peak concentrations are obtained at 20–30 min.

Not all drugs can be given intramuscularly due to solubility or irritant properties of the drug. Intramuscular diazepam and chlordiazepoxide show incomplete and erratic absorption presumably because of their lower water solubility resulting in crystallization at the injection site.

Rectal administration is used when oral dosing is not possible (e.g. due to vomiting) or when a local effect is required. Rectal absorption is less reliable than oral and can often be quite unpredictable. For many drugs, rectal administration shows poor bioavailability compared with oral use. Rectal administration of midazolam also shows rapid absorption with peak concentrations reached within 20 min.[53] However, diazepam shows erratic and incomplete absorption. The powerful narcotic oxycodone is given both rectally and orally, but the rectal suppository is often a 30 mg strength, while the tablet is a 5 mg strength. This difference in strength of formulation reflects the differing potencies and rates of absorption of these two routes.

Alprazolam is absorbed more rapidly sublingually than when given orally.[53] Buprenorphine, a potent narcotic opioid, is also given by this route.[54] Glyceryl trinitrate and other medications used for angina are administered this way resulting in rapid relief.

Other routes of administration, such as dermal, ocular and vaginal, are uncommon with drugs of abuse but are used for particular medical purposes when drug needs to be delivered to a local site. Usually any lipid-soluble drug can be absorbed at these other sites. The octanol–buffer partition coefficient (expressed as a logarithm, $\log K_P$) is a measure of lipid solubility. The higher the value, the greater the lipid solubility. $\log K_P$ values of greater than 1.0 reflect significant lipid solubility. These values, when known for a drug, are listed in the individual monographs for drugs in the Appendix.

## VOLUME OF DISTRIBUTION

All drugs once absorbed are transported throughout the body by the blood circulation. A hypothetical volume of distribution ($V_D$) defines the extent of this distribution. This term is the apparent volume of body fluids that drugs distribute to, and is calculated by dividing the total amount of drug in the body (absorbed dose) by the plasma concentration at time zero ($C_0$)

# Introductory aspects

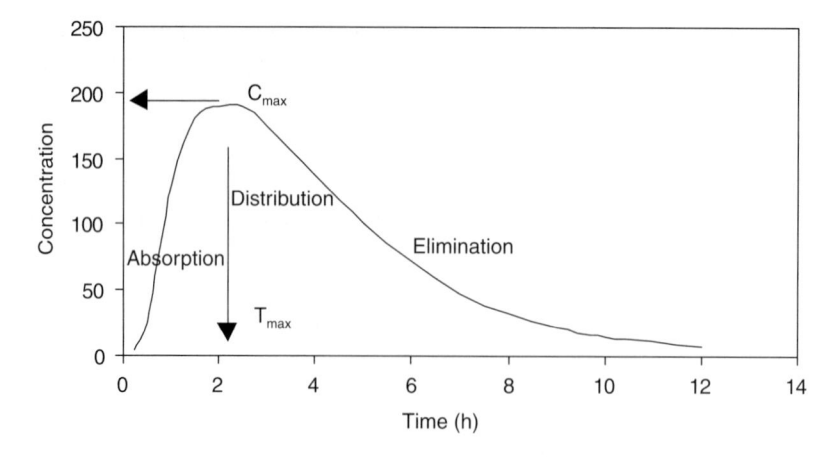

**Fig. 1.1** Pharmacokinetic characteristics of an orally absorbed drug

Blood concentration versus time curve following oral administration of a drug, showing time to maximum concentration ($T_{max}$), maximum concentration ($C_{max}$), and the absorption, distribution and elimination parts of the curve.

**Table 1.9** Dose, blood concentrations, bioavailability, half-life and volume of distribution for selected drugs

| Drug | Usual dose (mg)[a] | $C_{max}$[b] | Bioavailability (%)[c] | Half-life (h) | Volume of distribution (L/kg)[d] |
|---|---|---|---|---|---|
| Alprazolam | 0.5–4 | <0.1 | 90 | 6–22 | 0.7–1.3 |
| Amphetamine[f] | <40 | <0.1 | High | 4–30 | 3–5 |
| Amylobarbital | 30–600 | <12 | 95 | 8–40 | 1.0 |
| Cocaine[f] | <100 | <0.5 | Low | 0.6–2 | 1–3 |
| Diazepam | 5–40 | <1.5 | 100 | 20–50 | 0.5–2.6 |
| Ethanol | 8 g[e] | 0.015% | 50–80 | 0.015%/h | 0.53 |
| Ecstasy (MDMA)[f] | 100 | <0.3 | High | 8 | – |
| Flunitrazepam | 2 | <0.02 | 70 | 11–25 | 3.4–5.5 |
| GHB[f] | >200 | <150 | Moderate | <1 | – |
| LSD[f] | 50 µg | <0.01 | Moderate | 2–6 | 0.3 |
| Methamphetamine[f] | 50 | <0.1 | High | 10–30 | 3–4 |
| Morphine | 5–20 | <1 | 15–60 | 2–3 | 2–5 |
| Oxazepam | 15–60 | <1.5 | 93 | 4–15 | 0.5–2 |
| PCP[f] | 1–10 | <0.2 | Moderate | 7–46 | 6 |
| Temazepam | 10–30 | <1.2 | >80 | 5–15 | 0.8–1.4 |
| THC[f] | <50 | <100 | 6 | 19–96 | 9–11 |
| Pentobarbital | 100–200 | <10 | 95 | 15–48 | 0.7–1.0 |

[a] Usual recommended dose range; [b] maximum plasma concentration usually obtained from common doses; [c] oral bioavailability compared with an intravenous injection; [d] volume of distribution, ranges of published values; [e] standard drink of alcohol; [f] typical recreational dose or dose range.

before elimination has occurred (see Fig. 1.1). For intravenously administered drugs, the whole dose given is absorbed, whereas an amount less than the dose is available following oral administration. If the bioavailability is known, the apparent absorbed dose can be calculated.

$$V_D = \text{dose absorbed}/C_0$$
$$\text{Dose absorbed} = \text{dose} \times \text{bioavailability}/100$$

Drugs which do not distribute into other tissues or cellular water, but are only found in blood, will have a $V_D$ of ~0.05 L/kg; these include heparin (anticoagulant) and insulin (hormone that regulates blood glucose levels). Drugs which distribute into extracellular water (including the blood) will have a $V_D$ of ~0.2 L/kg; these include the antibiotic gentamicin and other large molecules which cannot easily penetrate cells.

The total body water volume is ~0.55 L/kg. Therefore drugs which are found in the body water compartment and are not bound to cellular structures will have values close to this. Examples of note are ethanol (alcohol) and phenytoin (anticonvulsant).

Drugs that are taken up into body fat or bind to cellular structures will have a higher $V_D$. It is not uncommon for volumes of distribution to be over 10. Morphine has a $V_D$ of 2–5 L/kg. A range of 0.5–5 is seen for most of the amphetamines and many of the benzodiazepines. The highly lipid-soluble THC has a volume of distribution of ~10. Drugs with high octanol–buffer partition coefficients will generally have high volumes of distribution. Examples of these parameters are contained in Table 1.9 and in the monographs for each drug in the Appendix.

## CLEARANCE

Clearance is a term that defines the ability of the body to remove a drug from one part of the body, i.e. kidneys, liver, etc. Total clearance is based on the sum total of all mechanisms operating to metabolize and excrete drug. Total clearance is usually defined in mL/min per body weight and can be calculated by a number of means. The most common are the two expressions shown below:

$$Cl = \text{dose}/AUC$$
$$Cl = k_0/C_{ss}$$

where Cl is clearance in mL/min; dose is actual dose absorbed by body; AUC is the area under the plasma concentration versus time curve; $k_0$ is the infusion rate of drug in a controlled clinical setting delivering the drug intravenously; and $C_{ss}$ is the steady-state plasma concentration of drug under these controlled conditions.

Clearance will vary depending on the physiological state of the organs, i.e. organ disease and organ damage. Advanced age will often reduce clearance. Total body clearances for selected drugs are shown in the Appendix monographs.

## HALF-LIFE

This is the most commonly used pharmacokinetic term in court. It defines the ability of the body to remove a drug. Half-life defines the time required for the body to remove half of the drug absorbed. Half-life is usually in hours (h), although some drugs have half-lives of minutes or weeks.

Half-life is estimated by calculating the slope of the terminal part of the plasma concentration versus time curve. At this stage it is assumed that no other competing process is operating, i.e. absorption is still taking place, distribution of drug into tissues is still taking place, and the decline in plasma concentration versus time is first order.

These assumptions are most important to remember, since they may seriously affect the calculation of half-life. The first-order decline in plasma concentration is often only assumed. The plot of the logarithm of the plasma concentration versus the time should be linear in this terminal region. If the half-life is not linear, then half-life cannot be calculated with any accuracy and almost certainly means that there are either multi-compartmental losses of drug, or the processes of absorption and tissue distribution are still occurring.

Half-life is calculated from the slope of this terminal region from:

$$\text{Half-life} = 0.693/\beta$$

where $\beta$ is the slope of the terminal part of the plasma concentration versus time curve.

The half-life is useful in estimating the concentration of drug in the past (back calculation). For example, a drug with a half-life of 12 h and a blood concentration of 2.0 mg/L will be expected to have a concentration of 1.0 mg/L 12 h later. This will reduce to 0.50 mg/L at 24 h and 0.125 mg/L after two days.

Half-lives of drugs vary enormously, from one hour for cocaine to over two days for nordiazepam. The half-life for intravenous heroin is only minutes. See Table 1.9 for half-lives for selected drugs and monographs (Appendix) for more pharmacokinetic data on each drug.

A half-life is not a constant of nature for a particular drug; rather it varies from person to person, and within a person. It is not uncommon for half-lives for a drug to vary 100%, even in healthy individuals. Consequently, where appropriate, any calculation involving half-life should take into account these factors.

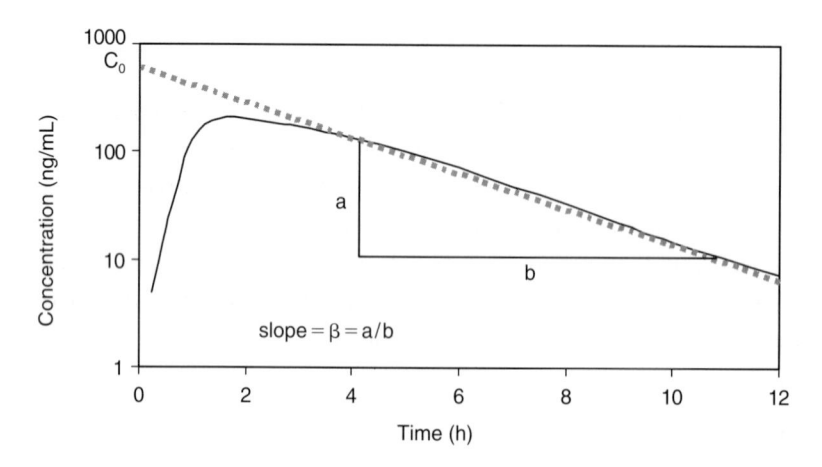

**Fig. 1.2** Calculation of half-life from terminal slope

Calculation of $\beta$ (slope), half-life and imaginary initial concentration ($C_0$) following an oral dose.

The half-life of commonly used drugs is usually measured in young and otherwise healthy persons. A number of factors will affect half-life and clearance of drugs generally. Congestive heart failure, kidney and liver disease are particularly important examples, others are advanced age (>64 years), very young children, obesity and other drugs. These issues will be explored for each of the main drug groups in later chapters, where information is available.

# METABOLISM

Essentially all drugs and chemical substances are broken down or converted to another substance, or substances, prior to excretion. This process is termed metabolism, or bioconversion.

The human body has evolved a number of mechanisms to metabolize chemicals, the primary purpose of which is to enable the substance to be more readily excreted by the body, thereby removing the substance. Metabolic processes can be divided into two or three main types. Phase 1 metabolism is an oxidative process modifying the molecule by changing the nature of a functional group or adding a functional group. Phase 2 metabolism is a conjugative process in which a sulphate or glucuronide ester is added to an existing functional group.

## Phase I processes

Phase 1 processes include hydroxylation, oxidation and dealkylation routes of metabolism. They are best typified by Fig. 1.3.

The enzyme system responsible for most of the dealkylation, hydroxylation and oxidation reactions are the cytochrome P450 series of enzymes which are found predominantly, but not exclusively, in the liver. One form, CYP3A, is responsible for hydroxylating and dealkylating many of the benzodiazepines, and the N-dealkylation of opioids. This form has two sub-types termed CYP3A3 and CYP3A4. Another form, CYP2D6, is responsible for the O-dealkylation of many of the opioids.

## Phase 2 processes

Conjugation reactions include formation of glucuronide and sulphate esters, as well as methyl, acetyl, glycyl and glutamyl conjugates (Fig. 1.4). The glucuronide is probably the most common conjugate and is seen with the benzodiazepine family of drugs, with morphine and related opioids as well as hydroxylated amphetamines.

Glucuronidation involves the enzyme uridine diphosphate glucuronide (UDP) glucuronyl transferase adding β-glucuronide acid to a nitrogen (N), oxygen (O) or sulphur (S) on a drug or drug metabolite. This enzyme is found predominantly in the liver but is also found in the lung, kidneys, brain and gastrointestinal tract. Glucuronides are mostly inactive, although a notable exception is the 6-glucuronide of morphine, which is more active than morphine itself as an analgesic.

Sulphate esters are also common with hydroxylated compounds, such as some asthma drugs ($β_2$-stimulants) and steroids. The other conjugates are not as common, and are not important metabolites for the drugs of abuse. The high polarity of the glucuronides and sulphates mean the kidneys are able to rapidly excrete them.

# Introductory aspects

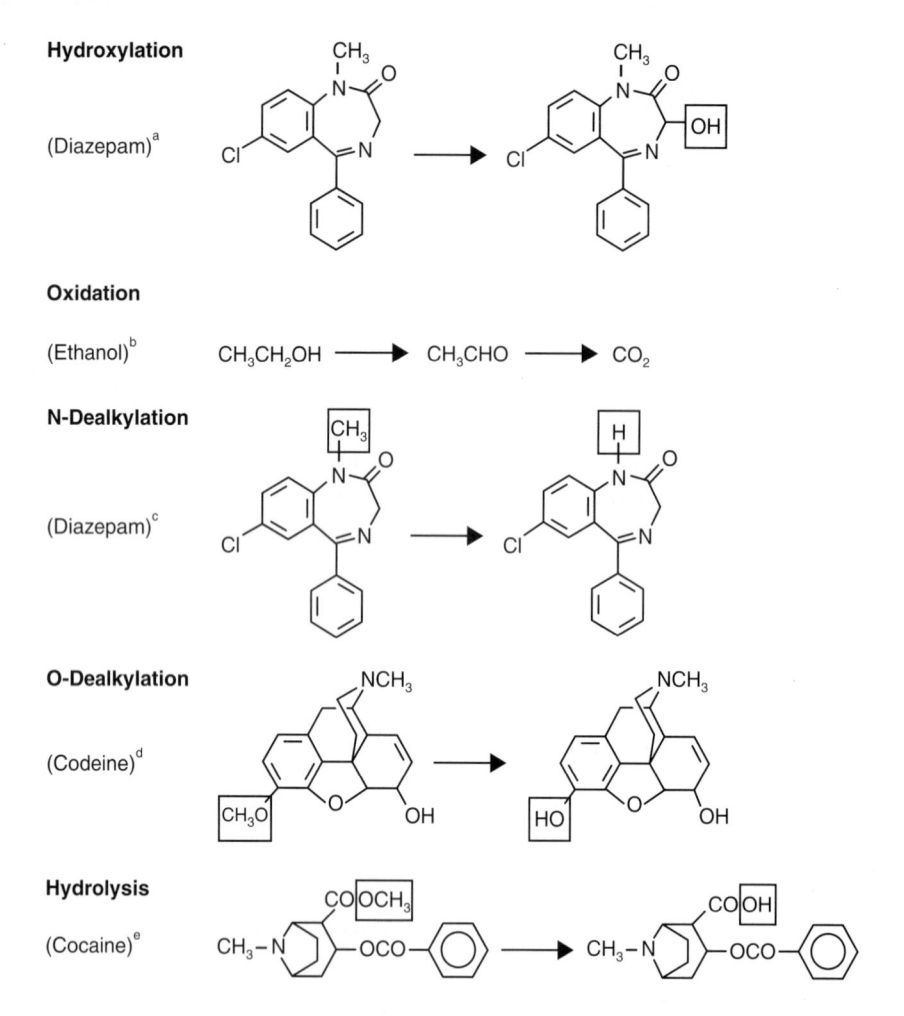

**Fig. 1.3** Phase I metabolic pathways

[a] Conversion of diazepam to temazepam; [b] conversion of ethanol to acetaldehyde and then to carbon dioxide; [c] conversion of diazepam to nordiazepam; [d] conversion of codeine to morphine; [e] conversion of cocaine to benzoylecgonine.

## EXCRETION

Elimination of metabolites and any unchanged drug occurs primarily in the urine. In fact the urine accounts for the majority of excreted drug, either unchanged or predominantly as a metabolite. Individual excretion data are shown in the monographs.

A significant amount of many drugs is excreted in the faeces. Amounts vary from a few per cent to over 30% of the administered dose. Faecal excretion derives from unabsorbed drug, or absorbed drug which is secreted in bile (from the liver) and which is not subsequently re-absorbed.

Biliary excretion is more important for molecules that have a higher molecular weight, such as conjugates. For example, PCP and the opioids are particularly good subjects for biliary excretion. Other drugs found in bile include the benzodiazepines, colchicine, cocaine and its metabolites, the tricyclic antidepressants (amitriptyline, dothiepin, imipramine,

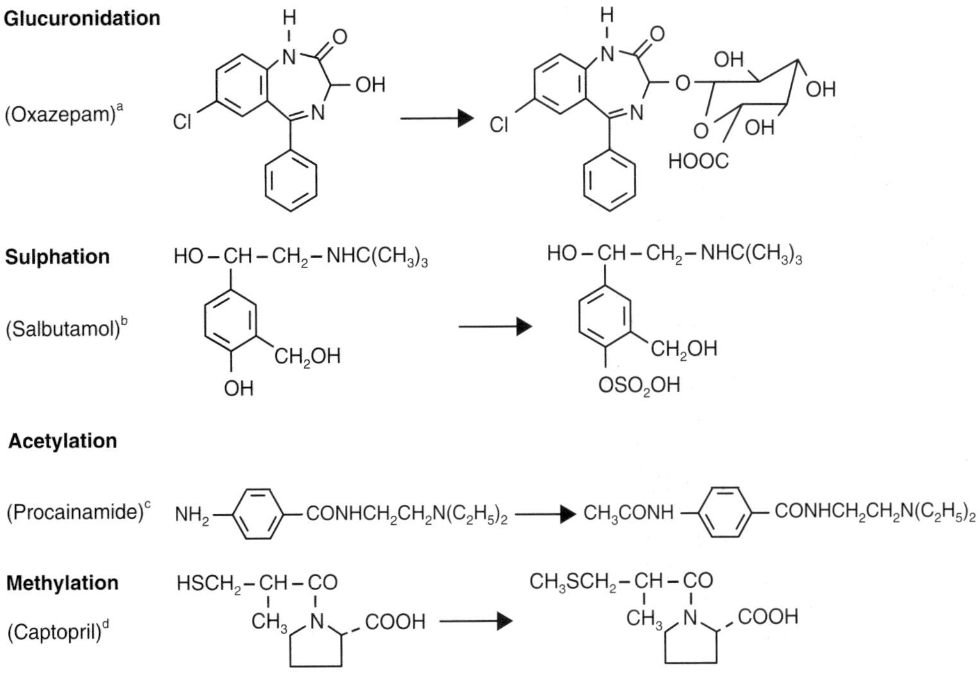

# Pharmacokinetics and duration of action

**Glucuronidation**

(Oxazepam)[a]

**Sulphation**

(Salbutamol)[b]

**Acetylation**

(Procainamide)[c]    $NH_2-\langle\rangle-CONHCH_2CH_2N(C_2H_5)_2 \longrightarrow CH_3CONH-\langle\rangle-CONHCH_2CH_2N(C_2H_5)_2$

**Methylation**

(Captopril)[d]

**Fig. 1.4** Phase 2 conjugation reactions

[a] Oxazepam (benzodiazepine) conversion to oxazepam-3-glucuronide; [b] $\beta_2$-stimulant salbutamol conversion to sulphate ester; [c] antiarrthymic procainamide conversion to N-acetyl metabolite; [d] antihypertensive drug captopril conversion to S-methyl metabolite.

doxepin, etc.), other psychiatric drugs (sertraline, trazodone, chlorpromazine, and thioridazine), as well as the sedatives ethychlorvynol and methaqualone, and many of the cardiovascular drugs.[10] Ethanol is present in bile. Other drugs are also likely to be present in bile.

As indicated in Chapter 1.2, drugs are excreted into saliva and sweat, although these are minor routes of excretion of drugs. Elimination of drugs in breath is a significant route for volatile drugs such as ethanol, volatile solvents, and gases.

## DURATION OF ACTION

In previous sections the term half-life was used to define the rate of removal of drug from the blood. This term is often misused to also mean duration of action of the drug. While in some cases the half-life does provide a reasonable correlation with biological effect, in many cases it does not. For the effect of a drug to be related directly to the blood concentration, it requires a direct correlation of the blood concentration with the tissue at which the drug is acting. For the drugs of abuse, the sites of action are the brain, or discrete sections of the brain.

For a drug to enter these brain regions, they will be subject to particular processes that allow entry into the brain. These are based on the physio-chemical properties of the drug, including the lipid-solubility characteristics (lipophilicity) and retentive ability of the brain region. Drugs with higher lipid solubility will tend to enter the brain quicker and to a greater degree than those that are water soluble. A measure of lipophilicity is the partition coefficient (expressed as

# Introductory aspects

log $K_P$). Benzodiazepines vary greatly in their lipophilicity (see monographs in Appendix). For example, clobazam has a log $K_P$ value of 0.9 and diazepam has a log $K_P$ value of 2.7. Since this is a logarithmic scale, diazepam has 63-fold greater lipid solubility than clobazam. This result would suggest much higher brain concentrations of diazepam than clobazam, if the same dose of drug were given, and would also show that the tissue concentrations of diazepam will be higher than the corresponding blood concentrations. Heroin has higher lipid solubility than morphine and therefore has a much quicker onset of action than morphine.

Another complicating factor when dealing with correlation between pharmacokinetic half-life and duration of action is the non-linear dose–response relationship for drugs. This means that a doubling of a dose does not necessarily mean a doubling of effect. In fact, for most drugs there is a threshold dose, the minimum effective concentration, below which no significant pharmacological effect can be observed; and a maximum dose, above which toxicity or serious side effects may develop, often with no additional therapeutic response.[51] These relationships are very important when the likely toxicological effects of drugs are considered. These relationships can best be seen in Fig. 1.5.

It is therefore unlikely that a direct correlation exists for the blood half-life and duration of action. This issue is dealt with in detail in later sections.

A further variable that confounds any relation between half-life and duration of action is the protein binding of drugs. Most drugs exist substantially in blood (and other tissues) bound to proteins and other macromolecules. Protein binding precludes that drug from eliciting an active response on a receptor. In other words, it is the non-protein-bound form that exhibits biological activity. Many of the benzodiazepines show protein binding of greater than 90%, leaving less than 10% to exert any biological activity. The extent of protein binding varies from one drug to another and may even vary depending on the concentration and the local tissue environment.[55] Protein binding is substantially affected by disease, particularly kidney and liver disease.

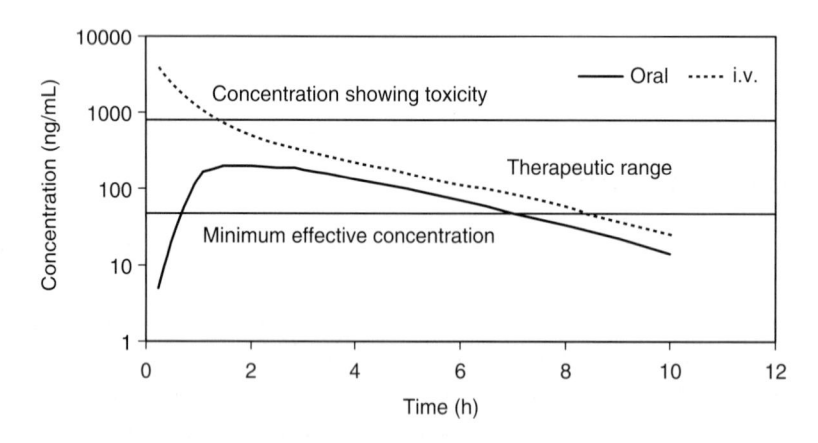

**Fig. 1.5** Diagrammatic representation showing a hypothetical pharmacological range of a drug

In this diagram the variation in blood concentration with time is shown for a drug following intravenous and oral administration. The threshold concentration is the minimum concentration at which the drug will exhibit a significant biological effect, and the toxic concentration is the concentration at which a toxic response is likely. The concentration range between a minimum effective concentration and a concentration likely to exhibit toxicity is known as the therapeutic range of a drug. Note that toxic responses are more likely with intravenous dosing in the early stages following an injection.

# Pharmacokinetics and duration of action

The monographs in the Appendix show the key pharmacokinetic properties of selected drugs, including their bioavailabilities, clearances, half-lives, partition coefficients and protein binding.

## METABOLIC INTERACTIONS

An important feature of the metabolism of many of the benzodiazepines is that other drugs may interfere with their metabolism. For example, cimetidine (an anti-ulcer drug),[56] and a number of the newer-generation antidepressants, inhibit the metabolism of alprazolam, and potentially many other benzodiazepines by CYP3A (see Table 1.10). This occurs either

Table 1.10  Significant metabolic drug interactions for drugs of abuse

| Drug class/type | Interacting drug of abuse |
| --- | --- |
| **Alcohol** Interacts with liver microsomal enzymes decreasing drug clearance, alcohol dehydrogenase and with chronic use increases clearance | Barbiturates, glutethimide, meprobamate  Chloral hydrate (affects ADH activity)  Benzodiazepines  Cocaine |
| **Barbiturates** Decreases blood concentrations by induction of P450 enzymes | Methamphetamine, MDMA, etc.  O-alkylated opioids, particularly pethidine (meperidine)[b]  Non-conjugated benzodiazepines |
| **Cimetidine** Increases blood concentrations by inhibition of P450 metabolism | Alcohol[c]  Non-conjugated benzodiazepines[a]  O-alkylated opioids, methadone  Other drugs metabolized by P450 enzymes |
| **MAOI inhibitors** (nialamide, phenelzine, tranylcypromine) Increase blood concentrations by inhibition of P450 enzymes, and interfere with serotonin metabolism | Alcohol[c]  Amphetamines and appetite suppressants, barbiturates  Pethidine (meperidine) and other opioids |
| **Propoxyphene** Increases blood concentrations by inhibition of P450 3A4 metabolism | Non-conjugated benzodiazepines  Other drugs metabolized by P450 3A4 |
| **Serotonin re-uptake inhibitors** (fluoxetine, paroxetine, sertraline, etc.) Increase blood concentrations by inhibition of P450 3A4 metabolism | Non-conjugated benzodiazepines  O-alkylated opioids  Other drugs metabolized by P450 3A4 |

[a] Refers to those benzodiazepines which are primarily metabolized by dealkylation and hydroxylation (alprazolam, chlordiazepoxide, diazepam, nordazepam analogues, triazolam, etc.), as opposed to those which are mainly conjugated (oxazepam, temazepam, lorazepam); [b] enhanced production of toxic norpethidine, cocaine O-alkylated opioids include codeine, ethylmorphine, dextromethorphan and oxycodone; [c] through microsomal metabolizing system.

by competitive inhibition of the enzyme(s) involved in their mutual metabolism or by inhibition of the enzyme(s) by the interfering drug. Many of the newer serotonin re-uptake inhibitors, including fluoxetine, paroxetine and sertraline, are relatively potent inhibitors of this enzyme.

A further variable is that drugs such as the barbiturates and the anticonvulsants phenobarbital and phenytoin enhance the production of the enzymes and therefore induce metabolism of drugs metabolized through this and related enzyme systems. In fact barbiturates also induce their own metabolism causing a time-dependent increase in clearance as the liver produces more enzyme.

Other drugs are also known to induce metabolism or inhibit metabolic processes. Table 1.10 provides some of the more notable interactions involving the drugs of abuse discussed in this book.[57,58] Texts describing adverse drug interactions are also available.[59,60]

Other types of interactions, such as pharmacodynamic where two or more drugs augment each other's effects, are described in the individual drug sections, where appropriate.

## PHARMACOKINETICS IN THE ELDERLY

Advanced age (>65 years old) will affect the clearance of drugs as a result of a general decline in the efficiency of all organs to carry out bodily functions including metabolic processes and excretory processes (Fig. 1.6). Advanced age usually results in altered body muscle to fat ratios, causing an increased volume of distribution. Drugs metabolized through the microsomal enzyme system are most affected by advancing age. Drugs affected usually require lower doses, sometimes less than one-half, in the elderly to compensate for the reduced clearance.[61–65]

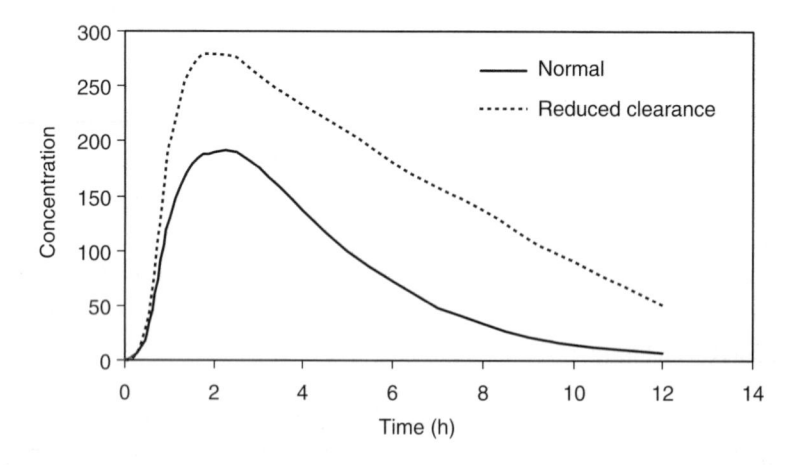

**Fig. 1.6** Diagrammatic representation of blood concentrations versus time in people with normal clearance and those with substantially impaired clearance

In this figure the total body clearance has been halved, causing a larger $C_{max}$, longer half-life and a larger AUC and consequently producing a larger biological effect. Clearance can be affected by advanced age, liver or kidney dysfunction, and even by heart failure (reduced heart function), or by a combination of these.

## PHARMACOKINETICS IN DISEASE STATES

### Liver disease

Liver disease, particularly cirrhosis and acute viral hepatitis, can affect clearance of drugs. This can occur by a number of mechanisms, including reduced metabolic capacity, alterations in the degree of protein binding, and an alteration in volume of distribution (Fig. 1.6).

Drugs that are conjugated, as opposed to those which are primarily metabolized by the microsomal system, are less affected by liver disease.[66–69]

### Kidney disease

Renal disease leading to severe insufficiency in creatinine clearance invariably produces profound changes in the pharmacokinetics of drugs (Fig. 1.6). For oxazepam and lorazepam, for example, renal insufficiency leads to an accumulation of the glucuronide conjugate (since kidneys are no longer able to excrete substances properly). Renal disease also leads to a change in protein binding, resulting in higher volumes of distribution and a prolongation of half-life.[68,70]

Drugs that are metabolized by the microsomal system are less affected by renal insufficiency since drug is still being metabolized by the liver. Metabolites, however, will accumulate, and if active pharmacologically, will exert an increased action. Changes in protein binding in renal disease can have a marked effect on increasing drug actions by making more drug available to the body.

### Critically ill persons

Persons dangerously ill, including those admitted to intensive care, are very much at risk of increased activity of sedatives due to a combination of haemodynamic and physiological imbalances.[57] Benzodiazepines and opioids (morphine, pethidine (meperidine), fentanyl, etc.) are widely used in intensive care settings in hospital and will exhibit an increased effect in these subjects. Those drugs with long half-lives, or that are metabolized to long-acting metabolites, e.g. nordiazepam, are most likely to cause problems in this group.

For example, midazolam, the most common benzodiazepine given in this setting, has a half-life of 2 h in normal adults; this increases to 10 h following cardiac surgery. As seen earlier, reduced function of the liver and kidneys will also increase the half-life.

## PHARMACOKINETICS IN OBESITY

Obesity tends to increase the volume of distribution of benzodiazepines primarily because of the increase in body fat. Absorption of drugs is unchanged due to obesity. Apparent volume of distribution is greatly increased for some drugs, including most benzodiazepines, thiopentone, phenytoin, verapamil and lignocaine (lidocaine). Drugs with the highest lipid solubility tend to show the largest increase. For example, the highly lipophilic drugs midazolam and diazepam show increases by a factor of 3. Less lipophilic drugs show a smaller net increase.[71]

# Introductory aspects

**Table 1.11** Comparative differences of children and elderly people in their pharmacokinetic handling

| Parameter | Children | Elderly |
|---|---|---|
| Metabolism | Limited capacity to metabolize drugs up to 5 months of age (oxidative processes and glucuronidation) | Reduced capacity to metabolize by oxidative processes with increasing age |
| Half-life | Increased up to approx. 5 months to 3 years | Decreased by approx. 2–3 fold for benzodiazepines subject to oxidative metabolism |
| | | Little change for others |
| Clearance | Reduced up to approx. 5 months to 3 years | Reduced by approx. 2–3 fold for benzodiazepines subject to oxidative metabolism |
| Volume of distribution | Lipophilic drugs probably affected more by proportional change in body fat | Increased with age |

Protein binding of drugs bound to albumin is not dramatically changed in obesity. Oxidative drug biotransformation is minimally changed in obesity, with the exceptions of ibuprofen and prednisolone, for which clearance increases with total bodyweight. Drug conjugation increases as a function of bodyweight in obesity for paracetamol (acetaminophen), lorazepam and oxazepam. High-clearance drugs, including midazolam, have no change in clearance in obese individuals compared with normal bodyweight controls.

## PHARMACOKINETICS IN CHILDREN

Children, particularly those under 3 years old and neonates, are known to have underdeveloped capacity to metabolize certain drugs.[72]

It is likely that drugs metabolized by microsomal oxidative processes are affected, although there are limited data in the literature to quantify the magnitude of the effects for individual drugs.[72–76]

Table 1.11 compares some pharmacokinetic parameters in children and elderly people.

## EFFECT OF BLOOD LOSS AND BLOOD REPLACEMENTS

In situations where extensive blood loss has resulted, e.g. injuries, and replacement fluids are given (fluids, blood transfusions and artificial products providing volume expansion), the blood concentration of drug may be affected if later analysis is carried out of blood taken under these circumstances.

The magnitude of the change is clearly dependent on a number of factors. A variable that is often difficult to define is to ensure that when blood is collected, sufficient time has elapsed to allow re-equilibrium of drug with the new fluids, and that the blood is not collected from the same line as the replacement fluids. For most situations, several minutes may be sufficient to allow such re-equilibrium, although each situation should be considered on its own merit.

Assuming equilibrium is established, the loss of drug from injuries is usually very small. The amount likely to have been lost can be calculated from the volume of distribution. A drug with a volume of distribution of 1.0 has ~4% of drug in the blood volume. Therefore loss of 1 L of blood will only result in the loss of ~1% of the body burden of drug (assuming a 4 L volume of blood). If the $V_D$ is 10 L/kg then 0.1% of drug would be lost in this situation. In the case of alcohol (ethanol), a loss of 1 L of blood would only result in a loss of ~2% of the total body burden. Consequently with these small losses there is little actual change in the blood concentration at equilibrium.

Often a greater effect on drug concentration is the impact of injuries and blood loss on organ function. Reduced blood pressures and blood flow through vital organs will slow the usual processes of metabolism and excretion, prolonging the duration of action of any drugs.

# 1.5 Tolerance and dependence

Drug dependency and tolerance are important components of those persons abusing drugs. For many users, drug dependency becomes a non-controllable disease and dictates their lives. Consequently, drug users become a common client of the medico-legal system because they develop high-risk activities to support their habits and because of the consequences of the drug effects on behaviour.

## DEFINING DRUG DEPENDENCY

Drug dependence can be defined as a state in subjects in which drugs have become part of their life and assume a greater importance than other activities in their life. For a person to be regarded as drug dependent they would normally be expected to meet at least three of the criteria shown in Table 1.12.

Drug dependence need not be a raging habit or compulsive drug-using behaviour; it can be just a subjective desire to use drugs. The development of neuroadaptation need not occur for a person to be considered drug dependent. Often the low-end dependent user of drugs will not have developed significant chemical dependence, but rather may be considered to be psychologically dependent. Addiction usually refers to the raging compulsive user who will have clearly developed neuroadaptation. However, it is not always possible to establish a quantitative measure of dependence, hence it is not usually possible to define accurately the extent of any chemical dependence.

It is also important to recognize that the more common situation is a pattern involving occasional or problematic use. This is less severe than a fully-fledged dependence. There are varying ways to define this behaviour. In this situation, repeated drug use leads to social, legal or medical problems but in the absence of compulsive drug-seeking behaviour. Such use can lead to actual physical or psychological harm. The binge alcohol drinker or the occasional user of heroin or amphetamines will often fit this pattern. Clearly drug abuse can readily lead to drug dependence.

**Table 1.12** Criteria for establishing drug dependence

- Show tolerance
- Exhibit withdrawal symptoms
- Show signs of drug-seeking behaviour
- Show neglect of personal hygiene and health
- The use of large amounts of drug or use over a longer period than intended
- A strong desire or compulsion to take drug

Adapted from the DSM-IV and ICD-10 criteria for diagnosing drug dependence.

Drug users who have developed drug dependence may develop physical (or chemical) dependence on cessation of drug that manifests by the appearance of recognizable groups of symptoms classed as an abstinence syndrome. The benzodiazepines, barbiturates, opiates, cannabis and the amphetamines all produce an abstinence syndrome on withdrawal of drug in persons who have developed neuroadaptation. Drug dependence is therefore a physiological state in which tolerance, withdrawal, drug-seeking behaviour, neglect of personal hygiene and health, use of larger than normal amounts, and strong desire or compulsion to use drugs are characteristic traits.

## TOLERANCE

Tolerance is a phenomenon in which a subject develops a neuroadaptation to a psychoactive drug requiring increasingly larger doses to achieve the same pharmacological effect. This occurs for most drugs, but occurs particularly easily for the amphetamines, barbiturates, cocaine and the opioid narcotics.

Tolerance appears to be caused by a reduction in the sensitivity of the receptor to the drug. This can be caused either by a reduction in the number of receptors or a reduction in the efficiency of coupling of the drug and its receptor to achieve a certain effect. This process usually takes place over days to weeks of use. Once this physiological change has occurred, it takes some weeks for the body to readjust back to a normal state.

Prescribed drug use can lead to tolerance or neuroadaptation to the drug, although this is relatively unusual and rarely leads to drug dependence as defined earlier. The most likely situation would be patients on long-term pain relief from morphine or another opiate, and patients prescribed benzodiazepines for anxiety-related conditions.

## SIDE EFFECTS AND ADVERSE REACTIONS

All drugs produce side effects. Side effects can range from minor discomfort, such as minor gastrointestinal disorders, headache, nausea, etc., to adverse reactions that are noxious and unintended and can be quite harmful to the person. Examples of such reactions include liver damage induced by an overdose of paracetamol or use of some antidepressants and antipsychotics, and the case of thalidomide, which causes fetal abnormalities leading to phocomelia.[v] These reactions can occur at normal therapeutic doses.

In some cases, adverse reactions cause profound behavioural changes that lead to, or form the background to, serious domestic and social situations. This may occur in persons using a legal drug in a prescribed manner, in persons using legal drugs in a non-prescribed manner, in persons using illegal drugs, or in persons using undesired combinations of drugs. These situations are brought up in court proceedings, and can become important issues. Unfortunately, there is often little information readily accessible to the courts that provides an overview of these drug-induced changes.

---

[v] Limb deformity characterized by the absence of the proximal portion of a limb or limbs, with the hands or feet attached to the trunk of the body by a single and often deformed bone.

# 1.6 Toxicology

Toxicity is defined as an unwanted drug response that is life threatening. This contrasts with side effects and adverse reactions, which are usually unwanted effects that produce a range of symptoms or reduce the effectiveness of the medication, but which rarely produce life-threatening reactions.

While a thorough understanding of the pharmacokinetic and pharmacological properties of drugs is essential, there are a number of processes that may affect the concentration of drugs, particularly in postmortem cases. These range from metabolic changes that are enzyme mediated, to artefacts caused by redistribution processes and contamination from neighbouring sites. Some substances are unstable in a biological matrix or when stored for some time before analysis is conducted.

Toxicologists and forensic pharmacologists assist in the interpretation of toxicological data in medico-legal proceedings.

## CHEMICAL INSTABILITY

Heroin, cocaine, acetylsalicylic acid (aspirin) and drugs administered as pro-drugs that are based on esters are hydrolysed after death. For example, postmortem deacetylation of heroin and 6-acetylmorphine will lead to an elevation of unconjugated morphine concentrations after death. It is extremely rare to detect heroin, or even 6-acetylmorphine, in blood following an injection of heroin.

The 7-amino metabolites of benzodiazepines show significant instability when frozen over prolonged periods of time.[77] Temazepam degrades in blood kept at 5°C, but not when stored frozen at −20°C.[78] Nordiazepam, chlordiazepoxide and demoxepam are unstable during storage at both 4°C and particularly 25°C. In the case of chlordiazepoxide, losses are observed within days.[79] In contrast, flurazepam and diazepam are relatively stable, as are the barbiturates.[80] Tranylcypromine concentrations in blood have also been shown to halve over 48 h at 37°C.[81]

Chemical instability is often hard to differentiate from those processes mediated by metabolic changes.

## METABOLIC CHANGES

The benzodiazepines are a particularly important example of a drug undergoing postmortem changes. Many of the benzodiazepines show losses that can be attributed to a combination of chemical degradation and metabolic attack. For example, the nitrobenzodiazepines, such as flunitrazepam, are rapidly converted to the 7-amino form.[77] This can occur in whole fresh blood over several days after bacteria invade the specimen, or in postmortem blood already contaminated by bacteria. This loss is only partly inhibited by fluoride, therefore a component

# Toxicology

**Table 1.13** Factors affecting postmortem blood concentrations of drugs

| | |
|---|---|
| Chemical instability | Hydrolytic reactions, e.g. hydrolysis of heroin, aspirin |
| | Sulfoxidation, e.g. thioridazine and dothiepin |
| Action of endogenous enzymes | Cofactor-mediated degradation of flunitrazepam |
| | Hydrolysis of heroin, 6-MAM through esterases |
| | Hydrolysis of acetylsalicylic acid and cocaine |
| Action of bacterial-derived enzymes | Activation of pro-drugs generally through esterases |
| | Nitro reduction |
| | Deconjugation of glucuronides |
| | S-oxidation of thioridazine, dothiepin |
| Redistribution | Changes in the blood concentration by diffusion of drug from neighbouring tissue |
| | Diffusion from gastric contents and aspirated material in lungs and trachea |
| Other processes | Contamination with other body fluids |
| | Incomplete tissue distribution |
| | Loss of tissue through putrefaction |
| | Embalming |

can also occur spontaneously. Similar changes occur for clonazepam, nitrazepam and possibly nitmetazepam.

The instability of other benzodiazepines is suspected, although the degree to which this occurs and the mechanism of loss are still poorly understood.[79,82]

Sulphur-containing drugs, such as thioridazine, are unstable postmortem and are converted, in part, to the sulphoxide and sulphone forms. This is particularly prominent in liver, although it also occurs in phosphate-buffered saline, presumably due to bacterial contamination.[83] This conversion is variable and not predictable, and leads to a change in the ratio of parent drug to metabolite that can lead to errors in differentiating acute from chronic exposure. This loss of thioridazine even occurs in blood samples stored frozen at $-20°C$ over one month. Similar changes are also possible for dothiepin.[84] While the sulphur atom is intrinsically more unstable chemically than many other moieties, prolonged incubation of amitriptyline in liver also results in significant losses.[83]

Substances capable of attack by esterases are rapidly altered postmortem. These include most pro-drugs, heroin and aspirin. The complete loss of heroin in deaths caused by this drug suggests that this process of deacetylation to 6-monoacetylmorphine and morphine occur very rapidly.

## POSTMORTEM REDISTRIBUTION

The observation that heart blood concentrations of digoxin were much higher than blood taken from peripheral sites, such as the leg (femoral), led to the discovery of the phenomenon of postmortem redistribution.[85] These authors postulated that digoxin was released from heart tissue after death and diffused into the pool of blood in the heart. The increase in concentration of digoxin in heart blood was substantial and easily exceeded the fatal concentrations associated with this drug, even though therapeutic (non-toxic) concentrations were present immediately prior to death.

Tricyclic antidepressants are also subject to postmortem redistribution and have become model drugs to study this phenomenon.[86-88] Increases in concentration of several-fold are known when concentrations in the heart are compared with either blood taken immediately after death, or blood that is taken peripherally at autopsy.

The diffusion of drug released from tissue-bound stores adjacent to blood vessels is the principal reason for this phenomenon. Figure 1.7 shows some examples of the degree this redistribution occurs for some commonly abused drugs.[87] One of the worst examples is propoxyphene, which shows three-fold increases from femoral blood to heart blood. In some cases, increases of 10-fold have occurred. Methamphetamine shows an increase, on average, of nearly two-fold, while diazepam and cocaine show only small increases. The increases for parent drugs are also accompanied by increases of their respective metabolites, e.g. norpropoxyphene, nordiazepam and benzoylecgonine (cocaine metabolite).

Methadone has also been shown to suffer from redistribution with ratios of heart to peripheral blood ranging from 0.3 to 4.0, with average increases of about 1.2–1.3.[87,89] There is a significant amount of site-to-site variability, suggesting other factors are also operating to affect blood concentrations. This may include a variable haematocrit with variable degree of haemolysis.

On the other hand, morphine appears to show little or no redistribution in man,[90,91] although increases have been observed in the rat.[92]

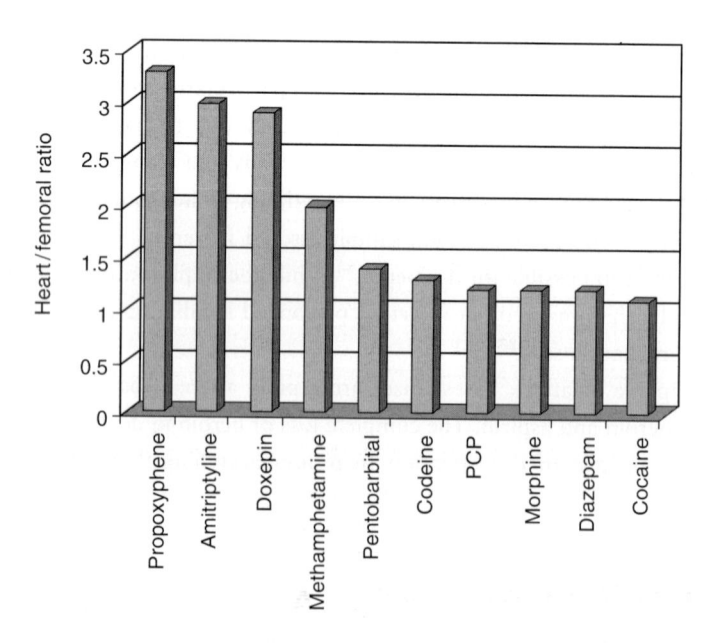

**Fig. 1.7** Heart blood to femoral blood concentration ratios for selected abused drugs (after a variety of sources including Refs 87 and 99)

While femoral blood (or other peripheral blood) shows the least change in postmortem drug concentrations, increases will also occur in femoral blood, particularly for drugs with large increases in heart blood. Increases of a factor of two are known for pethidine (meperidine) (and norpethidine metabolite) and amitriptyline (nortriptyline). Increases for other drugs are also likely, particularly those drugs that show higher muscle concentrations than blood concentrations.

Drugs that exhibit a moderate to high volume of distribution are likely candidates for postmortem redistribution, since these drugs will be extensively bound in tissues. Hydrophilic drugs such as paracetamol (acetaminophen), theophylline, barbiturates and morphine exhibit comparatively little redistribution compared with lipophilic antidepressants, opioids and antipsychotic drugs. Unexpected differences, even within a class of drugs, can occur. For example, the serotonin re-uptake inhibitor venlafaxine is much more subject to redistribution than paroxetine.[93]

Postmortem diffusion has been demonstrated by the instillation of alcohol, propoxyphene and paracetamol in the lungs (or trachea) to simulate aspiration of stomach contents containing drug. This results in significant concentrations of these drugs in a number of blood vessels, including the pulmonary and superior vena cava.[94]

Increases in heart blood concentrations and the liver immediately adjacent to the bowel are also more likely following oral overdoses due to perfusion of drug from the stomach contents and bowel. This has been observed for alcohol, tricyclic antidepressants and other drugs.[95–98] Similar phenomena are seen in the lungs where the left portions are more affected than the right.[97] There are significant differences in the concentrations of drugs in left and right lobes of the liver. These differences are highest for drugs that show the least redistribution, namely paracetamol (acetaminophen) and temazepam, in which increases of over three-fold occurred.

Unfortunately, these changes are not predictable, and show enormous variability from one case to another. The time from death to specimen collection and prevailing environmental conditions will significantly affect the degree to which blood concentrations have equilibrated to the new environment.

Table 1.14 summarizes the postmortem redistribution values of selected drugs.

## OTHER PROCESSES

The addition of formalin (5% and 8%) to blood and liver, such as in the embalming process, causes almost complete loss of carbon monoxide over one week. Substantial losses of diazepam and phenytoin occur in blood over 30 days in blood as well as substantial losses of phenobarbital and desipramine in liver.[100] The effects of formalin on barbiturate content in tissues is dependent on the tissue, with the greatest loss occurring in the liver and the least in the spleen, although drugs were still detectable after three years of storage.[101]

Toxicologists must therefore not only target the right substance to best account for these processes but also should aim to understand the mechanisms of any postmortem changes.

## INTERPRETATION OF TOXICOLOGICAL INFORMATION

The interpretation of drug data requires a good understanding of the basic pharmacology and pharmacokinetics of the drugs in question. Of course, the application of this knowledge

**Table 1.14** Summary of data on redistribution of drugs of abuse

| Drug | Degree of redistribution[a] (%) | Reference |
|---|---|---|
| **Opioids** | | |
| Morphine | <20 | 90, 91 |
| Methadone | 20–30 | 87, 89 |
| Pethidine (meperidine) | 90 | 87 |
| Propoxyphene | 300 | 87 |
| **Stimulants** | | |
| Amphetamine | 80 | 87 |
| Methamphetamine | 300 | 87, 99 |
| Cocaine/BE | 30 (50) | 87 |
| Phentermine | 60 | 87 |
| **Sedatives/hypnotics** | | |
| Amylobarbital | 40–200 | 86, 87 |
| Pentobarbital | 30–200 | 86, 87 |
| Secobarbital | 50–200 | 86, 87 |
| Diazepam (nordiazepam) | 30 (30) | 87 |
| Flunitrazepam | <20 | 77 |
| Temazepam | 50 | 87 |

[a] Increase in heart blood over femoral blood.

requires details of the subject under question, i.e. age and general health and where this is possible, and a knowledge of the drug-taking history. Without these data it will not usually be possible to provide sufficiently helpful comments on the likely effects of the drugs detected by the forensic toxicologists.

The ability to obtain detailed relevant circumstances of the case will often be difficult, yet without such data expert opinions will seriously suffer. Death further complicates the interpretation of toxicological data as this chapter has exposed. Issues of stability of drugs in an postmortem environment, as well as drug diffusion and redistribution, will need to be considered in such cases. Accordingly, the collection of appropriate specimens that will be least subject to artefactual changes are required.

The following chapters arranged by drug type focus on specific issues relating to each class of drug. Case reports illustrate issues at the end of each section. The final chapter focuses on clinical issues in forensic medicine and provides an overview of drug issues covered in each of the earlier drug sections.

# References for Section I

1. NIDA. *Prevalence of various types of drugs*. NIDA; 1995.
2. Commonwealth Department of Health and Family Services. *National Drug Strategy Household Survey: Survey Report*. Commonwealth Department of Health and Family Services; 1998.
3. International Narcotics Control Board. *Reports of the International Narcotics Control Board for 1995 and 1996*. International Narcotics Control Board; 1997.
4. ABCI. *Australian Illicit Drug Report 1998–99*. Canberra: Australian Bureau of Criminal Intelligence; March 2000.
5. Plueckhahn VD, Cordner SM, eds. *Ethics, legal medicine and forensic pathology*, 2nd edn. Melbourne: Melbourne University Press; 1991.
6. Forrest ARW. Obtaining samples at postmortem examination for toxicological and biochemical analyses. *J Clin Pathol* 1993; 46: 292–6.
7. Pounder DJ, Davies JI. Zopiclone poisoning: tissue distribution and potential for postmortem diffusion. *Forens Sci Internat* 1994; 65: 177–83.
8. Drummer OH, King CV, Kotsos AK, Peace A, Crockart H, McIntyre IM. The body burden of benzodiazepines in humans. In: Bernhard W, Sachs H, Jeger A, eds. *Proceedings of The International Association of Forensic Toxicologists*. Interlaken: Molina Press.
9. Robertson MR, Drummer OH. Postmortem distribution and redistribution of nitrobenzodiazepines in man. *J Forens Sci* 1998; 43(1): 9–13.
10. Agarwal A, Lemos N. Significance of bile analysis in drug-induced deaths. *J Anal Toxicol* 1996; 20: 61–2.
11. Park JI, Nakamura GR, Griesemer EC, Noguchi TT. Hydromorphone detected in bile following hydrocodone ingestion. *J Forens Sci* 1982; 27(1): 223–4.
12. McIntyre IM, Ruszkiewicz AR, Crump K, Drummer OH. Death following colchicine poisoning. *J Forens Sci* 1994; 39(1): 280–6.
13. Winek CL, Henry D, Kirkpatrick L. The influence of physical properties and lipid content of bile on the blood/bile ethanol ratio. *Forens Sci Internat* 1983; 22: 171–8.
14. Drummer OH. Use of vitreous humour in toxicology. *Analog* 1993; 15(2): 14–15.
15. McKinney PE, Phillips S, Gomez HF, Brent J, MacIntyre M, Watson WA. Vitreous humor cocaine and metabolite concentrations: do postmortem specimens reflect blood levels at the time of death? *J Forens Sci* 1994; 40: 102–7.
16. Yip CP, Shum BSF. A study on the correlation of blood and vitreous humour alcohol levels in the late absorption and elimination phases. *Med Sci Law* 1990; 30: 29–33.
17. Chatt A, Kataz S. *Hair analysis: application in the biomedical and environmental sciences*. New York: VCH; 1988.

18. Chattophhyay A, Roberts TM, Jervis RE. Scalp hair as a monitor of community exposure to lead. *Arch Environ Health* 1977; 30: 226–36.
19. Giovanoli-Jakubczak T, Berg GG. Measurement of mercury in human hair. *Arch Environ Health* 1974; 28: 139–44.
20. Kintz P, ed. *Drug testing in hair*, 1st edn. Boca Raton, Florida: CRC Press; 1996.
21. Sachs H. History of hair analysis. *Forens Sci Internat* 1997; 84: 7–16.
22. Couper FJ, McIntyre IM, Drummer OH. Extraction of psychotropic drugs from human scalp hair. *J Forens Sci* 1995; 40(1): 83–6.
23. *Forens Sci Internat* 1993; 63: 1–316.
24. *Forens Sci Internat* 1995; 70: 1–222.
25. *Forens Sci Internat* 1997; 84: 1–313.
26. General Directorate of Abu Dhabi Police. *Hair analysis in forensic toxicology*. Abu Dhabi: General Directorate of Abu Dhabi Police, UAE; 1995.
27. Moeller MR, Eser HP. The analytical tools for hair testing. In: Kintz P, ed. *Drug testing in hair*. Boca Raton, Florida: CRC Press; 1996. pp. 95–120.
28. Henderson GL. Mechanisms of drug incorporation in hair. *Forens Sci Internat* 1993; 63: 19–29.
29. Kidwell DA, Blank DL. Environmental exposure – the stumbling block of hair testing. In: Kintz P, ed. *Drug testing in hair*. Boca Raton, Florida: CRC Press; 1996. pp. 17–68.
30. Haley NJ, Hoffmann D. Analysis for nicotine and cotinine in hair to determine cigarette smoker status. *Clin Chem* 1985; 31: 1598–600.
31. Skopp G, Potsch L, Moeller MR. On cosmetically treated hair – aspects and pitfalls of interpretation. *Forens Sci Internat* 1997; 84(1–3): 43–52.
32. Green SJ, Wilson JF. The effect of hair color on the incorporation of methadone in hair in the rat. *J Anal Toxicol* 1996; 20: 121–3.
33. Rothe M, Pragst F, Spiegel K, Harrach T, Fischer K, Kunkel J. Hair concentrations and self-reported abuse history of 20 amphetamine and ecstacy users. *Forens Sci Internat* 1997; 89: 111–28.
34. Cirimele V, Kintz P, Mangin P. Drug concentration in human hair after bleaching. *J Anal Toxicol* 1995; 19: 331–2.
35. Welch MJ, Sniegoski LT, Allgood CC, Habram M. Hair analysis for drugs of abuse: evaluation of analytical methods, environmental issues, and development of reference materials. *J Toxicol* 1993; 17: 389–97.
36. Jurado C, Kintz P, Mendendez M, Repetto M. Influence of the cosmetic treatment of hair on drug testing. *Internat J Legal Med* 1997; 110: 159–63.
37. Baumgartner WA, Hill VA. Sample preparation techniques. *Forens Sci Internat* 1993; 63: 121–35.
38. Chiarotti M. Overview on extraction procedures. *Forens Sci Internat* 1993; 63: 161–70.
39. Dupont RL, Baumgartner WA. Drug testing by urine and hair analysis: complementary features and scientific issues. *Forens Sci Internat* 1995; 70: 63–76.
40. Ishiyama I, Nogai T, Nagai T, Komuro E, Monase T, Akimore N. The significance of the drug analysis in sweat in respect to rapid screening for drug abuse. *Zeitschr Rechtsmed* 1979; 92: 251–6.

# References

41. Cone EJ, Hillsgrove MJ, Jenkins AJ, Keenan RM, Darwin WD. Sweat testing for heroin, cocaine and metabolites. *J Anal Toxicol* 1994; 18: 298–305.
42. Kintz P, Tracqui A, Mangin P, Edel Y. Sweat testing in opioid users with a sweat patch. *J Anal Toxicol* 1996; 20: 393–7.
43. Schneyer LH, Young JA, Schneyer CA. Salivary secretion of electrolytes. *Physiol Rev* 1972; 52: 720–77.
44. Cone EJ. Saliva testing for drugs of abuse. *Ann New York Acad Sci* 1997: 91–127.
45. Höld KM, de Boer D, Zuidema J, Maes RAA. Saliva as an analytical tool in toxicology. *Internat J Drug Test* [serial online] 1996 [cited 21 December 2000]; 1: 1–33 [available from http://www.criminology.fsu.edu].
46. Danhof M, Breimer DD. Therapeutic drug monitoring in saliva. *Clin Pharmacokinet* 1978; 3: 39–57.
47. De la Torre R, Segura J, de Zeeuw R, Williams J. Recommendations for the reliable detection of illicit drugs in urine in the European Union, with special attention to the workplace. *Ann Clin Biochem* 1997; 34: 339–44.
48. Validation of assays. In: Society of Forensic Toxicologists; 1999. Internet source www.soft-tox.org.
49. ISO. *Guide to the expression of uncertainty in measurement*. Geneva: ISO; 1993.
50. Barwick VJ, Ellison SLR. The evaluation of a measurement uncertainty from method validation studies. *Accred Qual Assur* 2000; 5: 47–53.
51. Gibaldi M. *Biopharmaceutics and clinical pharmacokinetics*, 4th edn. Philadelphia: Lea and Febiger; 1991.
52. *Goodman and Gilman's the pharmacological basis of therapeutics*. Various edns. Basingstoke: Macmillan.
53. Garzone PD, Kroboth PD. Pharmacokinetics of the newer benzodiazepines. *Clin Pharmacokinet* 1989; 16: 337–64.
54. Bullingham RE, McQuay HJ, Porter EJ, Allen MC, Moore RA. Sublingual buprenorphine used postoperatively: ten hour plasma drug concentration analysis. *Br J Clin Pharmacol* 1982; 13: 665–73.
55. Jones DR, Hall SD, Jackson EK, Branch RA, Wilkinson GR. Brain uptake of benzodiazepines: effects of lipophilicity and plasma protein binding. *J Pharmacol Exp Therapeut* 1988; 245(3): 816–21.
56. Ruffalo RL, Thompson JF, Segal JL. Diazepam–cimetidine drug interaction: a clinically significant effect. *South Med J* 1981; 74(9): 1075–8.
57. Wagner BKJ, O'Hara DA. Pharmacokinetics and pharmacodynamics of sedatives and analgesics in the treatment of agitated critically ill patients. *Clin Pharmacokinet* 1997; 33(6): 426–53.
58. Bertz RJ, Granneman GR. Use of in vitro and in vivo data to estimate the likelihood of metabolic pharmacokinetic interactions. *Clin Pharmacokinet* 1997; 32: 210–58.
59. Griffin JP, D'Arcy PF, Speirs CJ. *A manual of adverse drug interactions*, 4th edn. London: Wright; 1988.
60. Tatro DS, ed. *Drug interaction facts*. St Louis: J.B. Lippincott; 1990.
61. Baillie SP. Age and the pharmacokinetics of morphine. *Age Aging* 1989; 18: 258–62.

62. Bandera R, Bollini P, Garattini S. Long-acting and short-acting benzodiazepines in the elderly: kinetic differences and clinical relevance. *Curr Med Res Opin* 1984; 4: 94–107.
63. Bentley JB, Borel JD, Nenand REJ, Gillespie TJ. Age and fentanyl pharmacokinetics. *Anaesthet Analges* 1982; 61: 968–71.
64. Closser MH. Benzodiazepines and the elderly. A review of potential problems. *J Subst Abuse Treat* 1991; 8(1–2): 35–41.
65. Vestal RE, McGuire EA, Tobin JD, Andres R, Norris AH, Mezey E. Aging and ethanol metabolism. *Clin Pharmacol Ther* 1977; 21(3): 343–54.
66. Greenblatt DJ, Shader RI, MacLeod SM, Sellers EM. Clinical pharmacokinetics of chlordiazepoxide. *Clin Pharmacokinet* 1978; 3(5): 381–94.
67. Ghabrial H, Desmond PV, Watson KJ, Gijsbers AJ, Harman PJ, Breen KJ, et al. The effects of age and chronic liver disease on the elimination of temazepam. *Eur J Clin Pharmacol* 1986; 30(1): 93–7.
68. Greenblatt DJ. Clinical pharmacokinetics of oxazepam and lorazepam. *Clin Pharmacokinet* 1981; 6: 89–105.
69. Dalhoff K, Poulsen HE, Garred P, Placchi M, Gammans RE, Mayol RF, et al. Buspirone pharmacokinetics in patients with cirrhosis. *Br J Clin Pharmacol* 1987; 24: 547–50.
70. Salva P, Costa J. Clinical pharmacokinetics and pharmacodynamics of zolpidem. Therapeutic implications. *Clin Pharmacokinet* 1995; 29(3): 142–53.
71. Abernethy DR, Greenblatt DJ. Drug disposition in obese humans. An update. *Clin Pharmacokinet* 1986; 11(3): 199–213.
72. Coffey B, Shader RI, Greenblatt DJ. Pharmacokinetics of benzodiazepines and psychostimulants in children. *J Clin Psychopharmacol* 1983; 3(4): 217–25.
73. Pokela ML, Olkkola KT, Seppala T, Koivisto M. Age-related morphine kinetics in infants. *Develop Pharmacol Therapeut* 1993; 20: 26–34.
74. Hughes J, Gill AM, Mulhearn H, Powell E, Choonara I. Steady-state plasma concentrations of midazolam in critically ill infants and children. *Ann Pharmacother* 1996; 30: 27–30.
75. Bost RO, Kemp P, Hnilica V. Tissue distribution of methamphetamine and amphetamine in premature infants. *J Anal Toxicol* 1989; 13: 300–2.
76. Barrett DA, Barker DP, Rutter N, Pawula M, Shaw PN. Morphine, morphine-6-glucuronide and morphine-3-glucuronide pharmacokinetics in newborn infants receiving diamorphine infusions. *Br J Clin Pharmacol* 1996; 41(6): 531–7.
77. Robertson MD, Drummer OH. Postmortem drug metabolism by bacteria. *J Forens Sci* 1995; 40(3): 382–6.
78. Al-Hadidi KA, Oliver JS. Stability of temazepam in blood. *Sci Justice* 1995; 35(2): 105–8.
79. Levine B, Blanke RV, Valentour JC. Postmortem stability of benzodiazepines in blood and tissues. *J Forens Sci* 1983; 28(1): 102–15.
80. Levine B, Blanke RV, Valentour JC. Postmortem stability of barbiturates in blood and tissues. *J Forens Sci* 1984; 29(1): 131–8.

81. Yonemitsu K, Pounder DJ. Postmortem changes in blood tranylcypromine concentration: competing redistribution and degradation effects. *Forens Sci Internat* 1993; 59(2): 177–84.
82. Stevens HM. The stability of some drugs and poisons in putrefying human liver tissues. *J Forens Sci* 1984; 24: 577–89.
83. Cerasuolo D, McIntyre IM, Drummer OH. Postmortem changes in drug concentration. In: *Proceedings of 31st International TIAFT meeting*. Leipzig; 1993. pp. 129–32.
84. Pounder DJ, Hartley AK, Watmough PJ. Postmortem redistribution and degradation of dothiepin. Human case studies and an animal model. *Am J Forens Med Patholol* 1994; 15: 231–5.
85. Vorpahl TE, Coe JI. Correlation of antemortem and postmortem digoxin levels. *J Forens Sci* 1978; 23(2): 329–34.
86. Pounder DJ, Jones GR. Postmortem drug redistribution – a toxicological nightmare. *Forens Sci Internat* 1990; 45: 253–63.
87. Prouty RW, Anderson WH. The forensic science implications of site and temporal influences on postmortem blood-drug concentrations. *J Forens Sci* 1990; 35(2): 243–70.
88. Bandt CW. Postmortem changes in serum levels of the tricyclic antidepressants. In: *Proceedings of the American Academy of Forensic Sciences*. Los Angeles; 1981.
89. Levine B, Wu SC, Dixon A, Smialek JE. Site dependence of postmortem blood methadone concentrations. *Am J Forens Med Pathol* 1995; 16(2): 97–100.
90. Logan BK, Snirnow D. Postmortem distribution and redistribution of morphine in man. *J Forens Sci* 1996; 41: 37–46.
91. Gerostamoulos J, Drummer OH. Postmortem redistribution of morphine and its metabolites. *J Forens Sci* 2000; 45: 843–5.
92. Sawyer WR, Forney RB. Postmortem disposition of morphine in rats. *Forens Sci Internat* 1988; 38: 259–73.
93. Jaffe P. The distribution and redistribution of four serotonin reuptake inhibitors in postmortem specimens. Melbourne: Monash University; 1997.
94. Pounder DJ, Yonemitsu K. Postmortem absorption of drugs and ethanol from aspirated vomitus – an experimental study. *Forens Sci Internat* 1991; 51: 189–95.
95. Pounder DJ, Smith DR. Postmortem diffusion of alcohol from the stomach. *Am J Forens Med Pathol* 1995; 16: 89–96.
96. Pounder DJ, Fuke C, Cox DE, Smith D, Kuroda N. Postmortem diffusion of drugs from gastric residue: an experimental study. *Am J Forens Med Pathol* 1996; 17(1): 1–7.
97. Pounder DJ, Adams E, Fuke C, Langford AM. Site to site variability of postmortem drug concentrations in liver and lung. *J Forens Sci* 1996; 41(6): 927–32.
98. Hilberg T, Bugge A, Beylich KM, Mørland J, Bjorneboe A. Diffusion as a mechanism of postmortem drug redistribution: an experimental study in rats. *Int J Legal Med* 1992; 105: 87–91.

99. Barnhart FE, Fogacci JR, Reed DW. Methamphetamine – a study of postmortem redistribution. *J Anal Toxicol* 1999; 23: 69–70.
100. Winek CL, Esposito FM, Cinicola DP. The stability of several compounds in formalin fixed tissues and formalin-blood solutions. *Forens Sci Internat* 1990; 44: 159–68.
101. Sunshine I, Hackett E. Chemical findings in cases of fatal barbiturate intoxications. *J Forens Sci* 1957; 2(2): 149–58.

# 2 Stimulants

| | | |
|---|---|---|
| **Foreword** | | 50 |
| 2.1 | Classification and sources of stimulants | 52 |
| 2.2 | Pharmacokinetics and duration of action | 60 |
| 2.3 | Mechanisms of action | 71 |
| 2.4 | Pharmacological actions and therapeutics | 74 |
| 2.5 | Adverse reactions, tolerance and dependence | 79 |
| 2.6 | Toxicology | 83 |
| 2.7 | Case reports | 93 |
| **References for Section 2** | | 96 |

# Foreword

Amphetamines have been known for over 70 years, and cocaine has been known for centuries as a herbal stimulant. Both drug types have limited medical uses, and are primarily drugs-of-abuse with the potential to cause profound behavioural effects that can lead to permanent physiological changes.

Amphetamines have enjoyed a rollercoaster-like empathy with drug users for many years. Waves of popularity in the USA and other countries have been replaced by the more fashionable cocaine. In recent years, the amphetamines have become more popular again. Whether this is due to changing perceptions of drug effectiveness or simply street availability is hard to discern. Whatever the reason, pharmacologically there is little to differentiate the two types of stimulant drugs. Both are well absorbed by a variety of means – smoking, nasal insufflation, oral and intravenous administration – and both produce an orgasm-like high following intravenous use or smoking. Their ability to enhance mood and energy characterizes their actions, as does their ability to cause depression, hypersomnolence and fatigue on withdrawal. Their association with homicidal and suicidal acts is a serious adverse consequence, which can become a significant issue in courts.

In Australia, surveys of young illicit drug users show 78% have used amphetamines and one-third have injected the drug.[1] Another survey of drug users in Sydney found that 5% were daily injectors.[2] Other sources indicate that amphetamines and ecstasy-like designer drugs have been used by ~8.7% and 4.7% of all Australians, respectively, and 3.6% and 2.4% have used them in the last 12 months. In contrast, the use of cocaine in Australia is estimated at 1.4% in the last 12 months and 4.3% lifetime use.[3] In Australia, amphetamine-like stimulants rank second to cannabis as the most used illicit drug, while in the USA cocaine is far more prevalent with a lifetime prevalence of ~10%. Cocaine is one of the most prevalent drugs mentioned in emergency admissions in the USA.[4] An estimated 4 million persons in the USA have used methamphetamine at least once and DAWN[i] data show that the number of methamphetamine-related deaths has nearly tripled over a number of medical examiner facilities across the USA from 1991 to 1994. This was also associated with a tripling of methamphetamine-related emergency department episodes in this period.[5]

These problems are not restricted to illegal drugs. The worldwide use of the legal stimulant methylphenidate is ~230 million daily doses, or 8.5 tonnes, of which 90% is used in the USA for the treatment of attention deficit disorder (ADD) in children. The United Nations through the International Narcotic Drug Control board estimate that methylphenidate, phentermine and amfepramone (diethylpropion) are the most common diverted legal stimulants.[6] There are many other legal stimulants obtained legally or diverted that are abused.

---

[i] Drug abuse warning network (USA).

## Foreword

This section provides an overview of the sources, pharmacology and pharmacokinetics of amphetamines, cocaine and other abused legal stimulants. This section also includes the relevance of their toxicology in forensic cases. A series of case reports are finally included to illustrate their behavioural and pharmacological effects and relevance to forensic cases.

# 2.1 Classification and sources of stimulants

The stimulants form a large family of drugs that includes the amphetamines, amphetamine-like hallucinogens such as ecstasy, drugs obtained from natural sources such as khat and mescaline, a range of ethical drugs such as the ephedrines and slimming tablets, and cocaine. Pharmacologically they are all related to the hormone adrenaline (epinephrine) and the neurotransmitter noradrenaline (norepinephrine).[ii] Except for cocaine, they are also related chemically to these endogenous substances.

The sources of these drugs vary greatly. Cocaine is chewed or extracted from the leaves of a plant, khat (cathine alkaloids) is simply present in leaves which are chewed or boiled, whereas the amphetamines are produced in clandestine laboratories from either simple chemical precursors or from ethical drugs such as ephedrine and pseudoephedrine.

This chapter provides an overview of the range of abused stimulants and details their chemical sources and pharmacological classification.

## HISTORICAL ASPECTS

Extracts of the suprarenal capsule (adrenal glands) were shown in 1895 to increase blood pressure (i.e. showed a pressor response).[7] In their paper to the *Journal of Physiology*, Oliver and Schaefer made the following conclusions:

> It appears established … the material which they form and which is found, at least in its fully active condition, only in the medulla of the gland, produces striking physiological effects upon the muscular tissue generally, and especially upon that of the heart and arteries. Its actions is to increase the tone of all muscular tissue …

The substance causing this effect was later identified as adrenaline. A few years later similarities were noted between the effects of these adrenal extracts and stimulation of sympathetic nerves.[iii] This led to the discovery of neurotransmitters as mediators of nerve function, and eventually led to the identification of the catecholamine noradrenaline as the primary sympathetic neurotransmitter (Fig. 2.1). This chemical differs from adrenaline by the absence of the N-methyl group. The β-phenylisopropylamine backbone is the structural basis for many of the sympathomimetic amines.

Amphetamine was first synthesized in 1887, but it was not until the late 1920s that its use to replace ephedrine as a nasal decongestant was recognized. In the 1930s, amphetamine was

---

[ii] Epinephrine and norepinephrine are North American names for adrenaline and noradrenaline.
[iii] A part of the peripheral autonomic nervous system that uses noradrenaline as neurotransmitter and that controls blood pressure, heart rate and distribution of blood flow.

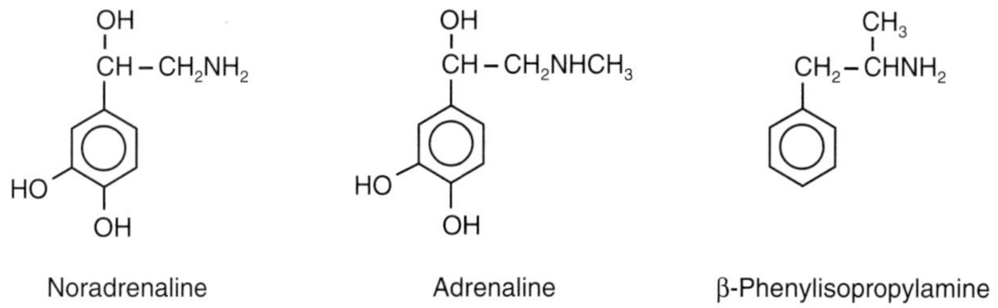

**Fig. 2.1** Structures of the precursors to stimulants

Both noradrenaline and adrenaline are catecholamines, and differ from phenylisopropylamine by the presence of the hydroxy groups.

marketed as Benzedrine inhaler for this purpose. A little while later, its ability to reduce appetite, to act as a general stimulant, and to treat narcolepsy and hyperactivity in children was recognized. By the time of the Second World War, its abuse potential was known. Despite this, the German, Japanese and allied armies used amphetamine to maintain alertness and battle fatigue. It is now classed as a drug of abuse with limited therapeutic value, and is appropriately scheduled.

It was not long after the discovery of sympathetic transmission that cocaine was found to affect sympathetic nerve transmission. The close relationship between the effects of cocaine and the amphetamines can be explained by their actions on the sympathetic nerve terminal (see Chapter 2.3).[iv]

Cocaine has been used by the Peruvian Indians for centuries for the well-being and increased endurance it produced after sucking the leaves of the plant *Erythroxylon coca* and related species. The plant thrives in hot and humid conditions at moderate elevation, although plants growing on the sides of mountains were favoured as producing the most cocaine. The leaves are plucked and left to dry in the sun before use. The Peruvians recognized that combining the leaves with lime increased its absorption and effects. This had the effect of liberating free cocaine. The free base is now used by drug addicts as 'freebasing'. The Incas made coca a royal emblem with a queen named 'Mama Cuca', and it was used by priests in various divine ceremonies.

Cocaine belongs to the tropane alkaloid family, which includes hyoscine, scopolamine and atropine from the deadly nightshade plants (*Datura stramonium* and *Atropa belladonna*). These belladonna alkaloids differ from cocaine pharmacologically, and are anticholinergic compounds.

Cocaine was first isolated in 1859 by the chemist Niemann. It was known as a drug that caused numbness of the tongue and was capable of insensitizing skin to pain. Sigmund Freud in Vienna studied its effects at length and was determined to find a medical use for the drug. In 1885 he wrote a review on cocaine, 'Über Coca',[8] which detailed not only the world knowledge on the drug at that time, but also his own personal experiences. A 50 mg oral dose

---

[iv] Sympathetic nerve terminals are the nerve endings from which neurotransmitters are released.

was described thus [pp. 58–60]:

> A few minutes after taking cocaine, one experiences a sudden exhilaration and feeling of lightness. One feels a certain furriness on the lips and palate, followed by a feeling of warmth in the same areas; if one now drinks cold water, it feels warm on the lips and cold in the throat. On other occasions the predominant feeling is a rather pleasant coolness in the mouth and throat.
>
> The psychic effect of cocaïnum muriaticum [cocaine hydrochloride] in doses of 0.05–0.10 g consists of exhilaration and lasting euphoria, which does not differ in any way from the normal euphoria of a healthy person.

A colleague, Dr Karl Koller, discovered cocaine's ability to cause anaesthesia in the eye. Within a short period, before the turn of the century, it was used in ophthalmology, dentistry and in general surgery as an anaesthetic. As early as 1905 an analogue of cocaine was produced chemically as an anaesthetic. Procaine is still used in medicine today, and analogues such as lignocaine (lidocaine) are well known.

In the late nineteenth century cocaine was freely available in drinks such as Coca Cola (25 mg/L) and Vin Mariani (267 mg/L),[9] and even as coca cordial, wine of coca, coca cheroots, cocaine cigarettes and cocaine inhalant.[9] Cocaine was considered at that time a herbal remedy for headache, neuralgia, melancholy, fatigue, hysteria, digestive disorders, syphilis, asthma and postnasal catarrh. Cocaine was removed from Coca Cola in 1905. By 1914 the Harrison Narcotics Act banned the free distribution of cocaine and limited its use by prescription. It was not until the late 1960s that the recreational use of cocaine became a significant social problem in the Western world.

A summary of this history can be found in several references.[8–12]

## STRUCTURES AND SOURCES OF AMPHETAMINE-LIKE STIMULANTS

### Legal stimulants

A selection of legally available stimulants are shown in Fig. 2.2. Amphetamine is included here because it has a limited range of medical indications (see Chapter 2.5) and readers can make comparisons with other drugs.

Ephedrine and pseudoephedrine are weak stimulants that occur naturally in the branches of a number of *Ephedra* species in concentrations up to ~1.2%. These two drugs are also stereoisomers around the carbon atom adjacent to the nitrogen and to which a methyl group is attached. Stereoisomerism[v] is common in the stimulant family. Drugs with the dextro (d) configuration are usually more active than those with the laevo (l) configuration. Ephedrine is more active centrally than pseudoephedrine, and d-amphetamine is much more

---

[v] Stereoisomerism occurs when a carbon atom has four different substituents bound to it. Depending on the relative spatial configuration of the substituents, the compound exists as isomers. These stereoisomers can have different pharmacological properties and should be considered as separate drugs. Most synthetic drugs exist as a mixture of stereoisomers, called racemates. Most of the amphetamine-like molecules have stereoisomers.

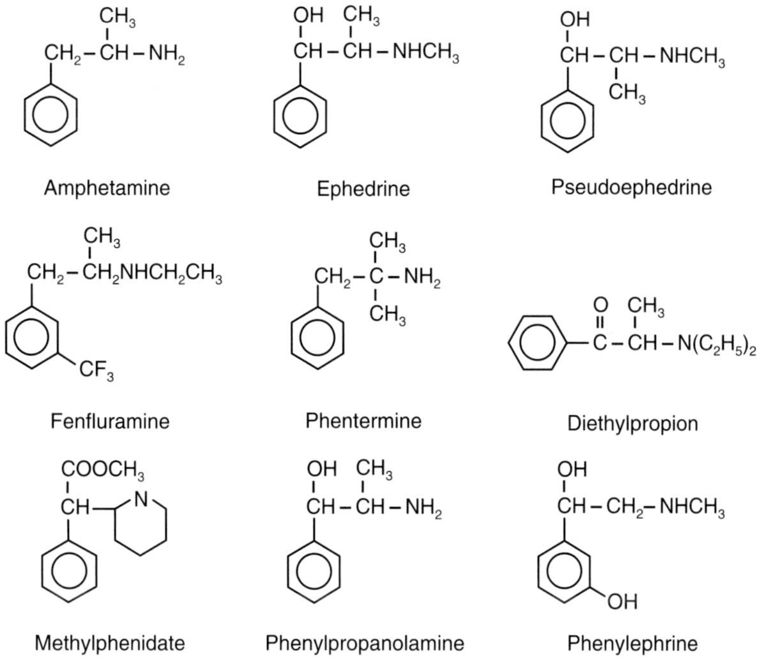

**Fig. 2.2** Structures of selected legal stimulants

active than the l-isomer.[vi] This has implications in analytical chemistry and forensic toxicology (see Chapter 2.6). For example, in the USA, the less active isomer l-amphetamine is marketed as a nasal decongestant (l-desoxyephedrine); the d-isomer, which has other medical uses, is the abused drug.

Phentermine, diethylpropion (amfepramone) and fenfluramine are all found in slimming tablets and are available as legally prescribed medicines. Other stimulant drugs not listed in Fig. 2.2 include benzphetamine, clobenzorex, fenproporex, fenetylline, mefenorex, mazindol, pemoline and propylhexedrine.

## Amphetamines

The amphetamines are related in structure to the legal stimulants (Fig. 2.3). Phenylisopropylamine is actually amphetamine and is the basic unit for other amphetamine analogues. Substitutions on the nitrogen and the ring system account for most of the structural variations.

The most common examples of amphetamines include methamphetamine and the designer amphetamines,[vii] 2-CB, DMA, MBDB, MDMA, MDA, PMA and MDE. MDE has also been

---

[vi] The active form of amphetamine is known chemically as S (+)-amphetamine, or d-amphetamine, or dexamphetamine. The less stereoisomer (enanitomer) is R (−)-amphetamine, or l-amphetamine or laevoamphetamine. The same nomenclature applies to the other amphetamines. The S and R refer to the absolute configuration, and the '+' or '−' (or d and l) refer to the direction light is rotated through a polariscope.

[vii] Designer amphetamines are those synthesized to mimic the actions of amphetamine, but have no medical use.

# Stimulants

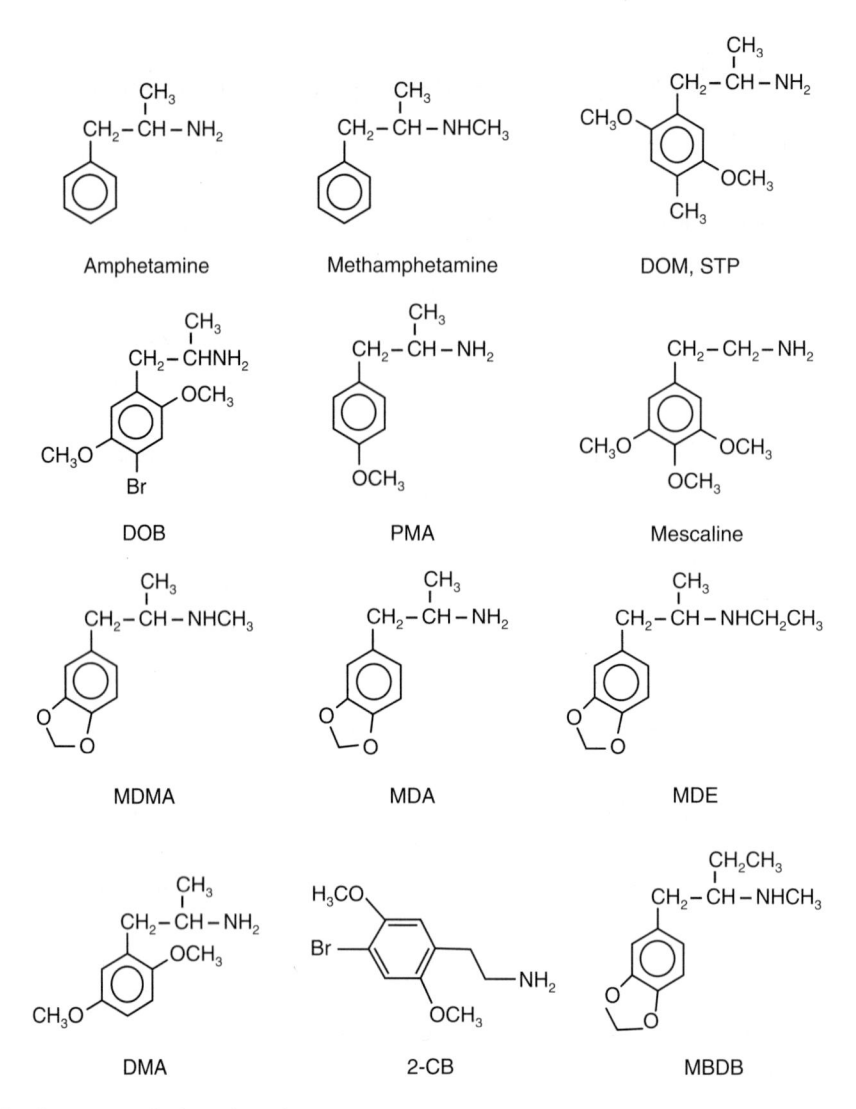

**Fig. 2.3** Structures of selected amphetamines

2-CB: 2,5-dimethoxy-4-bromophenethylamine; DOM: 4-methyl-2,5-dimethoxyamphetamine; DMA: 2,5-dimethoxyamphetamine; DOB: 4-bromo-2,5-dimethoxyamphetamine; MDA: methylenedioxyamphetamine; MDMA: methylenedioxymethamphetamine; MDE: methylenedioxyethylamphetamine; MBDB: N-methylbenzodioxazoylbutanamine; PMA: 4-methoxyamphetamine.

classified as an entactogen, a drug that enhances communication, understanding and empathy.[13] A bromo analogue of dimethoxyamphetamine (4-bromo-2,5-dimethoxyamphetamine, DOB) is reported to have 100 times the potency of MDA.[14]

The chemical variability of street dosage forms represented as 'ecstasy' is highlighted in a Zurich study, which found MDMA, amphetamine, MDE, cocaine, methamphetamine, caffeine, MDA, 2-CB, ephedrine and combinations of these in a 6-month period.[15]

Amphetamines listed in Fig. 2.3, with the exception of amphetamine and methamphetamine, have no medical use and are therefore not available as ethical drugs for purchase

Table 2.1  Common street names for amphetamines

| | |
|---|---|
| Amphetamine | Bennies, speed |
| Methamphetamine | Speed, crystal, crank, go, ice, meth, oxblood |
| 2-CB | Bromo, Nexus, Spectrum, Erox, XTC |
| DOM | Serenity, tranquillity, peace pill |
| MDA | Love pill, speed |
| MDMA | Adam, ecstasy, E, M&M, MDM, XTC |
| PMA | Ecstasy |
| MDE | Eve |

Note: street names vary from country to country and change over time.

or for prescription. They are produced by clandestine laboratories by a variety of chemical processes from a number of precursor molecules. A summary of these chemical reactions and precursors is available.[16] A common synthetic process is the conversion of legally available ephedrine and pseudoephedrine to methamphetamine. This synthetic process often leaves behind significant quantities of the starting drug, which is detectable in both the powder form sold on the streets and in specimens taken from amphetamine users. These impurities can be used to profile the source of the drug.

The stimulants related to amphetamine have attracted a number of street names. Speed and ecstasy are the most common. Table 2.1 summarizes some of the street names of common amphetamines. Oxblood is a deep red liquid form of methamphetamine derived from the crude reaction mixture (probably using a red phosphorous method) and has a purity of >70%. Note that acronyms are used for the designer amphetamines due to their long chemical names. Abbreviated chemical names are found in the legend to Fig. 2.3.

## Mescaline

Mescaline is the active alkaloid in the peyote cactus (*Lophophora williamsii*) originally found growing in northern Mexico and Southern USA. Mescaline is also present in other cactus species growing in sub-tropical and temperate areas of South America (*Trichocereus pachanoi*, 'San Pedro', and *Trichocereus peruvianus*, 'Aguacolla') (Fig. 2.4). Dried disk-shaped tops of the peyote cactus are called mescal buttons. Mescaline content varies from 0.5% to 1.5%.[17] Mescaline can also be made in clandestine laboratories with the right precursors.[16] A synthetic hallucenogenic analogue of mescaline is 2-CB (see Fig. 2.3).

## Cathinone

Cathinone (and other alkaloids found in khat, namely cathine, merucathinone, pseudomerucathinone and merucathine) is derived from the leaves of *Catha edulis* found growing in the highlands of the horn of Africa and the Arabian peninsula) (Fig. 2.3). Analysis of khat leaves also shows the presence of norpseudoephedrine and norephedrine. The leaves are only apparently active when fresh.[18] Common names include khat, qat, gad, tschat and miraa.

# Stimulants

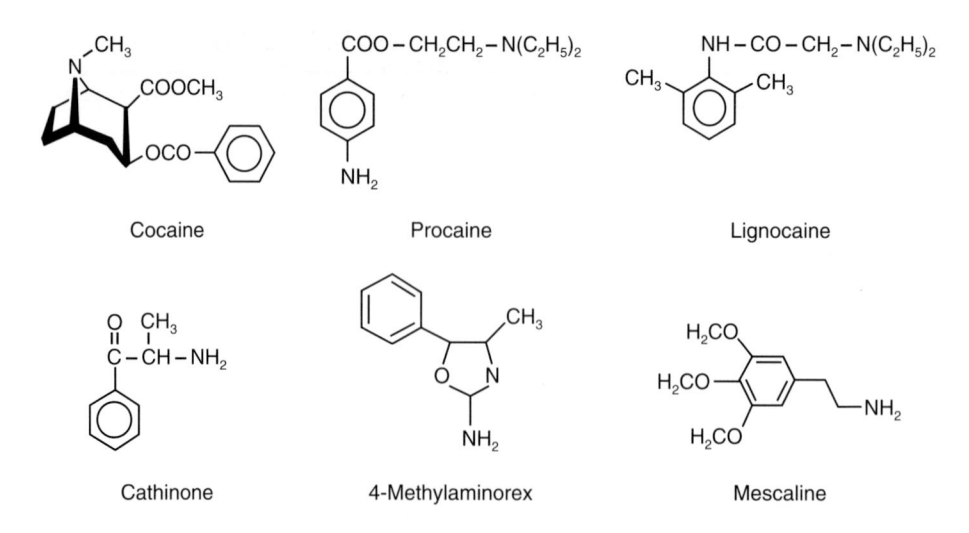

Fig. 2.4 Structures of cocaine and other selected stimulants

Methcathinone is the N-methyl analogue of cathinone and is prepared from ephedrine or pseudoephedrine.[16]

## 4-Methylaminorex

4-Methylaminorex (Fig. 2.4) is a potent stimulant drug previously used as a anorectic that has amphetamine-like properties. This drug has been available as a designer drug with the street names 'ice' and 'U4Euh'.[19] The desmethyl analogue, aminorex, has similar properties.

## Cocaine

Cocaine is derived by extraction of the leaves of *Erythroxylon coca*, where it occurs at concentrations of up to 2% by weight. The plant grows at 1000–2000 m elevations in the Andean mountains under warm tropical conditions. The alkaloid has an unusual structure (see Fig. 2.4) and is related to the tropane alkaloids. Cocaine is produced either as the base (crack, free base) or as the hydrochloride (HCl) salt.

Because of the similarity in anaesthetic properties, procaine and lignocaine[viii] have been used as cheap substitutes for cocaine (on the street) despite their lack of CNS-stimulating properties (Fig. 2.4).[20]

Cocaine availability and purity on the street are highly variable, as for any illegal drug. Street purity ranges from 1% to over 90%, with cocaine hydrochloride used mainly for intravenous injection and nasal insufflation, and the free-base 'crack' used in smoking (Fig. 2.5). Cutting agents are similar to heroin, and range from inert sugars, such as glucose, mannitol and lactose, to pharmacologically active drugs, such as caffeine, codeine and amphetamines. Mixed with heroin and injected it is known as a 'speedball'.[11]

---

[viii] Also known as lidocaine and xylocaine.

## Synopsis

### CLASSIFICATION AND SOURCES OF STIMULANTS

1 Stimulants are generally related pharmacologically to the hormone and neurotransmitter catecholamines, adrenaline (epinephrine) and noradrenaline (norepinephrine).
2 Amphetamine has been known for many decades, finding use as a nasal decongestant, an appetite suppressant and to combat fatigue. Its medical use now is limited to specialist indications, such as attention deficit syndrome (ADD) and narcolepsy.
3 A number of naturally occurring stimulants are known: the ephedrines (*Ephedra* spp.), the cathines (*Catha* spp.), mescaline (peyote cactus) and cocaine (*Erythroxylon coca*), which are, except for cocaine, structurally related to amphetamine.
4 Methamphetamine is one of the most common amphetamines, better known as 'speed', 'crank', 'crystal', 'ice', 'go', 'meth' and 'oxblood'.
5 Designer amphetamines related chemically to amphetamine include DOB, DOM, DMA, MDMA, MDA, MDE and PMA.
6 Street names of designer amphetamines include 'Adam', 'Eve', 'ecstasy', 'love pill', 'peace pill', 'serenity', 'speed' and 'tranquillity'.
7 Cocaine is not related chemically to amphetamines. Analogues of cocaine include procaine and lignocaine, both of which are legal anaesthetic drugs. Street names of cocaine include 'crack'; when mixed with heroin, it is known as a 'speedball'.

# 2.2 Pharmacokinetics and duration of action

The pharmacokinetics of stimulants are important to appreciate and understand since most of the acute effects of these drugs can be based on their pharmacokinetics. Since all members of this class have strongly basic properties, their pharmacokinetics and excretion will be markedly affected by physiological factors.

The structural diversity of this group of drugs (see previous chapter) leads to different pathways of biotransformation, some including formation of active metabolites. Cocaine belongs to a completely different family of drugs and has quite a different metabolic and pharmacokinetic profile to that of the amphetamines.

Since the most common amphetamine used illicitly is methamphetamine, this chapter will focus largely on this drug, together with cocaine. This chapter details some of the more important aspects of the absorption, bioavailability, half-life, metabolic fate and urine detection times.

## METABOLISM

### Amphetamine-like stimulants

The amphetamines are metabolized by similar pathways and involve a combination of hydroxylation of the ring and the side-chain carbon atom adjacent to the ring, and removal of the nitrogen (Fig. 2.5). Drugs with alkyl groups on the nitrogen are dealkylated (methamphetamine and MDMA) to other active amphetamines (amphetamine and MDA, respectively). Methylenedioxyethylamphetamine (ME) and MDMA are both metabolized to MDA[21] as well as other metabolites. MDE, in common with MDMA, MBDB and MDA, is transformed to dihydroxy compounds (catechols) following opening of the methylenedioxy ring.[22] These hydroxy metabolites are either mono-methylated or conjugated (as for the catecholamines adrenaline and noradrenaline). The side chain of the simpler amphetamines is oxidized to form benzoic acid derivatives (fenfluramine and amphetamine), which are excreted as the glycine conjugate (hippuric acid for amphetamine), or the sulphate or glucuronide conjugate. Amphetamine and PMA are also oxidized at the beta-carbon to form the pharmacologically active ephedrine analogues.

A number of legal stimulant drugs are metabolized to methamphetamine or amphetamine. The anti-parkinson drug selegiline is metabolized to the weakly active l-isomer of methamphetamine,[23] while fenethylline, clobenzorex,[24,25] mefenorex,[26,27] fenproporex[28] and benzphetamine are metabolized to d- and l-methamphetamine (l-desoxyephedrine) and/or d- and l-amphetamine (l-desoxynorephedrine). Urine specimens will test positive to amphetamines following use of these drugs by some standard immunoassays, HPLC and GC-MS techniques,

# Pharmacokinetics and duration of action

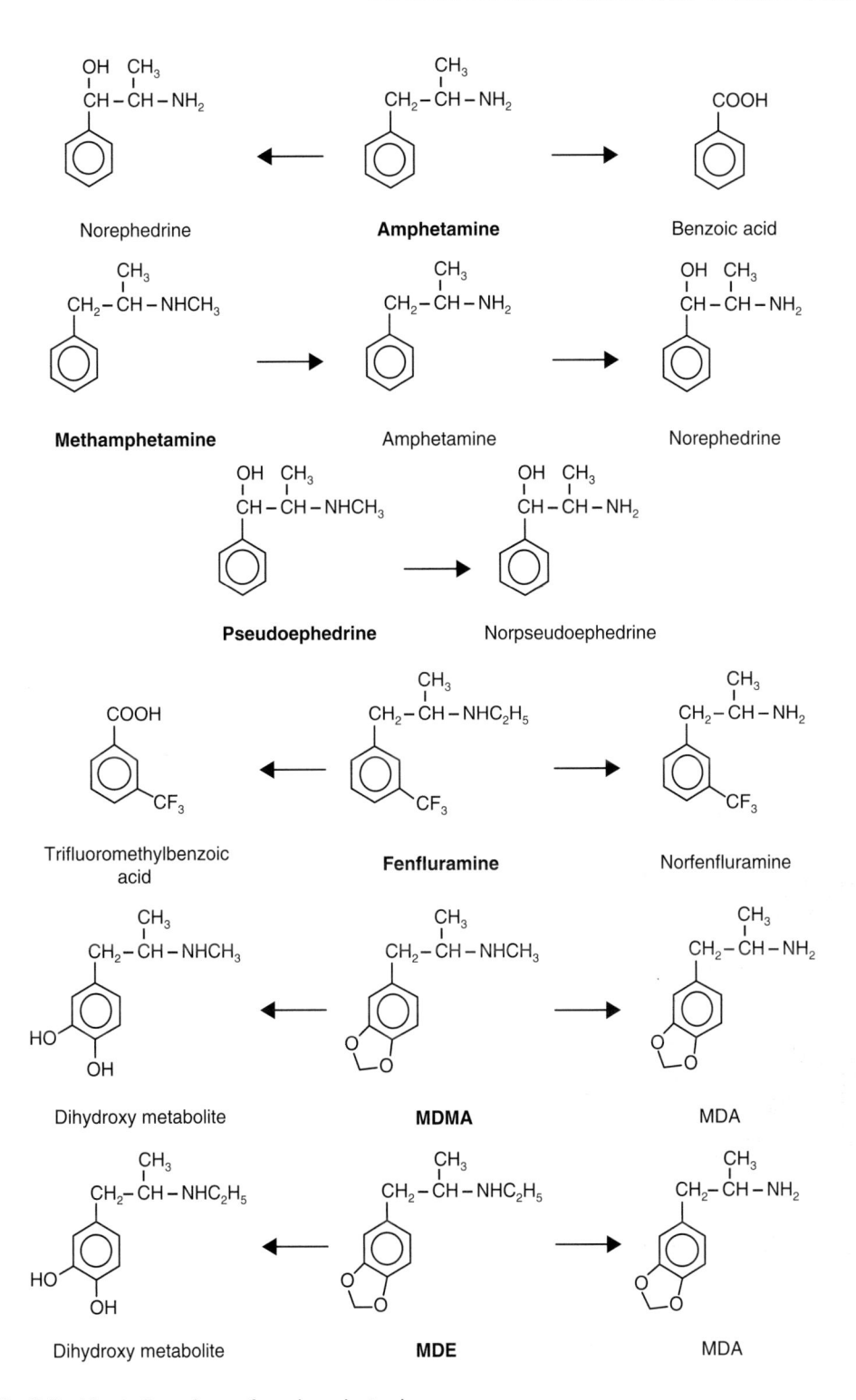

**Fig. 2.5** Metabolic pathways for selected stimulants

Only selected metabolites are shown for simplicity. All metabolites with hydroxyl (OH) groups would normally be conjugated with glucuronic acid. Benzoic acid and trifluoromethylbenzoic acid are excreted as sulphate esters or glycine conjugates.

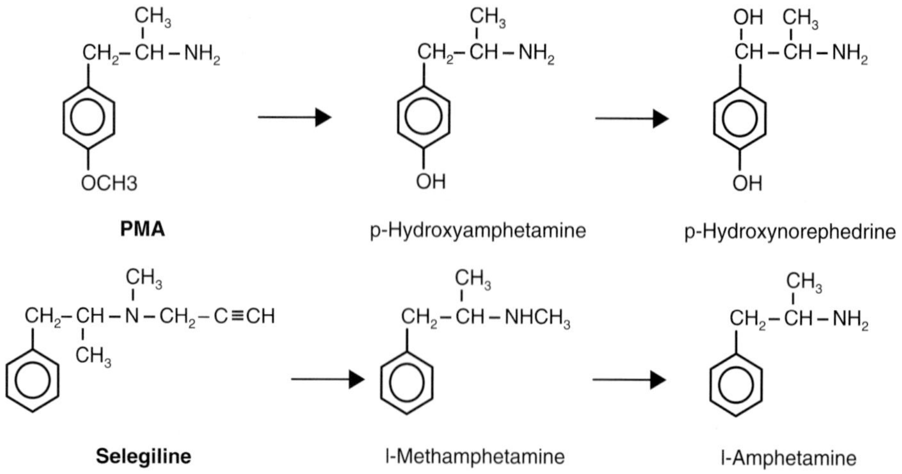

# Stimulants

**Fig. 2.5** (continued)

[Structures shown: PMA → p-Hydroxyamphetamine → p-Hydroxynorephedrine; Selegiline → l-Methamphetamine → l-Amphetamine]

unless chiral assays are used to discriminate the isomers and/or other metabolites unique to the parent drug are targeted (see Chapter 2.3).

Khat, or cathinone, the main alkaloid in this plant, is metabolized by oxidation of the keto-group at the alpha-position on the side chain to norephedrine and norpseudoephedrine (see pseudoephedrine metabolic profile).[29] A summary of the metabolism of some drugs is shown in Fig. 2.5 and in the monographs in the Appendix.

## Cocaine

The metabolism of cocaine has been thoroughly studied. The main metabolite of cocaine is benzoylecgonine, which is formed by chemical and enzymatic hydrolysis of the methyl ester. This is the main metabolite in both blood and urine. Other metabolites are norcocaine, ecgonine methyl ester and ecgonine (Fig. 2.6). Metabolism of cocaine to norcocaine allows the oxidation of the nitrogen to occur, forming N-hydroxynorcocaine. This metabolite or another product produced from its metabolism, such as N-nitrosonorcocaine, or the N-oxide, may be responsible for the hepatotoxicity of cocaine.[30]

Anhydroecgonine methyl ester (AEME, or methylecgonidine) is formed by smoking cocaine, and is produced by pyrolysis rather than metabolism. It is a unique marker for smoked cocaine.[9,31] Cocaethylene is also found as a metabolite, but only in persons consuming alcohol at the same time as using cocaine. Cocaethylene is active pharmacologically and is a unique marker of cocaine users consuming alcohol.[9]

## ABSORPTION AND HALF-LIFE

### Oral absorption and blood concentrations

The stimulant group of drugs, including legal stimulants and designer amphetamines, are generally well absorbed orally, which tends to be a major route of administration. Cocaine

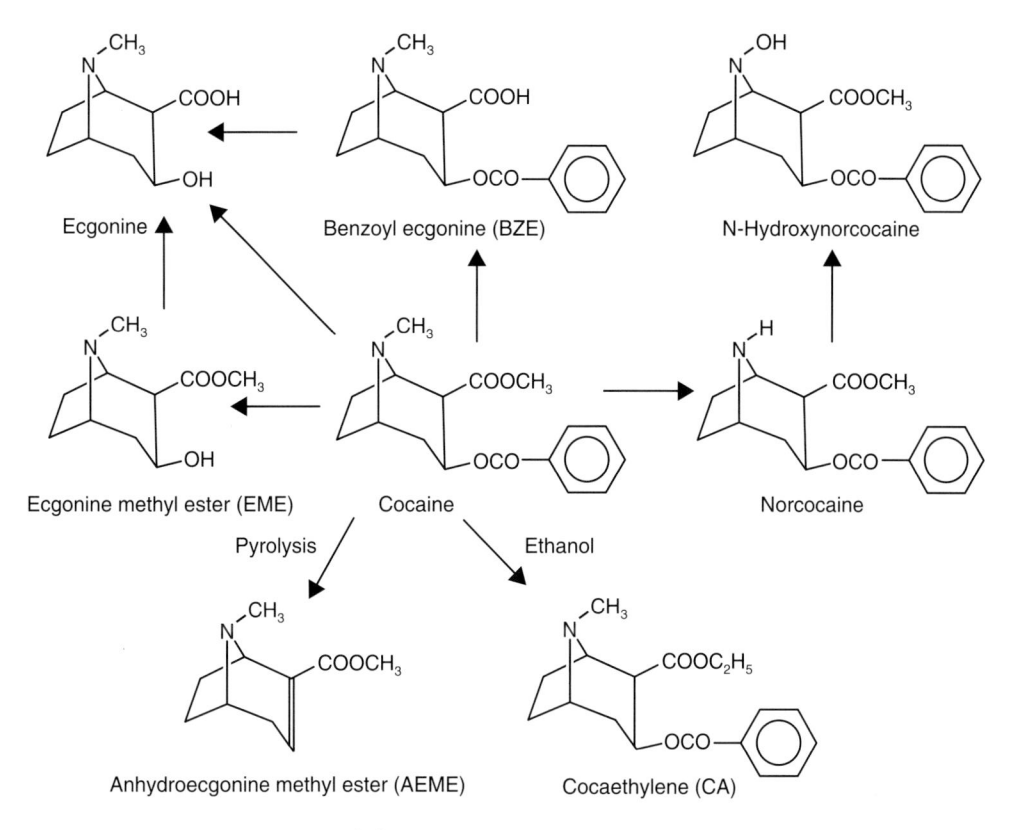

**Fig. 2.6** Metabolic pathways for cocaine

can also be taken orally, although this route is rarely used in practice since oral absorption produces relatively low blood concentrations compared with other routes of administration, and may subject the drug to significant first-pass metabolism to ecgonine methyl ester (EME).

Amphetamines are known to delay gastric emptying and decrease intestinal motility, hence they will delay their own absorption and the absorption of other drugs taken at the same time. Peak concentrations of amphetamines are generally within 1–2 h. Phentermine and fenfluramine tend to take longer to be absorbed, with time to maximum blood concentrations between 2 and 4 h.

Table 2.2 summarizes some pharmacokinetic data for these drugs, including likely blood concentrations following known oral doses. Note that the usual daily doses will vary widely when used recreationally and can easily exceed the doses mentioned in the table. For example, heavily drug-dependent users of amphetamine and methamphetamine can exceed 2000 mg daily and cocaine users are known to reach 5000 mg daily. While these doses are uncommon, they will accordingly generate higher blood (and tissue) concentrations.

There are little data, however, on the linearity of dose and blood concentrations of these drugs at high doses, hence predictions on blood concentrations from doses, or vice versa, will inevitably lead to large errors. This has been confirmed with controlled doses of MDMA[32] and diethylpropion. This may suggest that non-linearity will occur with other stimulant-like drugs.

# Stimulants

**Table 2.2** Selected pharmacokinetic data for some stimulants following oral administration

| Drug | Dose range (mg)[a] | Half-life (h)[b] | Dose[c] | Blood concentration (mg/L)[d] |
|---|---|---|---|---|
| Amphetamine | 5–60 | 4–30 | 30 (acute) | 0.1 |
| Methamphetamine | 5+ | 7–30 | 30 (acute) | 0.04 |
| MDMA | 50–150 | 8 | 100 (acute) | 0.4 |
| MDA | 50–250 | – | 100 (acute) | <0.4 |
| MDE | 50–250 | – | 50 (acute) | <0.2 |
| PMA | 50–100 | – | 100 (acute) | <0.4 |
| Phentermine | 15–40 | 7–24 | 30 (chronic) | 0.06–0.3 |
| Diethylpropion | 75 | 5–12 | 75 (acute) | 0.007 |
| Fenfluramine | 80–160 | 13–30 | 60 (acute) | 0.05–0.07 |
|  |  |  | 142 (chronic) | 0.04–0.3 |
| Ephedrine | 10–50 | 5–8 | 24 (acute) | 0.1 |
| Pseudoephedrine | Up to 240 | 3–16 | 60 (acute) | 0.2 |
|  |  |  | 360 (chronic) | 0.5–0.6 |
| Cathinone | 50+ | 2–5 | 50 (acute) | 0.2[e] |

[a] Usual dose range; [b] pharmacokinetic half-life of terminal elimination phase; [c] an example of a common dose associated with a blood concentration shown in next column; [d] peak blood concentration after dose described in previous column; [e] sum of peak norephedrine and norpseudoephedrine levels.

Oral dosing of methamphetamine produces maximum plasma concentrations approximately 3 h after administration. Peak concentrations following 18 mg and 30 mg are 0.02 µg/mL and 0.04 µg/mL, respectively.[33] MDMA produces peak levels of 0.4 mg/L at 2 h following a 1.5 mg/kg oral dose (~100 mg). Under conditions of a single oral dose, little MDA is detectable in blood.[22]

Oral administration of 0.25 mg/kg d-amphetamine shows maximum cardiovascular effects at 1 h, whereas maximum behavioural and subjective effects occur at 2 h. Subjective and behavioural effects decline thereafter, in spite of substantial amphetamine levels. Subjects receiving 0.5 mg/kg d-amphetamine orally show maximum plasma levels of 0.07 mg/L, which are twice those seen in the earlier group. In this case, plasma levels peak at 3–4 h, and blood pressure and subjective and behavioural effects are all maximal at 2–3 h and are declining by 4 h in spite of stable or rising plasma levels.[34]

The ephedrines (ephedrine and pseudoephedrine) are also well absorbed orally, although their potency as stimulants is substantially less than for the amphetamines. Since doses used are quite different (due to their different potencies), the expected plasma concentrations are accordingly quite different. Oral administration of 15–24 mg ephedrine produces a peak level of ~0.1 mg/L at 1–4 h post dose.[35,36] Oral administration of 180 mg pseudoephedrine gives peak plasma concentrations of 0.7–0.8 mg/L at ~1–2 h. The deliberate co-administration of sodium bicarbonate to increase urine pH slightly increases the peak plasma levels to 0.7–0.9 mg/L. Decreasing pH (ammonium chloride) slightly reduces the peak levels to 0.5–0.7 mg/L.[37]

Volunteers given khat leaves equivalent to 0.8 mg/kg body weight exhibit peak norephedrine and norpseudoephedrine concentrations of 0.11 mg/L and 0.09 mg/L, respectively at 2 h.[38]

Oral administration of 10–15 mg methylphenidate twice daily to hyperkinetic children (weights 21–38 kg) produces peak plasma concentrations of about 0.02 mg/L.[39]

Phentermine reaches peak blood concentrations of ~0.08 mg/L following a dose of 30 mg (of resin-bound form).[40] The steady-state plasma concentration ranges of phentermine following 30 mg of the HCl salt (Minobese forte), or 30 mg base encapsulated into a sustained-release formulation (Duromine), are 0.06–0.19 mg/L and 0.06–0.23 mg/L.[41]

Diethylpropion (amfepramone) produces much lower plasma concentrations. A single oral dose of 75 mg produces a peak concentration of 0.007 µg/mL, although the concentrations of phosphorescent metabolites approach 0.2 mg/L at 2 h.[42] This drug is subject to extensive first-pass metabolism, hence blood concentrations will be variable following a standard dose. High doses will produce a disproportionately higher concentration of parent drug.

### Cocaine

Oral administration of 120–200 mg cocaine hydrochloride produces peak plasma concentrations of 0.06–0.07 mg/L at ~1 h.[43] This route of administration is not traditionally favoured, but it is becoming more popular with naïve users and with women.

## Other routes of administration

Amphetamines and cocaine are most frequently administered in drug users by intravenous injection, nasal insufflation (snorting) or smoking. Intravenous dosing provides the most efficient and quickest way of administering the drug, and provided the drug is injected into a vein, all of the drug is delivered to the body almost immediately.

### Methamphetamine and amphetamine

Methamphetamine can be smoked as the hydrochloride salt by inhaling the vapours of a glass or aluminium pipe heated to around 200–400°C.[44] The efficiency of this process is high with yields of over 70%. Smoking produces a rapid absorption with peak blood concentrations within minutes. These concentrations are sustained for 3–4 h before declining. The blood concentration versus time profile for vaporized methamphetamine is very similar to intravenous administration. Blood concentrations of methamphetamine peak at close to 0.10 mg/L following a 30 mg smoke. Interestingly, saliva concentrations of methamphetamine are substantially higher than those in plasma. Amphetamine, the main metabolite of methamphetamine, is produced only in small amounts following intravenous dosing or smoking. Plasma concentrations peak at 12 h and are only 0.004 mg/L.[45]

The normal smoking of methamphetamine hydrochloride, or free base, such as with tobacco, produces a low and variable yield of methamphetamine (5–17%).[33] This is presumably due to the lower temperatures involved in cigarette smoking.

Amphetamines are also absorbed through mucosal surfaces. Insertion of a quantity of amphetamine into the vagina before intercourse is termed 'balling'.

## Cocaine

Cocaine base administered by smoking (volatilization with a glass pipe and heat) provides an almost equivalent absorption to intravenous dosing, with peak blood concentrations occurring within 5 min.[46] This process produces variable delivery of cocaine depending on the technique used and the temperature of the volatilization; however, yields (measured as bioavailability) will approach 70%. The salt form, cocaine hydrochloride, is substantially destroyed by the smoking process and is not an effective drug for this form of administration. As for the amphetamines, the smoking of cocaine base with tobacco produces a low yield of cocaine (~6%).[33]

Snorted cocaine is almost completely absorbed and made available to the body (bioavailability 94%), but the peak concentrations occur only after about 30 min and are much lower than for the other routes (Table 2.3). High doses produce delayed peak plasma concentrations taking 90 min after a 2 mg/kg dose (~140 mg).[43]

Figure 2.7 shows the pharmacokinetics of cocaine in the plasma of humans following intravenous injection, smoking and snorting. The delayed absorption following snorting is evident from this figure.

**Table 2.3** Plasma pharmacokinetic data for cocaine and benzoylecgonine following various routes of administration

| Dose | Peak plasma concentration (mg/L) | Time to peak (min) |
|---|---|---|
| **Intravenous** | | |
| 25 mg cocaine HCl (n=6)[a] | 0.1–0.35 | <5 |
|  | (0.06–0.16) | (70–160) |
| 23 mg cocaine HCl (n=4)[b] | 0.18±0.06 | 5 |
| 100 mg cocaine HCl (n=3)[c] | 0.5–1.1 | >5 |
| 200 mg cocaine HCl (n=2)[c] | 1.4–2.0 | <5 |
| **Smoking** | | |
| 42 mg free base (n=6)[a] | 0.05–0.35 | <5 |
|  | (0.05–0.17) | (80–150) |
| 50 mg cocaine HCl (n=6)[b] | 0.20±0.09 | 5 |
| **Snorting** | | |
| 32 mg cocaine HCl[a] | 0.05–0.12 | 20–50 |
|  | (0.09–0.16) | (170–230) |
| 106 mg cocaine HCl (n=6)[b] | 0.22±0.04 | 30 |
| 2 mg/kg (n=5)[d] | 0.17 | 90 |
| **Oral consumption** | | |
| 2 mg/kg (n=4)[d] | 0.06 | 60 |

[a] Cone, 1995 (Ref. 46); [b] Jeffcoat et al., 1989 (Ref. 51); [c] Barnett et al., 1991 (Ref. 47); [d] Wilkinson et al., 1980 (Ref. 43). Data in parentheses refer to benzoylecgonine.

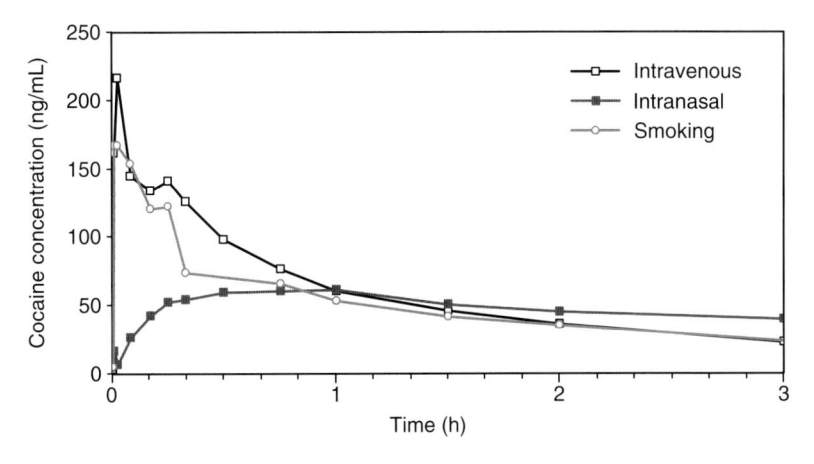

**Fig. 2.7** Plasma concentrations versus time profiles for cocaine taken by intravenous injection, intranasal insufflation and following smoking (after Cone, 1995)[46]

Cocaine plasma concentrations, following pharmacologically relevant doses, range up to about 0.35 mg/L after intravenous, smoking and intranasal routes,[46] although doses of 100 mg or higher will produce much higher levels.[47] Administration of two or more smoked or intravenous doses in rapid succession (total dose taken 121–332 mg) gives rise to plasma concentrations of cocaine ranging up to 1 mg/L.[48]

Cocaine is found in saliva in higher concentrations than in plasma.[49,50] Concentration ratios for saliva over plasma are approximately two, although they will be higher during active absorption due to contamination of the oral cavity (after smoking and nasal insufflation).[49] See Table 2.3 for a summary of pharmacokinetic parameters.

The plasma concentrations rise proportionally with dose from 0.19 mg/kg to 2.0 mg/kg when given intranasally.[43] The reported bioavailability following nasal insufflation ranges from 25% to 80%.

## HALF-LIFE

### Amphetamines

The half-lives of amphetamines vary from a few hours to more than a day (Table 2.2). Drugs with relatively long elimination half-lives will often show an accumulation of blood concentration with repeated dosing (chronic administration). Examples include phentermine and fenfluramine. An increasing pharmacological response will therefore occur with chronic dosing over the first few days of dosing.

The clearance of amphetamines is particularly sensitive to the pH of urine. This is due to the very basic nature of amphetamines, which are excreted rapidly if urine is acidic (increases ionization of drug), but only relatively slowly if urine is basic. Drug use and diet are two important variables that affect urinary pH. It is therefore very difficult to estimate half-life in amphetamine users, since urinary pH is rarely measured. The half-life of amphetamine is similarly affected by changing urinary pH. The half-life is normally 5–8 h, but is decreased to 3–6 h with low-pH (pH ~5) urine and increases to 9–16 h with high-pH urine (pH ~8).[37] A similar phenomenon is expected of the active components and metabolites of khat.

## Cocaine

The half-life of cocaine in the terminal elimination phase ranges from 40 min[48] to 4 h,[46] depending on how this elimination phase is estimated. Dose also markedly affects the pharmacokinetics of cocaine; higher doses increase the half-life.[47] Delayed elimination occurs in chronic users due to slow release from deep tissue sites, which is similar to that seen with cannabis (see Section 4).

## EXCRETION AND URINE DETECTION TIMES

### Amphetamines

The excretion of amphetamines and related stimulants in urine occurs largely by renal processes. In contrast to many other drugs of abuse, substantial amounts of unchanged drug are excreted in urine. Amphetamine is excreted almost completely unchanged when urine is kept acidic, while basic urine will retard elimination and allow substantial metabolism to occur. Under basic conditions, often only a few per cent is excreted unchanged. Similar phenomenon occur with other amphetamine analogues, including methamphetamine, phentermine, ephedrine and pseudoephedrine.

Under normal conditions (no alterations of urinary pH), methamphetamine is excreted largely as the parent drug (~40%) following smoked and intravenous single doses, while only 7% of the dose is excreted as its main metabolite, amphetamine.[45] Peak urine methamphetamine concentrations are almost 5 mg/L and are detectable for over 2 days following a 30 mg dose. The presence of amphetamine in the urine of methamphetamine users is often low and may even be absent in some persons.[52] Urine concentration ratios of amphetamine to methamphetamine are usually less than 0.1.

Abstinence from amphetamine can still result in detection in urine for 2 days. However, high-dose abusers can have urine positives for up to 9 days after last use using a 300 ng/mL-cut-off EMIT d.a.u. screening assay (polyclonal antibodies).[53] Some of these subjects have urinary amphetamine concentrations of 100 mg/L, and many have variable creatinine concentrations that cause substantial oscillation in urinary levels on serial collections.

MDMA is metabolized to the demethylated active analogue, MDA. The MDA to MDMA urine concentrations are 0.15 or less following consumption of MDMA. MDMA urine concentrations have been reported to range from 0.4 mg/L to 96 mg/L.[54] Following single oral doses of 1.5 mg/kg (~150 mg), little MDA is detectable in urine; the main metabolite is conjugated 4-hydroxy-3-methylmethamphetamine.[22]

MBDB can be detected in urine for 36 h after a single 100 mg oral dose, although MBDB is detectable for less than 24 h if urine cut-off concentrations are employed. MBD (demethylated metabolite) is present in all urine specimens to 36 h. The concentration ratio of MBD to MBDB ranged from slightly less than unity to less than 0.02 at the peak urine concentrations of 2–4 h.[55] These data will change with greater numbers of subjects and other dose regimens.

Ephedrine is substantially excreted into urine (not pH controlled) unchanged (~70% of dose). A single 25 mg dose would be detectable in urine for 24–36 h.[56]

The monographs of selected stimulants provide individual excretion data (Appendix).

## Cocaine

The amounts excreted in urine are cocaine (1–9%), benzoylecgonine (35–54%), and ecgonine methyl ester (EME) (32–49%).[57] Only small amounts of ecgonine are excreted in urine (<5%).[51] Similar relative amounts of these metabolites are excreted following nasal insufflation, intravenous injection or smoking. Larger amounts of EME are detected in urine following oral use.

Benzoylecgonine and EME are usually targeted in urine to establish cocaine use. The detection time of BE is ~1–4 days if a 300-ng/mL cut-off is used, but both BE and cocaine can be detectable for 15 days using sensitive assays.[58] The long detection time is probably related to slow leaching out of deep tissue sites, such as fatty tissues, in a similar way to cannabis.

## Synopsis

**PHARMACOKINETICS AND DURATION OF ACTION**

1. The amphetamine-like stimulants have good oral bioavailability and give maximum blood concentrations within 1–2 h, except for phentermine and fenfluramine, which may take up to 4 h. The maximum blood concentration for cocaine occurs at ~1 h.
2. Cocaine and the amphetamine-like stimulants are well absorbed by the intravenous route, nasal insufflation (snorting) and smoking through a heated pipe. Smoking produces rapid absorption similar to intravenous injection, while snorting produces a relatively slow absorption.
3. Cocaine is only absorbed by smoking when the free base is used, while both methamphetamine base and hydrochloride can be used for smoking.
4. Peak concentrations of methamphetamine and amphetamine usually peak at 0.1 mg/L or less following 30 mg doses. Proportionally higher concentrations are expected with higher doses.
5. Peak concentrations of cocaine following doses of 25–40 mg following oral or intravenous administration usually range up to 0.35 mg/L, and rise proportionally with dose.
6. The main metabolite of methamphetamine is amphetamine, which is present in urine in ratios up to ~10% of the methamphetamine concentration.
7. Other amphetamine-like stimulants are metabolized similarly if an alkyl group is present on the nitrogen, i.e. MDMA to MDA, MBDB to MBD, etc.
8. Detection times of stimulants in urine depend on dose used and pH of urine. The detection times of methamphetamine range up to 1–2 days following usual doses.

**Stimulants**

9 Cocaine is metabolized to benzoylecgonine (BE), ecgonine methyl ester (EME) and other metabolites. Cocaethylene is only present in co-consumers of alcohol, and anhydrococaine methyl ester (AEME) is only present in cocaine smokers.

10 Detection times of cocaine in urine are 1–4 days when conventional cut-off limits are used (300 ng/mL), but can extend to 15 days with sensitive assays (<1 ng/mL).

11 The duration of action of cocaine and the amphetamine-like stimulants usually parallel their blood plasma concentration.

# 2.3 Mechanisms of action

The amphetamine-like stimulants and cocaine modify the actions of endogenous substances such as adrenaline, noradrenaline and serotonin in functioning nerves in both the central nervous system (CNS) and in the periphery.

Articles and texts on the mechanisms of action of these drugs, and their neuropharmacology, are available.[9,59,60]

## AMPHETAMINES

Amphetamines interact with certain nerves to either replace the monoamine neurotransmitter in the nerve ending and act as a false transmitter, or facilitate the release of neurotransmitter from the nerve endings.[ix]

When amphetamines act as false transmitters, they substitute for noradrenaline or dopamine as neurotransmitter.[x] However, amphetamines are far weaker neurotransmitters (and stimulants) than noradrenaline (and other monoamines), hence the response elicited by amphetamines occurs at higher concentrations and is often not as intense as that elicited by endogenous neurotransmitters.

Facilitation of release of endogenous neurotransmitter is possibly the dominant mechanism of action. Amphetamines stimulate the release of noradrenaline and related neurotransmitters increasing the effect normally experienced by these agents. In the periphery, excessive stimulation of the heart may cause cardiac arrhythmias and sudden death. In the brain, disruption of nerve impulses occurs in areas affecting stereotyped and psychotic behaviour.

Peripherally, noradrenaline and adrenaline act on specific recognition sites (receptors) termed alpha- and beta-adrenoceptors. Activation of alpha-adrenoceptors mediates contraction of smooth muscle in blood vessels causing an increase in peripheral resistance and blood pressure. Activation of beta-adrenoceptors in the heart causes an increase in the rate and force of contraction. There are a number of sub-types of both adrenoceptors subserving different functions in the body.

Dopamine acts on its own receptor sites both in the periphery and in the CNS. Dopamine receptors in the brain (central receptors), along with serotonin receptors, are believed to be largely responsible for the behavioural changes associated with amphetamines.

The amphetamines, particularly methamphetamine and methylenedioxymethamphetamine (MDMA), are neurotoxic and cause long-lasting or permanent nerve damage to dopamine and serotonin-containing nerves in the brain. The mechanism for this neurotoxicity is not fully understood but may involve the formation of toxic metabolites.[61]

---

[ix] Nerve endings, or nerve terminals, are junctions like power switches that communicate with tissues or other nerves.

[x] Dopamine is a catecholamine related to noradrenaline, and is a neurotransmitter in the CNS.

# Stimulants

## COCAINE

Cocaine prevents the re-uptake[xi] of released neurotransmitter (noradrenaline, dopamine and serotonin[xii]) into the nerve terminal. Inhibition of this re-uptake has the effect of increasing the duration of action of the nerve impulse, or even disrupting the proper transmission from occurring. This impulse might be a signal to another nerve (in the brain) or to a muscle in the periphery (e.g. heart muscle, leg and arm muscles, etc.). In the brain, cocaine acts mainly on the dopamine-containing nerves preventing re-uptake and therefore prolonging the action of this neurotransmitter. Other nerve systems are also believed to be affected by cocaine.

Dopamine itself mediates its actions by affecting calcium ion transport. The caudate nucleus, nucleus accumbens and medial prefrontal cortex are the main regions affected by cocaine. Other brain areas affected are the dorsal raphé and locus coeruleus.

The dopamine system is too complex to simply review here. However, readers should be aware that there are a number of dopamine receptors that respond in different ways to dopamine. These include the $D_2$ receptor, whose activation appears to elicit many of the behavioural effects of cocaine, including stimulation of locomotor activity, generation of stereotyped behaviour, and positive reinforcing effects. Cocaine also affects the $D_1$ receptor-mediated responses, and possibly others.

Cocaine also disrupts neuronal transmission in nerves by blocking the movement of sodium ions through sensory neurons. This essentially explains its effect as an anaesthetic. This effect on nerve conduction can be dangerous in overdose when muscle conduction in the heart is affected, causing cardiac arrhythmias that may lead to sudden death.

Effectively the two types of stimulant drugs produce an increased response from endogenous monoamine neurotransmitters related to noradrenaline. The sudden 'rush' or 'high' experienced with intravenous injections, or smoking, of cocaine and amphetamines is caused by the sudden release of noradrenaline and related amines from nerve endings. This effect is similar to the rush of adrenaline experienced during a number of physiological states, including sexual orgasm, and nervousness associated with athletic events or public speaking. It is likely that cocaine also elicits neurotoxicity similar to the amphetamines.

## Synopsis

### MECHANISMS OF ACTION

1 Amphetamine-like stimulants and cocaine interact with nerves utilizing noradrenaline, dopamine and serotonin as neurotransmitters.

---

[xi] All nerves take up or absorb released neurotransmitter to terminate the action of the neurotransmitter on the adjacent nerve or muscle fibres. This re-uptake process also helps to replenish supplies of neurotransmitter for the next nerve function.

[xii] Serotonin, or 5-HT, is a neurotransmitter related to noradrenaline and is intimately involved in expression of behaviour and mood. Many antidepressants affect the actions of this chemical in the brain.

## Mechanisms of action

2. Amphetamines facilitate release of neurotransmitter at nerve terminals or replace the neurotransmitter itself and produce an adrenaline-like effect.
3. Cocaine prolongs the actions of nerves by preventing re-uptake of these neurotransmitters following release after a nerve impulse; the net effect is to produce a similar response to amphetamines.
4. Cocaine also acts as an anaesthetic by blocking the current of sodium ions through nerves. In high doses, this anaesthetic effect may cause cardiac arrhythmias and lead to sudden death.

# 2.4 Pharmacological actions and therapeutics

The stimulants have a number of legitimate medical uses. Amphetamines are still used for the treatment of attention deficit syndrome and narcolepsy, while the non-amphetamine stimulants are used as nasal decongestants and appetite suppressants. Cocaine is used as a local anaesthetic in ophthalmology and in minor ear, nose and throat surgery.

Obviously, both the amphetamines and cocaine also have a serious illicit use in many communities. The pharmacological effects of these drugs in both legal and abuse settings are reviewed in this chapter.

## AMPHETAMINES AND RELATED STIMULANTS

### Cardiovascular responses

One of the most prominent responses observed with amphetamines is the increase in blood pressure and alterations in heart function caused by the direct or indirect sympathomimetic activity on alpha-adrenoceptors.[xiii] Heart function is often increased as both the rate of contraction (heart rate or chronotropism) and force of contraction (inotropism). However, in some cases the heart rate may even decrease as a reflex due to the increase in blood pressure.

The smoking of 30 mg of methamphetamine produces an increase in heart rate of over 30 beats/min within 12 min of the start of inhalation. Systolic and diastolic blood pressures also increase by about 20 mm Hg. These effects are relatively transient. Within 60 min both heart rate and blood pressure usually return to normal.[45]

In some users amphetamines may precipitate myocarditis, a potentially fatal condition. Vascular complications are known, including vasospasm, oedema, necrosis, pain and loss of nerve function in the limbs (paraesthesia).

### Effects on smooth muscle

The effects of amphetamines on smooth muscle[xiv] are similar to those on the heart. Muscle tone is increased and may even cause tremor, e.g. hands and fingers develop a tremor in the same way as caused by nervousness. Other muscular effects include contraction of the bladder

---

[xiii] Adrenoceptors are receptors on which drugs such as noradrenaline act. The alpha sub-type causes constriction of blood vessels and increased peripheral resistance; the beta sub-type causes dilatation and a reduction in peripheral resistance.

[xiv] Smooth muscle includes those muscles normally used for body movements, i.e. trunk, legs and arms.

sphincter, which may cause difficulty in passing urine (see also section on opioids, p. 243). Amphetamines may also affect the gastrointestinal system by reducing motility and retarding drug absorption. These effects in the gut are not predictable and may even reverse, depending on the physiological state of the person. An increase in tone in the uterus is also seen.

One of the more serious conditions is rhabdomyolysis (liquefaction of muscles) caused by hyperthermia and characterized by large amounts of protein in urine. This leads to muscle necrosis and renal failure and is a very serious, potentially life-threatening condition.

## Central nervous system

One of the main effects sought by amphetamine users is euphoria, the high experienced with the amphetamine rush in the body. This high is associated with an elevation of mood and increased alertness. Increased confidence and increased mental and physical strength become part of this effect. This high may last for several hours depending on the pH of urine and dose.

Amphetamines produce other CNS effects, such as movement disorders (locomotor activity), and can produce a stereotyped behaviour. This behaviour will manifest itself as repeated movement or agitation, unusual facial expressions or grimacing, pacing and grooming, etc. Overt aggression and a feeling of increased strength are also frequent serious side effects of amphetamine use.

Amphetamine users experience methamphetamine psychosis. Recurrence of these psychotic episodes is called 'flashbacks' and appears to be mediated through hyperreactivity of noradrenaline-like nerve activity. It is likely that exposure to stressful events, threatening paranoid hallucinatory states, frightening experiences or a mild fear of other persons may induce occurrence of flashbacks.[62,63]

Improved mental and physical performance produced by amphetamines is sought by amphetamine users, although the improved performance may be more perceived than real. The reduction in fatigue is one of the more sought after effect by persons performing monotonous tasks of long duration (such as driving long-haul trucks), or where sleep deprivation occurs (e.g. studying for exams). This latter effect is also the basis for the treatment of narcolepsy with amphetamine-like stimulants. Oral doses of 10–30 mg of amphetamine or methamphetamine are capable of producing these effects.

Another effect associated with amphetamines is a reduction in appetite. This is clearly an important treatment for obese persons in whom excessive food intake is the cause of their problems. Because of the dependence-producing nature of amphetamines (see next chapter), the weaker stimulants are primarily prescribed for this use. Drugs such as phentermine, fenfluramine[xv] and diethylpropion are examples.

Amphetamines are unlikely to have a direct adverse effect on memory unless permanent neurological damage has occurred. In the short term, amphetamines, and cocaine, enhance concentration powers and endurance.

---

[xv] Fenfluramine and dexfenfluramine, on the advice of the United Nations International Narcotics Drug Control Board and national regulatory agencies, have been withdrawn from many countries, including Australia and the USA, because of serious adverse reactions.

# Stimulants

## Other effects

Some amphetamines, particularly many of the designer amphetamines (MDMA, MDA, PMA, etc.), also increase body temperature. Hyperthermia can be serious and lead to dangerous consequences including, rhabdomyolysis (see Chapter 2.6). Amphetamines are therefore capable of upsetting thermoregulatory settings in the brain stem.

# COCAINE

## Cardiovascular responses

The release of noradrenaline and other catecholamines by cocaine produces similar cardiovascular effects to the amphetamines. Blood pressure and heart rate are elevated following even moderate doses of cocaine. Increases in heart rate over 20 beats/min or increases in diastolic blood pressure over 10 mm Hg are common and occur at doses of 25 mg or greater.[46] The same actions will constrict coronary arteries, reducing blood supply to the heart itself. Some of the vasoconstrictor actions of cocaine are probably also due to the metabolite benzoylecgonine.

## Central nervous system

Cocaine produces euphoria, arousal, an elevation in mood and alertness, and an increased vigour. Anxiety and restlessness are necessary side effects of these actions. Larger doses may even produce tremor, minor seizures (tonic–clonic) and dysphoria. In many respects cocaine produces similar effects to those of the amphetamines. This euphoria generally last less than 45 min and is often much shorter. In order to achieve substantial and long-lasting highs, cocaine binges may involve several doses spaced only minutes apart.

Tactile hallucinations, such as the feeling of crawling under the skin, are well known. High body temperature is also a common experience with cocaine users.

## Effects on smooth muscle

These are less pronounced than for the amphetamines and are probably related to the greater effects of cocaine on dopamine-containing nerves in the brain than on noradrenaline-containing nerves in the peripheral parts of the body.

## Local anaesthetic activity

Cocaine blocks nerve conduction and is used as a topical anaesthetic for eye operations and other ophthalmological procedures, as well as those involving the ears, nose and throat (otolaryngology). Only cocaine solutions (50 and 100 mg/mL) are used for this purpose.

## Other activities

One of the better known effects of cocaine is rhinitis, or a runny nose. Chronic intranasal use can produce ulceration of the nasal cavity and even perforate the nasal septum.

## MEDICAL USES OF STIMULANTS

The most important additional effect of amphetamine-like stimulants is their ability to dilate bronchioles and reverse asthma and to reduce nasal congestion caused by the common cold and associated ailments. The weaker stimulants such as ephedrine and pseudoephedrine are used for this purpose. Pseudoephedrine, phenylephrine and l-amphetamine (l-desoxynorephedrine) are possibly the most common drugs used as nasal decongestants, while phenylephrine is also used as a mydriatic agent.

Amphetamine and methylphenidate are used to treat attention deficit syndrome (ADD). In fact, this is a relatively common condition with many children continuing their use of these drugs into adulthood. The dangers associated with abuse of these drugs should always be recognized.

The non-amphetamine stimulants are abused for the purposes of achieving an amphetamine-like effect, particularly by long-distance truck drivers. While this is hardly a medical use, their real purpose is often disguised as agents for weight reduction.

Since cocaine has stimulant activities similar to amphetamines, it can also be used to maintain alertness and reduce the effects of fatigue. Predominantly, amphetamines are considered more useful for this purpose.

There are no therapeutic concentrations for these stimulants. Drug concentrations in blood or plasma will of course depend on dose, volume of distribution, rate of metabolism, pH of urine for amphetamine-like stimulants, and the degree of tolerance.

Tolerance, while not affecting the pharmacokinetics of stimulants directly, will result in much higher doses being used after a period of regular use. For this reason, any notion of a therapeutic range would be misleading. However, Table 2.2 (Chapter 2.2) provides a guide as to expected blood/plasma concentrations of selected stimulants following standard doses in naïve users.

# Synopsis

## PHARMACOLOGICAL ACTIONS AND THERAPEUTICS

1  The main pharmacological uses of amphetamine-like stimulants are:
   (a) as nasal decongestants (pseudoephedrine, phenylephrine, l-amphetamine (l-desoxynorephedrine), phenylpropanolamine);
   (b) as bronchodilators (ephedrine);
   (c) in attention deficit hyperactivity disorders (d-amphetamine, methylphenidate);
   (d) in narcolepsy (d-amphetamine, methylphenidate);
   (e) in obesity and weight reduction (phentermine, diethylpropion, fenfluramine, clobenzorex, fenproporex, mefenorex, etc.).
2  The main effects sought by drug users are:
   (a) euphoria and elevation in mood;
   (b) increased energy, vigour and physical strength.

## Stimulants

3 Other effects of stimulants include:
   (a) high blood pressure (hypertension) and heart rate (tachycardia);
   (b) muscle tremor;
   (c) stereotyped behaviour, locomotor activity and aggression;
   (d) a reduction in appetite;
   (e) dilatation of bronchioles and reduced nasal congestion;
   (f) increased body temperature.
4 Cocaine has similar effects but also acts as an anaesthetic, and is used as a local anaesthetic in minor surgical procedures involving the ear, nose and throat.

# 2.5 Adverse reactions, tolerance and dependence

Both the amphetamines and cocaine are well known for their ability not only to cause profound behavioural changes, but also to produce chemical and psychological dependence. These drugs are therefore harmful and addictive, particularly to those regularly using the drugs. Estimates suggest that 20% of cocaine users are regular consumers of cocaine and 5% become dependent on the drug.[64] Similar figures are likely for amphetamine users.

This chapter explores the characteristics of adverse reactions associated with their use and the consequences of tolerance and dependence.

## ABUSE POTENTIAL

Some members of the stimulant family have a high potential for abuse leading to repeated use and a high probability of developing drug dependence. The amphetamines, and cocaine, cathinone and mescaline, are in this category. Other members of this family have less potential for abuse. The relative abuse potential of stimulants is categorized in Table 2.4.

## ADVERSE REACTIONS

The previous chapter already alerted readers to a number of serious side effects that limit the therapeutic use of these stimulants. Changes to the cardiovascular system, the development of hyperthermia and muscle tremor have already been discussed. The production of a psychotic state almost indistinguishable from paranoid schizophrenia is a major complication of amphetamine use.

**Table 2.4** Abuse potential of stimulants

| | |
|---|---|
| High | Amphetamine, cathinone, cocaine, 2-CB, MDMA, MDA, MDE, mescaline, methamphetamine, methcathinone, PMA |
| Medium | Ephedrine, phentermine, methylphenidate |
| Low | Pseudoephedrine, phenylpropanolamine, phenylephrine, diethylpropion, fenfluramine |

Abuse potential is defined as ability to lead to dependence after repeated use; abuse potential is relative.

# Stimulants

This psychotic state normally only develops in high dose, or binge settings, or with repeated longer-term use. The combination of volatility, aggression, disinhibition, impaired judgement, grandiosity, impulsiveness and hypersexuality are characteristics of such persons. Paranoid psychosis when combined with increased feelings of invincibility and aggression with delusions can be quite dangerous and lead to serious criminal offences. Murder and other violent attacks on people are known and are clearly exacerbated by amphetamine abuse. See Case Report 2.2 (p. 93).

Drivers of motor vehicles are more likely to drive erratically, drift out of a lane, speed, and show rapid and confused speech, rapid pulse, agitation, paranoia, dilated pupils, and violent and aggressive behaviour.[65]

Changes in perception and hallucinations can occur with both amphetamines and cocaine. These range from full-blown hallucinations, such as motor vehicle drivers seeing an object on their side of the road, to experiencing dream-like states in which space and time are altered. These effects are usually only seen with excessive use.

These effects are usually reversible, i.e. the person recovers after the drug has left the body, unless abstinence symptoms appear (see pp. 81–2). Delusions and paranoid tendencies tend to reduce in severity rather slowly and may take months to abate completely.

The amphetamine 'binge' cycle aptly describes the changing psychological and physiological status of an amphetamine user.[66] In this model, the binge is the phase in which the abuser injects (or smokes) more drug to maintain the euphoric state achieved after the initial 'high' and 'rush' phases. Hyperactivity, both mentally and physically, is associated with this state, as well as the other stimulant effects discussed earlier. Failure to inject repeatedly will produce the dysphoria, agitation and paranoia. A binge may last many days. 'Tweaking' occurs at the end of the binge and is the forerunner of the 'crash' phase in which increasing dysphoria and emptiness occur, but still there is the agitation and hyperactivity, quick speech, and rolling of the eyes (nystagmus). Nystagmus is not observed in persons using stimulant drugs, unless excessive abuse has occurred. The 'crash' is the last gasp associated with extreme fatigue and hypersomnolence. See Table 2.5 for a summary of drug effects.

## TOLERANCE

Repeated administration of cocaine results in the rapid development of tolerance. Within days of use, higher doses are required to achieve the same euphoric effect. Similarly, tolerance develops to the euphoric effects of amphetamines.

Tolerance to cocaine was not known early in its use late last century. Freud (in 1885) himself could not believe this was possible because he himself never became dependent on the drug [p. 348]:[8]

> I would ... advise without hesitation ... to give cocaine in subcutaneous experiments of 0.03 to 0.05 g per dose and not to shrink from an accumulation of doses.

Tolerance develops to most of the peripheral cardiovascular and smooth muscle effects of cocaine and amphetamine, although there is some dispute as to whether tolerance occurs for euphoric and hyperthermic effects of these stimulants. Tolerance does not seem to develop to

**Table 2.5** Symptoms associated with abstinence and stimulant abuse

| Symptoms of abstinence[a] | Symptoms of drug effects |
| --- | --- |
| Anhedonia | Aggression |
| Anergia | Cardiac arrhythmias |
| Craving | Compulsive behaviours |
| Depression | Disinhibition |
| Fatigue | Hallucinations (MDMA, etc.) |
| Lethargy | High heart rate (tachycardia) |
| Hypersomnolence | High blood pressure (hypertension) |
| Mood disorders | Hyperactivity |
| Suicidal behaviour | Hypersexuality |
|  | Impaired judgement |
|  | Impulsiveness |
|  | Nystagmus (high doses) |
|  | Paranoid psychoses (long-term use) |
|  | Volatility |
|  | Weight loss |

[a] Assuming the person has become physiologically dependent to a stimulant. Symptoms are organized alphabetically in each column.

the same extent with some of the central (CNS) effects, such as stereotyped behaviour and locomotor stimulation. This behaviour includes compulsive fidgeting, touching and picking of face and extremities, suspiciousness and other compulsive behaviours.

Tolerance is an effect caused by repeated administration of cocaine or amphetamines, and is very much dependent on the frequency and size of doses used. Occasional or binge users are unlikely to develop significant tolerance, unless repeated administration continues for 2 or 3 days. Most users of these drugs will not develop significant tolerance. Those that do develop significant tolerance can proceed from 20 mg amounts of methamphetamine or cocaine to a few grams of drug.

## DEPENDENCE AND ABSTINENCE

As defined earlier (Chapter 2.4), dependence is more than the expression of overt life-threatening withdrawal symptoms. Amphetamine and cocaine users exhibit drug-seeking behaviour, show neglect of personal hygiene and health, and show a strong desire to continue using these drugs.

Users will develop both chemical and psychological dependence. However, withdrawal symptoms on abstinence are not as characteristic as for the opioids. Users will tend to develop extreme fatigue and lethargy, and may even sleep intermittently for days ('crash' phase). Subjects will often become depressed and even show suicidal tendencies depending on the underlying psychiatric state of the person concerned (Table 2.5).

# Stimulants

The alteration in mood is a particularly important feature, since stimulants are primarily used to elevate mood. The rebound effect, in which mood is worsened on withdrawal, is associated with fatigue and is particularly dangerous in persons driving motor vehicles.

In its early use, persons becoming addicted to cocaine were those who were already addicted to morphine, or who had some underlying psychiatric problem.[8] In fact, one of the early uses for cocaine was to detoxify morphine addicts. Unfortunately for many, freed from dependence on morphine, cocaine was a worse scourge. In Freud's own words [p. 344]:

> ...that all reports on cocaine addiction refer to morphine addicts, individuals who had already succumbed to the demon, whose weakened will power and need for stimulus would abuse any stimulants offered to them...cocaine has taken no other victims of its own.

While this was a rather naïve view to say the least, there was an element of truth to his words. The view that addicts to one drug will become addicts to another is still a widely held view, and is almost certainly at least partly true. Early studies have suggested that mood disorders (affective disorders) increase susceptibility to stimulant abuse. Surveys of in-patient and out-patient cocaine abusers show that over 50% had pre-existing mood disorders, such as manic-depressive illness, cyclothymic disorders and attention deficit syndrome.[64]

The nature of long-term changes is less clear. There is evidence that amphetamines and cocaine produce degeneration of dopamine nerves in the brain. This may explain why long-term users develop mental deficits and mood dysfunction with time. Chronic drug-induced paranoid psychoses and panic-anxiety attacks are associated with abusers of these drugs. However, they occur relatively infrequently and may be associated with an pre-existing psychiatric disorder.

## Synopsis

**TOLERANCE AND DEPENDENCE**

1. Users of amphetamines, cocaine, cathinone and mescaline have a high potential to develop drug dependence, while phentermine, diethylpropion and pseudoephedrine have a relatively low abuse potential.
2. The main adverse reactions associated with stimulants include cardiovascular complications, hyperthermia, rhabdomyolysis, hallucinations and paranoid psychotic states.
3. Crimes of violence are associated with amphetamine and cocaine abuse.
4. Tolerance develops to the euphoric and many of the stimulatory effects of amphetamines following repeated use. Tolerance does not develop to the same extent for stereotyped behaviour, including fidgeting, touching and picking of face and extremities, suspiciousness and other compulsive behaviours.
5. Dependence is associated with amphetamine and cocaine users, although only a minority (~5%) develop overt drug dependence and express abstinence symptoms on withdrawal.
6. Abstinence is associated with lethargy, depression and extreme fatigue.
7. Paranoid psychosis, other mood disorders and aggression are the main behavioural problems associated with this class of drug, and can persist if permanent nerve damage has occurred.

# 2.6 Toxicology

Amphetamines and cocaine are toxic drugs. As the previous chapters have detailed, their abuse can lead to dramatic behavioural changes, which either endangers the life of an innocent family member or bystander from acts of violence, or leads directly to the death of the person consuming the drug. Frequently both circumstances occur together.

As with many other drugs of abuse, the actual concentrations of drugs determined by the laboratory in blood are rarely able on their own to predict the actual effects elicited by the drug, since tolerance develops rapidly to the effects of the drugs. Consequently, the background and circumstances of the case are critical to establishing the antecedent factors.

This section reviews the toxicology and pathology of amphetamine- and cocaine-associated cases.

## PREVALENCE IN FORENSIC CASES

Cocaine, methamphetamine or both are involved in approximately one-third of homicides in San Diego County (1987). When fatal accidental overdoses are included, cocaine is involved in twice as many cases as methamphetamine.[67] In Washington State, a large proportion of the deaths involving amphetamines result from homicidal (27%) or suicidal (15%) acts.[68]

DAWN[xvi] data show that the number of methamphetamine-related deaths has nearly tripled over a number of medical examiner facilities across the USA from 1991 to 1994. In Los Angeles and San Diego there were 134 and 115 deaths, respectively, associated with methamphetamine in 1994. This was also associated with a tripling of methamphetamine-related emergency department episodes in this period.[5] In other centres the amphetamine problem is less pronounced, although this is quite regionalized, depending on the geographic area.

A review of all autopsy and toxicology reports for persons dying in New York City in an 11-month period found 935 persons dying with cocaine in their bodies. Cocaine overdose was responsible for 4% of the deaths, and overdose with heroin and cocaine for 12% of the deaths. Violence was often the cause of death, with 38% dying from homicide, 7% from suicide and 8% from accidents.[69]

Cocaine has also been a major problem in Wayne County (Michigan), with 38% of all cases positive to cocaine and 50% of homicides positive for cocaine. In drug-related deaths, there was an incidence of 48%.[70]

The incidence of amphetamine and cocaine use in forensic cases is highly variable around the world depending on the availability of each drug.

---

[xvi] Drug abuse warning network (USA).

# Stimulants

## TOXICOLOGY AND PATHOLOGY OF STIMULANTS

### Amphetamines

Life-threatening reactions to amphetamines are well described. Initially, these can include agitation, fever, aggression and violence, and can rapidly lead to very high body temperatures, with elevated heart rate and blood pressures. The consequences of these effects are rhabdomyolysis (liquefaction of muscles leading to hyperkalaemia), intravascular coagulation, convulsions, profuse sweating, haemorrhages in the heart and blood vessels, and renal failure. Cases presenting some of these symptoms are described in Table 2.6.[14,71-77] In these cases other drugs have not contributed, except where shown.

Table 2.6  Summary of selected amphetamine-related deaths

| Reference | Amphetamine consumed | Drugs detected | (mg/L or mg/kg) | Circumstances/comments |
|---|---|---|---|---|
| 14 | Bromo-DMA | BrDMA | b = 0.9, l = 9.0 | 21-year-old female found dead in a car, partner was convulsing and remained comatose for several weeks |
| 75 | MDMA 7 deaths, 5 ingestions | MDMA | b = 0.1–1.3 | Consumption at parties/clubs/concert leading to hyperthermia, high pulse, seizures, rhabdomyolysis, renal failure |
| 71 | MDMA | MDMA | b = 2.8, l = 20 | Intoxicated 35-year-old male died in alley way |
|  |  | MDA | b = trace, l = 0 |  |
| 77 | MDMA, MDE, AM | MDMA | b = 2.1, sc = 96 | Found dead 7 h after consuming ecstasy at a party (male, 21 years) |
|  |  | MDA | b = 8.5, sc = 299 |  |
|  |  | MDE | b = 3.5, sc = 324 |  |
|  |  | AM | b = 256, sc < 0.1 |  |
| 76 | AM | AM | b = 1.5 (hospital) | Died several hours after ingestion of 120–160 mg amphetamine at a rave party, core temperature 40°C, hyperkalaemia, supraventricular tachycardia 180 beats/min, subendocardial haemorrhage (female, 18 years) |

## Toxicology

**Table 2.6** (continued)

| Reference | Amphetamine consumed | Drugs detected (mg/L or mg/kg) | | Circumstances/comments |
|---|---|---|---|---|
| 76 | MDE, MDMA | MDMA<br>MDA<br>MDE | b = 0.6<br>b = 0.2<br>b = 0.5 | Died ~20 h after consumption of cannabis, alcohol and ecstasy tablets; bizarre behaviour, violent shaking, vomiting, temperature 41.8°C, pulse 160 beats/min, intravascular coagulation, subendocardial haemorrhage (male, 22 years) |
| 86 | MDMA, cocaine, heroin | MDMA<br>BE<br>Morphine | b = 2.8<br>b = 0.97<br>b = 0.11 | Sudden death of 20-year-old male, petechial haemorrhages and pulmonary oedema at autopsy |
| 72 | MDE, MDMA | MDMA<br>MDE | b = 0.18, l = 13<br>b = 1.6, l = 11 | Death several hours after consuming many ecstasy tablets at a nightclub; felt feverish, intravascular coagulation |
| 82 | MDMA<br>7 deaths | MDMA | b = trace–4.2 | Characterized by varying degree of liver necrosis, myocardial necrosis, perivascular haemorrhage, hyperthermia; MDE and AM also seen in some cases |
| 74 | AM | AM | b = 2.4, sc = 0 | Death of 22-year-old male after an all-night dance; showed extreme aggressiveness, agitation and sleepiness |
| 78 | MDMA | No data | | Death of 15-year-old schoolgirl after ingestion of ecstasy and large volumes of water; died 3 days after admission to hospital; hyponatraemia and low other electrolytes, cerebral oedema |

## Table 2.6 (continued)

| Reference | Amphetamine consumed | Drugs detected | (mg/L or mg/kg) | Circumstances/comments |
|---|---|---|---|---|
| 87 | PMA | PMA | b = 5.7 | 21-year-old abuser, visceral shock lesions |
|  | AM | AM | b = 2.6 | 34-year old, hypertrophy, contraction bands |
|  | AM | AM | b = 1.2 | 56-year old, heart failure, convulsions |
| 73 | MDE | MDE | b = 12–22 | Consumed 10 ecstasy tablets over 8 h; began to sweat profusely, trembling, back spasms, aggressive, hallucinated; severe vascular congestion and petechial haemorrhages |
|  |  | MDA | b = 0.3 |  |
|  |  | MDMA | b = trace |  |
| 80 | PMA 10 deaths | PMA | b = 0.2–4.9 | Hyperpyrexia with rhabdomyolysis and haemorrhage a common finding, all bar one case involve other amphetamines (MA and/or AM, MDMA) |
| 68 | MA only (13) | MA | b = 0.09–18 (0.96)[a] | Review of Washington state methamphetamine-associated deaths, no apparent correlation with concentration and type of amphetamine death |
|  | MA and drugs (25) | MA | b = 0.05–69 (0.37) |  |
|  | MA and disease (14) | MA | b = 0.09–0.47 (0.36) |  |

b: blood or plasma; l: liver; u: urine; sc: stomach contents; BrDMA: 4-bromo-2,5-dimethoxyamphetamine. Other amphetamine abbreviations as used throughout book. [a] Median concentration in parentheses.

Death resulting from excessive water consumption (for hyperthermia) following ingestion of ecstasy tablets at a nightclub presents another mode of death for amphetamines.[78]

Postmortem findings in most intravenous addicts using stimulating amines and centrally depressive narcotics (opiates) exhibited myocardial lesions of varying age, consistent with various phases of myofibrillar degeneration, such as haemorrhages, contraction bands, focal necroses, granulation tissue, stromal condensation, and scarring, indicating an active chronic process in the myocardium and the subendocardium, with a bias toward the conduction system of the heart. Cardiac lesions in drug addicts seem to have a variety of causative factors: infections, toxic influence, hypersensitivity, influence of catecholamines and general hypoxia.[79]

# Toxicology

A series of 10 p-methoxyamphetamine (PMA)-related deaths in Australia are noteworthy due to their localization; most occurred in South Australia and all apparently involved oral ingestion ($n = 6$).[80,81] The cases presented typically with hyperthermia with core body temperatures well in excess of 40°C with one case recorded at 46.1°C! Death caused by hyperpyrexia and rhabdomyolysis was common, and in one case a massive intracerebral haemorrhage within the right frontal lobe occurred. Blood concentrations of PMA at death in the 10 cases ranged from 0.24 to 4.9 mg/L (mean 2 mg/L). The corresponding liver concentrations ranged from 1.4 to 21 mg/kg (mean 7.6 mg/kg). In eight of the cases, methamphetamine (blood 0.01–3.1 mg/L) and/or amphetamine (blood trace–1.6 mg/L) were also detected, and in five cases MDMA was also detected (trace–0.8 mg/L). Seized tablets containing PMA contained 50–90 mg of drug and were sold as ecstasy. During this cluster of deaths there were also a number of admissions to hospitals ($n = 14$) of PMA-related toxicity.

MDMA users, and probably amphetamine users, generally show changes in the liver, which vary from foci of individual cell necrosis to centrilobular necrosis and massive hepatic necrosis. Changes consistent with catecholamine-induced myocardial damage are also seen.[82] Ecstasy-associated hepatitis is known in which liver biopsies show acute hepatitis[83] and show biochemical evidence of severe hepatic damage.[84] Patients develop jaundice or have evidence of hepatic failure, particularly encephalopathy.

Corneal ulceration has also been reported in amphetamine users.[85]

In these cases the designer amphetamines such as PMA, MDMA, MDA, MDE and BrDMA are presented, as well as amphetamine and methamphetamine. For methamphetamine-related deaths there is no significant difference between mean tissue concentrations in accidental overdoses and in homicides.[67] This is also very likely for the other amphetamines. As a consequence, there are no fatal concentrations of amphetamines that would be consistent with causing death. Any blood concentration, in the right circumstance, can cause death. The manner and cause of death are only able to be determined after a thorough evaluation of the circumstances, and with the pathological and toxicological findings.

An examination of methamphetamine concentrations in drug-related deaths ($n = 92$) suggests that the range of concentrations in the recreational abusing population is substantial (0.05–9.30 mg/L) but with a median concentration of 0.42 mg/L. About 90% of that population had concentrations of less than 2.20 mg/L. There is substantial overlap in methamphetamine concentration between drug-related deaths and drug-associated deaths,[xvii] although the highest concentrations are seen in the unintentional drug-related deaths.[68]

Maternal methamphetamine abuse can lead to fetal death.[88,89] The mean fetal blood concentration of methamphetamine in eight cases ranged from 0.03 to 1.20 mg/L. The fetal concentrations tend to be higher than those detected in the mother.[89]

Deaths in neonates have been attributed to exposure to amphetamine from the mother's breast milk. While amphetamines are excreted in breast milk in amphetamine-using mothers this is unlikely to produce significant exposure to the neonate.[90]

---

[xvii] Drug-associated death is defined as a death in which a drug of a particular type was detected, but did not directly cause or contribute to death, whereas in a drug-related death the drug in question directly caused or contributed to death.

# Stimulants

**Table 2.7** Summary of selected non-amphetamine deaths

| Reference | Stimulant consumed | Drugs detected (mg/L or mg/kg) | Circumstances/comments |
|---|---|---|---|
| 93 | Fenfluramine 2 cases | FE b = 16, l = 136<br>FE b = 6.5, l = 48 | Two children (2 and 6 years old) accidentally ingested large amounts of drug, convulsions, twitching, coma and asystolic cardiac arrest |
| 94 | Fenfluramine | FE b = 6.5, l = 49 | Ingestion of 2 g in a 13-year-old boy, twitches, convulsions, hyperthermia, coma |
| 95 | Fenfluramine | FE l = 24 | 5-year-old girl swallowed slow-release tablets, drowsy, fine nystagmus, tonic–clonic convulsions, dilated pupils and cardiac arrest |
| 96 | Benzphetamine | BN b = 14, l = 106 | 16-year-old depressed male found dead on bedroom floor |
| 97 | Phentermine | PE b = 0.5–7.6 | Review of seven phentermine-related deaths |
| 98 | Methylphenidate | MP b = 2.8, l = 2.1 | Intravenous injection of 40 mg methylphenidate; shortness of breath, nausea, vomiting and hypertensive |
| 99 | Pseudoephedrine 2 cases | PS b = 19, l = 33<br>PS b = 66 | No details provided<br>Two-year-old child ingested seven 60 mg tablets |
| 99 | Ephedrine | EP b = 25, l = 15 | Ingestion of 2.1 g ephedrine and 7 g caffeine |
| 99 | Diethylpropion | DP b = 5.4, l = 0.9 | Intravenous injection in 25-year-old male |
| 100 | Pseudoephedrine | PS b = 21, h = 24, v = 11 | Suicide of 37-year-old female diabetic, therapeutic levels of codeine, pentobarbital and chlorpheniramine also detected |
| 101 | Fenfluramine | FE b = 7.5, l = 155 | Apparent suicide in obese woman |

b: blood or plasma; l: liver; h: bile; v: vitreous humour; PE: phentermine; BN: benzphetamine; MP: methylphenidate; FE: fenfluramine; DP: diethylpropion; EP: ephedrine; PS: pseudoephedrine.

## Non-amphetamine stimulants

The amphetamine-like stimulants are also capable of causing death. Table 2.7 summarizes some of those reported. Symptoms associated with their abuse include many of those reported for the amphetamines, such as convulsions and twitching, high temperature, anxiety, tremor, psychoses with paranoid or manic features, delusions, hallucinations and hostile behaviour. Death normally occurs from heart failure, possibly because of fatal cardiac arrhythmias and/or blood pressure disturbances. However, complications from hyperthermia are also likely, at least in some cases.

Fenfluramine (or dexfenfluramine) and phentermine, and other weight-reducing agents, have been associated with pulmonary hypertension and heart valve damage. Use of the combination of fenfluramine and phentermine appears to increase the risk of pulmonary hypertension in young persons.[91,92] The combination 'fen-phen' (fenfluramine and phentermine) is particularly dangerous.

Table 2.7 also provides a guide to blood and liver concentrations capable of causing death. These tend to be higher than for the amphetamines because of their weaker stimulant activities. Nevertheless, caution should also be exercised in the interpretation of deaths involving these drugs since multiple mechanisms operate and tolerance will occur. Tolerance is less likely to be a factor than with the amphetamines. A thorough evaluation of the circumstances and pathology are of course essential.

Based on these reports and others from the author's own laboratory, approximate minimum fatal concentrations of non-amphetamine stimulants are summarized in Table 2.8. Clearly, the presence of natural disease, including cases presenting in the elderly, and the presence of other significant drugs will contribute to any toxicity elicited by these stimulants.

## TOXICOLOGY AND PATHOLOGY OF COCAINE

Cocaine is a toxic drug, and abusers present similar features to those using amphetamines. Intense paranoia, bizarre and violent behaviour, hyperthermia and sudden collapse are characteristic of these cases. The pathology of cocaine deaths shows that cocaine can cause serious pathological changes in a number of organ systems.[102,103] An early summary of the USA experience with cocaine, including forensic toxicological aspects, is useful reading.[104]

**Table 2.8** Fatal concentrations of selected stimulants[a]

| Stimulant | Minimum peripheral blood concentration (mg/L)[b] | Minimum liver concentration (mg/kg)[b] |
|---|---|---|
| Diethylpropion | 5 | 0.9 |
| Fenfluramine | 5 | 50 |
| Phentermine | 0.5 | 1 |
| Methylphenidate | 3 | 2 |
| Pseudoephedrine | 19 | 15 |

[a] Assuming no significant influence from another drug, nor natural disease or injuries;
[b] rounded data from references in Table 2.7 and data from the author's own laboratory.

# Stimulants

Cardiovascular damage is relatively common in young cocaine addicts.[105] Ischaemic events have been reported regularly, and there appears to be a strong relationship between cocaine use, heart contraction bands, and sudden arrhythmic death. Associations have also been made with myocarditis, cardiomyopathy and valvular heart disease.

Cocaine use is a significant risk factor for fatal brain haemorrhage, and is a consequence of the pharmacodynamic effect of cocaine, not a cocaine-induced vasculopathy.[106] Cerebral vasculitis had also been associated with cocaine abuse.[107,108]

The degree of periglomerular fibrosis and interstitial cellular infiltration in the kidney is significantly higher in cocaine addicts than in controls. Mononuclear cell infiltrate in the medullary region, arteriolar sclerosis and vascular changes in the kidneys were consistently noted in cocaine-related deaths.[109]

Chronic interstitial pneumonia with extensive accumulation of free silica within histiocytes associated with mild pulmonary fibrosis causing death in a crack cocaine user has also been published.[110]

There have been recent reports of rhabdomyolysis associated with cocaine abuse, including hyperpyrexia, acute renal failure, and disseminated intravascular coagulation without evidence of vasculitis, polarizable foreign crystals, or other specific lesions. The mechanism of cocaine-associated rhabdomyolysis is unclear, but potentially includes ischaemia due to vasoconstriction, direct toxicity, hyperpyrexia, and increased muscle activity from agitation or seizure. Adulterants may also play a role. In unexplained cases of rhabdomyolysis, toxicological evidence of cocaine should be sought. In those cases of rhabdomyolysis associated with acute renal failure, the presence of cocaine in blood may be prolonged because of impaired renal clearance.[111]

In a study of 99 cocaine deaths, blood cocaine concentrations in cocaine-related deaths were indistinguishable from postmortem concentrations in recreational users, although benzoylecgonine concentrations were higher in cocaine-related deaths. Consequently, isolated measurements of postmortem cocaine and BE blood concentrations cannot be used to assess or predict toxicity.[112] Mean tissue concentrations of cocaine and benzoylecgonine are significantly higher in accidental overdoses than in homicides, except for cocaine concentrations in liver, which do not differ significantly between the two groups.[67]

As a consequence, there are no fatal concentrations of cocaine and metabolites that would be consistent with causing death. Any blood concentration, in the right circumstance, can cause death. The manner and cause of death are only able to be determined after a thorough evaluation of the circumstances, and the pathological and toxicological findings. This is complicated by the presence of other toxic drugs, usually in the classes covered in this book.

In almost 1000 cocaine-positive fatalities in New York, other drugs were also detected: heroin and other opiates (39%), ethanol (33%) and barbiturates and minor tranquillizers (2%). Cocaine toxicity was responsible for 4% of the deaths, and heroin and cocaine toxicity for 12% of the deaths. Violence was often the cause of death. Thirty-eight per cent died of homicide, 7% of suicide, and 8% from accidents. Of particular interest were six persons who died of acute cardiac events directly related to cocaine, as well as four cases of ruptured dissections of the ascending aorta, and nine cases of cerebral haemorrhage.[69] In Wayne County (Michigan) most of the cocaine-positive cases also involved use of other toxic drugs, such as heroin.

Cocaine death as a sole cause was unusual and represented 2–10% of all drug-related fatalities.[70] This is likely to be a feature of cocaine-associated deaths in other parts of the world.

## REDISTRIBUTION

The redistribution of many of these drugs after death is unknown. However, since most are relatively lipid soluble it is likely that blood concentrations will increase after death due to diffusion from neighbouring tissue containing higher concentration of drug.

MDMA has been shown to have elevated levels in heart compared with femoral blood by approximately four-fold.[71] A two-fold increase has been observed for MDE.[73]

Cocaine has declining postmortem concentrations due to continuing hydrolysis to benzoylecgonine. Studies in swine have shown little postmortem change in cocaine and benzoylecgonine concentrations in femoral blood at 8 h post death. However, ecgonine methyl ester concentration increases substantially. Interestingly, vitreous humour concentrations of cocaine, but not benzoylecgonine, increase almost three-fold after death.[113]

An interesting phenomenon occurs when cocaine is ingested with alcohol. Cocaethylene, an active metabolite of cocaine, is produced only when alcohol is present, and is formed postmortem in the liver (when both cocaine and ethanol are present). This will result in a lowering of the postmortem liver concentration of cocaine and cause an elevation of cocaethylene concentrations.[114]

## TISSUE CONCENTRATIONS

There are few data to suggest that measuring tissue concentrations of amphetamine or cocaine provides any more useful information than peripheral blood concentrations.

Liver concentrations of MDE and MDMA following death were some two- to three-fold higher than femoral blood.[71,73] Much higher concentrations were observed in another case report involving MDMA and MDE.[72] Similar findings have been observed for methamphetamine and amphetamine.[115] Liver concentrations in PMA-related deaths averaged at 3.6 times higher than blood concentrations, but ranged from 0.6- to six-fold.[80] Bile has also been shown to contain higher concentrations than blood.[72,115] Vitreous humour contains comparable concentrations to peripheral blood. Similar findings have also been reported for benzphetamine,[96] methylphenidate[98] and phentermine.[97] Liver concentrations of cocaine appear to be similar to those in blood.[99]

## Synopsis

### TOXICOLOGY

1 Cocaine and/or amphetamines are involved in a large proportion of homicidal or suicidal deaths in the USA.
2 Amphetamine-like stimulants are present in a relatively large proportion of all cases of sudden and unexpected death. The highest incidence is in drug-related deaths and homicides.

**Stimulants**

3 Amphetamines cause death from hyperthermia leading to rhabdomyolysis, intravascular coagulation, convulsions, and excessive fluid intake, and excessive heart stimulation and blood pressure leading to fatal arrhythmias, minor and major haemorrhages, and cellular necrosis.
4 Cocaine produces a similar pathology to amphetamines, including hyperthermia, tissue ischaemia, haemorrhage, and sudden cardiovascular collapse.
5 Postmortem redistribution of the designer amphetamines occurs with two-fold increases being observed from femoral to heart blood. Cocaine shows little redistribution.
6 Bile, vitreous humour and liver show significant amounts of drug. However, tissue concentrations provide little meaningful additional concentration to peripheral blood concentrations.
7 There is considerable overlap in the non-toxic and toxic concentrations of amphetamines and cocaine, hence there is no meaningful blood concentrations that define a toxic response.

# 2.7 Case reports

## CASE REPORT 2.1 AMPHETAMINE- AND COCAINE-INDUCED SELF-DEFENCE

This case involved the shooting murder of a chronic amphetamine and cocaine user by his stepfather. The deceased had a long history of drug use associated with violent and confrontational behaviour with his family. This stepfather, in trying to protect his family and himself from another violent attack, shot the man dead.

Toxicology testing on the deceased showed benzoylecgonine in urine (7 mg/L), methamphetamine in blood 0.6 mg/L with amphetamine, as well as a small amount of alcohol (BAC 0.01%).

The stepfather was charged with murder, but was acquitted by a jury.

This case illustrates the violence and irrational behaviour often associated with chronic amphetamine use. This behaviour had not always been associated with the deceased and was clearly caused by his drug usage. The benzoylecgonine in urine indicates prior use of cocaine. Amphetamine is usually present in lower concentrations than methamphetamine as a consequence of normal metabolism of methamphetamine.

## CASE REPORT 2.2 SPEED AND VIOLENCE

This 38-year-old man was a long-term user of amphetamines and had developed a $130-a-day habit, although he only used the drug orally with Coca-Cola. On the day of his death, he apparently used 4 g of methamphetamine. To support this habit he committed burglaries; as many as 135 were attributed to him.

He was known to be violent and aggressive to his friends and acquaintances, suffered from mood swings, and was often agitated. His friends considered him paranoid and unstable.

He was shot after threatening a police officer with a knife during an attempted burglary.

Toxicology showed methamphetamine at 1.4 mg/L, amphetamine at 0.2 mg/L and a trace of ephedrine 0.06 mg/L. This case highlights the dangers associated with confronting a person with a raging amphetamine habit. Paranoia to the police is common; however, violence, aggression and unpredictable behaviour rarely lead to non-confrontational situations. Persons abusing amphetamines are also far more likely to act out their aggression, or display energy and muscular power beyond their normal capabilities.

## CASE REPORT 2.3 RAVE TO THE GRAVE

A previously well 21-year-old male had attended a rave party. The following day his behaviour became increasingly bizarre, and due to his suicidal behaviour he was admitted to a psychiatric hospital. A diagnosis of acute paranoid psychosis was made. This condition resolved itself after 48 h and he was discharged.

A week later he was observed to drive off the central pier of a jetty, accelerating along the pier and making no effort to escape after the car landed in the water.

Toxicology testing revealed no drugs except for a therapeutic concentration of paracetamol.

This case illustrates a possible connection with ecstasy use and alteration in serotonin function in the brain causing paranoid psychosis and depression.

After Cox, 1993.[116]

## CASE REPORT 2.4 AMPHETAMINE-INDUCED FATIGUE

This 34-year-old male was a long-distance truck driver and had been driving from Brisbane to Melbourne, via Sydney (a total distance of some 1900 km). He had stopped briefly in Sydney to off-load some cargo and had continued on to Melbourne.

At approximately 150 km from his destination his rig had left the road, overturned and crashed into a plantation of trees. The driver was killed. The accident occurred in the early hours of the morning.

The autopsy showed no evidence of natural disease. Toxicology showed low concentrations of methamphetamine and amphetamine in urine at 0.4 mg/L and 0.1 mg/L, respectively. No drugs were detected in blood.

Examination of the wreck produced a few tablets later identified as methamphetamine. Logbook entries show driving for seven days without a day off. Accident scene investigation suggested fatigue as a likely factor.

This case illustrates the perennial problem of long-distance truck drivers driving long distances without adequate rests. This leads to chronic sleep deprivation and fatigue. The use of amphetamines to counteract this problem is well documented, as is the rebound fatigue when the effects of the drug wear off.

In this case, evidence of amphetamines in urine, but not in blood, strongly suggests use of methamphetamine several hours earlier. Amphetamine-induced fatigue is most likely at this time, particularly at night when bodily processes expect sleep.

## CASE REPORT 2.5 COCAINE INTOXICATION LEADING TO DEATH

A 25-year-old male was observed to be screaming irrationally on the street. He attempted to forcibly enter several homes and knock down passing citizens. Police responded, restrained him with handcuffs, and transported him to the county hospital. Upon arrival, he was unresponsive and in ventricular fibrillation, and had a temperature of 41.8°C, with no spontaneous respiration. All efforts to resuscitate him were unsuccessful and he was pronounced dead 4 h after being apprehended.

Toxicology showed a blood and brain cocaine concentration of 0.4 mg/L and 0.37 mg/kg, cocaethylene blood and brain concentrations of 0.21 mg/kg and 0.15 mg/kg, respectively, and a trace of alcohol in the blood (0.02%).

This case illustrates the behaviour associated with extreme cases of cocaine intoxication as well as the classical sympathetic overstimulation caused by cocaine. Extremely high body temperatures and arrhythmias are features of many cocaine deaths.

In this case consumption of alcohol in combination with cocaine has contributed to the behavioural changes and produced cocaethylene, which shares most of its toxic features with cocaine.

Taken from Hime *et al.*, 1991.[117]

## CASE REPORT 2.6 DETECTION OF AMPHETAMINE USE AT THE WORKPLACE

A 25-year-old woman died from injuries sustained in her workplace while operating machinery.

Blood and urine specimens were taken and sent to a forensic laboratory for routine analysis of drugs.

The report indicated no drugs were detected.

Investigations by authorities revealed a possible history of amphetamine use by the deceased.

The medical examiner requested a re-analysis specifically targeting amphetamines. This revealed the presence of methamphetamine at 170 ng/mL and a trace of amphetamine in urine but not in blood.

This information now confirmed previous use of speed. The laboratory had originally used a cut-off of 500 ng/mL for amphetamines and had not reported a presumptive amphetamine result below the cut-off. In this situation, the proof of amphetamine usage suggests the possibility that rebound fatigue or other amphetamine-induced behaviours may have contributed to her death.

The use of cut-offs is not recommended in forensic cases unless prior agreement with the client has been obtained.

# References for Section 2

1. Spooner C, Flaherty B, Homel P. *Results of a street intercept survey of young illicit drug users in Sydney*. Sydney: Drug and Alcohol Directorate, NSW Health Department; 1992.
2. Hall W, Darke S, Ross M, Wodak A. Patterns of drug use and risk-taking among opioid and amphetamine injecting drug users in Sydney. *Addict* 1993; 88: 509–16.
3. Commonwealth Department of Health and Family Services. National Drug Strategy Household Survey: Survey Report. Commonwealth Department of Health and Family Services; 1998.
4. United Nations. *United Nations World Drug Report*. New York: Oxford University Press; 1997.
5. Increasing morbidity and mortality associated with abuse of methamphetamine, United States, 1991–1994. *MMWR* 1995; 44(47): 882–6.
6. International Narcotics Drug Control Board Annual Report. Vienna: United Nations; 1997.
7. Oliver G, Schaefer EA. The physiological effects of extracts of suprarenal capsules. *J Physiol* 1895; 18: 230–76.
8. Byck R, ed. *Cocaine papers: Sigmund Freud*. New York: Stonehill; 1975.
9. Benowitz NL. Clinical pharmacology and toxicology of cocaine. *Pharmacol Toxicol* 1993; 72: 3–12.
10. *Goodman and Gilman's the pharmacological basis of therapeutics*. Various edns. Basingstoke: Macmillan; 1998.
11. Barceloux *et al. Medical toxicology*. Baltimore: Williams Wilkins; 1996.
12. Karch SB. *The pathology of drug abuse*, 2nd edn. Boca Raton, Florida: CRC Press; 1996.
13. Nichols DE. Differences between the mechanism of action of MDMA, MBDB, and the classic hallucinogens: identification of a new therapeutic class: entactogens. *J Psychoactive Drugs* 1986; 18: 305–13.
14. Winek CL, Collom WD, Bricker JD. A death due to 4-bromo-2,5-dimethoxyamphetamine. *Clin Toxicol* 1981; 18(3): 267–71.
15. Brenneisen R, Bourquin D, Bracher K, Helmlin HJ, Vonlanthen D. Methamphetamine: synthesis, pharmacology, analysis, and toxicology. In: *American Academy of Forensic Sciences Workshop*. San Francisco: AAFS; 1998.
16. United Nations. *Clandestine manufacture of substances under international control*. New York: United Nations; 1996.
17. United Nations. *Recommended methods for testing peyote cactus (mescal buttons)/mescaline and psilocybe mushrooms/psilocybin*. New York: United Nations; 1989.
18. Kalix P, Geisshusler S, Brenneisen R, Koelbing U, Fisch HU. Cathinone, a phenylpropylamine alkaloid from khat leaves that has amphetamine effects in humans. *NIDA Res Monogr* 1991; 105: 289–90.

19. Brewster ME, Davis FT. Appearance of aminorex as a designer analog of methylaminorex. *J Forens Sci* 1991; 36: 587–92.
20. Pricone MG, Drummer OH. Deaths caused by lignocaine. *Analog* 1995; 17(5).
21. Ensslin HK, Maurer HH, Gouzoulis E, Hermle L, Kovar K-A. Metabolism of racemic 3,4-methylenedioxyethylamphetamine in humans. *Drug Metab Disposit* 1996; 24: 813–20.
22. Helmlin HJ, Bracher K, Bourquin D, Vonlanthen D, Brenneisen R. Analysis of 3,4-methylenedioxymethamphetamine (MDMA) and its metabolites in plasma and urine by HPLC-DAD and GC-MS. *J Anal Toxicol* 1996; 20(6): 432–40.
23. Romberg RW, Needleman SB, Snyder JJ, Greedan A. Methamphetamine and amphetamine derived from the metabolism of selegiline. *J Forens Sci* 1995; 40(6): 1100–2.
24. Tarver JA. Amphetamine-positive drug screens from use of clobenzorex hydrochlorate [letter]. *J Anal Toxicol* 1994; 18(3): 183.
25. Maurer HH, Kraemer T, Ledvinka O, Schmitt CJ, Weber AA. Gas chromatography–mass spectrometry (GC–MS) and liquid chromatography–mass spectrometry (LC–MS) in toxicological analysis. Studies on the detection of clobenzorex and its metabolites within a systematic toxicological analysis procedure by GC–MS and by immunoassay and studies on the detection of alpha- and beta-amanitin in urine by atmospheric pressure ionization electrospray LC–MS. *J Chromatogr B Biomed Sci Appl* 1997; 689(1): 81–9.
26. Rendic S, Slavica M, Medic-Saric M. Urinary excretion and metabolism of orally administered mefenorex. *Eur J Drug Metab Pharmacokinet* 1994; 19(2): 107–17.
27. Kraemer T, Vernaleken I, Maurer HH. Studies on the metabolism and toxicological detection of the amphetamine-like anorectic mefenorex in human urine by gas chromatography-mass spectrometry and fluorescence polarization immunoassay. *J Chromatogr B Biomed Sci Appl* 1997; 702(1–2): 93–102.
28. Cody JT, Valtier S. Detection of amphetamine following administration of fenproporex. *J Anal Toxicol* 1996; 20(6): 425–31.
29. Mathys K, Brenneisen R. Determination of (S)-(−)cathinone and its metabolites (R,S)-(−)norephedrine and (R,R)-(−)norpseudoephedrine in urine by high-performance liquid chromatography with photodiode array detection. *J Chromatogr* 1992; 593: 1–2.
30. Boyer CS, Petersen DR. Pharmacokinetic analysis of the metabolism of cocaine to norcocaine and N-hydroxynorcocaine in mice. *Drug Metab Disposit* 1992; 20: 863.
31. Martin BR, Lue LP, Boni JP. Pyrolysis and volatilization of cocaine. *J Anal Toxicol* 1989; 13: 158–62.
32. De la Torre R, Farre M, Ortuno J, Mas M, Brenneisen R, Roset PN, et al. Non-linear pharmacokinetics of MDMA ('ecstasy') in humans. *Br J Clin Pharmacol* 2000; 49(2): 104–9.
33. Cook CE. Pyrolytic characteristics, pharmacokinetics, and bioavailability of smoked heroin, cocaine, phencyclidine, and methamphetamine. *NIDA Res Monogr* 1991; 115: 6–23.
34. Angrist B, Corwin J, Bartlik B, Cooper T. Early pharmacokinetics and clinical effects of oral d-amphetamine in normal subjects. *Biol Psychiatry* 1987; 22(11): 1357–68.

35. Pickup ME, Patterson JW. The determination of epehedrine plasma levels by a gas chromatographic method. *J Pharm Pharmacol* 1974; 26: 561–2.
36. Midha KK, Cooper JK, McGilveray IJ. Simple and specific electron capture GLC assay for plasma and urine ephedrine concentrations following single doses. *J Pharmaceut Sci* 1979; 68: 557–60.
37. Kuntzman RG, Tsai I, Brand L, Mark LC. The influence of urinary pH on the half-life of pseudoephedrine in man and dog and a sensitive assay for its determination in human plasma. *Clin Pharmacol Therapeut* 1971; 12: 62–7.
38. Widler P, Mathys K, Brenneisen R, et al. Pharmacodynamics and pharmacokinetics of khat: a controlled study. *Clin Pharmacol Therapeut* 1994; 55(5): 556–62.
39. Hungrund BL, Perel JM, Hurvic MJ. Pharmacokinetics of methylphenidate in hyperkinetic children. *Br J Clin Pharmacol* 1979; 8: 571–6.
40. Hinsvark ON, Truant AP, Jenden DJ, Steinborn JA. The oral bioavailability and pharmacokinetics of soluble and resin-bound forms of amphetamine and phentermine in man. *J Pharmacokinet Biopharmaceut* 1973; 1: 319–28.
41. Groenewoud G, Schall R, Hundt HKL, Muller FO, van Dyk M. Steady-state pharmacokinetics of phentermine extended-release capsules. *Internat J Clin Pharmacol Ther Toxicol* 1993; 31: 368–72.
42. Wright GJ, Lang JF, Lemieux RE, Goodfriend MJ. The objective and timing of drug disposition studies, appendix III. Diethylpropion and its metabolites in the blood plasma of the human after subcutaneous and oral administration. *Drug Metab Rev* 1975; 4: 267–76.
43. Wilkinson P, van Dyke C, JAtlow P, Barash P, Byck R. Intranasal and oral cocaine kinetics. *Clin Pharmacol Therapeut* 1980; 27: 386–94.
44. Cook CE, Jeffcoat AR, Perez-Reyes M, Sadler BM, Hill JM, White WR, et al. Plasma levels of methamphetamine after smoking of methamphetamine hydrochloride. *NIDA Res Monogr* 1991; 105: 578–9.
45. Cook CE, Jeffcoat AR, Hill JM, Pugh DE, Patetta PK, Sadler BM, et al. Pharmacokinetics of methamphetamine self-administered to human subjects by smoking S-(+)-methamphetamine hydrochloride. *Drug Metab Dispos* 1993; 21(4): 717–23.
46. Cone EJ. Pharmacokinetics and pharmacodynamics of cocaine. *J Anal Toxicol* 1995; 19(6): 459–78.
47. Barnett G, Hawks R, Resnick R. Cocaine pharmacokinetics in humans. *J Ethnopharmacol* 1981; 3: 353–66.
48. Isenschmid DS, Fischman MW, Foltin RW, Caplan YH. Concentration of cocaine and metabolites in plasma of humans following intravenous administration and smoking of cocaine. *J Anal Toxicol* 1992; 16: 311–14.
49. Cone EJ, Oyler J, Darwin WD. Cocaine disposition in saliva following intravenous, intranasal, and smoked administration. *J Anal Toxicol* 1997; 21(6): 465–75.
50. Kato K, Hillsgrove M, Weinhold L, Gorelick DA, Darwin WD, Cone EJ. Cocaine and metabolite excretion in saliva under stimulated and nonstimulated conditions. *J Anal Toxicol* 1993; 17(6): 338–41.

51. Jeffcoat AR, Perez-Reyes M, Hill JM, Sadler BM, Cook CE. Cocaine disposition in humans after intravenous injection, nasal insufflation (snorting), or smoking. *J Exp Pharmacol Therapeut* 1989; 17: 153–9.
52. Valentine JL, Kearns GL, Sparks C, Letzig LG, Valentine CR, Shappell SA, et al. GC-MS determination of amphetamine and methamphetamine in human urine for 12 hours following oral administration of dextro-methamphetamine: lack of evidence supporting the established forensic guidelines for methamphetamine confirmation. *J Anal Toxicol* 1995; 19(7): 581–90.
53. Smith-Kielland A, Skuterud B, Mørland J. Urinary excretion of amphetamine after termination of drug abuse. *J Anal Toxicol* 1997; 21: 325–9.
54. Kunsman GW, Levine B, Kuhlman JJ, Jones RL, Hughes RO, Fujiyama CI, et al. MDA–MDMA concentrations in urine specimens. *J Anal Toxicol* 1996; 20(7): 517–21.
55. Kintz P. Excretion of MBDB and BDB in urine, saliva, and sweat following single oral administration. *J Anal Toxicol* 1997; 21(7): 570–5.
56. Welling PG, Lee KP, Patel JA, Walker JE, Wagner JG. Urinary excretion of ephedrine in man without pH control following oral administration of three commercial ephedrine sulfate preparations. *J Pharmaceut Sci* 1971; 60: 1629–34.
57. Inaba T, Stewart DJ, Kalow W. Metabolism of cocaine in man. *Clin Pharmacol Therapeut* 1978; 23: 547–52.
58. Cone EJ, Weddington WW, Jr. Prolonged occurrence of cocaine in human saliva and urine after chronic use. *J Anal Toxicol* 1989; 13(2): 65–8.
59. Rang HP, Dale MM, Ritter JM. *Pharmacology*, 3rd edn. London: Churchill Livingstone; 1995.
60. Woolverton WL, Johnson KM. Neurobiology of cocaine abuse. *Trends Pharmacol Sci* 1992; 13: 193–200.
61. Seiden LS, Sabol KE. Methamphetamine and methylenedioxymethamphetamine neurotoxicity: possible mechanisms of cell destruction. In: Majewska MD, ed. *NIDA Research Monograph* 163. Rockville, Maryland: NIDA; 1996.
62. Yui K, Ishiguro T, Goto K, Ikemoto S. Precipitating factors in spontaneous recurrence of methamphetamine psychosis. *Psychopharmacology* 1997; 134(3): 303–8.
63. Yui K, Goto K, Ikemoto S, Ishiguro T. Methamphetamine psychosis: spontaneous recurrence of paranoid-hallucinatory states and monoamine neurotransmitter function. *J Clin Psychopharmacol* 1997; 17(1): 34–43.
64. Gawin FH, Ellinwood EH. Cocaine and other stimulants. *N Engl J Med* 1988; 318: 1173–82.
65. Logan BK. Methamphetamine and driving. *J Forens Sci* 1996; 41: 457–63.
66. Stalcup SA. Binge amphetamine use. In: American Academy of Forensic Sciences Amphetamine Workshop; 1998; San Francisco: AAFS.
67. Bailey DN, Shaw RF. Cocaine- and methamphetamine-related deaths in San Diego County (1987): homicides and accidental overdoses. *J Forens Sci* 1989; 34(2): 407–22.
68. Logan BK, Fligner CL, Haddix T. Cause and manner of death in fatalities involving methamphetamine. *J Forens Sci* 1998; 43(1): 28–34.

69. Tardiff K, Gross E, Wu J, Stajic M, Millman R. Analysis of cocaine-positive fatalities. *J Forens Sci* 1989; 34(1): 53–63.
70. Hood I, Ryan D, Monforte J, Valentour J. Cocaine in Wayne county medical examiner cases. *J Forens Sci* 1990; 35: 591–600.
71. Rohrig TP, Prouty RW. Tissue distribution of methylenedioxymethamphetamine. *J Anal Toxicol* 1992; 16: 52–3.
72. Fineschi V, Masti A. Fatal poisoning by MDMA (ecstasy) and MDEA: a case report. *Int J Legal Med* 1996; 108(5): 272–5.
73. Weinmann W, Bohnert M. Lethal monointoxication by overdosage of MDEA. *Forens Sci Internat* 1998; 91: 91–101.
74. Meyer E, van Bocxlaer JF, Dirinick IM, Thienpont L, de Leenheer AP. Tissue distribution of amphetamine isomers in a fatal overdose. *J Anal Toxicol* 1997; 21: 236–9.
75. Henry JA, Jeffreys KJ, Dawling S. Toxicity and deaths from 3,4-methylene-dioxymethamphetamine ('ecstasy'). *Lancet* 1992; 340: 384–7.
76. Cox DE, Williams KR. 'ADAM' or 'EVE'? – a toxicological conundrum. *Forens Sci Internat* 1996; 77(1–2): 101–8.
77. Forrest AR, Galloway JH, Marsh ID, Strachan GA, Clark JC. A fatal overdose with 3,4-methylenedioxyamphetamine derivatives. *Forens Sci Internat* 1994; 64(1): 57–9.
78. Parr MJA, Low HM, Botterill P. Hyponatraemia and death after 'ecstasy' ingestion. *Med J Australia* 1997; 166: 136–7.
79. Rajs J, Falconer B. Cardiac lesions in intravenous drug addicts. *Forens Sci Internat* 1979; 13(3): 193–209.
80. Felgate HE, Felgate PD, James RA, Sims DN, Vozzo DC. Recent paramethoxyamphetamine deaths. *J Anal Toxicol* 1998; 22: 169–72.
81. Byard RW, Gilbert J, James R, Lokan RJ. Amphetamine derivative fatalities in South Australia – is 'Ecstasy' the culprit? *Am J Forens Med Pathol* 1998; 19(3): 261–5.
82. Milroy CM, Clark JC, Forrest AR. Pathology of deaths associated with 'ecstasy' and 'eve' misuse. *J Clin Pathol* 1996; 49(2): 149–53.
83. Fidler H, Dhillon A, Gertner D, Burroughs A. Chronic ecstasy (3,4-methylene-dioxymetamphetamine) abuse: a recurrent and unpredictable cause of severe acute hepatitis. *J Hepatol* 1996; 25(4): 563–6.
84. Ellis AJ, Wendon JA, Portmann B, Williams R. Acute liver damage and ecstasy ingestion. *Gut* 1996; 38(3): 454–8.
85. Poulsen EJ, Mannis MJ, Chang SD. Keratitis in methamphetamine abusers. *Cornea* 1996; 15(5): 477–82.
86. Moore KA, Mozayani A, Fierro MF, Poklis A. Distribution of 3,4-methylene-dioxymethamphetamine (MDMA) and 3,4-methylenedioxyamphetamine (MDA) stereoisomers in a fatal poisoning. *Forens Sci Internat* 1996; 83: 111–19.
87. Lora-Tamayo C, Tena T, Rodriguez A. Amphetamine derivative related deaths. *Forens Sci Internat* 1997; 85: 149–57.
88. Bost RO, Kemp P, Hnilica V. Tissue distribution of methamphetamine and amphetamine in premature infants. *J Anal Toxicol* 1989; 13: 300–2.

89. Stewart JL, Meeker JE. Fetal and infant deaths associated with maternal methamphetamine abuse. *J Anal Toxicol* 1997; 21(6): 515–17.
90. Steiner E, Villen T, Hallberg M, Rane A. Amphetamine secretion in breast milk. *Eur J Clin Pharmacol* 1984; 27(1): 123–4.
91. Mark EJ, Patalas ED, Chang HT, Evans RJ, Kessler SC. Fatal pulmonary hypertension associated with short-term use of fenfluramine and phentermine. *N Engl J Med* 1997; 337(9): 602–6.
92. Connolly HM, Crary JL, McGoon MD, Hensrud DD, Edwards BS, Edwards WD, *et al.* Valvular heart disease associated with fenfluramine-phentermine. *N Engl J Med* 1997; 337(9): 581–8.
93. Gold RG, Gordon HE, da Costa RWD, Porteous IB. Fenfluramine overdosage. *Lancet* 1969 (13 December): 1306.
94. Fleisher MR, Campbell DB. Fenfluramine overdosage. *Lancet* 1969 (13 December): 1306–7.
95. Simpson H, McKinley I. Poisoning with slow-release fenfluramine. *BMJ* 1975 (22 November): 462–3.
96. Brooks JP, Phillips M, Stafford DT, Bell JS. A case of benzphetamine poisoning. *Am J Forens Med Pathol* 1982; 3: 245–7.
97. Levine B, Caplan YH, Dixon AM. A fatality involving phentermine. *J Forens Sci* 1984; 29(4): 1242–5.
98. Levine B, Caplan YH, Kauffman G. Fatality resulting from methylphenidate overdose. *J Anal Toxicol* 1986; 10: 209–10.
99. Baselt RC, Cravey RH. *Disposition of toxic drugs and chemicals in man*, 3rd edn. Year Book Medical Publishers; 1990.
100. McIntyre IM, Drummer OH. A case of pseudoephedrine toxicity. *Analog* 1992; 15(2): 14–15.
101. Kintz P, Mangin P. Toxicological findings after fatal fenfluramine self-poisoning. *Hum Exp Toxicol* 1992; 11(1): 51–2.
102. Wetli CV. Fatal cocaine intoxication. *Am J Forens Med Pathol* 1987; 8: 1–2.
103. Karch SB. Introduction to the forensic pathology of cocaine. *Am J Forens Med Pathol* 1991; 12(2): 126–31.
104. Finkle BS, McCloskey KL. The forensic toxicology of cocaine (1971–1976). *J Forens Sci* 1977; 23: 173–89.
105. Roh LS, Hamele-Bena D. Cocaine-induced ischemic myocardial disease. *Am J Forens Med Pathol* 1990; 11(2): 130–5.
106. Nolte KB, Brass LM, Fletterick CF. Intracranial hemorrhage associated with cocaine abuse: a prospective autopsy study. *Neurology* 1996; 46(5): 1291–6.
107. Morrow PL, McQuillen JB. Cerebral vasculitis associated with cocaine abuse. *J Forens Sci* 1993; 38(3): 732–8.
108. Case Records of the Massachusetts General Hospital. Weekly clinicopathological exercises. Case 27-1993. A 32-year-old man with the sudden onset of a right-sided headache and left hemiplegia and hemianesthesia [clinical conference]. *N Engl J Med* 1993; 329(2): 117–24.

109. Di Paolo N, Fineschi V, Di Paolo M, Wetly CV, Garosi G, Del Vecchio MT, et al. Kidney vascular damage and cocaine. *Clin Nephrol* 1997; 47(5): 298–303.
110. O'Donnell AE, Mappin FG, Sebo TJ, Tazelaar H. Interstitial pneumonitis associated with 'crack' cocaine abuse. *Chest* 1991; 100(4): 1155–7.
111. Nolte KB. Rhabdomyolysis associated with cocaine abuse. *Hum Pathol* 1991; 22(11): 1141–5.
112. Karch SB, Stephens B, Ho CH. Relating cocaine blood concentrations to toxicity – an autopsy study of 99 cases. *J Forens Sci* 1998; 43(1): 41–5.
113. McKinney PE, Phillips S, Gomez HF, Brent J, MacIntyre M, Watson WA. Vitreous humor cocaine and metabolite concentrations: do postmortem specimens reflect blood levels at the time of death. *J Forens Sci* 1994; 40: 102–7.
114. Moriya F, Hashimoto Y. The effect of postmortem interval on the concentrations of cocaine and cocaethylene in blood and tissues: an experiment using rats. *J Forens Sci* 1996; 41: 129–33.
115. Logan BK, Weiss EL, Harruff RC. Case report: distribution of methamphetamine in a massive fatal ingestion. *J Forens Sci* 1996; 41(2): 322–3.
116. Cox DE. 'Rave' to the grave. *Forens Sci Internat* 1993; 60: 5–6.
117. Hime GW, Hearn WL, Rose S, Cofino J. Analysis of cocaine and cocaethylene in blood and tissues by GC-NPD and GC-ion trap mass spectrometry. *J Anal Toxicol* 1991; 15: 241–5.

# 3 Benzodiazepines and related drugs

| | | |
|---|---|---|
| **Foreword** | | 104 |
| 3.1 | **Source and structures** | 105 |
| 3.2 | **Pharmacokinetics and duration of action** | 116 |
| 3.3 | **Mechanisms of action** | 130 |
| 3.4 | **Pharmacological actions and therapeutics** | 134 |
| 3.5 | **Adverse reactions and tolerance** | 141 |
| 3.6 | **Toxicology** | 151 |
| 3.7 | **Case reports** | 163 |
| | **References for Section 3** | 166 |

# Foreword

The benzodiazepines are a particularly large family of drugs that possess anti-anxiety, hypnotic, and other properties that have made them one of the most prescribed classes of drug. They act to facilitate neurotransmission of γ-aminobutyric acid (GABA), an important inhibitory neurotransmitter involved in regulation of mood, behaviour and consciousness. Well over 50 members are probably in active use throughout the world, although many are restricted to individual countries. They have surprisingly similar pharmacological properties, although there are differences that are exploited medically. Their pharmacokinetics and metabolism provide important criteria for their use. They are used in the treatment of a variety of anxiety-related conditions, and, not surprisingly, this has also led to their abuse by various sections of the community. While substantially safer than the barbiturates they replaced, the benzodiazepines do cause physiological dependence on repeated use, and are associated with abstinence symptoms on withdrawal.

Benzodiazepines are strongly associated with opioid users and in drug-related deaths, and are one of the main drug classes found in poisoning-related hospital admissions. Because of the illicit trafficking in these drugs, the United Nations has controlled 12 barbiturates and 35 benzodiazepines.[1] While benzodiazepines themselves have a relatively wide therapeutic index, they can cause death by themselves, particularly in elderly persons and in persons with compromised cardio-respiratory function. When combined with heroin and other opioids, or with other depressants of the central nervous system (CNS), they will often contribute to a toxic response. Their ability to modify behaviour, and occasionally to produce profound paradoxical or bizarre behaviour, causes the benzodiazepines to appear prominently in court proceedings involving violent crime, such as assault, sexual abuse and homicide.

In recent years, other drugs that interact at the same, or a related, binding site of the benzodiazepine receptor on the GABA$_A$ complex have become available which show more selective actions and often have less CNS depressant actions. These include drugs such as buspirone, zopiclone, zolpidem and zaleplon. These are included in this section due to their similar actions to benzodiazepines. Older sedatives and hypotics are only mentioned in passing.

This section reviews the pharmacology of the main members of these classes of drugs, as well as providing a summary of the classification of benzodiazepines and related sedatives and hypnotics, their pharmacokinetic properties, their medical uses and adverse effects, and finally aspects of their toxicology with applications in forensic cases.

# 3.1 Source and structures

The benzodiazepines are all synthetically derived drugs whose chemical structures are quite diverse and cover a range of substitutions that impart a range of physio-chemical and pharmacological properties. Recent pharmaceutical developments now include drugs that are no longer benzodiazepines, but share close structural and pharmacological similarity with this family of drugs. Over 50 benzodiazepines are in use throughout the world; however, usually no more than a dozen are available in any given country.

The structures of the newer sedatives and hypnotics are quite different to the benzodiazepines and barbiturates, although they share a common site of action with the benzodiazepines and possess similar pharmacological properties. They tend to have a higher degree of selectivity to one or more important pharmacological properties.

The structural features of the barbiturates are included for comparison, although they are used little in modern medicine today except for specialist situations in neurology for epilepsy and in anaesthesia, and in some developing countries. Consequently, their abuse is largely limited to these developing countries.

## STRUCTURAL FEATURES OF BENZODIAZEPINES

The benzodiazepines are based on the fusion of a benzene ring (ring A) with the diazepine ring (ring B). The subsequent molecule known as a benzodiazepine is characterized by two nitrogens on the diazepine ring B. These nitrogens are usually in the 1 and 4 positions of the ring. Figure 3.1 shows the main structural base of benzodiazepines. The numbering conventions of atoms around the molecules are shown in the structures.

Differences in the benzodiazepines are based on the presence of additional structures on the 1, 2, 3, 5 and 7 positions of the molecule. Variations in these substituents lead to a change in their pharmacological potencies and efficacies, variations in the physio-chemical properties, and of course variations in the range of activities. For example, diazepam,[i] one of

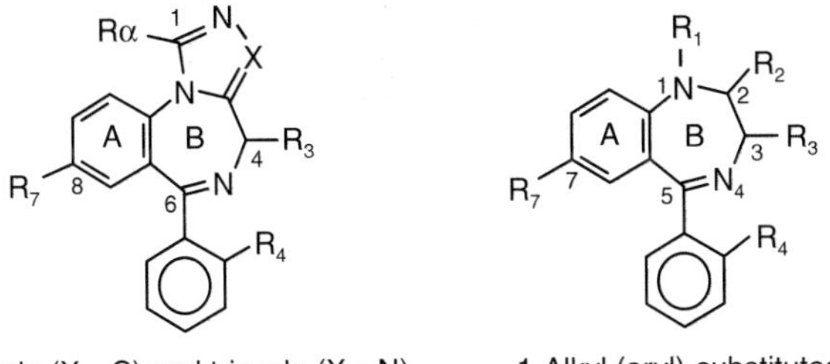

Diazolo (X = C) and triazolo (X = N) 1,4-benzodiazepines

1-Alkyl (aryl)-substituted-1,4-benzodiazepine

**Fig. 3.1** Basic structure of a benzodiazepine

---

[i] Diazepam is marketed as Valium, although many other registered names exist.

# Benzodiazepines

**Fig. 3.2** Chemical structures of triazolam and diazepam

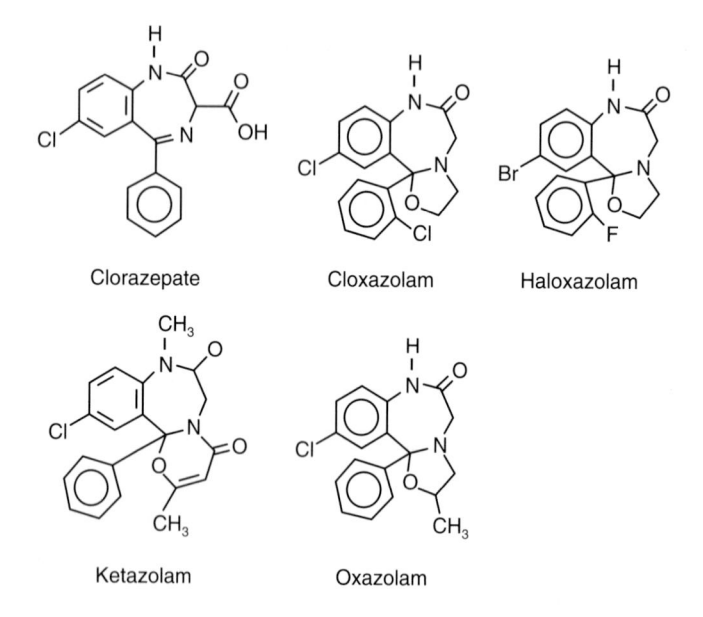

**Fig. 3.3** Structures of benzodiazepines acting as pro-drugs

On administration clorazepate and oxazolam are converted to nordazepam; ketazolam is converted to diazepam; cloxazolam and haloxazolam are converted to 2-chloro- and 2-bromo- derivatives of nordazepam.

the most common benzodiazepines, contains a methyl-group on the 1 position, an oxo group on the 2 position, a phenyl group (benzene) on the 5 position and a chlorine on the 7 position (Fig. 3.2). Details of the properties of this class are described in Chapter 3.5.

The diazolo and triazalo group of benzodiazepines (Fig. 3.1) differs from the diazepam group in that another ring system has been added on the 1 and 2 positions of the benzodiazepine nucleus. This leads to a sub-class of highly potent benzodiazepines such as triazolam[ii] (Fig. 3.2). Details of the properties of this class as described later in Chapter 3.5.

The original benzodiazepines were based on the nordazepam[iii] structure, which was formed from the first benzodiazepine, chlordiazepoxide (Fig. 3.3). Diazepam, which has

---

[ii] In many countries triazolam is marketed as Halcion, although many other registered names exist.
[iii] Also known as nordiazepam.

nordazepam as the main metabolite, appeared on the market shortly after chlordiazepoxide. Analogues of diazepam and its principal active metabolite, nordazepam, are most numerous among this family. On administration, many of these analogues are converted either to diazepam or to nordazepam, and owe many of their properties to these two drugs. In turn, all of those drugs metabolized to nordazepam are further bioconverted to oxazepam, which is also a well-known short-acting benzodiazepine. In fact, for many of these drugs the presence of oxazepam in urine (e.g. in drug screening) can be linked to the administration of at least several discrete benzodiazepines.[1] The more common 1,4-benzodiazepines related to diazepam are shown in Table 3.1.

Table 3.1  Structures of selected 1,4-benzodiazepines

| Benzodiazepine | $R_1$ | $R_2$ | $R_3$ | $R_5$ | $R_7$ |
|---|---|---|---|---|---|
| Bromazepam | H | =O | H | 2'-Pyridyl | Br |
| Camazepam | $CH_3$ | =O | $R_B$ | Phenyl | Cl |
| Clonazepam | H | =O | H | 2-Cl-phenyl | $NO_2$ |
| Clorazepate | H | =O | COOH | Phenyl | Cl |
| Chlordiazepoxide[a] | – | $CH_3NH$ | H | Phenyl | Cl |
| Delorazepam | H | =O | H | 2-Cl-phenyl | Cl |
| Diazepam | $CH_3$ | =O | H | Phenyl | Cl |
| Doxfazepam | OH-Et | =O | OH | 2-F-phenyl | Cl |
| Ethyl loflazepate | H | =O | $CH_3CH_2COO$ | 2-F-phenyl | Cl |
| Flunitrazepam | $CH_3$ | =O | H | 2-F-phenyl | $NO_2$ |
| Flurazepam | $R_A$ | =O | H | 2-F-phenyl | Cl |
| Halazepam | $CF_3CH_2$ | =O | H | Phenyl | Cl |
| Lorazepam | H | =O | OH | 2-Cl-phenyl | Cl |
| Lormetazepam | $CH_3$ | =O | OH | 2-Cl-phenyl | Cl |
| Medazepam | $CH_3$ | H | H | Phenyl | Cl |
| Nordazepam | H | =O | H | Phenyl | Cl |
| Nitrazepam | H | =O | H | Phenyl | $NO_2$ |
| Oxazepam | H | =O | OH | Phenyl | Cl |
| Pinazepam | $CH\equiv C-CH_2$ | =O | H | Phenyl | Cl |
| Prazepam | △—$CH_2$ | =O | H | Phenyl | Cl |
| Quazepam | $CF_3CH_2$ | =S | H | 2-F-phenyl | Cl |
| Temazepam | $CH_3$ | =O | OH | Phenyl | Cl |
| Tetrazepam | $CH_3$ | =O | H | $R_C$ | Cl |

[a] $N_4$: N-oxide and double bond at $C_1-C_2$; $R_A$: N-diethylaminoethylene; $R_B$: N-dimethylaminocarbonyloxy; $R_C$: 1,2-dehydrocyclohexyl; Et: ethyl.

# Benzodiazepines

Alprazolam

Adinazolam

Brotizolam

Clinazolam

Estazolam

Etizolam

Flumazenil

Imidazenil

Midazolam

Loprazolam

Triazolam

Bretazenil

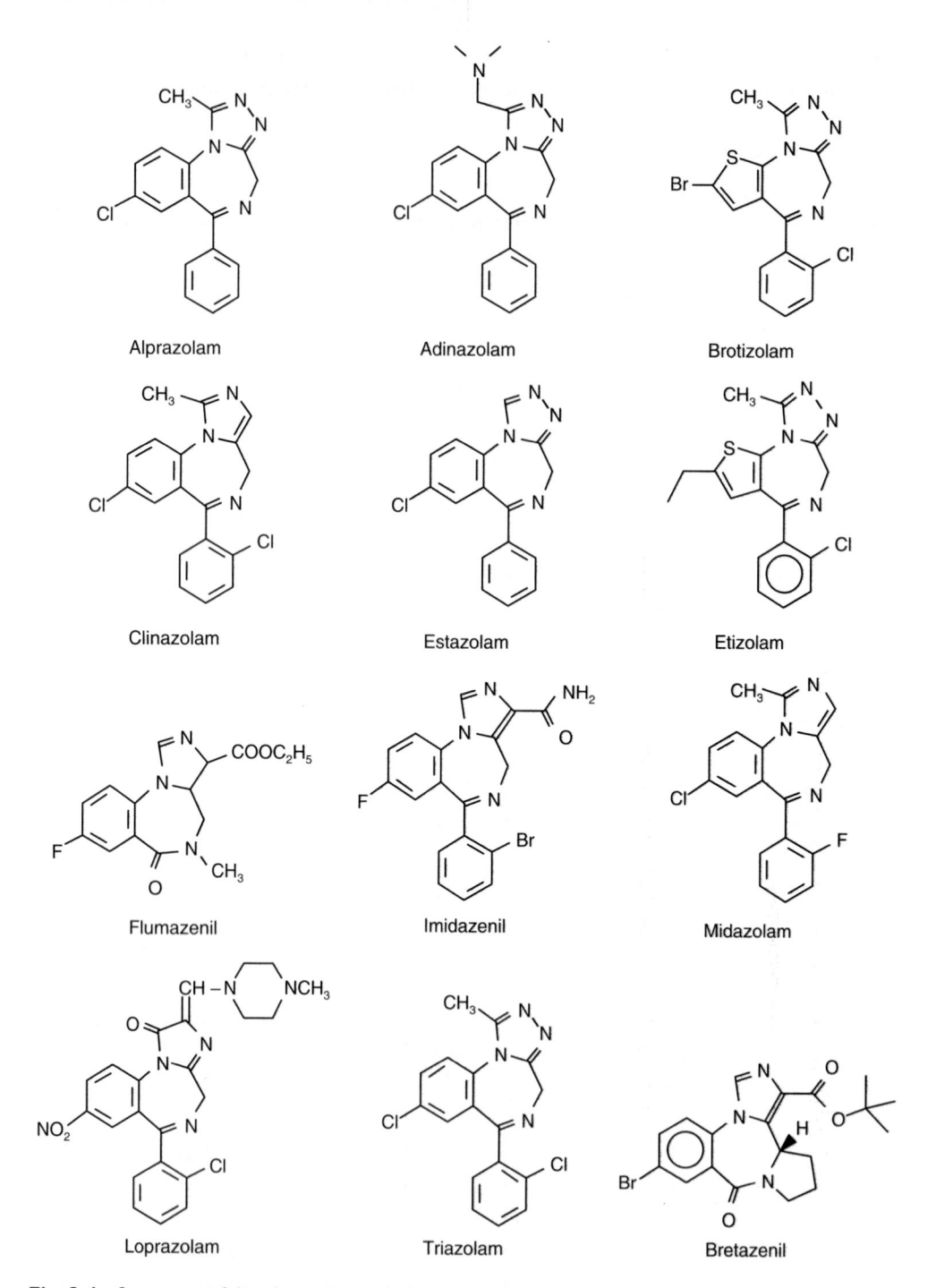

**Fig. 3.4** Structures of diazolo- and triazolo-benzodiazepines

Flumazenil, imidazenil and bretazenil are partial agonists or antagonists at the benzodiazepine receptor.

# Source and structures

There is a special type of benzodiazepine that shows little or no pharmacological activity itself, but is rapidly converted to an active benzodiazepine following administration. These are known as pro-drugs. Examples of pro-drugs of diazepam, or nordazepam analogues, are shown in Fig. 3.3.

A number of drugs belonging to the benzodiazepine family are active but are metabolized to an even more active form. Examples include ethyl loflazepate, pinazepam and prazepam. Nordazepam (the main metabolite of diazepam) is the most common 'active' metabolite of these benzodiazepines.

In more recent times ring-substituted benzodiazepines were developed (based on the triazolam-like structure), which generally showed much higher potency than the first-generation benzodiazepine based on chlordiazepoxide and diazepam. These include the diazolo- and triazolo-benzodiazepines typified by midazolam and alprazolam, respectively. For example, triazolam is the most potent member in active use with daily doses starting at 0.125 mg. By comparison, a typical dose for diazepam is 5–10 mg, and for chlordiazepoxide 100 mg. These closed-ring analogues are also metabolized by different routes than the first-generation benzodiazepines. Rather than oxazepam, or a structural variant, being the main metabolite, a side-chain α-hydroxyl metabolite is usually the dominant product (Fig. 3.4).

Other sub-types of benzodiazepines can be recognized. The 7-nitro group of 5-aryl-1,4-benzodiazepine (e.g. clonazepam, flunitrazepam, nitrazepam) shows unusual metabolic features in that extensive metabolism occurs postmortem to a 7-amino metabolite (see Chapter 3.2).[2] This metabolite is the target species for analysis, although it is not biologically active.

Recent analogues have had the 'benzo' moiety of the benzodiazepine nucleus replaced by a thienyl ring (bentazepam, brotizolam, clotiazepam) (see individual monographs in the Appendix and Figs 3.4 and 3.5). These compounds are, strictly speaking, no longer benzodiazepines, but

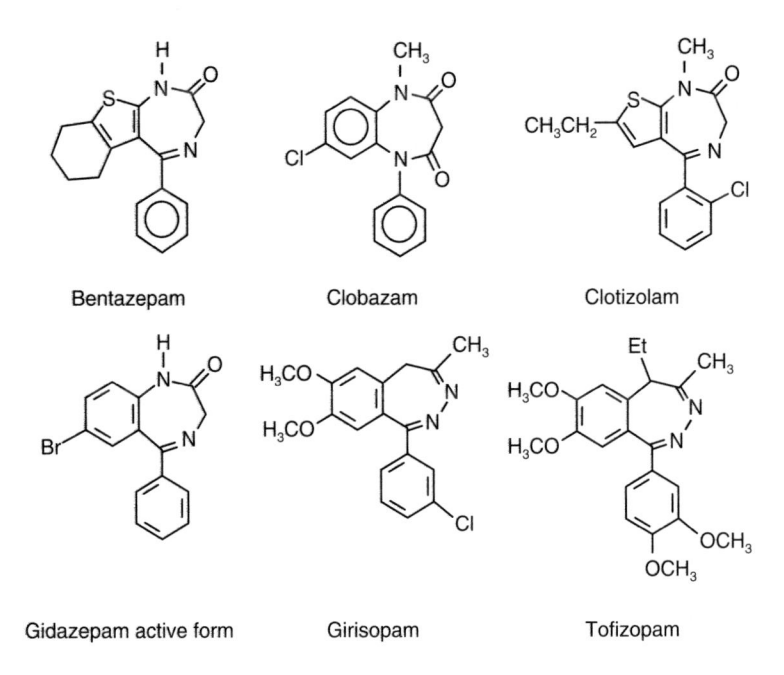

**Fig. 3.5** Structures of miscellaneous benzodiazepines

thienyldiazepines. However, because of their similarity in pharmacological properties it is convenient to include these in the benzodiazepine family.

One member of the family is actually a 1,5-benzodiazepine, namely clobazam. This drug is mainly used to treat various forms of epilepsy and is also used as an anxiolytic, but it has similar properties to the classical 1,4-benzodiazepines (Fig. 3.5). Other benzodiazepine analogues are shown in Fig. 3.5. Two of these are 2,3-benzodiazepines, which show a quite different range of pharmacological activities than the conventional benzodiazepine (see Chapter 3.4).

Readers are referred to the individual monographs to the benzodiazepines (Appendix) for more details and to the references cited in these monographs.

## CLASSIFICATION OF BENZODIAZEPINES

Benzodiazepines are orally active, i.e. they can be absorbed and exhibit activity when taken by mouth. Benzodiazepines can also be administered by other routes, such as intravenously or intramuscularly. See Chapter 3.2 for more details.

The pharmacokinetic half-life of benzodiazepines is largely used to determine their principal medical use. Benzodiazepines with a relatively short half-life (short-acting) are used predominantly as hypnotics and as supplements to pre-operative anaesthesia, whereas the longer-acting benzodiazepines are used as anxiolytics (or minor tranquillizers).

**Table 3.2** Classification of benzodiazepines

| Short-acting (<24 h) | Long-acting (≥24 h) |
|---|---|
| $N_1$-substituted 5-aryl-1,4-benzodiazepines | |
| Bentazepam,[a] bromazepam, clotiazepam,[a] delorazepam, doxefazepam, haloxazepam, lorazepam, lormetazepam, oxazepam, temazepam, tetrazepam | Cloxazolam, diazepam, ethyl loflazepate, flurazepam, flutoprazepam,[d] nordazepam, quazepam, tetrazepam |
| Precursors or pro-drugs of nordazepam and nordazepam analogues | |
| – | Camazepam, clorazepate, chlordiazepoxide, halazepam, ketazolam, medazepam, prazepam, oxazolam, pinazepam |
| 7-Nitro-1,4-benzodiazepines | |
| Flunitrazepam | Clonazepam, nitrazepam, nimetazepam |
| Triazolo-5-aryl-1,4-benzodiazepines | |
| Alprazolam, adinazolam, brotizolam,[a] estazolam, etizolam,[a] triazolam | – |
| Diazolo-5-aryl-1,4-benzodiazepines | |
| Midazolam, Loprazolam | – |
| Other members | |
| Girisopam,[b] tifizopam[b] | Clobazam[c] |

[a] Thienyl-substituted diazepines; [b] 2,3-benzodiazepine; [c] 1,5-benzodiazepine; [d] pro-drug.

Other classifications of the benzodiazepine half-life have included an intermediate-acting group, such as bromazepam, clonazepam, delorazepam, estazolam, flunitrazepam and tetrazepam. These have been used as anxiolytics, hypnotics or both, and in specialized situations such as treatment of some types of epilepsy (clonazepam) (see Chapter 3.4).

Some references have used the term ultra-short-acting for midazolam and triazolam. The mean half-lives for these two drugs are 2 and 3 h, respectively. Since their duration of action is often much longer,[3] the author has chosen to use only two classifications – short- and long-acting. See Chapter 2.3 for a discussion on duration of action.

Short-acting refers to benzodiazepines with mean half-lives of less than 24 h, whereas long-acting refers to benzodiazepines with half-lives of 24 h or longer.

The classification of some benzodiazepines is shown in Table 3.2, showing groupings of benzodiazepines by their pharmacokinetic half-life and their chemical structure.

## OTHER RELATED ANXIOLYTICS AND HYPNOTICS

There are numerous other anxiolytics and hypnotics available throughout the world. Many of the older drugs are now either restricted in their availability, or have been surpassed by safer alternatives.

### Barbiturates

The barbiturates are undoubtably the largest and most significant group to be superseded by the benzodiazepines. These include amylobarbital, butobarbital, phenobarbital, pentobarbital, secobarbital, and many others. The United Nations controls some 12 barbiturates through the 1971 Convention on Psychotropic Substances,[1] although about 50 are still in clinical use around the world. It is interesting to note that some 2500 barbiturate derivatives have been synthesized since their discovery at the turn of the twentieth century.

There is a significant world market for these drugs, particularly in some of the less developed countries.

Barbiturates are based on the barbituric acid structure and are usually di-substituted at the 5 position of the ring. A notable deviation from this structure is thiopental, which is a 2-thio analogue. Thiopental and other thiobarbiturates possess a higher lipid solubility and a quicker onset of action than the barbiturates. In fact, thiopentone is a short-acting anaesthetic often used for minor surgical procedures, and as an induction agent.

The structural features of some selected barbiturates are shown in Fig. 3.6. The barbiturates have a number of synonyms, including replacing the '-al' ending with '-one', i.e. pentobarbitone for pentobarbital. Other synonyms are listed in Fig. 3.6 alongside the respective compounds.

### Azapirones

A relatively new class of drugs, the azapirones – buspirone, gepirone, ipsapirone and zalospirone – are selective agonists at the $5HT_{1A}$ receptor sub-type of 5HT (serotonin) receptors.[4] These are potent hypnotics and are structurally quite different to the barbiturates and the benzodiazepines. They have in common the pyrimidinyl–piperazine structure, which appears on the right of the structures (two rings in series) in Fig. 3.7.

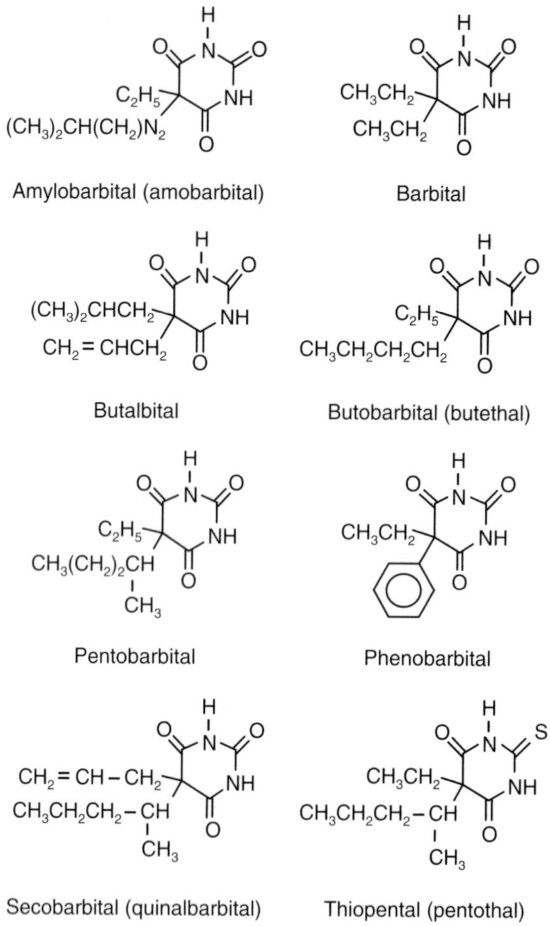

# Benzodiazepines

Fig. 3.6 Structures of selected barbituates

## Imidazopyridines

Alpidem represents another class of drug related pharmacologically to the benzodiazepines, but having a quite different structure (Fig. 3.7). Alpidem is an imidazopyridine (left-hand fused ring system).

## Cyclopyrrolones

A further structural variant is the cyclopyrrolone, represented by suriclone and zopiclone (Fig. 3.7). These drugs have some similarity with the imidazopyridines in that they have a fused ring system on the left of structure (as drawn) with a substituted phenyl (aryl) group and another group projecting to the right of the structure. However, they are generally considered a new class of hypnotics.

## Pyrazolopyrimidines

A new non-benzodiazepine hypnotic binding to the ω1-sub-type of the $GABA_A$ complex is Zaleplon. The structure is shown in Fig. 3.7.

Source and structures

Buspirone (an azapirone)

Gepirone (an azapirone)

Alpidem (an imidazopyridine)

Zaleplon

Zolpidem (an imidazopyridine)

Zopiclone (a cyclopyrrolone)

**Fig. 3.7** Structures of non-benzodiazepine sedatives/hypnotics

Chloral hydrate
(sedative and hypnotic)

Ethchlorvynol
(sedative and hypnotic)

Doxylamine
(sedative and hypnotic)

Ethinamate
(hypnotic)

Glutethimide
(sedative and hypnotic)

Meprobamate
(anxiolytic)

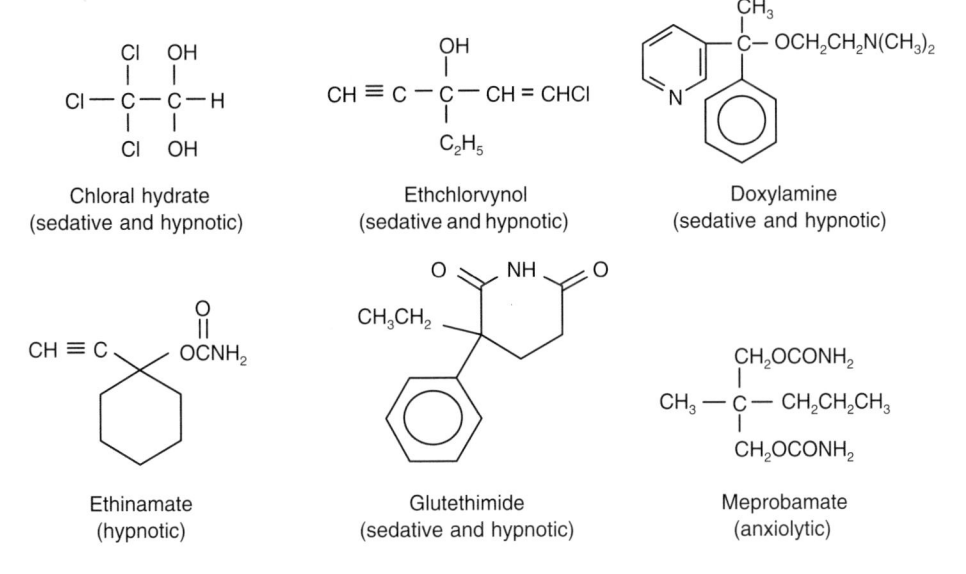

**Fig. 3.8** Structures of miscellaneous sedatives/hypnotics

113

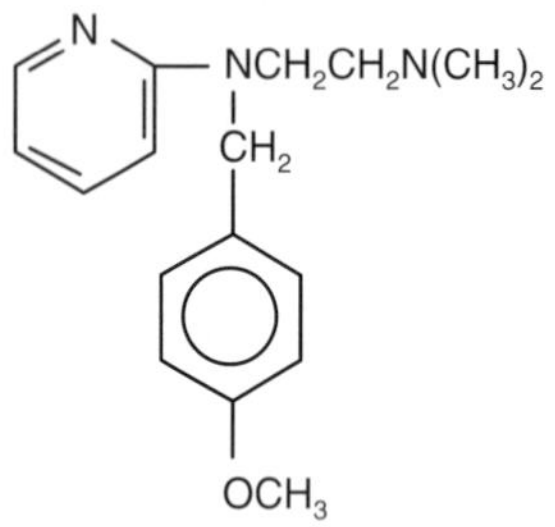

# Benzodiazepines

**Mepyramine**
(sedative and hypnotic)

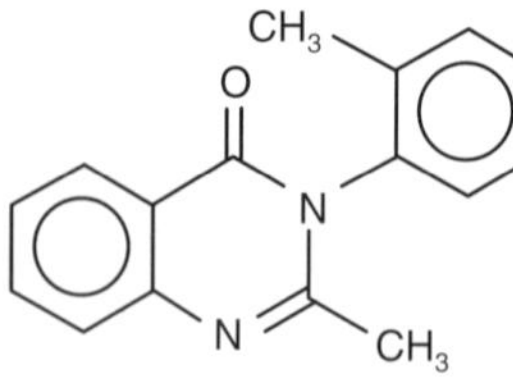

**Methaqualone**
(sedative and hypnotic)

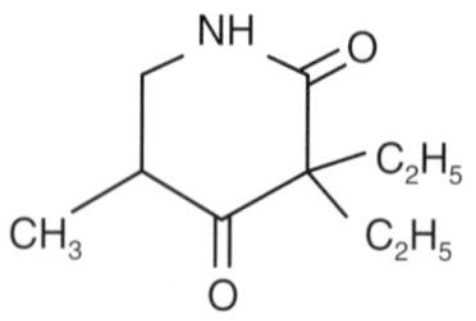

**Methyprylon**
(sedative and hypnotic)

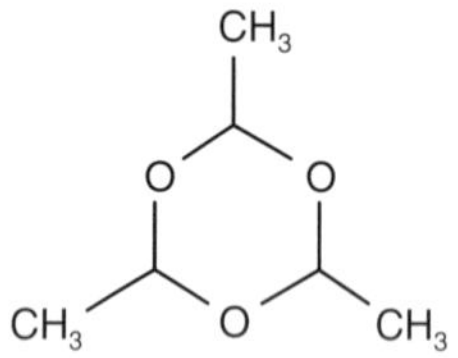

**Paraldehyde**
(sedative and hypnotic)

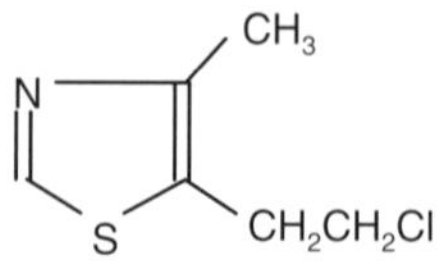

**Chlormethiazole**
(sedative and hypnotic)

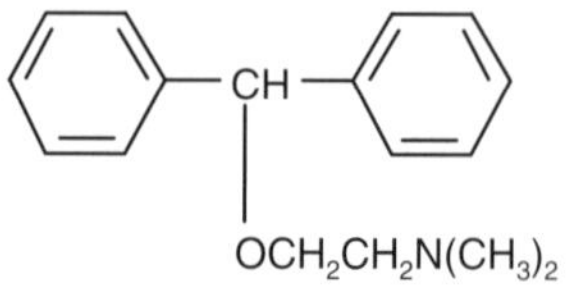

**Diphenhydramine**
(sedative and hypnotic)

**Fig. 3.8** (continued)

## Other unrelated sedatives and hypnotics

During the course of this century a number of other substances have been used – some still are – as sedatives and hypnotics. These include chloral hydrate, glutethimide, meprobamate and methaqualome. A selection of these structurally diverse drugs is listed in Fig. 3.8, including two sedating anti-histamines, doxylamine and mepyramine. Many other anti-histamines have been used for their sedative properties, such as in sweetened over-the-counter syrups.

## Synopsis

### STRUCTURE AND CLASSIFICATION

1. The benzodiazepines are based on the diazepine ring fused to benzene, with the nitrogens usually in the 1,4 positions. Substitution leads to varying degrees of metabolic stability, pharmacological potency and lipid solubility. The diazepam, the diazolo (midazolam) and triazolo (alprazolam) sub-groups are special variations. The nitrobenzodiazepines, the thienyldiazepines and the 2,3-benzodiazepines are further sub-groups. Over 50 benzodiazepines are in clinical use.

2. Many of the 1,4-benzodiazepines are either converted metabolically to nordazepam and/or oxazepam as pro-drugs or are metabolized to another active species.

3. The benzodiazepines can be classified both by their structural features and by their pharmacokinetic half-lives. Benzodiazepines with a half-life of less than 24 h can be classified as short-acting; the remainder can be classified as long-acting. This classification aligns more with their duration of action,

which is usually much longer than their pharmacokinetic half-life. The shortest half-life is 3 h (triazolam) and the longest half-lives are days (nordazepam, desalkylflurazepam).
4 Barbiturates are generally a more homologous series based on the barbital structure. They generally involve substitution of the two 5 positions on the ring, alkylation of one of the nitrogens, or, in the case of thiopental, replacement of one of the oxygen atoms with sulphur.
5 The remaining older sedatives have diverse structural features and include well-known drugs such as chloral hydrate, ethchlorvynol, glutethimide, meprobamate, methaqualone, paraldehyde and the sedating anti-histamines doxylamine, diphenhydramine and mepyramine.
6 The new-generation hypnotics and sedatives belong to three completely different structural classes – the azapirones (buspirone), the imidazopyridines (alpidem, zolpidem), the cyclopyrrlone class (suriclone, zopiclone) and the pyrazolopyrimidine zaleplon.

# 3.2 Pharmacokinetics and duration of action

The pharmacokinetics of benzodiazepines are one of the most important characteristics and define many of the uses of this class of drugs.

This chapter details some of the more important aspects of the pharmacokinetics of benzodiazepines and related drugs, including the barbiturates and the newer hypnotics and sedatives alpidem, zolpidem, buspirone, zopiclone and zaleplon.

Readers are directed to review articles,[1,5-7] and others, listed in the monographs for each drug.

## ABSORPTION AND BIOAVAILABILITY

### Oral absorption and bioavailability

All the benzodiazepines are generally well absorbed orally and reach peak plasma concentrations within a few hours of oral administration. For example, diazepam gives peak concentrations in plasma at ~0.5 and 2 h after an oral dose. However, there are significant variations in their bioavailability and blood concentrations. See Table 3.3 for time-to-peak concentrations ($C_{max}$) for selected drugs.

For example, adinazolam and triazolam have absolute bioavailabilities of ~40%, i.e. only 40% of the drug taken orally ever appear in the blood stream. Other benzodiazepines, such as diazepam, have bioavailabilities close to 100%, which means effectively all drug is absorbed and delivered to the circulating blood. Other drugs have bioavailabilities between these two extremes (Table 3.3).

For oral administration, food can often affect the absorption process in terms of both rate and extent, leading to either an enhanced or a reduced bioavailability. The time-to-maximum plasma concentration for alprazolam in fasted subjects is 1.6 h, but 2.5 h when taken with a standard meal.[8] However, this does not affect the amount of alprazolam absorbed. Similar results are obtained with triazolam and other benzodiazepines. Food is therefore not a significant factor with these drugs in terms of affecting the amount absorbed, although it may have a relatively small effect in delaying absorption.

### Other routes of administration

Occasionally other routes of administration are used for these drugs. Intramuscular administration is the most common alternative site. Absorption from this site is somewhere between that of intravenous and oral administration. For example, midazolam is rapidly absorbed intramuscularly with drug detectable after 5 min. Peak concentrations are reached at

**Table 3.3** Dose, time to maximum, bioavailability and clearance for selected hypnotics and sedatives

| Drug | Usual dose (mg)[a] | $T_{max}$ (h)[b] | Bioavailability (%)[c] | Clearance (mL/min/kg)[d] |
|---|---|---|---|---|
| Alprazolam | 0.5–4 | 1–2 | 90 | 1.2 |
| Chlordiazepoxide | 100 | 0.5–6 | 100 | 0.5 |
| Diazepam | 5–40 | 0.5–2 | 100 | 0.5 |
| Flunitrazepam | 0.5–2 | 2 | 70 | n/a |
| Lorazepam | 1–4 | 1–2 | 90 | 1.0 |
| Oxazepam | 15–60 | 0.5–8 | 93 | 1.2 |
| Temazepam | 10–30 | 0.25–5 | >80 | 1.2 |
| Triazolam | 0.125–0.250 | 0.3–4 | 44 | 3–8 |
| Amylobarbital | 30–600 | ~1 | 95 | 0.5 |
| Pentobarbital | 100–200 | ~1 | 95 | 0.3–0.5 |
| Zaleplon | 5–10 | ~1 | 30 | 0.9 |
| Zopiclone | 7.5–15 | 0.5–1.5 | 80 | 3.3 |
| Zolpidem | 10–20 | 0.5–3 | 70 | 0.25 |

[a] Usual recommended dose range; [b] time to peak plasma concentration; [c] absolute availability compared with an intravenous injection; [d] total plasma clearance.

20–30 min. Lorazepam also shows excellent bioavailability intramuscularly (>90%) with peak blood concentrations within 3 h of administration. In contrast, intramuscular diazepam and chlordiazepoxide show incomplete and erratic absorption, presumably because of their lower water solubility resulting in crystallization at the injection site.[9]

Rectal administration of midazolam also shows rapid absorption with peak concentrations reached within 20 min.[8] However, diazepam shows erratic and incomplete absorption. Alprazolam is absorbed more rapidly sublingually than when given orally.[8]

Other routes of administration, such as dermal, ocular and vaginal, are unlikely to be of significance in the use of benzodiazepines and related drugs. However, given the generally high lipid solubility of benzodiazepines, it would be expected that significant absorption from these other routes is quite likely.

## Half-life

Half-lives of benzodiazepines vary enormously, from 3 h for triazolam to over 2 days for nordazepam. See Table 3.4 for a summary of the half-lives of commonly used benzodiazepines in otherwise young and healthy persons. The table has been separated into those benzodiazepines with half-lives of less than 24 h and those with half-lives that are equal to or greater than 24 h. Clearly, as the data show, some benzodiazepines overlap these two categories. Similar details are shown in Table 3.5 for other hypnotics and sedatives.

In addition, see monographs (Appendix) for more data on each individual benzodiazepine.

# Benzodiazepines

Table 3.4 Half-lives and principal metabolites of selected benzodiazepines

| Benzodiazepine | Half-life (h) | Key active metabolite(s) |
|---|---|---|
| **Short-acting benzodiazepines (<24 h)** | | |
| Adinazolam | 1–3 | N-Desmethyl adinazolam |
| Alprazolam | 6–22 | α-Hydroxy alprazolam |
| Bromazepam | 8–19 | None |
| Brotizolam | 4–10 | α-Hydroxy and 4-hydroxy brotizolam |
| Clinazolam | n/a | α-Hydroxy and 4-hydroxy clinazolam |
| Clotiazepam | 3–18 | Desmethyl and 3-hydroxy clotiazepam |
| Cloxazolam | 8–25[b] | Lorazepam |
| Delorazepam | 8–22[b] | Lorazepam |
| Estazolam | 10–24 | 4-Hydroxy estazolam |
| Etizolam | 3 | α-Hydroxy etizolam |
| Flunitrazepam | 11–25 | None |
| Lormetazepam | 8–25[b] | Lorazepam |
| Lorazepam | 8–25 | None |
| Loprazolam | 3–15 | Possibly none |
| Midazolam | 1.5–2.5 | α-Hydroxy midazolam |
| Oxazepam | 4–15 | None |
| Temazepam | 5–15 | Oxazepam |
| Tetrazepam | 10–44 | 3-Hydroxy and desmethyl tetrazepam |
| Triazolam | 1.5–5.5 | α-Hydroxy triazolam |
| **Long-acting benzodiazepines (≥24 h)** | | |
| Chlorazepate | 30–100[a] | Nordazepam |
| Chlordiazepoxide | 5–30 | Nordazepam |
| Clobazam | 10–44 | Desmethyl clobazam |
| Clonazepam | 18–60 | None |
| Diazepam | 20–50 | Nordazepam |
| Flurazepam | 40–200[c] | Desalkyl flurazepam |
| Halazepam | 50–99[a] | Nordazepam |
| Ethyl loflazepate | 50–100[c] | Desalkyl flurazepam |
| Flutoprazepam | 90[d] | Desalkyl flutoprazepam |
| Ketazolam | 50–99[a] | Nordazepam |
| Medazepam | 50–99[a] | Nordazepam |
| Nitrazepam | 16–48 | None |
| Nordazepam | 50–99 | Oxazepam |
| Oxazolam | 50–99[a] | Nordazepam |
| Pinazepam | 50–99[a] | Nordazepam |
| Prazepam | 50–99[a] | Nordazepam |
| Quazepam | 39–53 | N-dealkylated and 2-oxo metabolite |

[a] As nordazepam; [b] as lorazepam; [c] as desalkylflurazepam; [d] as desalkyl metabolite.
Note: nordazepam is metabolized to oxazepam.

**Table 3.5** Half-lives and principal metabolites of related drugs

| Benzodiazepine | Half-life (h) | Key active metabolite(s) |
|---|---|---|
| **Barbiturates** | | |
| Amylobarbital | 8–40 | None |
| Barbital | 48 | None |
| Butalbital | 30–88 | None |
| Butobarbital | 40 | None |
| Pentobarbital | 48 | None |
| Phenobarbital | 50–150 | None |
| Secobarbital | 19–34 | None |
| Thiopental | 12 | Weak activity from pentobarbital |
| **Newer types of sedatives** | | |
| Buspirone | 1–7 | Weak activity from 1-pyrimidinylpiperazine metabolite |
| Zaleplon | 1 | None |
| Zopiclone | 3.5–6 | Weak activity from N-oxide |
| Zolpidem | 2 | None |
| **Older types of sedatives** | | |
| Chloral hydrate | 6–10 | Trichloroethanol |
| Chlormethiazole | 3–5 | Probably none |
| Ethchlorvynol | 19–32 | None |
| Diphenhydramine | 3–8 | No significant metabolite |
| Doxylamine | 10 | None |
| Ethinamate | 2–3 | None |
| Glutethimide | 5–22 | None |
| Meprobamate | 6–17 | None |
| Methaqualone | 20–60 | None |
| Methyprylon | 7–11 | Some activity from metabolites |
| Paraldehyde | 3–10 | None |

# ROUTES OF METABOLISM

## Benzodiazepines

Benzodiazepines are generally extensively metabolized with often little unchanged benzodiazepine detected in the urine. For this reason, analytical procedures targeting benzodiazepines in urine detect different substances to those found in the blood (plasma).[1,10]

Individual metabolic pathways and metabolites are described for each benzodiazepine and related drug in the relevant monographs presented in the Appendix. The metabolic pathways for many of the benzodiazepine family are shown in Fig. 3.9.

The most common metabolites are hydroxylated and dealkylated analogues, which are often also biologically active, e.g. nordazepam from diazepam, oxazepam from temazepam, and desalkyl flurazepam from flurazepam.

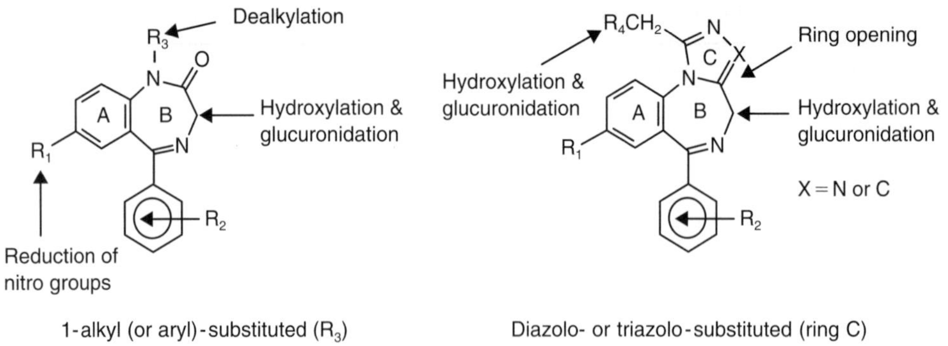

# Benzodiazepines

**Fig. 3.9** Metabolic schema for 1,4-benzodiazepines

Benzodiazepines that do not belong to these two classes are still likely to be metabolized by the same routes, except where functional groups at (R) are capable of metabolism, e.g. methyl, methoxy, etc.

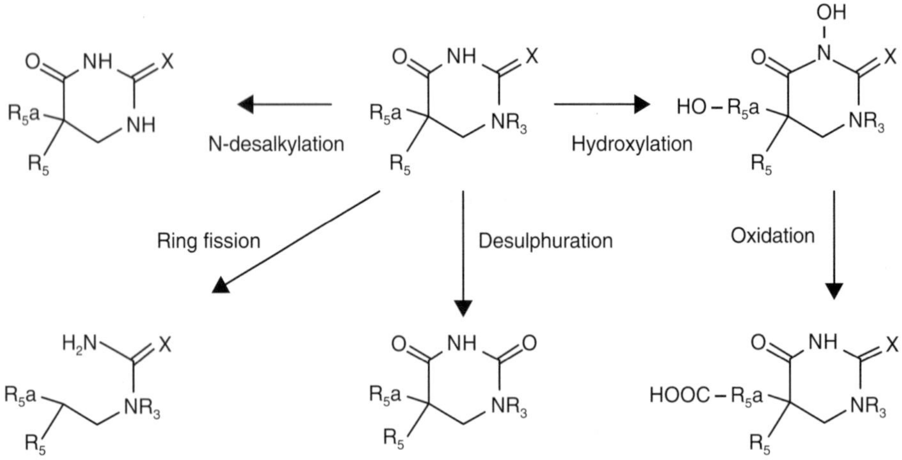

**Fig. 3.10** General metabolic schema for barbiturates

X: S (thiopental) or O for most other barbiturates.

## Barbiturates

Barbiturates undergo extensive metabolism to a number of metabolites. A general schema is shown in Fig. 3.10, showing hydroxylation and oxidation reactions on one or more of the side-chain (5-position) alkyl groups, N-dealkylation on the nitrogen, ring cleavage and, for thio-barbiturates, desulphuration of the sulphur at position 2 to an oxygen (e.g. thiopental).

Examples of actual metabolic routes for selected barbiturates are shown in Fig. 3.10. Pentobarbital is metabolized to an N-hydroxy compound, and the isopentyl group at the 3 position is successively converted to hydroxy, keto and carboxylic acid metabolites.

Butalbital, which has a vinylic group on the 5 position (double bond attached to a carbon), is converted to a diol on this moiety, whereas the other alkyl group is hydroxylated.

A range of other metabolites involving these routes is found with most of the barbiturates. With few exceptions, metabolites are inactive pharmacologically. A notable exception is thiopentone, which is metabolized, in part, to pentobarbital, which of course is biologically active. Pentobarbital probably accounts for much of the sedative effects of thiopental. Approximately 10% of thiopental is converted to pentobarbital.

## Other non-benzodiazepines

Buspirone is metabolized primarily by hydroxylation to the 5-hydroxy form and a cleavage product known as 1-pyrimidinylpiperazine (1-PP). The 5-hydroxy metabolite is further metabolized to the glucuronide conjugate. The 1-PP metabolite has some biological activity (Fig. 3.11). Other metabolites have also been identified and include the despyrimidinyl, despyrimidinylpiperazine, four hydroxyglucuronide isomers, methoxyglucuronide and two hydroxymethoxyglucuronide isomers of buspirone.[11]

Zolpidem is converted to a range of pharmacologically inactive metabolites. These include the carboxy metabolites at both methyl positions on the phenyl and imidazopyridine rings.[12]

Zopiclone is extensively metabolized by the P450 enzymes with less than 10% excreted unchanged in urine. The main metabolites are the N-oxide and the N-desmethyl forms (Fig. 3.11). The N-oxide has some pharmacological activity.[13,14]

Zaleplon is metabolized by aldehyde oxidase to 5-oxo-zaleplon and by P-450 enzymes (CYP3A4) to desethyl-zaleplon. The 5-oxo-desethyl metabolite is also known.

## ENZYME SYSTEMS INVOLVED IN METABOLISM

The enzyme system responsible for most of the hydroxylation reactions of benzodiazepines is the cytochrome P450 series of enzymes. One form, CYP3A, is responsible for hydroxylating and dealkylating many of the benzodiazepines and related drugs. This form has two sub-types termed CYP3A3 and CYP3A4.

The activity of these enzymes can be affected by other drugs, including the benzodiazepines themselves, and, depending on the drug concerned, can either lead to a higher or a lower incidence of side effects. Table 3.6 shows benzodiazepines and related drugs that are known to be metabolized, in part or exclusively, by this system, and those not believed to be metabolized by this system.

Those drugs that are metabolized by CYP3A are likely to have an altered metabolism when two or more of these drugs are co-administered. Consequently, this may affect the duration of action, and determine whether side effects are elicited.

## EXCRETION

Elimination of these metabolites and any unchanged drug occurs primarily in the urine. Again, individual excretion data are shown in the monographs. A significant amount is excreted in the faeces. Amounts vary from a few per cent to ~30% of the administered dose. Faecal excretion derives from unabsorbed drug, or absorbed drug that is secreted in bile (from the liver) and is not subsequently re-absorbed.

All benzodiazepines and related sedatives are likely to be excreted into breast milk of lactating mothers; however, the likely exposure to the infant will only be a fraction of the

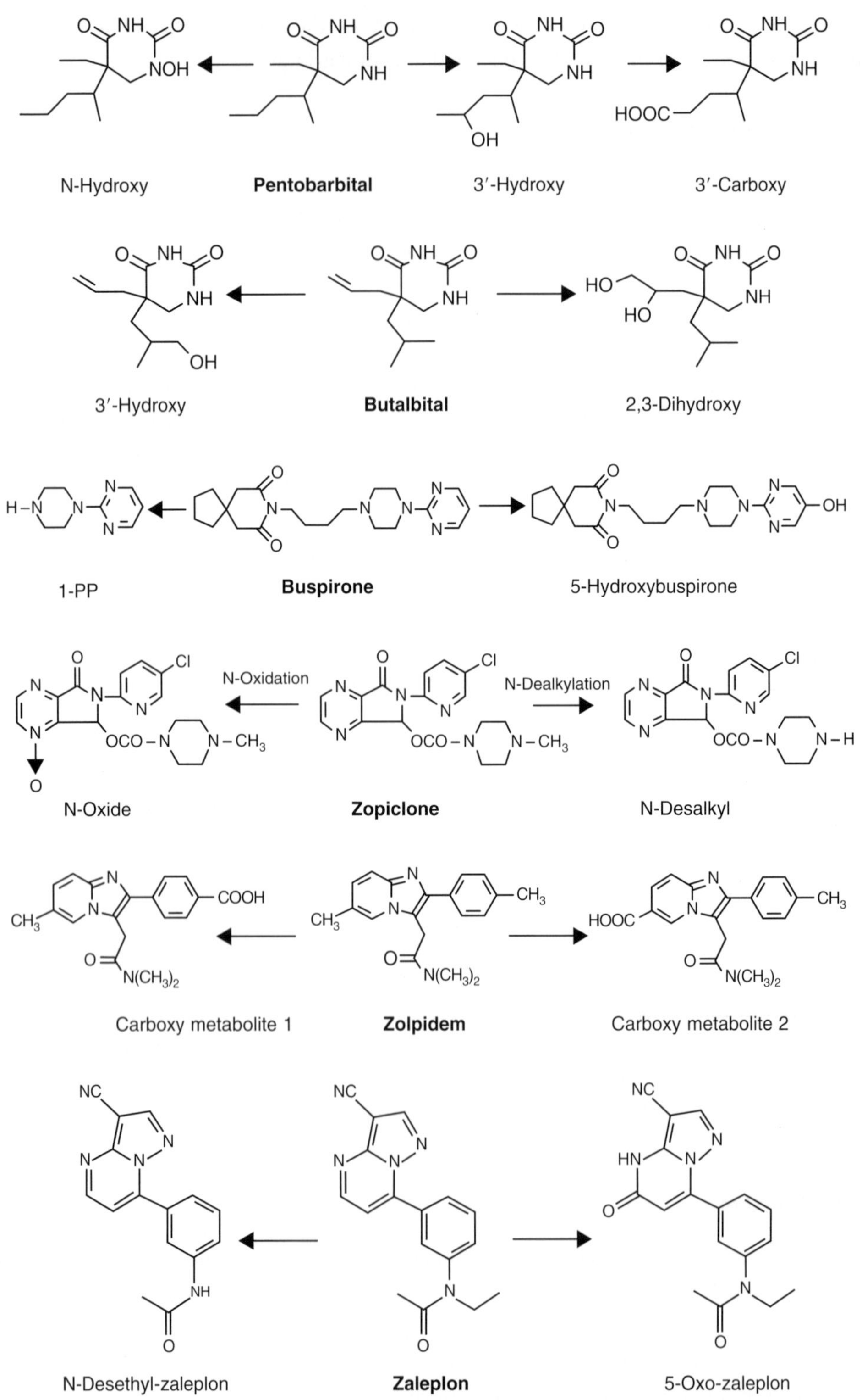

# Benzodiazepines

Fig. 3.11 Metabolic schema for selected non-benzodiazepines

**Table 3.6** Sedative substrates for CYP3A (3 or 4)

| Substrate | Not substrate |
|---|---|
| Alprazolam | Temazepam |
| Adinazolam | Oxazepam |
| Bromazepam | Lorazepam |
| Brotizolam (likely) | Lormetazepam |
| Buspirone (likely) | |
| Chlordiazepoxide | |
| Clobazam | |
| Clinazolam | |
| Clonazepam (likely) | |
| Clorazepate | |
| Diazepam | |
| Estazolam (likely) | |
| Flunitrazepam | |
| Flurazepam (likely) | |
| Midazolam | |
| Nitrazepam | |
| Nordazepam (and all drugs metabolized to this drug) | |
| Tofisopam (likely) | |
| Triazolam | |
| Zaleplon | |
| Zolpidem | |

From manufacturers' product information and Martindale 31st edition (Ref. 15).

maternal dose. Consequently, exposure of infants to sedatives through breast milk is not likely to be clinically significant.[16,17]

## DURATION OF ACTION

In previous sections, the term half-life has been used to define the rate of removal of drug from the blood. This term is frequently confused to also mean duration of action of the drug. While in some cases the half-life does provide a reasonable correlation with biological effect, in many cases it does not. For the effect of a drug to be related directly to the blood concentration, it requires a direct correlation of the blood concentration with the tissue at which the drug is acting. For a benzodiazepine, for example, the site of action is the brain (see Chapter 3.3), or discrete regions of the brain.

For a benzodiazepine to enter these brain regions, it will be subject to particular processes that allow entry into the brain. These are based on the physio-chemical properties of the drug, including the lipid solubility characteristics (lipophilicity) and retentive ability of the brain region. Drugs with higher lipid solubility will tend to enter the brain quicker and to a greater degree than those that are more water soluble. A measure of lipophilicity is the partition coefficient (expressed as $\log_P$). Benzodiazepines vary greatly in their lipophilicity (see monographs in the Appendix). For example, clobazam has a $\log_P$ value of 0.9 and diazepam has a $\log_P$ value of 2.7. Since this is a logarithmic scale, diazepam has 63 times greater lipid solubility than clobazam. This result would suggest much higher brain concentrations of diazepam than clobazam, if the same dose of drug were given. One would also expect a higher tissue concentration of diazepam than the corresponding blood concentration.

There is generally a poor correlation between blood half-life of benzodiazepine and duration of action. In practice there is a tendency for low-potency benzodiazepines (e.g. oxazepam) to have a shorter duration of action compared with their half-lives, and for high-potency benzodiazepines (e.g. triazolam) to have a longer duration of action than predicted from their half-lives. This probably relates to the greater receptor occupancy of highly potent drugs even at low blood concentrations, and because of their higher affinity for the benzodiazepine receptor, a slower dissociation rate from the sites of action.[3] For low-potency drugs, concentrations may drop below an effective concentration well before the drug is no longer measurable.

Highly lipid-soluble benzodiazepines are also more likely to enter the brain quicker than more water-soluble drugs. This is illustrated by quazepam, which has the highest lipid solubility for a benzodiazepine. Quazepam with a $\log_P$ of 4.0 has a rapid onset of action (sleep induction) due apparently to the rapid oral absorption and uptake into the brain. Quazepam also has a rapid offset of its action due to its rapid and extensive distribution into other tissues, reducing the incidence of adverse reactions to the drug.[18,19] This rapid offset in its effects is seemingly at odds with its long half-life of approximately two days. In these respects, quazepam is similar to thiopental, one of the barbiturates used in anaesthesia. It is not a coincidence that both drugs have a sulphur group as a replacement to an oxygen atom in their structures. The fentanyls (see opioids section, p. 219) are also quick acting due to their high tissue uptake.

Most of the benzodiazepines exist substantially in blood (and other tissues) bound to proteins and other macromolecules. Protein binding precludes that drug from eliciting an active response on a receptor. In other words, it is the non-protein-bound form that exhibits biological activity. Many of the benzodiazepines show protein binding of greater than 90%, leaving less than 10% to exert any biological activity. The extent of protein binding varies from one drug to another and may even vary depending on the concentration and the local tissue environment.[20] Protein binding is substantially affected by disease, particularly kidney and liver disease (see p. 127).

The monographs in the Appendix show the important pharmacokinetic properties of benzodiazepines and related drugs, including their bioavailabilities, clearances, half-lives, partition coefficients and protein binding.

## METABOLIC INTERACTIONS

A number of drugs interfere with the metabolism of many of the benzodiazepines. For example, cimetidine (Tagamet®, anti-ulcer drug)[21] and several of the newer-generation antidepressants inhibit the metabolism of alprazolam and potentially many other benzodiazepines by CYP3A (see Table 3.7). This occurs either by competitive inhibition of the enzyme(s) involved in their mutual metabolism or by direct inhibition of the enzyme(s) by the interfering drug.

Cimetidine (400 mg b.d.), for example, increases the half-life of diazepam (0.1 mg/kg over 7 days) by 39%, decreases clearance by 38%, and slows the formation of the active metabolite nordiazepam. Cimetidine (1 g daily) also increases half-life and blood concentrations of adinazolam by ~30% and enhances the decrement in performance to adinazolam on psychopharmacological tests. Omeprazole (20 mg once daily), which is also an inhibitor of gastric acid secretion and used in treating ulcers, has similar effects to cimetidine.[21]

Serotonin re-uptake inhibitor antidepressants include fluoxetine and fluvoxamine. These are potent inhibitors of the CYP3A enzymes. Fluvoxamine has been shown to enhance blood concentrations of alprazolam and, importantly, increase the psychomotor effects caused by alprazolam. This interaction is quite significant given that many patients are likely to be prescribed both an antidepressant and an anti-anxiety or hypnotic drug.[22] Fluvoxamine is a more potent inhibitor of the metabolism of alprazolam in isolated human liver microsomes than fluoxetine, paroxetine or sertraline.[23] Triazolam and midazolam have had similar interactions observed in the presence of ketoconazole (antifungal) and erythromycin (antibiotic).[24]

Zopiclone is also affected by inhibitors of CYP3A. In healthy volunteers, itraconazole (antifungal) increases the plasma concentrations by almost 30% and increases half-life from 5 to 7 h.[25]

A further variable is that drugs such as the barbiturates enhance the production of the enzymes and therefore induce metabolism of benzodiazepines. Barbiturates also induce their

**Table 3.7** Drugs affecting clearance of benzodiazepines

| Known inhibitors | Potential inhibitors | Inducers |
|---|---|---|
| Disulfiram | Sertraline | Barbiturates |
| Cimetidine | Propoxyphene | Carbamazepine |
| Clarithromycin | Propranolol | Phenytoin |
| Diltiazem | Metronidazole | Rifampacin |
| Erythromycin | Contraceptive steroids | |
| Fluoxetine | | |
| Fluvoxamine | | |
| Itraconazole | | |
| Paroxetine | | |
| Ketoconazole | | |
| Verapamil | | |
| Diltiazem | | |
| Saquinavir | | |

own metabolism causing a time-dependent increase in clearance as the liver produces more enzyme. Other drugs are also known to induce metabolism (see Table 3.7).[24,26]

## PHARMACOKINETICS IN VARIOUS PHYSIOLOGICAL STATES

### In the elderly

Advanced age (>65 years old) will affect the clearance of benzodiazepines, particularly those metabolized through the microsomal enzyme system. Benzodiazepines affected include chlordiazepoxide and all benzodiazepines metabolized to diazepam or nordiazepam, the triazolobenzodiazepines triazolam, alprazolam and adinazolam, and a number of other drugs including brotizolam. Reviews on the clinical pharmacokinetics of benzodiazepines with age are available.[7,22,27–29]

#### Benzodiazepines undergoing oxidative pathways

Age reduces the clearance of adinazolam, a triazolo-benzodiazepine, by ~30% and increases half-life by ~40%. The change in the kinetics in the elderly is mirrored by an increased decrement in psychomotor performance.[30] Age also reduces the clearance of the related drug, alprazolam. The half-life increases from a mean of 11 h in young males to 19 h in elderly volunteers.[31] Similar changes are also observed for loprazolam including a more pronounced effect on performance tests.[32] In some cases lower doses are recommended, often half the dose prescribed to a young individual.

#### Benzodiazepines undergoing conjugation

Age does not significantly affect the clearance and half-life of oxazepam[9] or temazepam.[33] This is not surprising since oxazepam and temazepam are metabolized primarily by conjugation. Similar findings are found with lorazepam (also metabolized by conjugation), although one study found a small reduction in clearance and volume of distribution.[9] Some reduction in clearance is expected even for those drugs that are conjugated due to normal reductions in body fat, and loss of some cardiovascular, renal and liver functions with advanced age.

Nitrazepam is metabolized by a combination of nitro reduction, acetylation, ring cleavage and conjugation reactions. Clinical studies have shown increases in half-life with advanced age of 50%[34] and 38%[35] with no change in total plasma clearance. This age effect is caused by an increase in volume of distribution in the elderly. Ageing has little apparent effect on the pharmacokinetics of flunitrazepam.[36]

These results show that most of the significant changes in half-life and clearance are associated with the oxidative metabolic processes leading to an increased impairment of psychomotor function.

#### Non-benzodiazepine hypnotics and sedatives

Age reduces the clearance of zolpidem, although the effect is only marked over the age of 70 years. In these persons plasma concentrations are higher by at least two-fold, although there is little change in half-life.[37] Reductions in dose to 5 mg nightly are recommended in persons over 65 years. Halving the dose of suriclone when treating elderly subjects is also recommended.[38]

## Barbiturates

Barbiturates, in common with the benzodiazepines undergoing oxidative pathways, are affected by advanced age, as a result of an increased volume of distribution, reduced liver function and the general decline in bodily functions.

## In children

Children, particularly young children (under 3 years old) and neonates, are known to have underdeveloped capacity to metabolize certain drugs.[39] Most of the studies on the pharmacokinetics of benzodiazepines in children relate to midazolam, since this drug is frequently used as a premedication during anaesthesia.

Studies have shown that the plasma concentrations of midazolam in children 3 years and older were half than those of younger children. This is attributed to an increased clearance in children 3 years and older. Mean clearance rates in older children, children between 1 and 2 years of age, and infants (<1 year) were 19.7, 4.7 and 6.0 mL/min/kg, respectively.[40,41]

It is likely that other benzodiazepines and related drugs metabolized by microsomal oxidative processes are similarly affected, although there are little data in the literature to quantify the magnitude of the effects for individual drugs.

## In liver disease

Liver disease, particularly cirrhosis and acute viral hepatitis, can affect clearance of benzodiazepines and barbiturates. This can occur by a number of mechanisms, including reduced metabolic capacity, alterations in the degree of protein binding, and an alteration in volume of distribution.

There is no significant effect of liver cirrhosis on the half-life and total clearance of nitrazepam, although there is an increase in unbound fraction in plasma. Alprazolam and buspirone are markedly affect by cirrhosis. Buspirone peak plasma concentrations are increased by 1500% compared with normal subjects.[42] A three-fold increase in half-life occurs with zolpidem in liver disease. The fraction of unbound drug also increases significantly.[37]

Drugs that are conjugated, as opposed to those that are primarily metabolized by the microsomal system, are little affected by liver disease. Oxazepam and lorazepam are both conjugated for elimination and neither is substantially affected by liver disease,[9] although small reductions in clearance are observed due to a reduction in protein binding and an increase in volume of distribution.

## In kidney disease

Renal disease leading to severe insufficiency in creatinine clearance invariably produces profound changes in the pharmacokinetics of benzodiazepines. For oxazepam and lorazepam, for example, renal insufficiency leads to an accumulation of the glucuronide conjugate (since kidneys are no longer able to excrete substances properly). Renal disease also leads to a change in protein binding resulting in higher volumes of distribution and a prolongation of half-life.[9]

Drugs that are metabolized by the microsomal system are less affected by renal insufficiency since drug is still being metabolized by the liver. Metabolites, however, will accumulate, and if active pharmacologically, will exert an increased action. Changes in protein binding in renal disease can have a marked effect on increasing drug actions by making more drug available to the body.[31]

Similar patterns are seen with zolpidem in kidney disease. The fraction of unbound drug increases significantly, and the volume of distribution and half-life double.[37]

## In critically ill persons

Persons dangerously ill, including those admitted to intensive care, are very much at risk of increased activity of sedatives, due to a combination of haemodynamic and physiological imbalances. Benzodiazepines are widely used in intensive care settings in hospital and will exhibit an increased effect in these subjects. Those drugs with long half-lives or those that are metabolized to long-acting metabolites, e.g. nordiazepam, are most likely to cause problems in this group.[26]

For example, midazolam, the most common benzodiazepines given in this setting, has a half-life of 2 h in normal adults, which increases to 10 h following cardiac surgery. As seen earlier, reduced function of the liver and kidneys will also increase the half-life.

Since most members of the sedative and hypnotic classes of drug have relatively high volumes of distribution, blood loss following injuries and subsequent replacement with fluids and blood products will not significantly affect the blood concentration after re-equilibrium has occurred.

## In obesity

Obesity tends to increase the volume of distribution of benzodiazepines primarily because of the increase in body fat. Drugs with the highest lipid solubility tend to show the largest increase. For example, the highly lipophilic drugs midazolam and diazepam show increases in volume of distribution by a factor of three. Less lipophilic drugs show a smaller net increase.[43] In contrast, obesity has little effect on the kinetics of zolpidem.[37]

There are few data to quantify the effect of obesity on other benzodiazepines at this stage. However, it is likely that the change in the volume of distribution is a significant factor for these drugs, although competing factors may minimisze the effects of any change in volume of distribution.

## Gender differences

Gender differences in the pharmacokinetics of benzodiazepines have been observed with a tendency for women to have a slightly longer half-life than men.[44]

# Synopsis

**PHARMACOKINETICS AND DURATION OF ACTION**

1. Benzodiazepines are generally well absorbed orally and reach peak blood concentrations within a few hours. Oral bioavailability ranges from 40 to100%. Food has generally little effect on the amount of drug absorbed.
2. Intramuscular absorption is only useful for the more water-soluble drugs. Because of their relatively high lipid solubility, benzodiazepines are likely to be absorbed from all other routes, including ocular, rectal, sublingual and vaginal.
3. The metabolism of benzodiazepines and barbiturates proceeds either through the oxidative microsomal enzyme system or by conjugation with glucuronic acid. Hydroxylated or dealkylated metabolites of benzodiazepines are often also biologically active and may substantially increase the duration of action of the drug.
4. Benzodiazepines are classified depending on their pharmacokinetic half-lives in plasma. Short-acting benzodiazepines extend up to 24 h, while long-acting extend for periods in excess of 24 h. Barbiturates are generally long acting, with the exception of the anaesthetic thiopental.
5. The clearance of barbiturates and benzodiazepines is decreased by liver disease, although the greatest effects occur with those drugs metabolized by the microsomal oxidative system. Lorazepam and other similar drugs metabolized by glucuronidation are least affected. Kidney disease particularly affects drugs metabolized to active drugs and those showing a high degree of protein binding.
6. Advanced age has similar effects to liver and kidney disease due to the reduction in output of major organs and changes in the volume of distribution. Doses of sedatives are usually halved in the elderly (>65 years), although oxazepam, lorazepam and temazepam are least affected by age.
7. The elimination of benzodiazepines metabolized by the CYP3A microsomal oxidation system is reduced by a number of drugs, including other benzodiazepines, cimetidine, omeprazole, the serotonin re-uptake inhibitors, antifungal agents, some blood pressure drugs, and some antibiotics. Barbiturates enhance metabolism of themselves and the benzodiazepines.

# 3.3 Mechanisms of action

Benzodiazepines bind with high affinity to specific receptors in the central nervous system of mammals. These receptors are functionally linked to the γ-aminobutyrate (GABA) receptor, in particular the $GABA_A$ sub-type that regulates the flow of chloride through an ion channel.

GABA is the main inhibitory neurotransmitter in the CNS; it is found particularly in the cerebellum, cerebral cortex, hippocampus and striatum. Nerves that rely on GABA for the transmission of impulses are involved in a number of behavioural features, and are linked to nerves that are modulated by opioids and other psychotropic drugs sensitive to another important neurotransmitter, serotonin. Drugs that affect GABA activity are important therapeutic agents, and include not only the benzodiazepines but also barbiturates and other sedatives and hypnotics, some anticonvulsants, some anaesthetics such as propofol and thiopental, hypnotic steroids, some anthelmintic and insecticidal compounds, and even alcohol.[45]

## BENZODIAZEPINES

The functional interaction of benzodiazepines with the GABA receptor causes a mutual augmentation of binding, such that benzodiazepines increase the affinity of GABA to their binding site, and GABA increases the affinity of benzodiazepines at adjacent binding sites on the receptor ion channel. At this site, the interaction of a benzodiazepine causes an allosteric change in the complex leading to an increase in affinity for GABA. This has the net effect of increasing the number of ion channels open to allow chloride ($Cl^-$) transport through the ion channels (ionophores). This process ultimately inhibits the activity of neurones thereby reducing the arousal of the cortical and limbic systems in the CNS. Benzodiazepines also reduce emotion by depressing the electrical after-discharge in the amygdala, hippocampus and septum components of the limbic system.

The $GABA_A$ $Cl^-$ receptor is now regarded as involving either a four- or five-unit complex. Six isoforms and 15 sub-types are now known.[46] GABA binds mainly to the α-subunit, while benzodiazepines bind to the β-subunit, called the (BZ-ω) binding site. The γ-subunit is essential to allow functional modulation of the channels by benzodiazepines.

A number of isotypes are now known in the brain, and elsewhere, which show different sensitivities to the benzodiazepines and related drugs.

A benzodiazepine can bind to the β-subunit as:

- a full agonist, i.e. it can elicit a full positive response;
- a partial agonist, i.e. elicits a less than maximal response;
- an antagonist, i.e. it blocks the action of agonists;
- an inverse agonist, i.e. by eliciting a negative (or inverse) response.

## Mechanisms of action

This detail is important in understanding differences in activity between benzodiazepine and non-benzodiazepine sedative/hypnotic drugs. This also explains why some benzodiazepines and related analogues have different activities, and a different profile of side effects.

Bretazenil, an experimental benzodiazepine, produces anticonflict (anxiolytic) and anticonvulsant effects at much lower doses than diazepam, whereas sedation occurs at much higher doses. Similar separation of typical benzodiazepine activities have been reported for other analogues (e.g. clonazepam). The non-benzodiazepine, alpidem, is an anxiolytic and anticonvulsant drug without effects on sedation and muscle relaxation. The dose–response curve for bretazenil and other partial agonists is shallower than for diazepam, and the maximum protection against chemically-induced convulsion is lower. Bretazenil also acts as a partial antagonist, blocking some of the effects of diazepam. This is an expected effect of a partial agonist. There are a number of useful reviews on this topic.[4,45–48]

Further knowledge of the complexity of the mechanism of action of benzodiazepines comes from studies which show that benzodiazepines bind with different affinity to receptor sub-types. For example, alpidem and zolpidem bind with high affinity to the $\omega_1$-sub-type (BZ-$\omega_1$), but have very low affinity for the $\omega_2$-sub-type (BZ-$\omega_2$). Benzodiazepines with selectivity for the $\omega_1$-sub-type include quazepam and lormetazepam. Zaleplon binds selectively to the BZ-$\omega_1$ sub-type with full agonist activity. The $\omega_2$-sub-type is found mainly in the sensorial and motor cortical and subcortical structures of the brain, whereas $\omega_2$-sub-types are found mainly in the limbic system, striatum and spinal cord.

The exact significance of this complex mechanism of action is still unclear, but it does suggest that not all benzodiazepines and their analogues are the same. Some will show selectivity as anxiolytics, but show few sedative actions including loss of co-ordination, loss of memory and, importantly, little ability to elicit tolerance. Others may be more useful as muscle relaxants.

Many of the newer types of anxiolytics and hypnotics mentioned in this book have these more selective actions, while still binding to the β-subunit of the GABA receptor complex. Atypical benzodiazepines such as imidazenil show promise as partial agonists, causing an anxiolytic and anticonvulsant effect, but have minimal disruptive effects on learning and sedation and are virtually devoid of tolerance potential.[48]

Benzodiazepines also have an apparent effect on serotonin pathways causing a reduction in serotonergic activity.[4] Serotonin (5-HT) is a key neurotransmittor involved in regulation of mood and behaviour. Drugs that affect serotonin activity in critical regions of brain are used as antidepressants and antipsychotics.

The GABA$_A$ receptor also responds to a large number of drugs including the CNS depressants, alcohol, anaesthetic steroids and barbiturates. It is not surprising, therefore, that these drugs have similar effects to the benzodiazepines and augment the activity of benzodiazepines when co-administered.[45]

## Biochemical changes

Benzodiazepines also affect a number of other key areas of the brain involved in either neuromodulation or neurotransmission. These include decreasing $K^+/Na^+$ ratios and increasing membrane-associated nucleic acids, decreasing catecholamine uptake in some brain regions, reducing the turnover of serotonin (5-HT) in the cortex, and increasing the levels of acetylcholine in the brain.

Alprazolam (1.5 mg single dose) has been shown to lower plasma levels of a metabolite of noradrenaline, namely 3-methoxy-4-hydroxyphenylethylene glycol (MHPG), lower plasma levels of cortisol and lower systolic blood pressure by as much as 10 mmHg. In contrast, diazepam (10 mg) does not affect plasma MHPG levels, nor does it affect blood pressure.[49] These data suggest a selective effect on noradrenergic neurones and the hypothalamus (site of ACTH production).

## BARBITURATES

Barbiturates have a similar site of action to the benzodiazepines in that they augment the actions of GABA in the CNS. However, in contrast to the benzodiazepines, they increase the duration of the Cl$^-$ channel opening. The binding site at the GABA receptor is different to that of the benzodiazepines, but sufficiently close to affect each other's actions. At higher doses they tend to activate the channels, depress the actions of other neurotransmitters and exert some membrane effects. These other effects are the likely cause of barbiturates' adverse reactions as general CNS depressants, and explain their use as surgical anaesthetics.

## ZOLPIDEM AND THE IMIDAZOPYRIDINES

The non-benzodiazepine zolpidem belongs to the imidazopyridine family of drugs. This drug has been available now for several years in Europe and the USA.

The actions resemble the benzodiazepines with strong sedative and hypnotic actions. It does not have anticonvulsant activity and tends not to produce tolerance to its sedative effect. As a hypnotic, it shortens sleep latency, but tends not to have the same problems as the benzodiazepines on stages of sleep.

The drug binds selectively to the $BZ_1$-$\omega_1$ receptor of the GABA complex and facilitates GABA-mediated neuronal inhibition, as do the benzodiazepines.[50] The related drug alpidem has similar properties.

## ZOPICLONE AND THE CYCLOPYRROLONES

At least two drugs of this type are known, suriclone and zopiclone. These drugs also act on the benzodiazepine-binding site of the $GABA_A$ receptor (BZ-$\omega$) but bind non-selectively to this site in contrast to zolpidem and some of the benzodiazepines. Zopiclone appears to act as a partial agonist on the $GABA_A$ receptor complex, while suriclone has more intrinsic activity.[51]

## BUSPIRONE AND THE AZAPIRONES

A relatively new class of drugs, the azapirones (or pyrimidinyl-piperazines), buspirone, gepirone, ipsapirone, tandospirone and zalospirone are selective agonists at the $5HT_{1A}$ receptor sub-type of 5HT receptors.[4] The $5HT_{1A}$ sub-type is found in the hippocampus and other parts of the limbic system. One part of the hippocampus, the septo-hippocampal region, is implicated in the control of anxiety and affective states. These drugs are anxiolytics and have a similar efficacy to the benzodiazepines, but do not have the same sedative, anticonvulsant and muscle relaxant properties. Consequently, these drugs do not show any impairment of motor skills and cognitive functions, a well-known side effect of the benzodiazepines.

## Synopsis

**MECHANISMS OF ACTION**

1 Benzodiazepines bind to a $\omega$-subunit of the GABA receptor and modulate the movement of chloride through an ion channel in discrete areas of the brain. This process ultimately inhibits the activity of neurones, thereby reducing the arousal of the cortical and limbic systems in the amygdala, hippocampus and septum components of the limbic system. A range of anxiolytic and behavioural effects are caused by this interaction.
2 Nerves that rely on GABA for the transmission of impulses are involved in a number of behavioural features and are linked to nerves that are modulated by opioids and to a range of antidepressant and antipsychotic drugs.
3 The range of activities of benzodiazepines depends on the affinity to this receptor, their selectivity to sub-types of this receptor ($BZ-\omega_1$ or $BZ-\omega_2$), and whether they act as partial agonists, full agonists or antagonists.
4 A range of drugs affect or interfere with the actions of benzodiazepines, including many other sedatives and hypnotics, opioids, alcohol, some anaesthetics and barbiturates.
5 Barbiturates bind to a neighbouring site of the GABA receptor complex and prolong the opening of the chloride channel.
6 Zolpidem and the imidazopyridine family of drugs have strong sedative and hypnotic actions and bind selectively to the $BZ-\omega_1$ receptor of the GABA complex. Zaleplon has a similar mechansim of action.
7 Zopiclone and the cyclopyrrolones also act on the benzodiazepine binding site of the GABA receptor ($BZ-\omega$) but bind non-selectively and with less intrinsic activity.
8 Buspirone and the azapirones act at a completely different site in the CNS to the benzodiazepines. They are selective agonists at the $5HT_{1A}$ receptor sub-type of 5HT (serotonin) receptors.

# 3.4 Pharmacological actions and therapeutics

All benzodiazepines and related drugs in clinical use possess a variety of pharmacological and physiological properties. The strength of these properties varies between the benzodiazepines, although many share a number of medical uses.

One of the most prescribed drug in these classes, diazepam, is indicated for the treatment of anxiety and insomnia, for the relief of muscle spasticity, and for the management of status epilepticus, and is used intravenously before endoscopies, for regional surgical procedures, for cardioversion and for induction of general anaesthesia.

Other benzodiazepines will find use in some or all of these indications (see Table 3.8). Their use is usually dictated by the relevant national regulatory authorities and marketing by individual drug companies. Readers should refer to the relevant jurisdictional prescribing authority for indications, contraindications and recommended doses.

This chapter reviews the therapeutic actions of these drugs. Useful reviews and texts are listed.[28,37,50,52–60]

## INDICATIONS FOR BENZODIAZEPINES

### Anxiety

Benzodiazepines are used for the treatment of a wide variety of anxiety disorders, including generalized anxiety disorder, and panic attacks associated with phobias.

Anxiety is a broad term that encompasses a number of disorders or conditions. In most cases, anxiety is a normal human emotion caused by life experiences, which is not pathological nor necessarily requires drug therapy. Anxiety can manifest itself as worry and feelings of anxiousness and irritability, and can also lead to sleep disorders, chest pains, dizziness, light-headedness, dry mouth, elevated heart rate (tachycardia), frequent urination, insomnia, irritability, nausea and diarrhoea, sweating, and obsessive and compulsive acts. In severe cases an anxiety disorder can be a serious condition and will require medical attention.

Anxiety can manifest itself as a recognized medical disorder, such as:

- panic disorder
- agoraphobia and other phobias
- obsessive–compulsive disorder
- post-traumatic stress disorder
- generalized anxiety disorder.

## Pharmacological actions and therapeutics

Table 3.8  Medical uses of benzodiazepines

| Indication | Example of benzodiazepine |
| --- | --- |
| As hypnotics | Adinazolam, brotizolam, flunitrazepam, flurazepam, loprazolam, lorazepam, oxazepam, quazepam, temazepam, triazolam |
| As anxiolytics | Chlordiazepoxide, diazepam, lorazepam, temazepam, alprazolam, prazepam, halazepam, ketazolam, tetrazepam |
| As anti-depressants | Adinazolam, alprazolam |
| As muscle relaxants | Bromazepam, diazepam, tetrazepam |
| As anti-convulsants | Brotizolam, diazepam, clobazam, clonazepam |
| For pre-operative sedation and induction of anaesthesia | Midazolam, diazepam, flunitrazepam |
| For acute alcohol withdrawal | Chlordiazepoxide, diazepam, oxazepam |
| For panic attacks | Alprazolam, clobazam, clonazepam, etizolam |

Panic attacks may occur alone or may be associated with certain phobias, such as agoraphobia which is defined as a fear of being in places or situations from which escape might be difficult or embarrassing, or in which help might not be available in the event of an attack. Symptoms associated with panic attacks include shortness of breath, palpitations, trembling, sweating, choking, nausea and abdominal distress, depersonalization, numbness and tingling sensations, flushes and chills, and fear of doing something wrong. For a review of the diagnosis and treatment of anxiety disorders readers are referred to references 55 and 61.

Alprazolam and a number of other benzodiazepines are useful in these conditions. Other drugs such as antidepressants are also used to treat panic attacks. Benzodiazepines are not recommended in most cases of anxiety disorders where cognitive behaviour therapy and/or pharmacotherapy is required.[62]

## Insomnia

The treatment of insomnia, and sleep difficulties in general, is one of the main uses of benzodiazepines, particularly with the shorter-acting drugs.

All of the benzodiazepines and those other drugs classified as sedatives and hypnotics induce sleep. The pattern and the duration of sleep characterize the various members of the hypnotic drugs. Normal sleep consists of non-rapid eye movements (NREM) and rapid eye movement (REM) stages. The REM stage is the most important and provides the best-quality sleep and the most recallable dreams. The NREM stage consists of a number of sub-stages of which stage 2 represents about 50% of sleep time. This is followed by slow-wave sleep (stages 3 and 4). Hypnotics tend to decrease latency time to fall asleep, increase stage 2 of NREM, decrease the REM stage and reduce the duration of slow-wave sleep.

Benzodiazepines tend to reduce sleep latency (enable a quicker onset of sleep), but decrease REM and slow-wave sleep. Barbiturates have similar effects to the benzodiazepines but are more pronounced, whereas zolpidem tends to interfere with sleep patterns least. Depending on the duration of action of drug, hypnotic effects may last for a few to several hours. Tolerance develops to the hypnotic effects relatively rapidly.

### Other therapeutic uses

Benzodiazepines have been shown to have a large range of uses other than for anxiety and insomnia. These include depression, muscle spasm, convulsions, acute alcohol withdrawal and preoperative sedation (see Table 3.8).

Lorazepam (2 mg parenteral) has been found useful as a tranquillizer in patients with agitated, assaultive or psychotic behaviour.[63]

Benzodiazepines reduce nocturnal gastric secretion and partially protect against stress ulcers. Benzodiazepines may also improve a variety of anxiety-related gastrointestinal disorders.[64]

Benzodiazepine antagonists have been shown to enhance pain control achieved by opioids. Flumazenil, a benzodiazepine receptor antagonist, enhanced morphine analgesia and decreased post-discharge side effects and need for post-discharge analgesia.[65] Alternatively, benzodiazepines such as midazolam appear to antagonize the effects of morphine.[66] Benzodiazepines themselves do not exhibit any significant analgesic activity.[67]

Readers are referred to the monographs on individual benzodiazepines in the Appendix for more information on recommended uses of these drugs.

## OTHER HYPNOTICS AND SEDATIVES

### Zopiclone and the cyclopyrrolones

Zopiclone has similar properties to the benzodiazepines, including use in insomnia and anxiety, and has amnesic, anticonvulsant and muscle relaxant properties. Zopiclone is usually used in the short-term treatment of insomnia. Usual doses are 7.5 mg at night. Higher doses to 15 mg are possible, but lower doses (3.75 mg) are advised in the elderly. Reviews are available.[37,58,68,69]

### Buspirone and the piperidinyl-piperazines

Buspirone has a similar ability to act as an anti-anxiety agent as the benzodiazepines.[54] The usual dose range is 15–30 mg per day, with doses up to 60 mg per day possible. Lower doses are recommended in elderly subjects due to a reduced clearance.

The piperidinyl-piperazines such as buspirone do show some side effects, such as nausea, dizziness, headache and restlessness in approximately 10% of subjects, but these are rarely severe.

These drugs are anxiolytics and have a similar efficacy to the benzodiazepines, but they do not have the same sedative, anticonvulsant and muscle relaxant properties. Consequently, these drugs do not show any significant impairment of motor skills and cognitive functions, a well-known side effect of the benzodiazepines. Buspirone also differs from the benzodiazepines in that it is not effective in the treatment of panic attacks. As for the antidepressants, the maximum effect of these drugs takes approximately 1 month to develop.

The concomitant use of serotonin re-uptake inhibitors (antidepressants) can lead to a serotonergic syndrome characterized by hypomania, confusion, agitation, incoordination, tremulousness, myoclonic jerks and decreased level of consciousness.[70] Serotonin re-uptake inhibitors include sertraline, citalopram, fluoxetine, fluvoxamine, paroxetine and venlafaxine. Many of the older tricyclic antidepressants also exhibit some inhibition of serotonin uptake. These include imipramine and clomipramine. Buspirone should not be administered with monoamine oxidase inhibitors. In contrast to benzodiazepines, concomitant use of ethanol does not show increased CNS depressant activity.

## Zolpidem and the imidazopyridines

The non-benzodiazepine zolpidem belongs to the imidazopyridine family of drugs. This drug has been available now for several years in Europe, and more recently in the USA.

The actions resemble the benzodiazepines with strong sedative and hypnotic actions. It does not have anticonvulsant activity and tends not to produce tolerance to its sedative effect. As a hypnotic, it shortens sleep latency, but tends not to have the same problems as the benzodiazepines on stages of sleep. Reports suggest that its action as a hypnotic persist for some days after cessation of dosing.

In contrast to the benzodiazepines, zolpidem does not produce respiratory depression in overdose, nor does it increase the CNS depressant effects of co-administered alcohol.

Therapeutic doses are 10–20 mg, although half these doses are recommended in the elderly. Zolpidem is rapidly absorbed from the gastrointestinal system with an oral bioavailability of ~70%. The elimination half-life is ~2 h in normal persons but will be elevated in persons with advanced age, in hepatic insufficiency such as cirrhosis, and in renal disease.

## Zaleplon

This new hypnotic resembles triazolam in its short action, but has similar selectivity to zolpidem.[71] Recommended doses range from 5 to 10 mg. There is less potential for hangover effects the next morning after a normal hypnotic dose. Zaleplon also produces comparable dose-dependent decrements on several performance tasks, including balance, circular lights, digit-enter and recall, digital substitution test, picture recall/recognition and repeated acquisition.[72]

## BENZODIAZEPINES IN THE ELDERLY

As discussed in previous chapters the elderly are more sensitive to benzodiazepines than their younger counterparts. The reasons for this include altered pharmacokinetics (see Chapter 3.2), and possibly altered pharmacodynamic responses leading to significant cognitive and psychomotor impairment in persons with already reduced or compromised cerebral function. Consequently, if benzodiazepines are prescribed to the elderly lower doses are recommended to reduce these adverse effects.[22,28,29,57,73]

# Benzodiazepines

## NON-MEDICAL USES OF SEDATIVES

Non-medical use of benzodiazepines is widespread in the Western world. The uses generally are based on relief of anxiety and insomnia consequent to misuse of other drugs such as heroin, amphetamines, cocaine and alcohol. Benzodiazepines are most associated with opioid users. Doses may range from that recommended therapeutically to many times the recommended dose. The use of several flunitrazepam (Rohypnol® etc.) tablets at once is well known in a drug abuse setting.

The type of benzodiazepines used will depend more on the availability within a legal jurisdiction, rather than necessarily a strict preference for a particular drug (see Chapter 3.5 for further details).

## THERAPEUTICS

Therapeutic concentrations of benzodiazepines and related drugs vary widely depending on their potency (and consequently dose), protein binding, volume of distribution and rate of

**Table 3.9** Therapeutic concentrations of benzodiazepines and newer sedatives/hypnotics

| Drug | Therapeutic concentration range in blood (mg/L) |
|---|---|
| **Benzodiazepines** | |
| Alprazolam | 0.02–0.06 |
| Bromazepam | 0.08–0.17 |
| Chlordiazepoxide | 0.7–2.0 (0.3–2.8)[a] |
| Clobazam | 0.1–0.4 |
| Clonazepam | 0.02–0.06 |
| Diazepam | 0.1–1.0 |
| Flunitrazepam | 0.005–0.02 |
| Flurazepam | 0.001–0.028 (0.04–0.15)[b] |
| Lorazepam | 0.02–0.25 |
| Nitrazepam | 0.02–0.2 |
| Nordazepam | 0.1–1.0 |
| Oxazepam | 0.1–1.0 |
| Temazepam | 0.1–1.0 |
| Triazolam | 0.002–0.02 |
| **Newer sedatives and hypnotics** | |
| Buspirone | 0.0009–0.005 |
| Zaleplon | ~0.01–0.1 |
| Zolpidem | 0.08–0.15 |
| Zopiclone | 0.01–0.05 |

[a] Demoxepam in parentheses; [b] desalkylflurazepam in parentheses.

metabolism. The notion of therapeutic concentration refers to a concentration normally seen in persons taking recommended doses of a drug. Tables 3.9 and 3.10 show the concentration range at which a significant effect is expected at recommended doses.

Therapeutic concentrations will be expected to produce a significant physiological response in most persons, particularly those not tolerant to the drug. However, these data should only be used a guide since in some patients much higher doses are sometimes prescribed for legitimate medical purposes.

Concentrations below the minimum are unlikely to produce any significant pharmacological response in most subjects. This is of relevance in toxicology when considering the combined effects of drugs; concentrations of drugs at or below an effective concentration are not likely to produce any significant physiological response.

The use of sedatives such as benzodiazepines in drug-naïve persons can result in significant drowsiness, dizziness, and short latency period to sleep, and is likely to cause amnesia. Mixing benzodiazepines with alcohol will exacerbate the effects.

**Table 3.10** Therapeutic concentrations of barbiturates and older sedatives

| Drug | Therapeutic concentration range in blood (mg/L) |
|---|---|
| **Barbiturates** | |
| Amylobarbital | 1–5 |
| Barbital | 10–40 |
| Butalbital | 1–10 |
| Butobarbital | 5–15 |
| Hexobarbital | 4–10 |
| Pentobarbital | 1–3 |
| Phenobarbital | 10–40 |
| Secobarbital | 1–5 |
| Thiopental | 5–50 |
| **Older sedatives** | |
| Chloral hydrate[a] | 2–10 |
| Chlormethiazole | 0.1–1.0 |
| Diphenhydramine | 0.02–0.1 |
| Doxylamine | 0.07–2 |
| Ethchlorvynol | 0.5–8 |
| Ethinamate | 5–10 |
| Glutethimide | 2–10 |
| Meprobamate | 10–25 |
| Methaqualone | 0.5–3 |
| Methyprylon | 5–15 |
| Paraldehyde | 30–300 |

[a] As trichloroethanol.

# Benzodiazepines

## Synopsis

### COMMON USES AND THERAPEUTICS

1 Benzodiazepines are used in the treatment of various forms of anxiety and insomnia, for the relief of muscle spasticity, for the management of some forms of epilepsy and status epilepticus, in minor depression, in panic disorders associated with agoraphobia, intravenously for preoperative sedation and induction of anaesthaesia, and for acute alcohol withdrawal.
2 Benzodiazepines, but not zolpidem or buspirone, upset normal sleep patterns reducing REM and slow-wave sleep duration.
3 Benzodiazepines, while useful in treating some forms of anxiety, are not advocated in disorders where cognitive-behaviour therapy and/or pharmacotherapy is required.
4 Benzodiazepines themselves do not produce analgesia; however, they reduce opioid-induced analgesia, while antagonists augment opioid-induced analgesia.
5 Zopiclone is used primarily for the short-term treatment of insomnia in doses of 3.75–15 mg taken at night before sleep.
6 Buspirone is used to treat anxiety in doses of 15–30 mg daily.
7 Zolpidem is used largely as a hypnotic in doses of 10–20 mg at night.
8 Zaleplon is used as a hypnotic in doses of 5–10 mg at night.
9 Concentrations achieved during therapeutic use are known for these drugs and range from a minimum effective concentration to the concentrations achieved with high therapeutic doses.

# 3.5 Adverse reactions and tolerance

Despite their relative safety in low prescribed doses, benzodiazepines can elicit significant adverse reactions when used in high doses or in an abuse setting. Their involvement in forensic cases is often compounded when they are used in conjunction with alcohol, heroin and other drugs.

In some situations benzodiazepines cause profound behavioural changes. When these occur in cases of serious physical and sexual assault, or in road traffic crashes, courts need to understand the basis and extent of these adverse reactions.

This chapter presents a review of the behavioural and other relevant side effects associated with the use of benzodiazepines and related sedatives. The development of dependence and how this affects the response to these drugs is also discussed.

Useful reviews on this subject are listed.[73–76]

## BENZODIAZEPINES

### Effects on the central and autonomic nervous systems

The side effects of benzodiazepines of most significance are those related to sedation, or a seemingly non-specific depression of the central nervous system (CNS). These symptoms include tiredness or drowsiness, an inability to fully concentrate, and slowing of reflexes and thought patterns. In more severe cases, difficulties with balance control and even ataxia may occur.

Side effects for the benzodiazepines involving the autonomic nervous system include dry mouth, blurred vision, urinary retention and excessive perspiration. These usually subside in the first week of therapy and are rarely serious. The dose of drug can be reduced if the side effect is intolerable. Other less frequent side effects include nausea, vomiting, constipation, rashes, blurred vision and weight gain.

Some benzodiazepines are less sedating than others. There is evidence that clobazam, a 1,5-benzodiazepine, is less sedating than other benzodiazepines at equivalent doses reducing anxiety,[77] and does not produce subjective or objective impairment of performance and alertness seen with other benzodiazepines.[78]

Benzodiazepines that have a long pharmacokinetic half-life will produce less residual CNS sedation the morning after a night-time hypnotic dose. Drugs such as oxazepam, temazepam and triazolam are preferred over diazepam or flurazepam, or drugs converted to nordazepam and flurazepam or desalkylflurazepam. This is particularly important in persons driving motor vehicles or those operating machines during their working life (see p. 146).

## EFFECT ON MEMORY AND COGNITIVE FUNCTIONS

Another side effect commonly associated with benzodiazepines is amnesia. The loss of memory occurs during the influence of the drug effects, and is therefore called anterograde amnesia. This is largely caused by impairment of the acquisition of newly learned information into long-term episodic storage. Patients will therefore often forget, or only record partial memory, during the duration of drug action. This is commonly seen in day-surgery patients given a short-acting benzodiazepine such as midazolam to assist in the anaesthesia. This property is apparently shown by all members of the family, although the duration and extent of the response will depend on the dose used and duration of action of the benzodiazepine.[59] Midazolam will show little effect some hours after drug administration, whereas diazepam, a long-acting benzodiazepine, will show these effects for much longer, often for more than 1 day.

The amnesic effects occur following both intravenous and oral administration, and decay at similar rates depending on the half-life of the drug.[79] Diazepam impairs acquisition of new information, while leaving retrieval processes intact. There is evidence that patients given diazepam show signs of an enhancement of recall for material learned before the drug was given. Impairment caused by diazepam is similar for a variety of cognitive tasks and is proportional to the magnitude of the memory component required.

Cognition (speech patterns and content) is adversely affected by single doses of a number of benzodiazepines including chlordiazepoxide, lorazepam, triazolam and flurazepam.

These decrements in memory and psychomotor and cognitive functions are likely to occur for all other benzodiazepines.[80] It is therefore important that persons taking benzodiazepines on a long-term basis are warned of these side effects. Persons operating machinery, driving motor vehicles or involved in situations where constant learning is required are most at risk of impairment and reduced work output.

The elderly are particularly prone to memory loss, partly because of the reduced ability to inactivate these drugs (reduced clearance) and the ageing process of the brain. Benzodiazepines will exacerbate underlying dementia. The effect of benzodiazepines, such as diazepam, on the elderly ($>65$ years old) is probably no greater than on the young. The apparent increased effect of benzodiazepines on the elderly is due to their already lower baseline performance. This has the net effect of making some benzodiazepine-induced loss of cognitive or psychomotor performance more noticeable.[81]

### Effects on respiration

Benzodiazepines have little effect on breathing when used therapeutically in healthy persons. When used as pre-anaesthetics, a slight depression of alveolar ventilation occurs causing respiratory acidosis. In doses used for endoscopy, benzodiazepines also decrease alveolar ventilation and $P_{O_2}$, increase $P_{CO_2}$, and may cause $CO_2$ narcosis in patients with chronic obstructive airways disease (COAD). An increased effect including apnoea is seen with co-administration of opioids and other CNS depressant drugs such as alcohol.

Benzodiazepines may worsen sleep-related breathing disorders, especially in patients with chronic obstructive pulmonary disease or cardiac failure. Long-term use may induce sleep apnoea in predisposed persons or in people with recent myocardial infarction.[82]

In overdose, benzodiazepines are most toxic if some form of compromised airways function exists, such as in the elderly, or if another CNS depressant drug is present in significant concentrations.

## Effects on the cardiovascular system

Benzodiazepines have little effect on cardiovascular function at therapeutic doses. In anaesthetic doses, benzodiazepines decrease blood pressure and increase heart rate. This may be related to a decrease in peripheral resistance and/or reduction in cardiac output. In large doses, midazolam decreases considerably both cerebral blood flow and oxygen assimilation. In persons with compromised cardiovascular function the use of large doses of benzodiazepines may further compromise cardiovascular function, particularly if pre-existing respiratory disease exists.

## Effects on behavioural aggression

A number of benzodiazepines have been shown to elicit an increase in aggression, particularly on provocation. Although these reactions are relatively rare, they can be accompanied by suicidal and homicidal behaviour. Benzodiazepines known to show these effects include alprazolam, chlordiazepoxide, clonazepam, diazepam and lorazepam, but seemingly not oxazepam.[83-87]

This reaction to the use of benzodiazepines has been termed behavioural toxicity, as distinct from the traditional biochemical or pharmacological toxicity causing a life-threatening response.[88]

Behavioural toxicity has been defined as those pharmacological reactions of a drug that produce alterations in perceptual and cognitive functions, psychomotor performance, motivation, mood and interpersonal relationships to the degree that they interfere with, or limit the capacity, of the individual to function within his setting, or constitute a hazard to his physical well-being. The doses used must be within those normally used therapeutically.

Paradoxical rage reactions are known to be associated with use of benzodiazepines. Paradoxical rage reactions occur infrequently in the general population, but there is evidence that this is a disinhibitory phenomenon and occurs more frequently in persons with underlying anxiety and depression. Interestingly, aggression is not recognized as any violent behaviour by the patient. This would suggest subjects have no conscious control over their actions.

This is typified by alprazolam, which can cause agitation, depersonalization, and perceptual disorder in patients on withdrawal from this drug. Mania, amnesia, and aggressive and assaultative behaviour have also been connected with use of alprazolam. Dangerously aggressive behaviour when taken to excess is illustrated in Case Report 3.2 (p. 163). This case report highlights potential problems associated with high doses of alprazolam, particularly in persons with depression and some underlying brain damage.

Behavioural aggression associated with alprazolam has also been reported in patients with panic disorder and agoraphobia. Alprazolam reduces hostility and anxiety, but patients show an increase in aggression in response to provocation in a behavioural test.[89]

The incidence of aggression or hostility with alprazolam has varied from 10% in a mixed diagnostic group[90] to 58% in patients with borderline personality disorder.[91] Aggression may be more likely in patients with panic disorder, or agarophobia with panic attacks with a secondary major depressive episode.[89,92]

Eleven per cent of children receiving clobazam for refractory epilepsy develop a severe behaviour disorder characterized by aggressive agitation, self-injurious behaviour, insomnia and incessant motor activity after initiation of therapy with this drug.[93] These children are disabled developmentally, display an average age of 6.4 years, and receive between 0.4 and 1.4 mg/kg per day of clobazam. This behavioural change can be reversed on cessation of clobazam therapy.

Some children given flunitrazepam as pre-anaesthetic show aggression following doses ranging from 1 to 2 mg.[94]

Triazolam has been associated with a greater number of side effects, including behavioural effects, compared with other benzodiazepines. This led to its withdrawal in the UK.[95] However, triazolam is probably not associated with any more behavioural disturbances than temazepam in psychiatric patients and in normal volunteers; rather, these effects were due to the relatively high dose being prescribed.[96,97] The use of a 0.25 mg dose is approximately of similar potency to 30 mg temazepam, with 0.125 mg doses now widely recommended as starting doses. It is therefore important that when comparisons are made with other drugs, comparative doses are used.

Disinhibition has also been reported with midazolam (an imidazole benzodiazepine).[98] Typical drug responses include uncooperativity, hallucination, aggression, hostility and violent movement leading to assault.[99] Non-drinking alcoholics may exhibit disinhibitory behaviour without any demonstrable signs of clinical sedation after moderate doses of midazolam. This reaction may be exacerbated by alcohol-induced changes in sensitivity to benzodiazepines in the brain.[99]

These effects are dose dependent. Midazolam only demonstrates adverse reactions such as agitated excitement, restlessness and irritation with higher doses (0.35 and 0.45 mg/kg rectally) in children given the drug as a premedication for surgery.[100]

Similar reports have appeared with clonazepam when used in the treatment of epileptics. Hyperactivity, shouting, aggression and belligerence to other patients is dose related and disappears on cessation of drug.[85]

This increase in aggression tends to occur with the more potent benzodiazepines, such as alprazolam, triazolam, lorazepam and clonazepam, and tends to increase with dose of drug.

The use of benzodiazepines as a first-line treatment in the elderly with dementia is not recommended due to their sedating activity causing impairment of motor activity leading to higher incidence of falls and bone breaks. In these patients, benzodiazepines are also likely to increase in aggression in already aggressive persons.[73]

### Reversal of disinhibitory effects

These disinhibitory reactions to benzodiazepines can be predictably reversed by the administration of the benzodiazepine antagonist, flumazenil, and by physostigmine.[101] Flumazenil is a valuable antidote to treat toxic reactions to benzodiazepines. Physostigmine is a reversible inhibitor of cholinesterase, and although it has effects on cholinergic receptors, it has possible antagonist activity at the benzodiazepine GABA receptor chloride ionophore complex.

Consequently, physostigmine also reverses paradoxical excitement, respiratory depression, delirium and coma caused by overdosage to benzodiazepines, thus also acting as an antidote.[101,102] Flumazenil also reverses any adverse or toxic effects of zopiclone.

The actions of opioid antagonists and physostigmine to reverse the effects of benzodiazepines suggest a complex interplay between a number of brain and receptor functions.

Combination with alcohol

The combination of alcohol and therapeutic doses of alprazolam (1 mg) has been shown to increase aggressiveness in response to provocation in a competitive reaction time task in moderate social drinkers.[103] This increase is greater than predicted from alcohol and alprazolam alone, suggesting synergistic effects of this combination on behavioural control. It is noteworthy that these drugs show typical effects of sedation and intoxication, together with increased feelings of anxiety.

Case Report 3.3 (p. 164) illustrates the behavioural toxicity associated with the combination of benzodiazepine and alcohol. It is noteworthy that the subject in this case report had not shown this behaviour before when only alcohol was consumed, or even when alcohol and one of the tricyclic antidepressants was used, indicating the special properties of the benzodiazepines.

## Effects on sexual behaviour

Excitement can occur as a behavioural state following benzodiazepine usage. This can manifest itself as an increase in sexual fantasies. In this situation, a number of complaints of sexual assault following medical or dental treatment in hospitals or surgeries have proven to be fictitious. In most cases, the benzodiazepine midazolam was used. The reasons for some of the complaints are not clear but have involved medical procedures that seemingly caused the patient to believe that sexual assault had occurred while under the influence of midazolam. Difficulties associated with recall of events (see section on memory and cognitive functions, p. 142) are undoubtedly a major reason.

On the other hand, cases of sexual assault have been proven against health professionals. These have occurred during minor surgical procedures, or by drugging the person with a benzodiazepine spiked in a soft drink or coffee. To guard against false accusations, and to protect individuals from actual sexual assault, recommendations have been made for dentists (and medical practitioners) to administer sedative drugs only in the company of a second appropriate person, i.e. another health professional.

A number of case reports have also described sexual disinhibition with clonazepam, a high-potency benzodiazepine used in the treatment of mania, panic disorder and epilepsy.[104–106] See Case Reports 3.4 and 3.5 (pp. 164–5).

Case Report 3.5 shows the appearance of sexual disinhibition following transfer from alprazolam to clonazepam. This profile has similarities with behavioural aggression developing with benzodiazepines. During the time the benzodiazepine is acting, the patient develops a new 'out-of-character' behaviour, and only becomes fully aware of his/her actions after withdrawal of the drug. In this context, benzodiazepines may be contraindicated in individuals with a history of provocative and inappropriate behaviours during adolescence, and in persons with a history of alcohol or drug abuse.

## OTHER ANXIOLYTICS

The barbiturates and many of the older sedatives cause significant sedation and other effects related to depression of the CNS. Again, those barbiturates with longer half-lives will have longer residual effects than the shorter-acting analogues.

The new-generation hypnotics tend to show less sedative actions. This applies particularly to the anxiolytic buspirone, which is less sedating than the benzodiazepines and does not appear to potentiate the adverse effects of alcohol. Buspirone is particularly useful in the elderly since it reduces the risk of hip fractures and other falls.[57] Zolpidem also has little effect on psychomotor function and is therefore relatively safe the morning after a night-time dose,[50] but it does adversely affect learning and memory.[107] Zopiclone is most similar to the benzodiazepines, although significant impairment of psychomotor performance is usually seen at doses of 7.5 mg or higher. Zaleplon appears to act similarly to triazolam.[72,108]

Barbiturates have had a similar profile of behavioural reactions to the benzodiazepines with aggression and rage reactions reported. Barbiturates do have more CNS depressant activity than the benzodiazepines, consequently the profiles of persons taking barbiturates tend to have more side effects and adverse reactions. The barbiturates are largely obsolete in modern practice and are no longer considered a major drug of abuse in developed countries.

Buspirone does not adversely affect cognitive function and there is no evidence of any significant impairment of short-term memory.[57] Zolpidem shows a small variable effect on memory that appears to be dose related and is only of significance at doses of 20 mg.[50] Buspirone has little effect on the cardiovascular system although rare events (<1 in 1000 subjects) have been noted, such as myocardial infarction, cardiomyopathy and hypotension. Their connection to use of buspirone is unclear. Buspirone is now regarded as a far safer drug in the elderly.[57] Neither buspirone nor zolpidem shows any significant reduction in respiratory function, unlike benzodiazepines.[50,57]

Zopiclone, however, appears to show similar effects on memory as the benzodiazepines, although memory impairment is less than for many of the benzodiazepines.[58,107,109] Zopiclone appears to have similar disinhibitory actions as the benzodiazepines; however, these are absent with zolpidem and buspirone.

## EFFECT ON DRIVING

A particularly important adverse reaction to benzodiazepines, and indeed many of the other related sedatives, is their ability to adversely affect driving skills.

Impairment of skills associated with driving motor vehicles occurs leading to increased lateral road movement and slowed reaction times. For example, diazepam at 10 mg increases lateral position variability in drivers. The increase is deemed dangerous, since one-third of subjects reach impairment levels leading to movement into the next lane or into the shoulder of the road.[110] Except for clobazam, similar results have been found for other benzodiazepines.[78,111]

Epidemiological studies show less clear effects on risks of crashes. Hospital admission data show that people who used minor tranquillizers in the previous 3 months had a five-fold higher risk of a serious traffic accident.[111] The increase in risk has been estimated at 1.5-fold[112,113] and four-fold, respectively.[114] The highest-risk groups are the youngest age group and males. An increased risk is also found for benzodiazepine-like anxiolytics (2.5-fold).

There is evidence that long-half-life benzodiazepines (such as diazepam) increase the risk of being involved in an accident by approximately 50%. In contrast, short-acting benzodiazepines are not associated with an increase in risk.[115]

Benzodiazepines have not always been linked to increased accident risk. Case–control studies of older drivers who were involved in crashes found that current use of benzodiazepines had little association with increased risk for injurious collisions.[116,117] Useful reviews are found in references 118–122.

Whatever the risk, there is sufficient evidence to show a potential for benzodiazepines to interfere with cognitive and psychomotor functions at therapeutic doses. It is therefore much more likely that misuse, use by the elderly, and use with other psychoactive drugs have a potential to contribute to accidents.

## DRUG INTERACTIONS

It has long been known that the combination of benzodiazepines with other CNS depressant drugs increases the likelihood of significant side effects or toxic responses. The co-administration of alcohol is probably the most important single-drug interaction seen in forensic cases. While perhaps obvious, the use of two or more benzodiazepines will increase the combined drug effect. This is a relatively common situation in forensic cases.

Co-administration of zopiclone with alcohol enhances psychomotor impairment caused by each alone. The effects dissipate on removal of the alcohol.[58] In rat studies the co-administration of alcohol and the benzodiazepine chlordiazepoxide causes an additive interaction of both drugs on their depressant effects and in their aggression-heightening effects.[123]

## TOLERANCE AND DEPENDENCE

### Benzodiazepines

Tolerance develops readily to the sedative effects of the benzodiazepines. This usually manifests in a reduction of sedative-like side effects (drowsiness etc.) within the first week of treatment. However, tolerance to the anxiolytic effects is not demonstrable in the short term, particularly if 'therapeutic doses' are used. Abuse of benzodiazepines is more likely to cause tolerance, particularly in persons not using the drug for a relevant clinical condition but rather for recreational reasons. In these situations, doses used may be many times those recommended for therapeutic use.

It is of interest that some benzodiazepines are more likely to be abused than others. For example, structured interviews with methadone-maintenance patients indicate that diazepam is a preferred benzodiazepine, which is often used in high dose.[124] In countries where flunitrazepam is available, this drug is often preferred.[125–127] Comparative controlled clinical psychology studies have shown diazepam as producing barbiturate-like subjective effects (38%) more frequently than oxazepam (14%), and that high-dose diazepam had a higher abuse liability than oxazepam.[128] Flunitrazepam (2 mg) produces more disruptive effects on all performance tasks compared with triazolam (0.5 mg) and produces a greater sense of 'liking' and 'highs' than triazolam.[129] However, extensive reviews on the relative abuse liability of benzodiazepines suggest that diazepam has a higher abuse liability,[128] although no one member of this class is clearly more liable to abuse.[130] These apparent differences may relate more to availability on the street than distinct pharmacological differences.

Physical dependence to benzodiazepines can lead to withdrawal symptoms. Mild withdrawal symptoms include anxiety, apprehension and fearfulness, dizziness, headache, muscle stiffness, insomnia and sensitivity to light and sound. More severe symptoms include intense rebound anxiety, nausea, vomiting, delirium, hallucinations, hyperthermia, sweating, panic attacks, confusional or paranoid psychoses, high heart rate and increased blood pressure and occasionally seizures (see Table 3.11).

In general, the patient experiences a rebound phenomenon that produces symptoms, which may be more severe than before therapy started. The longer-half-life benzodiazepines often produce withdrawal symptoms several days after cessation of drug use. On the other hand, short-acting benzodiazepines will produce an abstinence syndrome within a day or two of cessation. The patient will eventually return to normal, although this may take several weeks.

Table 3.11 lists some factors that lead to physical dependence and withdrawal of benzodiazepines. The potent short-acting benzodiazepines such as alprazolam, clonazepam, flunitrazepam, lorazepam and triazolam are more likely to cause a patient to develop drug dependence than longer-acting and less potent benzodiazepines. Oxazepam appears to show least dependence-producing liability. Long-term use is probably a bigger risk factor as is use of higher than recommended doses.

Table 3.11  Withdrawal reactions and benzodiazepines

Factors most likely to cause withdrawal reactions
- Short-half-life benzodiazepines (short-acting benzodiazepines)
- High-potency benzodiazepines, e.g. alprazolam, triazolam, lorazepam
- Duration of continuous benzodiazepine use (>3 months)
- High relative dose

Mild withdrawal reactions
Anxiety, apprehension, dizziness, headache, insomnia, muscle stiffness, sensitivity to light and sound

Strong withdrawal reactions
Intense rebound anxiety, nausea, vomiting, delirium, hallucinations, hyperthermia, sweating, panic attacks, confusional or paranoid psychoses, high heart rate, increased blood pressure, occasionally seizures

After MacKinnon and Parker, 1982.[131]

# Adverse reactions and tolerance

This abstinence syndrome can be minimized, or even prevented, by slow and gradual reduction in dose over weeks. The actual rate of reduction will depend on the half-life of drug, the dose used, and, of course, the seriousness of the dependence. Barbiturates, such as pentobarbital, show cross-tolerance with the benzodiazepines and can be used to minimize withdrawal reactions.

## BARBITURATES

Persons using barbiturates regularly will develop tolerance rapidly. The magnitude of the tolerance can lead to an escalation of doses several-fold. Abstinence leads to symptoms not unlike those experienced with benzodiazepines.

## BUSPIRONE, ZOLPIDEM AND ZOPICLONE

Buspirone produces physical dependency and is effective in long-term studies without loss of efficacy.[57]

Zolpidem has also not been shown to produce symptoms of dependence or show any obvious loss in efficacy with long-term use.[50]

Neither buspirone nor zolpidem show any evidence of cross-tolerance to benzodiazepines, i.e. replacing benzodiazepines with these drugs will elicit an abstinence syndrome similar to benzodiazepines.

On the other hand, persons using zopiclone long term do appear to develop dependence similar to the benzodiazepines.[109] This appears to be less frequent and less severe than with the benzodiazepines.[58]

## Synopsis

### BEHAVIOURAL AND OTHER SIDE EFFECTS

1 Benzodiazepines produce a number of recognizable side effects, including amnesia and reduced concentration powers, dry mouth, drowsiness and tiredness, nausea, decreased visual accommodation, slurred speech, and balance problems.
2 These effects are dose dependent, last for longer with the longer-acting benzodiazepines, and are magnified in the elderly and those persons requiring use of fine motor skills, e.g. operating machinery and driving motor vehicles.
3 Benzodiazepines have little adverse effect on respiration and the cardiovascular system, except in overdose, and often only in clinically compromised persons such as the aged.
4 Barbiturates also cause significant sedation and other side effects associated with non-specific depression of the CNS.
5 Zolpidem and buspirone show fewer side effects due to their more specific actions.
6 Behavioural aggression is a well-known adverse reaction with the benzodiazepines and barbiturates. This disinhibitory reaction can be quite profound and causes bizarre and often aggressive involuntary changes in personality.

## Benzodiazepines

7   Behavioural aggression is more likely with longer-acting, high-potency benzodiazepines, situations when high doses are used, in persons with depression or borderline personalities, or in persons with some form of brain damage.
8   Alcohol increases the likelihood of disinhibition and CNS depression reactions, and is contraindicated in persons using barbiturates, benzodiazepines, and the older non-specific sedatives and zopiclone, but not buspirone or zolpidem.
9   Benzodiazepines adversely affect driving skills and are likely to increase the risk of a motor vehicle accident.
10  Barbiturates and benzodiazepines may produce tolerance and dependence on repeated long-term use, particularly if used long term or high or intravenous doses are used to achieve euphoria.
11  Arguably, the abuse liability of certain benzodiazepines appears higher, with diazepam and flunitrazepam often cited.
12  Withdrawal reactions following abstinence can produce significant symptoms, including excessive anxiety, apprehension and fearfulness, nausea, vomiting, panic attacks, psychoses, delirium, hallucinations, blood pressure changes and seizures in extreme cases.
13  The potent shorter-acting benzodiazepines are more likely to cause drug dependence and produce abstinence symptoms.
14  Zopiclone appears to have somewhat less sedative effects than the benzodiazepines, and is less likely to produce dependence.
15  Neither zolpidem nor buspirone are known to produce drug dependence.

# 3.6 Toxicology

The benzodiazepines are often characterized as having a wide therapeutic index[iv] with a low risk of serious adverse reactions and toxicity. This contrasts with the barbiturates, which are known to have a narrow therapeutic index. Previous chapters have defined the difference between the expected therapeutic properties as those classed as adverse or unwanted.

This chapter reviews the toxicology of this group of drugs, as well as reviewing the blood concentrations (and, where relevant, tissue concentrations) in cases where toxicity has been implicated to these drugs, and discusses factors that can affect the interpretation of such data.

Suitable review articles on the toxicology of benzodiazepines and related drugs are listed.[132–139]

## USE OF BENZODIAZEPINES BY DRUG USERS

The intravenous use of benzodiazepines is generally less common than oral use. However, intravenous use is widespread, with survey estimates showing that about half inject benzodiazepines.[140] In Britain, temazepam was the most common injected benzodiazepine.[141] Overall, the use of benzodiazepines by drug users in Britain may be more than one-third. Injection of temazepam gel-filled capsules has been associated with increased morbidity and mortality caused by the development of vascular lesions.[142–145] Flunitrazepam has been a commonly abused drug in Europe, Australia and in the southern USA.[146]

Clearly, the manner and dose of the drug are important factors in determining whether a toxic response will occur. In most cases, toxicity is associated with concomitant use of other CNS depressant drugs, particularly alcohol and the opioids.

## TOXIC REACTIONS TO BENZODIAZEPINES

The depression of the CNS is the single most important feature associated with minor tranquillizers, particularly the benzodiazepines and barbiturates.

### General symptoms

Sedation, which is usually an unwanted effect of these drugs, becomes a major feature of excessive use of the barbiturates and benzodiazepines. Gross ataxia (failure of muscular

---

[iv] Therapeutic index refers to the dose range between expected therapeutic properties and unwanted toxic reactions. A narrow therapeutic index for a drug implies a narrow margin of safety between a recommended therapeutic dose and toxicity, while a wide therapeutic index implies a wide margin between the two.

co-ordination) and speech impediments will occur with excessive sedation. Depression of breathing reflex accompanied by a respiratory acidosis is known to occur in cases of toxicity.

In anaesthetic doses, benzodiazepines decrease blood pressure and increase heart rate. This may be related to a decrease in peripheral resistance and/or reduction in cardiac output. In large doses, benzodiazepines are likely to decrease both cerebral blood flow and oxygen assimilation.

## Hospital admissions

Subjects presenting to hospital accident and emergency units following an overdose of benzodiazepines typically exhibit somnolence, diplopia (double vision), dysarthria (slurred speech), ataxia and impairment of a range of intellectual functions. The benzodiazepines have less effect on cardiovascular function than other drugs; however, low blood pressure (hypotension) and low heart rate (bradycardia) can occur. Effects on breathing are seen occasionally in cases presenting to hospital, although this is more likely to present in cases where death is imminent. Coma, particularly deep-cyclic coma (stages 3–4) occurs in 5–49% of cases.[133]

The use of supportive care to maintain adequate breathing and adequate blood pressure and heart rate are therefore important features of treatment.

In many cases, presentations to hospital are the result of mixed drug ingestions with other CNS depressant drugs, such as alcohol, narcotic analgesics, antipsychotic drugs and the tricyclic antidepressants. Since these other drugs are usually stronger depressants of the CNS, they are often primarily responsible for the toxic symptoms.

## Flumazenil antidote to poisoning

Flumazenil, the benzodiazepine antagonist, rapidly reverses the effects caused by benzodiazepines and is therefore the drug of choice in such cases. Doses titrated slowly to a total dose of 2–5 mg will reverse benzodiazepine-induced coma within 1–2 min.

Flumazenil has a short duration of action (~1 h), hence overdoses to benzodiazepines will normally involve additional top-up doses to protect against redevelopment of toxic reactions. This is most important in benzodiazepines with longer half-lives. Flumazenil is also effective in reversing toxicity of zopiclone and zolpidem.

## Death associated with benzodiazepines

Deaths associated with toxicity of benzodiazepines alone are comparatively rare considering the large number of prescriptions dispensed throughout the world.

Linking mortality statistics with national prescribing data showed that there were 5.9 deaths per million prescriptions for benzodiazepines alone or with alcohol only.[138] In comparison, the barbiturate-related death rate was 118 per million prescriptions.[139]

There have been, however, a number of deaths described in the literature. These are summarized in Table 3.12. These data show that most of the benzodiazepines in common use throughout the world are capable of causing death. These cases have been selected on the

Table 3.12  Reported cases of death due to benzodiazepines alone

| No. of cases | Gender, age | Benzodiazepine | Concentration (mg/L) | Cause and manner of death, and comments | Reference |
|---|---|---|---|---|---|
| 1 | 69 | Alprazolam | No concentration data | Suicide, no details provided | 158 |
| 1 | | Alprazolam | | | 159 |
| 1 | F42 | Alprazolam | b = 0.18 AM | Suicidal death due to alprazolam; died after several days | 166 |
| 1 | F61 | Alprazolam | b = 0.38, l = 2.2 | Suicidal death due to alprazolam, therapeutic trazodone (b = 0.6) | 170 |
| 1 | F32 | Alprazolam | b = 0.18, l = 0.8 | Suicidal death due to alprazolam | 170 |
| 1 | M30 | Alprazolam | b = 0.08, l = 0.39 | Toxic effects of alprazolam, plus low levels of hydromorphone | 170 |
| 4 | Unknown | Alprazolam | b = 0.12–0.39 | Four cases with no details | 172 |
| 1 | F44 | Alprazolam | b = 2.3, l = 9.2, v = 0.6 | Suicidal death in a woman with psychiatric problems | 178 |
| 1 | F60 | Bromazepam/diazepam | b = 5.0 and b = 0.5 | Death due to bromazepam toxicity with therapeutic diazepam | 169 |
| 1 | F? | Bromazepam | b = 5.0 | Death apparently due to an overdose of bromazepam, no details | 172 |
| 1 | M75 | Chlordiazepoxide (750 mg) | b = 29 | Suicide, congestive heart failure, mitral valve deficiency | 158 |
| 1 | ? | Chlordiazepoxide | b = 26, l = 10 | Death apparently due to chlordiazepoxide alone, no details | 172 |
| 1 | M35 | Clobazam/diazepam | b = 1.5 and b = 1.1 | Suicidal death due to benzodiazepines; pneumonia at autopsy | 132 |

**Table 3.12** (continued)

| No. of cases | Gender, age | Benzodiazepine | Concentration (mg/L) | Cause and manner of death, and comments | Reference |
|---|---|---|---|---|---|
| 3 | ? | Diazepam | Mean b = 4.8 | Death apparently due to diazepam alone; no details provided | 173 |
| 2 | 63, F66 | Diazepam (F66 = 1.6 g) | F66 b = 1.6 | Suicides, F66 had severe chronic lung disease | 160 |
| 2 | M20s, M40s | Diazepam | b = 5, 19 | No natural disease or injuries, full autopsy | 161 |
| 1 | 35 | Diazepam (280 mg) | No concentration measured | Died from hypoxic brain damage and pneumonia 7 days later | 137 |
| 1 | M25 | Diazepam | b = 3.7 | Suicidal death due to benzodiazepines plus natural disease | 168 |
| 1 | F65 | Diazepam/flunitrazepam/ temazepam | b = 2.6, b = 0.07 and b = 0.1 | | 132 |
| 2 | ~80 | Flunitrazepam | k = 0.5 | 28 mg flunitrazepam taken; no pathological abnormality | 162 |
| 4 | M23, M45, M58, M71 | Flunitrazepam | b = 0.47, 0.27, 0.77, 0.37 | | 163 |
| 44 | Not given | Flunitrazepam | b = 0.16–0.64 | No details given, no other drugs | 156 |
| 1 | F22 | Flunitrazepam/oxazepam | b = 0.3 and b = 0.8 | Suicidal death due to benzodiazepines | 132 |
| 1 | F56 | Flunitrazepam/temazepam | b = 0.2 and b = 0.3 | Death due to benzodiazepines, also traces of other drugs | 132 |
| 1 | — | Flunitrazepam/nitrazepam | b = 0.2 and b = 0.02 | Benzodiazepine toxicity with chronic bronchitis and emphysema | 132 |
| 1 | M47 | Flurazepam (~2.6 g) | b = 0.5 (1.9) | Death apparently due to flurazepam alone, decomposed body | 174 |

**Table 3.12** (continued)

| No. of cases | Gender, age | Benzodiazepine | Concentration (mg/L) | Cause and manner of death, and comments | Reference |
|---|---|---|---|---|---|
| 2 | 39, F67 | Flurazepam (F67 = 3.6 g) | No concentration data | Suicides, F67 died after 3 days of bowel necrosis | 158 |
| 1 | F52 | Flurazepam | b = 5.5 (0.73), l = 130 (3.2) | | 164 |
| 1 | | Flurazepam/nitrazepam | b = 1.4 and b = 0.94 | Suicidal death due to benzodiazepines and left ventricular hypertrophy | 132 |
| 1 | 6 | Lorazepam | b = 2.8 | Accidental overdose to lorazepam, no details | 172 |
| 1 | F69 | Nitrazepam | b = 1.1 | Suicidal death due to nitrazepam, also trace of temazepam | 132 |
| 1 | F83 | Nitrazepam | b = 0.56 | Suicidal death due to nitrazepam, also significant natural disease | 132 |
| 1 | M69 | Nitrazepam | b = 0.75 | Nitrazepam toxicity in a man with ischaemic heart disease | 132 |
| 1 | M25 | Nitrazepam/temazepam | b = 0.7 and b = 0.8 | Suicidal death plus significant natural disease, trace of dothiepin | 132 |
| 1 | F48 | Nitrazepam/temazepam | b = 1.3 and b = 2.0 | Suicidal death due to benzodiazepines | 132 |
| 1 | M75 | Nitrazepam | b = 1.2, l = 0.7 | Nitrazepam toxicity | 175 |
| 16 | No ages given | Nitrazepam | b = 0.5–2.8 | No details given, no other drugs | 156 |
| 1 | F? | Nitrazepam | u = 6 | Possible overdose, no blood toxicology | 177 |
| 1 | M85 | Oxazepam | b = 5.0 | Suicidal death due to oxazepam plus coronary atherosclerosis | 132 |
| 1 | M60 | Oxazepam | b = 2.4 AM | Oxazepam toxicity plus emphysema, bronchitis, heart disease | 132 |

**Table 3.12** (continued)

| No. of cases | Gender, age | Benzodiazepine | Concentration (mg/L) | Cause and manner of death, and comments | Reference |
|---|---|---|---|---|---|
| 1 | M76 | Oxazepam | b = 4.6 | Oxazepam toxicity plus coronary atherosclerosis | 132 |
| 1 | M34 | Oxazepam | b = 3.0 | Oxazepam toxicity plus ketoacidosis | 132 |
| 1 | M63 | Oxazepam/temazepam | b = 0.4 and b = 0.1 | Suicidal death due to benzodiazepines and pneumonia – delayed death | 132 |
| 2 | No data | Oxazepam | b = 4.4, 6.1 | No details given, no other drugs | 156 |
| 2 | M77, F77 | Temazepam | b = 7.0, 3.8; l = 107, 39 | Suicidal deaths from ingestion of temazepam alone | 165 |
| 1 | 39 | Temazepam | No concentration data | Suicide, no data provided | 159 |
| 3 | 58, 67, 58 | Triazolam | No concentration data | Suicides | 158, 159, 158 |
| 1 | F76 | Triazolam | b = 0.016 | Suicidal death due to triazolam plus early pneumonia and chronic bowel obstruction | 167 |
| 1 | F75 | Triazolam | b = 0.02 | Suicidal death due to triazolam (120 × 0.25 mg) and coronary artery disease | 167 |
| 4 | ?, M63, M71, M31 | Triazolam | b = 0.01, 0.04, 0.04, 0.04 | 2 suicides, details of case histories unavailable | 171 |
| 2 | F79, F45 | Triazolam | b = 0.11, no result | Both suicides, F79 had enlarged heart, F45 putrefied case | 176 |

AM: antemortem; b: blood; k: kidney; l: liver; u: urine; v: vitreous humour.

basis that benzodiazepines have been attributed as the principal cause of death and no other drug (other than one or more benzodiazepines) was found to be the predominant cause of death. In particular, cases involving alcohol have been excluded. The most frequent benzodiazepines reported as causing death were alprazolam, diazepam, triazolam, flunitrazepam, nitrazepam, flurazepam and oxazepam.

Unfortunately, in many of the cases the age, gender and circumstances including the pathology findings are not available, hence the accuracy of the conclusions reached, i.e. benzodiazepine toxicity, could often not be verified.

The ages of the cases ranged from young adults to the elderly, with most cases being in the >50 years age group. Since a number of deaths have occurred in persons who are elderly, it is likely that natural disease processes have played a role in the death. Indeed, in many of the cases for which details are available, significant natural disease was present at the time of death. This is not surprising; the toxicity of all drugs will be higher in persons with compromised cardiovascular, respiratory and metabolic functions. However, it is important to note that death has occurred with benzodiazepines alone in young persons with no significant natural disease (see Case Report 3.6, p. 165).

Estimates of the relative toxicity potential of benzodiazepines have been made based on the incidence of poisonings and their relative prescription rates. An evaluation of deaths attributed to benzodiazepines in Victoria over 5 years showed that flunitrazepam had a higher toxicity index (9.2 deaths per million prescriptions) than all other benzodiazepines. The next ranking benzodiazepine was nitrazepam at 1.7 deaths per million prescriptions.[132] Another study showed that temazepam was the most toxic and gave the highest sedation index.[134] In a British study, flurazepam and temazepam are apparently more toxic with rates of 9.8 and 7.1 deaths per million prescriptions, respectively.[131] These differences probably relate to differences in how deaths to drugs are attributed and the relative abuse of members of this class of drugs in the various jurisdictions.

With the benzodiazepines, and indeed other drugs subject to abuse, the manner of use is critical in terms of toxic potential. Intravenous use of drugs is clearly more toxic than oral use, primarily because of the more rapid onset of action and higher bioavailability. Some of the benzodiazepines have been subject to intravenous abuse, in particular temazepam, which has been available as a liquid in a soft gelatin capsule. See Case Report 3.6.

## TOXIC REACTIONS TO BARBITURATES

Barbiturates have had a well-documented history of toxicity. Their mechanism of action is significant, and severe depression of CNS occurs when used in an abuse setting or following an overdose. Table 3.15 summarizes the blood concentrations reported as causing death in absence of other significant factors.

## TOXIC REACTIONS TO ZOLPIDEM

Only mild symptoms are observed in acute single-drug poisonings with zolpidem in doses up to 0.6 g. Subjects mainly suffer from drowsiness and somnolence, although coma is possible

Table 3.13 Selected cases of death due to other newer sedatives

| No. of cases | Gender, age | Drug | Concentration (mg/L) | Cause and manner of death, and comments | Reference |
|---|---|---|---|---|---|
| 1 | M81 | Zopiclone | b = 3.5, l = 0.8 | Suicidal death due to zopiclone, also therapeutic quinine | 154 |
| 1 | F26 | Zopiclone/pentazocine | b = 1.2, l = 5.1 and b = 41, l = 12 | Suicidal death due to zopiclone and pentazocine | 157 |
| 1 | F29 | Zopiclone/ethanol | b = 1.2, l = 1.8/ BAC = 0.15% | Suicidal death due to zopiclone and ethanol | 155 |
| 4 | No details | Zopiclone | b = 0.6–1.8 | No details given, no other drugs | 148 |
| 1 | M39 (obese) | Zolpidem Hydrocodone Morphine | b = 1.4, hb = 2.9, l = 4.7, u = 2 hb = 0.16, u = 2.8 hb = 0.04 | Overdose to ~1g (max.) of zolipdem in 164-kg man with fatty hepatomegaly, moderate cardiomegaly and clinical hypertension | 152 |
| 1 | F49 | Zolpidem/ethanol | b = 0.52–0.80, hb = 0.75, u = 1.3/BAC = 0.22% | Ingestion of unknown amount of zolpidem and alcohol, no significant natural disease | 153 |
| 2 | F36 | Zolpidem/ risperidone | b = 4.5, l = 23, v = 1.6 b = 5.6 as 9-OH metabolite | Found dead in bed, history of paranoid disorder, depression with panic, and post-traumatic stress disorder | 148 |
|   | F58 | Zolpidem | b = 1.6, l = 12, v = 0.5 | Found dead in bed, history of hypertension and mental illness, and had cardiomegaly, hepatomegaly, mild coronary atherosclerosis |   |

BAC: blood alcohol concentration; b: peripheral blood; hb: heart blood; l: liver; u: urine; v: vitreous humour.

after ingestion of 0.6 g zolpidem. Other symptoms include agitation, dizziness, hypotonia, mydriasis, arterial hypotension, tachycardia and vomiting. The acute toxicity of zolpidem is markedly less pronounced than that of the short-acting benzodiazepines, triazolam and midazolam. No severe symptoms may occur in subjects with zolpidem single-drug poisonings at 40-fold therapeutic dose. Combined intoxications with other CNS active drugs or ethanol can induce coma in some patients, even if the amount of the additionally ingested drugs in itself would not have caused a comatose state. Flumazenil was an effective antidote in mono- and combined intoxications involving zolpidem.[135,147]

There are reports of acute zolpidem overdose, although these have involved either significant amounts of disease or other drugs.[148–153] Selected cases are summarized in Table 3.13. Liver concentrations of zolpidem range from approximately 5 to 33 mg/L of peripheral blood concentrations in cases of suspected overdose, and heart blood concentrations may be slightly elevated over peripheral blood.

## TOXIC REACTIONS TO ZOPICLONE

Zopiclone is relatively well tolerated. However, when misused CNS depression is the most common reported event. Some cases have had high plasma potassium concentrations (hyperkalaemia), high plasma glucose (hyperglycaemia) and a slightly elevated bilirubin. However, cardiovascular disturbances are uncommon.

Death has been reported following overdosage both alone and with alcohol. In the absence of other significant drugs, femoral blood concentrations of zopiclone of 3.5 mg/L can cause death.[154] Lower blood concentrations may be toxic, but insufficient details of the cases have been described. Cases involving alcohol have also been described.[154,155]

Zopiclone is found in highest concentrations in bile (10-fold higher than blood),[155] although liver concentrations are similar to peripheral blood concentrations.[155–157] Little postmortem redistribution is observed for zopiclone.[155]

## TISSUE DISTRIBUTION OF SEDATIVES

With few exceptions, the drugs listed in this section show relatively low lipid solubility. Consequently, concentrations in most organs including liver are similar or only slightly higher than blood. Certain tissues deserve particular mention.

While there are few data for many of the benzodiazepines, studies have shown that benzodiazepines, including alprazolam, clonazepam, chlordiazepoxide, diazepam, flunitrazepam, flurazepam and nitrazepam, are present in bile in concentrations ranging from ~1 to 26 times that of femoral blood. Bile is therefore a potentially useful specimen for detecting use of benzodiazepines beyond when blood levels are detectable. Of course, urine has traditionally been of value for this purpose, but it is not always available in postmortem cases. Benzodiazepines are found in vitreous humour. However, in contrast to many other drugs, blood concentrations are substantially less than for blood.[164,165,179,180]

Most of the major benzodiazepines have been detected in hair, including diazepam, nordazepam, alprazolam, flunitrazepam, lorazepam, oxazepam and temazepam. Concentrations

Table 3.14 Fatal concentrations of benzodiazepines and newer sedatives/hypnotics

| Drug | Minimum fatal concentration in blood (mg/L)[a] |
|---|---|
| **Benzodiazepines** | |
| Alprazolam | 0.1 |
| Bromazepam | 2.8 |
| Chlordiazepoxide | 26 |
| Clobazam | None reported |
| Clonazepam | None reported |
| Diazepam | 5 |
| Flunitrazepam[b] | 0.16 |
| Flurazapam | 1.8 |
| Lorazepam | 2.8 |
| Nitrazepam[b] | 0.5 |
| Nordazepam | See diazepam |
| Oxazepam | 4.4 |
| Temazepam | 3.8 |
| Triazolam | 0.04 |
| **Newer sedatives and hypnotics** | |
| Buspirone | None reported |
| Zolpidem | None reported |
| Zopiclone | 0.6 |

[a] No other significant drug or significant natural disease contributing to cause of death; [b] postmortem data for nitrazepam, clonazepam and flunitrazepam include sum total of parent and corresponding 7-amino metabolite.

are generally low, rarely being above 10 ng/mg hair.[181–184] Isolation conditions vary widely, with some favouring ball milling with extraction with methanol or buffer. Alkaline digestion with NaOH and dilute HCl acid have been described. However, strong base degrades the benzodiazepines markedly reducing recoveries,[184] although alprazolam is apparently stable to dilute NaOH.[183]

Benzodiazepine metabolites are also detected in hair. This applies particularly to diazepam and temazepam, in which nordazepam and oxazepam should be targeted, and to the 7-nitro-benzodiazepines, in which the respective 7-amino metabolites should also be targeted. Their presence in hair will be helpful in distinguishing consumption from external contamination.

Benzodiazepines have been detected in sweat,[185] and are found in saliva at relatively low concentrations. Consequently, sensitive assays are required to measure benzodiazepines in saliva.[186,187]

**Table 3.15** Fatal concentrations of barbiturates and other sedatives

| Drug | Minimum fatal concentration in blood (mg/L)[a] |
| --- | --- |
| **Benzodiazepines** | |
| Amylobarbital | 5 |
| Barbital | 100 |
| Butalbital | 5 |
| Butobarbital | 5 |
| Pentobarbital | 10 |
| Phenobarbital | 50 |
| Secobarbital | 5 |
| Vinbarbital | 10 |
| **Newer sedatives and hypnotics** | |
| Chloral hydrate | 40 |
| Chlormethiazole | 10 |
| Diphenhydramine | 2 |
| Doxylamine | 1.2 |
| Ethchlorvynol | 20 |
| Ethinamate | 100 |
| Glutethimide | 20 |
| Meprobamate | 50 |
| Mepyramine | None reported alone |
| Methaqualone | 10 |
| Methyprylon | 30 |
| Paraldehyde | 400 |

[a] No other drug or significant natural disease contributing to cause of death.

# Synopsis

## TOXICOLOGY

1 While benzodiazepines exhibit a wide therapeutic index, in abuse situations they can produce profound and life-threatening reactions. These include gross ataxia, coma, cardiovascular disturbances and depression of breathing.

2 The toxic effects of benzodiazepines, as well as those of zopiclone and zolpidem, can be reversed by the antagonist flumazenil.

3 Death can occur from benzodiazepines alone, with most reported cases involving alprazolam, diazepam, triazolam, flunitrazepam, nitrazepam, flurazepam and oxazepam.

4 Toxic reactions are more likely in the aged, those with compromised cardiovascular or respiratory function, and those mixing benzodiazepines with other CNS depressant drugs, particularly alcohol.

## Benzodiazepines

5. Buspirone and zolpidem appear relatively safe in overdose when not mixed with CNS depressant drugs.
6. Zopiclone has toxicity similar to benzodiazepines and has led to death from misuse.
7. Benzodiazepines are found in higher concentrations in bile than blood, but have much lower concentrations in vitreous humour and saliva.
8. Despite the instability of benzodiazepines and their lability to certain chemical reagents, they can be extracted from hair. Hair analysis provides a longer detection window than other tissues.

# 3.7 Case reports

## CASE REPORT 3.1 NEGATIVE DRUG RESULT

A young woman was taken to the police claiming to have been drugged at a nightclub the previous evening.

Blood and urine specimen were collected and were sent to the local forensic laboratory for testing for drugs of abuse, including benzodiazepines.

The result was weakly positive for benzodiazepines in urine, but negative for these drugs (and others) in blood.

The complainant asked for a re-analysis by another laboratory. This laboratory used much lower cut-off limits on hydrolysed urine and tested the blood for sedative drugs using targeted GC-MS. The report showed the presence of lorazepam at 0.01 ng/mL in blood. Lorazepam was also detected in urine.

These results now supported the allegation made by the woman and resulted in a continuing investigation. Lorazepam is not readily detectable by most initial screening techniques. Even GC or GC-MS analysis would not detect this potent benzodiazepine unless this drug was targeted using selected ion monitoring of a derivatized extract. Many of the potent benzodiazepines are poorly detected by conventional analytical techniques. This also includes zopiclone.

In other cases, the specific targeting of metabolites in urine or the use of hair may prove useful to identify drugs given to innocent victims.

## CASE REPORT 3.2 PARADOXICAL REACTION TO BENZODIAZEPINES

A 34-year-old man with no history of bipolar disorder, aggression or violent behaviour, and with a stable work environment, had developed some minor difficulties organizing his thoughts some 6 months after an episode of minor head trauma following an accident with a baseball bat.

He had been treated with a low dose of amitriptyline (25 mg) for depression for 1 month and subsequently with alprazolam. Following an episode of marital discord he had taken 10 mg of alprazolam and had slept for about 8 h. On awakening he had an argument with his wife and started throwing rocks at the windows of their truck. He then drove his vehicle at high speed. He was chased by police officers. The episode culminated with him driving directly at several police cars.

Some months later the subject presented with no clinical reasons for his behaviour.

After French *et al.*, 1989.[188]

## CASE REPORT 3.3 BEHAVIOURAL AGGRESSION

This middle-aged man had no previous history of violence or aggressive behaviour. He lived by himself and would occasionally have drinking binges with his mates at a local hotel. He had recurring episodes of depression for which his general medical practitioner had prescribed nortriptyline 150 mg nocte. He was also taking temazepam 20 mg nocte when required for sleep. He had complained of an inadequate response to nortriptyline and, on advice of a friend, had requested a prescription for clonazepam. The doctor obliged and prescribed 4 mg as required.

A few days later he was charged for assault following an alleged incident at a local hotel that he regularly frequented. The victim, his best friend, with whom he was drinking, was attacked without obvious provocation and had his skull fractured. The defendant claimed no memory of the incident and was quite shocked by the allegation.

At trial, the defence through the assistance of an expert pharmacologist claimed that the memory loss was quite possibly a result of the use of clonazepam, particularly in combination with excessive alcohol. Witnesses estimated his alcohol consumption at up to 20 glasses of beer over several hours. It was argued that he suffered the effects of disinhibitory behaviour and therefore had no conscious control over his actions and harboured no malice and should therefore not be found guilty.

The general practitioner, when questioned in court, gave no rational reason for the prescription of clonazepam and appeared not to have warned the defendant about possible dangers if used with alcohol, although he was aware of his drinking habits.

The 12-person jury acquitted the defendant.

## CASE REPORT 3.4 SEXUAL AND AGGRESSIVE FANTASIES

A 28-year-old mother sought psychiatric help due to chronic depression. The patient was started on the antidepressant imipramine at a stabilized dose of 100 mg.

Her depression responded poorly to this drug and the patient exhibited anxiety and tension symptoms. She was started on 5 mg diazepam to be taken as needed up to four times daily. During this phase, she developed a marked increase in sexual and aggressive fantasies, and anger at her husband, her therapist and her young daughter. She also exhibited uncharacteristic physical abusive tendencies toward her daughter and herself.

On cessation of diazepam, these dysphoric symptoms subsided and her impulse control improved greatly.

After Gardos, 1980.[105]

## CASE REPORT 3.5 SEXUAL DISINHIBITION DUE TO BENZODIAZEPINES

A 22-year-old woman presented with anxiety, panic attacks and depression. In childhood she had two traumatic experiences: her parents divorced and she was threatened with a knife by a stranger who also exposed himself. She developed a variety of symptoms, including night terrors and panic attacks, for which she saw a counsellor. As a teenager she became involved in serious drug (stimulants) and alcohol abuse and was sexually promiscuous. At age 17 she became a born-again Christian, stopped abusing drugs and alcohol, and became sexually abstinent. At age 22, she again developed panic attacks particularly when she was in close proximity to men.

She subsequently was treated with alprazolam 0.5 four times daily and nortriptyline 75 mg, which resulted in a marked decrease in anxiety, depression and frequency and intensity of her panic attacks. Since anxiety was still present, alprazolam was replaced by clonazepam. This stopped the occurrence of panic attacks and her anxiety disappeared. However, within a few days she began to feel sexually disinhibited and began to behave in a sexually promiscuous manner. She quit her job and started work as a striptease dancer. On questioning, the patient enthusiastically denied that there was anything wrong. Her general behaviour was otherwise normal.

Soon after, she stopped clonazepam and abruptly terminated her new vocation. In subsequent weeks, the patient was quite disturbed by her actions.

After Fava and Borofsky, 1991.[106]

## CASE REPORT 3.6 DEATH DUE TO FLUNITRAZEPAM

A 23-year-old Asian man, with a prior history of intravenous drug use and abuse of flunitrazepam, was found dead on the couch in the morning. He had been observed to leave a toilet in a social club the previous night staggering and slurring his speech.

Postmortem examination showed no significant natural disease, although lungs were congested with moderately severe oedema. Toxicology showed flunitrazepam and 7-amino-flunitrazepam in peripheral blood at 0.07 and 0.4 mg/L, respectively. No other drugs were detected following an extensive toxicological examination.

The cause of death was given as 'flunitrazepam toxicity'.

This case shows substantial elevations of flunitrazepam and metabolite blood concentrations from those expected following normal therapeutic doses, and shows that death due to flunitrazepam abuse is possible in the absence of other factors (after Drummer *et al.*, 1993[163]). The consumption of other CNS depressant drugs will further increase the toxicity and lead to lower fatal doses of flunitrazepam (and other benzodiazepines).

# References for Section 3

1. United Nations. *Recommended methods for the detection and assay of barbiturates and benzodizepines in biological specimens*. New York: United Nations; 1997.
2. Robertson MD, Drummer OH. Postmortem drug metabolism by bacteria. *J Forens Sci* 1995; 40(3): 382–6.
3. Colburn WA, Jack ML. Relationships between CSF drug concentrations, receptor binding characteristics, and pharmacokinetic and pharmacodynamic properties of selected 1,4-substituted benzodiazepines. *Clin Pharmacokinet* 1987; 13: 179–90.
4. Traber J, Glaser T. 5-HT1A receptor-related anxiolytics. *Trends Pharmacol Sci* 1987; 8: 432–7.
5. Greenblatt DJ. Benzodiazepine hypnotics: sorting the pharmacokinetic facts. *J Clin Psychiat* 1991; 52(9, suppl.): 4–10.
6. Breimer DD, Jochemsen R, von Albert HH. Pharmacokinetics of benzodiazepines. *Arzneimittelforschung* 1980; 30: 875–81.
7. Bandera R, Bollini P, Garattini S. Long-acting and short-acting benzodiazepines in the elderly: kinetic differences and clinical relevance. *Curr Med Res Opin* 1984; 4: 94–107.
8. Garzone PD, Kroboth PD. Pharmacokinetics of the newer benzodiazepines. *Clin Pharmacokinet* 1989; 16: 337–64.
9. Greenblatt DJ. Clinical pharmacokinetics of oxazepam and lorazepam. *Clin Pharmacokinet* 1981; 6: 89–105.
10. Huang W, Moody DE. Immunoassay detection of benzodiazepines and benzodiazepine metabolites in blood. *J Anal Toxicol* 1995; 19: 333–42.
11. Kerns EH, Rourick RA, Volk KJ, Lee MS. Buspirone metabolite structure profile using a standard liquid chromatographic-mass spectrometric protocol. *J Chromatogr B* 1997; 698: 133–45.
12. Hempel G, Blaschke G. Direct determination of zolpidem and its main metabolites in urine using capillary electrophoresis with laser-induced fluorescence detection. *J Chromatogr B Biomed Appl* 1996; 675(1): 131–7.
13. Houghton GW, Dennis MJ, Templeton R, Martin BK. A repeated dose pharmacokinetic study of a new hypnotic agent, zopiclone (Imovane). *J Clin Pharmacol Ther Toxicol* 1985; 23(2): 97–100.
14. Hempel G, Blaschke G. Enantioselective determination of zopiclone and its metabolites in urine by capillary electrophoresis. *J Chromatogr B Biomed Appl* 1996; 675(1): 139–46.
15. Martindale W. *Martindale's: the complete drug reference*, 32nd edn. Pharmaceutical Press; 1999.

16. Darwish M, Martin PT, Cevallos WH, Tse S, Wheeler S, Troy SM. Rapid disappearance of zaleplon from breast milk after oral administration to lactating women. *J Clin Pharmacol* 1999; 39(7): 670–4.
17. Fernandez C, Martin C, Gimenez F, Farinotti R. Clinical pharmacokinetics of zopiclone. *Clin Pharmacokinet* 1995; 29(6): 431–41.
18. Arnold J. Determinants of pharmacological effects and toxicity of benzodiazepine hypnotics: role of lipophilicity and plasma elimination kinetics. *J Clin Psychiat* 1991; 52(9, suppl.): 11–14.
19. Kales A. Quazepam: hypnotic efficacy and side effects. *Pharmacotherapy* 1990; 10(1): 1–12.
20. Jones DR, Hall SD, Jackson EK, Branch RA, Wilkinson GR. Brain uptake of benzodiazepines: effects of lipophilicity and plasma protein binding. *J Pharmacol Exp Therapeut* 1988; 245(3): 816–21.
21. Ruffalo RL, Thompson JF, Segal JL. Diazepam-cimetidine drug interaction: a clinically significant effect. *South Med J* 1981; 74(9): 1075–8.
22. Ozdemir V, Fourie J, Busto U, Naranjo CA. Pharmacokinetic changes in the elderly. Do they contribute to drug abuse and dependence? *Clin Pharmacokinet* 1996; 31(5): 372–85.
23. Von Moltke LL, Greenblatt DJ, Court MH, Duan SX, Harmatz JS, Shader RI. Inhibition of alprazolam and desipramine hydroxylation in vitro by paroxetine and fluvoxamine: comparison with other selective serotonin reuptake inhibitor antidepressants. *J Clin Psychopharmacol* 1995; 15(2): 125–31.
24. Bertz RJ, Granneman GR. Use of in vitro and in vivo data to estimate the likelihood of metabolic pharmacokinetic interactions. *Clin Pharmacokinet* 1997; 32: 210–58.
25. Jalava KM, Olkkola KT, Neuvonen PJ. Effect of itraconazole on the pharmacokinetics and pharmacodynamics of zopiclone. *Eur J Clin Pharmacol* 1996; 51: 331–4.
26. Wagner BKJ, O'Hara DA. Pharmacokinetics and pharmacodynamics of sedatives and analgesics in the treatment of agitated critically ill patients. *Clin Pharmacokinet* 1997; 33(6): 426–53.
27. Kanto J, Maenpaa M, Mantyla R, Sellman R, Valovirta E. Effect of age on the pharmacokinetics of diazepam given in conjunction with spinal anesthesia. *Anesthesiology* 1979; 51(2): 154–9.
28. Greenblatt DJ, Harmatz JS, Shader RI. Clinical pharmacokinetics of anxiolytics and hypnotics in the elderly. Therapeutic considerations (Part I). *Clin Pharmacokinet* 1991; 21(3): 165–77.
29. Closser MH. Benzodiazepines and the elderly. A review of potential problems. *J Subst Abuse Treat* 1991; 8(1–2): 35–41.
30. Fleishaker JC, Hulst LK, Ekernas S-A, Grahen A. Pharmacokinetics and pharmacodynamics of adinazolam and N-desmethyladinazolam after oral and intravenous dosing in healthy, young and elderly volunteers. *J Clin Psychopharmacol* 1992; 12(6): 403–14.
31. Greenblatt DG, Wright CE. Clinical pharmacokinetics of alprazolam. *Clin Pharmacokinet* 1993; 24(6): 453–71.

32. Swift CG, Swift MR, Ankier SI, Pidgen A, Robinson J. Single dose pharmacokinetics and pharmacodynamics of oral loprazolam in the elderly. *Br J Clin Pharmacol* 1985; 20(2): 119–28.
33. Ghabrial H, Desmond PV, Watson KJ, Gijsbers AJ, Harman PJ, Breen KJ, et al. The effects of age and chronic liver disease on the elimination of temazepam. *Eur J Clin Pharmacol* 1986; 30(1): 93–7.
34. Jochemsen R, Van Beusekom BR, Spoelstra P, Janssens AR, Breimer DD. Effect of age and liver cirrhosis on the pharmacokinetics of nitrazepam. *Br J Clin Pharmacol* 1983; 15(3): 295–302.
35. Kangas L, Iisalo E, Kanto J, Lehtinen V, Pynnonen S, Ruikka I, et al. Human pharmacokinetics of nitrazepam: effect of age and diseases. *Eur J Clin Pharmacol* 1979; 15(3): 163–70.
36. Seppälä M, Alihanka J, Himberg JJ, Kanto J, Rajala T, Sourander L. Midazolam and flunitrazepam: pharmacokinetics and effects on night time respiration and body movements in the elderly. *Int J Clin Pharmacol Ther Toxicol* 1993; 31(4): 170–6.
37. Salva P, Costa J. Clinical pharmacokinetics and pharmacodynamics of zolpidem. Therapeutic implications. *Clin Pharmacokinet* 1995; 29(3): 142–53.
38. Crome P, Wijayawardhana P, Ankier SI, Dowell P, Chevalier P, Guillet P. The pharmacokinetics of suriclone after single- and multiple-dose administration in healthy elderly volunteers. *Drugs Aging* 1993; 3(5): 436–40.
39. Coffey B, Shader RI, Greenblatt DJ. Pharmacokinetics of benzodiazepines and psychostimulants in children. *J Clin Psychopharmacol* 1983; 3(4): 217–25.
40. Jacqz-Aigrain E, Burtin P. Clinical pharmacokinetics of sedatives in neonates. *Clin Pharmacokinet* 1996; 31(6): 423–43.
41. Jacqz-Aigrain E, Wood C, Robeix I. Pharmacokinetics of midazolam in critically ill neonates. *Eur J Clin Pharmacol* 1990; 39: 191–2.
42. Dalhoff K, Poulsen HE, Garred P, Placchi M, Gammans RE, Mayol RF, et al. Buspirone pharmacokinetics in patients with cirrhosis. *Br J Clin Pharmacol* 1987; 24: 547–50.
43. Abernethy DR, Greenblatt DJ. Drug disposition in obese humans: an update. *Clin Pharmacokinet* 1986; 11(3): 199–213.
44. Fletcher CV, Acosta EP, Strykowski JM. Gender differences in human pharmacokinetics and pharmacodynamics. *J Adolesc Health* 1994; 15: 619–29.
45. Sieghart W. GABAA receptors: ligand-gated Cl ion channels modulated by multiple drug-binding sites. *Trends Pharmacol Sci* 1992; 13: 446–50.
46. Sigel E, Buhr A. The benzodiazepine binding site of $GABA_A$ receptors. *Trends Pharmacol Sci* 1997; 18: 425–9.
47. Haefely W, Martin JR, Schoch P. Novel anxiolytics that act as partial agonists at benzodiazepine receptors. *TIPS* 1990; 11: 452–6.
48. Doble A, Martin IL. Multiple benzodiazepine receptors: no reason for anxiety. *TIPS* 1992; 13: 76–81.
49. Charney DS, Breier A, Jatlow PI, Heninger GR. Behavioral, biochemical, and blood pressure responses to alprazolam in healthy subjects: interactions with yohimbine. *Psychopharmacology* 1986; 88: 133–40.

50. Langtry HD, Benfield P. Zolpidem. A review of its pharmacodynamic and pharmacokinetic properties and therapeutic potential. *Drugs* 1990; 40(2): 291–313.
51. Concas A, Serra M, Santoro G, Maciocco E, Cuccheddu T, Biggio G. The effect of cyclopyrrolones on GABAA receptor function is different from that of benzodiazepines. *Naunyn Schmiedebergs Arch Pharmacol* 1994; 350(3): 294–300.
52. Greenblatt DJ. Pharmacology of benzodiazepine hypnotics. *J Clin Psychiat* 1992; 53(6, suppl.): 7–13.
53. Rang HP, Dale MM, Ritter JM. *Pharmacology*, 3rd edn. London: Churchill Livingstone; 1995.
54. Napoliello MJ, Domantay AG. Buspirone: a worldwide update. *Br J Psychiat* 1991; 12(suppl.): 40–4.
55. Shader RI, Greenblatt DJ. Use of benzodiazepines in anxiety disorders. *New Engl J Med* 1993; 328: 1398.
56. Soderpalm B. Pharmacology of the benzodiazepines; with special emphasis on alprazolam. *Acta Psychiat Scand* 1987; 76(suppl. 335): 39–46.
57. Steinberg JR. Anxiety in elderly patients. *Drugs Aging* 1994; 5(5): 335–45.
58. Wadworth AN, McTavish D. Zopiclone. A review of its pharmacological properties and therapeutic efficacy as an hypnotic. *Drugs Aging* 1993; 3(5): 441–59. [Published erratum appears in *Drugs Aging* 1994 Jan; 4(1): 62.]
59. Barbee JG. Memory, benzodiazepines, and anxiety: integration of theoretical and clinical perspectives. *J Clin Psychiat* 1993; 54(10, suppl.): 86–101.
60. Greenblatt DJ, Miller LG, Shader RI. Neurochemical and pharmacokinetic correlates of the clinical action of benzodiazepine hypnotic drugs. *Am J Med* 1990; 88(suppl. 3A): 18S–24S.
61. Sheikh JI. Anxiety disorders and their treatment. *Clin Geriatr Med* 1992; 8(2): 411–26.
62. Norman TR, Ellen SR, Burrows GD. Benzodiazepines in anxiety disorders: managing therapeutics and dependence. *Med J Australia* 1997; 167: 490–5.
63. Salzman C, Solomon D, Miyawaki E, Glassman R, Rood L, Flowers E, et al. Parenteral lorazepam versus parenteral haloperidol for the control of psychotic disruptive behaviour. *J Clin Psychiat* 1991; 52: 177–80.
64. Hobbs WR, Rall TW, Verdoorn TA. Hypnotics and sedatives: ethanol. In: Goodman Gilman A, Goodman LS, eds. *The pharmacological basis for therapeutics*, 9th edn. New York: Macmillan; 1996.
65. Gear RW, Miaskowski C, Heller PH, Paul SM, Gordon NC, Levine JD. Benzodiazepine mediated antagonism of opioid analgesia. *Pain* 1997; 71(1): 25–9.
66. Daghero AM, Bradley EL, Jr., Kissin I. Midazolam antagonizes the analgesic effect of morphine in rats. *Anesth Analg* 1987; 66(10): 944–7.
67. Reddy S, Patt RB. The benzodiazepines as adjuvant analgesics. *J Pain Symptom Manage* 1994; 9(8): 510–14.
68. Goa KL, Heel RC. Zopiclone. A review of its pharmacodynamic and pharmacokinetic properties and therapeutic efficacy as an hypnotic. *Drugs* 1986; 32: 48–65.
69. Hajak G. A comparative assessment of the risks and benefits of zopiclone. *Drug Safety* 1999; 21: 457–69.

70. Baertz M, Malcolm D. Serotonin syndrome from fluvoxamine and buspirone. *Can J Psychiat* 1995; 40(7): 428–9.
71. Danjou P, Paty I, Fruncillo R, Worthington P, Unruh M, Cevallos W, et al. A comparison of the residual effects of zaleplon and zolpidem following administration 5 to 2 h before awakening. *Br J Clin Pharmacol* 1999; 48(3): 367–74.
72. Rush CR, Frey JM, Griffiths RR. Zaleplon and triazolam in humans: acute behavioral effects and abuse potential. *Psychopharmacology* 1999; 145(1): 39–51.
73. Yudofsky SC, Silver JM, Hales RE. Pharmacologic management of aggression in the elderly. *J Clin Psychiat* 1990; 51(10, suppl.): 22–8.
74. Woods JH, Katz JL, Winger G. Abuse liability of benzodiazepines. *J Pharmacol Exp Therapeut* 1987; 39(4): 254–413.
75. Van Der Bijl P, Roelofse JA. Disinhibitory reactions to benzodiazepines: a review. *J Oral Maxilofacial Surg* 1991; 49: 519–23.
76. Rush CR, Higgins ST, Bickel WK, Hughes JR. Abuse liability of alprazolam relative to other commonly used benzodiazepines: A review. *Neurosci Biobehav Rev* 1993; 17(3): 277–85.
77. Hindmarch I. A preliminary study of the effects of repeated doses of clobazam on aspects of performance, arousal and behaviour in a group of anxiety rated volunteers. *Eur J Clin Pharmacol* 1979; 16: 17–21.
78. Hindmarch I, Gudgeon AC. The effects of clobazam and lorazepam on aspects of psychomotor performance and car handling ability. *Br J Clin Pharmacol* 1980; 10: 145–50.
79. Ghoneim MM, Mewaldt SP, Hinrichs JV. Behavioral effects of oral versus intravenous administration of diazepam. *Pharmacol Biochem Behav* 1984; 21: 231–6.
80. Mewaldt SP, Ghoneim MM, Hinrichs JV. The behavioral actions of diazepam and oxazepam are similar. *Psychopharmacology* 1986; 88: 165–71.
81. Hinrichs JV, Ghoneim MM. Diazepam, behavior, and aging: increased sensitivity or lower baseline performance? *Psychopharmacology* 1987; 92: 100–5.
82. Guilleminault C. Benzodiazepines, breathing, and sleep. *Am J Med* 1990; 88(suppl. 3A): 25S.
83. Salzman C, Shader RI, Harmatz JS. Responses of the elderly to psychotropic drugs: predictable or idiosyncratic? *Psychopharmacol Bull* 1975; 36: 30–2.
84. Bond A, Lader M. Differential effects of oxazepam and lorazepam on aggressive responding. *Psychopharmacology* 1988; 95: 369–73.
85. Binder RL. Three case reports of behavioral disinhibition with clonazepam. *Gen Hosp Psychiat* 1987; 9: 151–3.
86. Wilkinson CJ. Effects of diazepam (Valium) and trait anxiety on human physical aggression and emotional state. *J Behav Med* 1985; 8(1): 101.
87. Cole JO, Kando JC. Adverse behavioral events reported in patients taking alprazolam and other benzodiazepines. *J Clin Psychiat* 1993; 54(10, suppl.): 49–61.
88. Ramaekers JG. Behavioural toxicity of medicinal drugs. *Pharmacoepidemiology* 1998; 18: 189–208.
89. Bond AJ, Curran HV, Bruce MS, O'Sullivan G, Shine P. Behavioral aggression in panic disorder after 8 weeks' treatment with alprazolam. *J Affect Disord* 1995; 35: 117–23.

# References

90. Rosenbaum JF, Woods SW, Groves JE, Klerman GL. Emergence of hostility during alprazolam treatment. *Am J Psychiat* 1984; 141: 792–3.
91. Gardner DL, Cowdry RW. Alprazolam-induced dyscontrol in borderline personality control. *Am J Psychiat* 1985; 142: 98–100.
92. Pyke RE, Kraus M. Alprazolam in the treatment of panic attack patients with and without major depression. *J Clin Psychiat* 1988; 49: 66–8.
93. Sheth RD, Goulden KJ, Ronen GM. Aggression in children treated with clobazam for epilepsy. *Clin Neuropharmacol* 1994; 17(4): 332–7.
94. Cozanitis DA, Lautsila A. Adverse behaviour in children following flunitrazepam administration for anaesthetic premedication. *Ann Francaises Anesthesie Reanim* 1987; 6(6): 537–8.
95. The sudden withdrawal of triazolam – reasons and consequences. *Drug Therapeut Bull* 1991; 29(23): 89.
96. Rothschild AJ, Bessette MP, Carter-Campbell J, Murray M. Triazolam and disinhibition. *Lancet* 1993; 341: 186.
97. Rush CR, Higgins SR, Hughes JR, K. BW. A comparison of the acute behavioural effects of triazolam and temazepam in normal volunteers. *Psychopharmacology* 1993; 112: 407–14.
98. Lobo BL, Miwa LJ. Midazolam disinhibition reaction. *Drug Intell Clin Pharm* 1988; 22: 725.
99. Fiset L, Milgrom P, Beirne OR, Roy-Byrne P. Disinhibition of behaviors with midazolam: report of a case. *J Oral Maxillofacial Surg* 1992; 50: 645–9.
100. Roelofse JA, Stegman DH, Hartshorne J, De V. Joubert JJ. Paradoxial reactions to rectal midazolam as premedication in children. *Internat J Oral Maxillofacial Surg* 1990; 19: 2–6.
101. Blitt CD, Petty WC. Reversal of lorazepam delirium by physostigmine. *Anesthes Analges* 1975; 54(5): 607.
102. Milam SB, Bennett CR. Physostigmine reversal of drug-induced paradoxical excitement. *Internat J Oral Maxillofacial Surg* 1987; 16: 190–3.
103. Bond AJ, Silveira JC. The combination of alprazolam and alcohol on behavioral aggression. *J Stud Alcohol* 1993(suppl. No. 11): 30–9.
104. Kubacki A. Sexual disinhibition on clonazepam. *Can J Psychiat* 1987; 32: 643–5.
105. Gardos G. Disinhibition of behaviour by antianxiety drugs. *Psychosomatics* 1980; 21(12): 1025.
106. Fava M, Borofsky GF. Sexual disinhibition during treatment with a benzodiazepine: A case report. *Internat J Psychiat Med* 1991; 21(1): 99–104.
107. Mattila MJ, Vanakoski J, Kalska H, Seppälä T. Effects of alcohol, zolpidem, and some other sedatives and hypnotics on human performance and memory. *Pharmacol Biochem Behav* 1998; 59(4): 917–23.
108. Sanger DJ, Benavides J, Perrault G, Morel E, Cohen C, Joly D, *et al*. Recent developments in the behavioural pharmacology of benzodiazepine (w) receptors: evidence for the functional significance of receptor subtypes. *Neurosci Biobehav Rev* 1994; 18(3): 355–72.

109. Zopiclone (Zimovane) and neuro-psychiatric reactions. Committee on Safety of Medicines. *Current Problems*; 1990.
110. O'Hanlon JF, Volkerts ER. Hypnotics and actual driving performance. *Acta Psychiatr Scand* 1986; 332(suppl.): 95–104.
111. Skegg DCG, Ricards SM, Doll R. Minor tranquillisers and road accidents. *Br Med J* 1979; 1: 917–19.
112. Ray WA, Fought RL, Decker MD. Psychoactive drugs and the risk of injurious motor vehicle crashes in elderly drivers. *Am J Epidemiol* 1992; 136(7): 873–83.
113. Barbone F, McMahon AD, Davey PG, Morris AD, Reid IC, McDevitt DG, et al. Association of road-traffic accidents with benzodiazepine use. *Lancet* 1998; 352: 1331–6.
114. Neutel CI. Risk of traffic accident injury after a prescription for a benzodiazepine. *Ann Epidemiol* 1995; 5(3): 239–44.
115. Hemmelgarn B, Suissa S, Huang A, Boivin JF, Pinard G. Benzodiazepine use and the risk of motor vehicle crash in the elderly. *JAMA* 1997; 278(1): 27–31.
116. Leveille SG, Buchner DM, Koepsell TD, McCloskey LW, Wolf ME, Wagner EH. Psychoactive medications and injurious motor vehicle collisions involving older drivers. *Epidemiology* 1994; 5(6): 591–8.
117. Jick H, Hunter JR, Dinan BJ, Masen S, Stergachis A. Sedating drugs and automobile accidents leading to hospitalization. *Am J Public Health* 1981; 71: 1399–400.
118. Mørland J. Driving under the influence of non-alcohol drugs. *Forens Sci Rev* 2000; 12: 79–105.
119. Christophersen AS, Morland J. Drugged driving, a review based on the experience in Norway. *Drug Alcohol Depend* 1997; 47(2): 125–35.
120. Christophersen AS, Ceder G, Kristinsson J, Lillsunde P, Steentoft A. Drugged driving in the nordic countries – a comparative study between five countries. *Forens Sci Internat* 1999; 106: 173–90.
121. Ferrara SD. Alcohol, drugs and traffic safety. *Br J Addict* 1987; 82(8): 871–83.
122. Parliament of Victoria. Inquiry into the effects of drugs (other than alcohol) on road safety in Victoria: final report. Melbourne: Parliament of Victoria; 1996.
123. Miczek KA, O'Donnell JM. Alcohol and chlordiazepoxide increase suppressed aggression in mice. *Psychopharmacology* 1980; 69: 39–44.
124. Stitzer ML, Griffiths RR, McLellan AT, Grabowski J, Hawthorne JW. Diazepam use among methadone maintenance patients: patterns and dosages. *Drug Alcohol Depend* 1981; 8: 189–99.
125. Barnas C, Rossman M, Roessler H, Reimer Y, Fleishacker WW. Benzodiazepines and other psychoactive drugs abused by patients in a methadone maintenance program: familiarity and preference. *J Clin Psychopharmacol* 1992; 12: 397–402.
126. Navaratnam V, Foong K. Adjunctive drug use among opiate addicts. *Curr Med Res Opin* 1990; 11: 611–19.
127. San L, Tato J, Torrens M, Castillo C, Farre M, Cami J. Flunitrazepam consumption among heroin addicts admitted for inpatient detoxification. *Drug Alcohol Depend* 1993; 32: 281–6.

128. Griffiths RR, Wolf B. Relative abuse liability of different benzodiazepines in drug abusers. *J Clin Psychopharmacol* 1990; 10(4): 237–43.
129. Farre M, Teran M-T, Cami J. A comparison of the acute behavioral effects of flunitrazepam and triazolam in healthy volunteers. *Psychopharmacology* 1996; 125: 1–12.
130. Woods JH, Winger G. Abuse liability of flunitrazepam. *J Clin Psychopharmacol* 1997; 17(3 suppl. 2): 1S–57S.
131. MacKinnon GL, Parker WA. Benzodiazepine withdrawal syndrome: a literature review and evaluation. *Am J Drug Alcohol Abuse* 1982; 9(1): 19–33.
132. Drummer OH, Ranson DL. Sudden death and benzodiazepines. *Am J Forens Med Pathol* 1996; 17(4): 336–42.
133. Gaudreault P, Guay J, Thivierge RL, Verdy I. Benzodiazepine poisoning. *Drug Safety* 1991; 6(4): 247–65.
134. Buckley NA, Dawson AH, Whyte IM, O'Connell DL. Relative toxicity of benzodiazepines in overdose. *Br Med J* 1995; 310(6974): 219–21.
135. Garnier R, Guerault E, Muzard D, Azoyan P, Chaumet-Riffaud A-E, Efthymiou M-L. Acute zolpidem poisoning – analysis of 344 cases. *Clin Toxicol* 1994; 32(4): 391–404.
136. Ellenhorn MJ. *Medical toxicology*. Baltimore: Williams Wilkins; 1996.
137. Höjer J, Baehrendtz S, Gustafsson L. Benzodiazepine poisoning: experience of 702 admissions to an intensive care unit during a 14-year period. *J Intern Med* 1989; 226: 117–22.
138. Serfaty M, Masterton G. Fatal poisonings attributed to benzodiazepines in Britain during the 1980s. *Br J Psychiat* 1993; 163: 386–93.
139. Johns MW. Self-poisoning with barbiturates in England and Wales during 1959–74. *Br Med J* 1977; i: 1128–30.
140. Darke SG, Ross JE, Hall WD. Benzodiazepine use among injecting heroin users. *Med J Australia* 1995; 162: 645–7.
141. Strang J, Griffiths P, Abbey J, Gossop M. Survey of injected benzodiazepines among drug users in Britain. *Br Med J* 1994; 308: 1082.
142. Rubin SM, Morrison CL. Temazepam misuse in a group of injecting drug users. *Br J Addict* 1992; 87: 1387–92.
143. Bhabra MS, Meshikhes AN, Thomson GJ, Craig P, Parrott NR. Intraarterial temazepam: an important cause of limb ischaemia in intravenous drug abusers. *Eur J Vasc Surg* 1994; 8(2): 240–2.
144. Russell ID, Kane GG, Royle CA, Jackson DS. Aggressive management of intra-arterial temazepam injection. *J R Army Med Corps* 1994; 140(2): 93–4.
145. Carnwath T. Drug injectors in Glasgow: a community at risk? A report from a multidisciplinary group (the Possilpark Group). Temazepam tablets as drugs of misuse [letter; comment]. *Health Bull* 1993; 51(6): 418–29.
146. ABCI. Australian Illicit Drug Report 1998-99. Canberra: Australian Bureau of Criminal Intelligence; March 2000.
147. Wyss PA, Radovanovic D, Meier-Abt PJ. Acute overdose of zolpidem (Stilnox). *Schweiz Med Wochenschr* 1996; 126(18): 750–6.
148. Gock SB, Wong SHY, Nuwayhid N, Venuti SE, Kelley PD, Teggatz JR, *et al*. Acute zolpidem overdose – report of two cases. *J Anal Toxicol* 1999; 23: 559–62.

149. Tracqui A, Kintz P, Mangin P. A fatality involving two unusual compounds – zolpidem and acepromazine. *Am J For Med Pathol* 1994; 14: 309–12.
150. Winek C, Whaba W, Janssen J, Rozin L. Acute overdose of zolpidem. *J Anal Toxicol* 1996; 78: 165–8.
151. Debailleul G, Abi Khalil F, Lhereux P. HPLC quantification of zolpidem and prothipendyl in a voluntary intoxication. *J Anal Toxicol* 1991; 15: 35–7.
152. Meeker JE, Som CW, Macapagal EC, Benson PA. Zolpidem tissue concentrations in a multiple drug related death involving Ambien®. *J Anal Toxicol* 1995; 19: 531–4.
153. Keller T, Schneider A, Tutsch-Bauer E. GC/MS determination of zolpidem in postmortem specimens in a voluntary intoxication. *Forens Sci Int* 1999; 106: 103–8.
154. Boniface PJ, Russell SGG. Two fatal cases of fatal zopilcone overdose. *J Anal Toxicol* 1996; 20: 131–3.
155. Pounder DJ, Davies JI. Zopiclone poisoning: tissue distribution and potential for postmortem diffusion. *Forens Sci Internat* 1994; 65: 177–83.
156. Druid H, Holmgren P. A compilation of fatal and control concentrations of drugs in postmortem femoral blood. *J Forens Sci* 1997; 42(1): 79–87.
157. Van Bocxlaer J, Meyer E, Clauwaert K, Lambert W, Piette M, De Leenheer A. Analysis of zopiclone (Imovane) in postmortem specimens by GC-MS and HPLC with diode-array detection. *J Anal Toxicol* 1996; 20: 52–4.
158. Litovitz TL, Schmitz BF, Holm KC. 1988 Annual Report of the American Association of Poison Control Centers National Data Collection System. *Am J Emerg Med* 1989; 7: 495–545.
159. Litovitz TL, Schmitz BF, Holm KC. 1986 Annual Report of the American Association of Poison Control Centers National Data Collection System. *Am J Emerg Med* 1987; 5: 405–45.
160. Litovitz TL, Schmitz BF, Matyunas N, Holm KC. 1987 Annual Report of the American Association of Poison Control Centers National Data Collection System. *Am J Emerg Med* 1988; 6: 479–515.
161. Finkle BS, McCloskey KL, Goodman LS. Diazepam and drug associated death. *J Am Med Assoc* 1979; 242: 429–34.
162. Heyndrickx B. Fatal intoxication due to flunitrazepam. *J Anal Toxicol* 1987; 11: 278.
163. Drummer OH, Syrjanen ML, Cordner SM. Deaths involving the benzodiazepine flunitrazepam. *Am J Forensic Med Pathol* 1993; 14(3): 238–43.
164. McIntyre IM, Syrjanen ML, Lawrence KL, Dow CA, Drummer OH. A fatality due to flurazepam. *J Forens Sci* 1994; 39(6): 1571–4.
165. Martin CD, Chan SC. Distribution of temazepam in body fluids and tissues in lethal overdose. *J Anal Toxicol* 1986; 10: 77–8.
166. Edinboro LE, Backer RC. Preliminary report on the application of a high performance liquid chromatographic method for alprazolam in postmortem blood specimens. *J Anal Toxicol* 1985; 9: 207–8.
167. Sunter JP, Bal TS, Cowan WK. Three cases of fatal triazolam poisoning. *Br Med J* 1988; 297: 719.

168. Goenechea S, Brzezinka H, Holtz J. A fatal case involving diazepam. *TIAFT Bull* 1988; 20(1).
169. Brehmer C, Iten PX. A fatal bromazepam poisoning. *TIAFT Bull* 1992; 22(4).
170. Fitzgerald RL. Alprazolam: medical examiner case reports and review of human exposure. *TIAFT Bull* 1994; 24(2).
171. Joynt BP. Triazolam blood concentrations in forensic cases in Canada. *J Anal Toxicol* 1993; 17: 171.
172. Baselt RC, Cravey RH. *Disposition of toxic drugs and chemicals in man*, 3rd edn. Foster City, CA: Year Book Medical Publishers; 1990.
173. Dinovo EC, Gottschalk LA, Mc Guire FL, Birch H, Heiser JF. Analysis of results of toxicological examinations performed by coroners' or medical examiners' laboratories in 2000 drug-involved deaths in nine major U.S. Cities. *Clin Chem* 1976; 22: 847–50.
174. Aderjan R, Mattern R. Eine toedlich verlaufene monointoxikation mit Flurazepam (Dalmadorm). *Arch Toxicol* 1979; 43: 69–75.
175. Guisti GV, Chiarotti M. Lethal nitrazepam intoxications. *Zeitschr Rechtsmed* 1979; 84: 75–8.
176. Steentoft A, Worm K. Cases of fatal triazolam poisoning. *J Forens Sci Soc* 1993; 33: 45–8.
177. Oliver JS, Smith H. Determination of nitrazepam in poisoning cases. *Forens Sci Internat* 1974; 4: 183–6.
178. Jenkins AJ, Levine B, Locke JL, Smialek JE. A fatality due to alprazolam intoxication. *J Anal Toxicol* 1997; 21: 218–20.
179. Agarwal A, Lemos N. Significance of bile analysis in drug-induced deaths. *J Anal Toxicol* 1996; 20: 61–2.
180. Kintz P, Boukhabza A, Tracqui A, Mangin P, Lugnier A, Chaumont A. Tissue disposition after bromazepam, secobarbital and amobarbital poisoning. *TIAFT Bull* 1991; 21(2).
181. Cirimele V, Kintz P, Staub C, Mangin P. Testing human hair for flunitrazepam and 7-amino-flunitrazepam by GC/MS- NCI. *Forens Sci Internat* 1997; 84: 189–200.
182. Yegles M, Mersch F, Wennig R. Detection of benzodiazepines and other psychotropic drugs in human hair by GC/MS. *Forens Sci Internat* 1997; 84: 211–18.
183. Höld KM, Crouch DJ, Wilkins DG, Rollins DE, Maes RA. Detection of alprazolam in hair by negative ion chemical ionization mass spectrometry. *Forens Sci Internat* 1997; 84: 201–9.
184. Couper FJ, McIntyre IM, Drummer OH. Extraction of psychotropic drugs from human scalp hair. *J Forens Sci* 1995; 40(1): 83–6.
185. Kintz P, Tracqui A, Mangin P, Edel Y. Sweat testing in opioid users with a sweat patch. *J Anal Toxicol* 1996; 20: 393–7.
186. Sharp ME, Wallace SM, Hindmarsh KW, Peel HW. Monitoring saliva concentrations of methaqualone, codeine, secobarbital, diphenhydramine and diazepam after single doses. *J Anal Toxicol* 1983; 7: 11–14.
187. United Nations. *Guidelines for testing drugs under international control in hair, sweat and saliva*. United Nations, 1998 ST/NAR/30.
188. French AP. Dangerously aggressive behavior as a side effect of alprazolam. *Am J Psychiat* 1989; 146(2): 276.

# 4 Cannabis

| | |
|---|---|
| **Foreword** | 178 |
| 4.1 Source and structures of cannabinoids | 179 |
| 4.2 Pharmacokinetics and duration of action | 183 |
| 4.3 Mechanisms of action | 197 |
| 4.4 Pharmacological actions and therapeutics | 198 |
| 4.5 Tolerance and dependence | 203 |
| 4.6 Toxicology | 205 |
| 4.7 Case reports | 209 |
| **References for Section 4** | 212 |

# Foreword

Cannabis, or marijuana, is one of the most frequently used illicit drugs in the Western world. Surveys in the USA show 31% of respondees admit to using marijuana during their college year and 19% admit to using within the month.[1] Estimates show that 39% of Australians have used this drug and almost 20% have used it in the last 12 months.[2,3] A high level use of cannabis and other illicit drugs was found in British medical students.[4] There also is a strong relationship between frequent cannabis use by juveniles and participation in crime. The United Nations estimate 1100 million tonnes were produced in 1995 with a further 3000 tonnes for herbal use. Worldwide annual use has been estimated at 141 million people, or 2.45% of the world population.[5]

This substance is therefore a widely used illicit drug and has attracted a vast amount of attention from scientists, enforcement agencies, health professionals and many other groups. Since behavioural changes are only transient and may not be permanent in occasional users, this has produced enormous differences of opinion among professionals and politicians over the dangers of marijuana consumption and the value of drug testing. On the other hand, chronic frequent use is associated with increased adverse health outcomes, including lung disease, cancers, and mental disease such as psychoses and schizophrenia.

Recent studies show humans have endogenous cannabinoid receptors and that tetrahydrocannabinol (THC) mimics the action of endogenous endocannabinoids. While the physiological role of these substances and the receptors they act on are unclear, there is strong evidence to suggest that cannabinoids are at least involved in pain control. Cannabis is therefore likely to have a more significant role when used in combination with drugs that affect analgesia, notably opioids and the benzodiazepines.

This section provides a review of the pharmacology, pharmacokinetics and toxicology of cannabis in a forensic context.

# 4.1 Source and structures of cannabinoids

*Cannabis sativa* is the plant that produces the material referred to as marijuana. This is the main source of marijuana, although many different varieties of this plant are now known, which grow under various conditions. The cannabis plant produces a whole family of related substances called cannabinoids, of which tetrahydrocannabinol (THC) is the most important.

## HISTORICAL ASPECTS AND SYNONYMS

The first recorded mention of cannabis dates back to 2737 BC from the Chinese emperor Shen-Nung who, in his writings, mentioned its properties against malaria and rheumatism. The word hemp apparently derives from ancient Chinese. The use of the stalk for the manufacture of clothing was known for well over 2000 years. Cannabis was known in the Indian subcontinent and the Arabian Peninsula well before the birth of Christ as an herbal remedy. The remains of cannabis seeds in an archaeological dig in Germany have been dated back to 500 BC. Its properties as a narcotic drug producing tranquillity were known. Much later cannabis was used as an aphrodisiac to treat impotence, as a carminative (for flatulence), and as a remedy to treat upset stomachs and headaches. Cannabis extracts were also used to clear ear canals and in combination with opium to produce sleep.[6]

Early names for cannabis include Ma-yo (Chinese), Qunuba, Qunabu, Kannapu (Assyrian), and bhang (Indian). 'Soma' was a drink made from cannabis in the Indian subcontinent used in religious ceremonies to liberate sins and to aid in meditation and concentration. The word marijuana (or marihuana) may stem from the Indian name 'Malihua' or the Portuguese 'Maranguano', although the Greek 'kannabis' is another derivation. Hashish (the dried oily resin) may derive from Arabic and literally means weed. In southern Africa, it is called 'dagga'.

Sinsemilla is a seedless more potent form produced from unfertilized flowering tops of female cannabis plants, often found in the USA. Other forms of cannabis include Thai sticks, hashish (resin) and the oil (hash oil). Modern names used to describe cannabis include 'weed', 'grass', 'dope' and 'pot'.

## CANNABIS SPECIES

This perennial self-seeding plant originates from central Asia and is now grown in every populated continent. There are various sub-species of *Cannabis sativa*, including Indica, Americana, Mexicana and Ruderalis. Modern hybridization methods have produced numerous cultivars and strains, including 'skunk weed' which has a $\Delta^9$-THC content of over 20% (dried). However, most forms of cannabis have THC yields of 2–8%. Sinsemilla cannabis with the flowering heads has a typical THC content of 7–14%.

# Cannabis

The cannabis plant is dioecious, i.e. male and female flowers are borne on separate plants. The female plant is more robust with larger flowers and, importantly, contains a higher content of THC. The plant has a characteristic growth habit with serrated leaves (5–11 serrations) and unusual flower heads and can reach 2–5 m tall. The plants prefer a warm humid climate, although they will grow in most climates. However, indoor and glasshouse cultivation are required for the cooler climates.

All parts of the female plant contain THC, including flowers, leaves, seeds and stalks. Oil is produced from the seeds and flower heads, and even biscuits (cookies) have been made from the plant.

The hemp variety of cannabis is used to produce long fibres for rope, paper and textile manufacturers, and contains a much lower THC content, typically less than 0.5%.

## ACTIVE CONSTITUENTS OF *CANNABIS SATIVA*

The main active constituent of the various parts of the cannabis plant is $\Delta^9$-tetrahydrocannabinol (THC). This exists as the $(-)$-*trans* isomer. There are, however, other constituents in significant amounts, including cannabidiol (CBD) and cannabinol (CBN), which vary depending on growing conditions and strains.[7]

Over 400 substances have been isolated from the cannabis plant, of which more than 60 are cannabinoids, or chemical compounds containing 21 carbon atoms related to THC. The overall effects of this plant on humans are the result of the sum total of all of their activities. The structures of THC, CBD and CBN and some other cannabinoids are shown in Fig. 4.1. It is important to note that some references refer to $\Delta^9$-THC and some to $\Delta^1$-THC. These refer to the same substance. The numbering system of the ring system has led to some confusion in the literature. The term $\Delta^9$-THC is regarded as correct.

The only cannabinoids that show significant activity are $\Delta^9$-THC, $\Delta^8$-THC, the propyl analogue of THC, called $\Delta^9$-tetrahydrocannabivarol, and CBN (see Fig. 4.1). However $\Delta^8$-THC

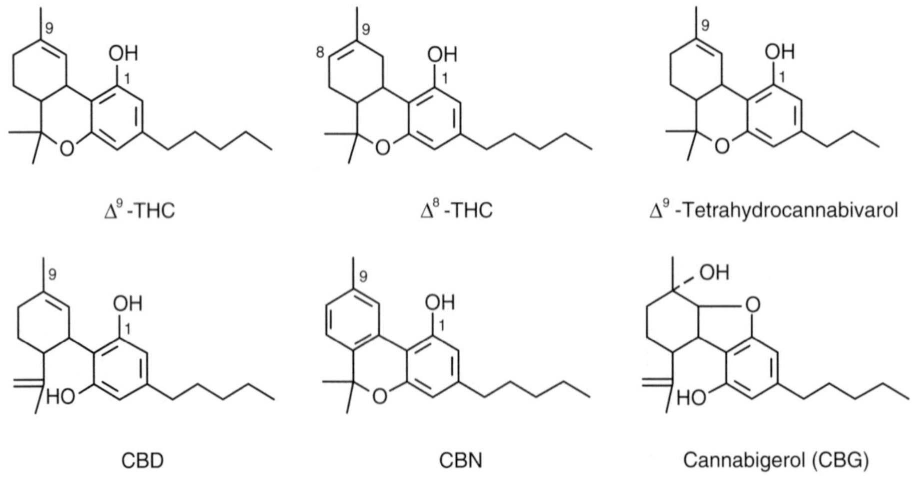

**Fig. 4.1** Structures of various cannabinoids

and Δ⁹-tetrahydrocannabivarol are minor constituents of cannabis and are not expected to contribute to the effects of cannabis. CBN is a degradative product of cannabis and is not found in fresh cannabis. Its activity is only a fraction of that of THC. When cannabis is smoked, the natural 2- and 4-carboxylated analogues of THC are converted by pyrolysis to THC.

## CANNABIS PRODUCTS

Cannabis plant products include the dried resin called hashish, which contains 6–10% THC, and the chopped flowering top of the plant rolled into cigarettes called marijuana (1–6%). Hash oil, an oily extract from the flowering tops, contains 15–60% THC. The typical marijuana cigarette contains 5–20 mg THC.

Sinsemilla is a crude drug extract from the flowering tops of female cannabis plants that have not been pollinated.[8]

Hemp is the stalk of the plant and is used in production of paper, ropes and twine and in textiles. Low-THC-containing seeds and oil are used in cosmetics and numerous types of health foods and shampoos.

## OTHER SUBSTANCES WITH THC-LIKE ACTIVITY

Four types of synthetic derivatives of THC have also been developed. These are based on the dibenzopyran THC nucleus, the bi- and tri-cyclic analogues of THC that lack the pyran ring, aminoalkylindoles (pravodoline derivatives) and the eicosanoid group. Nabilone (a benzopyran derivative of THC) is available clinically as a synthetic cannabinoid.

The latter is the group related to arachidonic acid derivatives, and includes anandamide and 2-arachidonyl glycerol (Fig. 4.2).[9]

More recently, research substances have become available that show selectivity for the $CB_1$ and $CB_2$ receptor subtypes. In addition, antagonists of the action of THC have been discovered.[9]

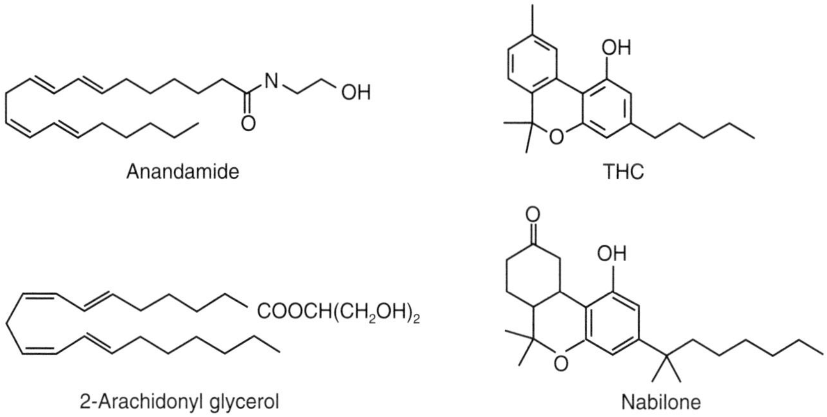

**Fig. 4.2** Structures of cannabinoid-like substances

# Cannabis

## Synopsis

### SOURCES AND STRUCTURES OF CANNABINOIDS

1. Cannabis was known for centuries before the birth of Christ to treat malaria, rheumatism, flatulence, headaches and stomach aches, for use as an aphrodisiac and to induce a state of pleasantness or bliss.
2. Cannabis derives from the perennial *Cannabis sativa* and its sub-species; hundreds of cultivars have been produced to increase yield, growth and other characteristics.
3. The dioecious plant grows in warm, humid to temperate climates reaching heights of 2–5 m, and has serrated leaves and characteristic flower heads. The plant can be cultivated indoors under controlled climatic conditions.
4. The female plant is most vigorous and produces the highest yield of the main active constituent, $\Delta^9$-tetrahydrocannabinol (THC).
5. All parts of the plant are active, particularly the flower heads and seeds; yields of THC typically range from 1% to 6%.
6. The only cannabinoids that show significant activity in the plant are $\Delta^9$-THC, $\Delta^8$-THC and $\Delta^9$-tetrahydrocannabivarol.
7. Cannabis products include hashish (dried resin), hash oil (from flowering tops), sinsemella (unpollinated flowers), hemp (stalk), marijuana (plant material), and hash cookies (seeds).
8. Modern names for cannabis include 'weed', 'grass', 'dope', 'dagga' and 'pot'.
9. Low-THC-yielding varieties are used to produce fibres for ropes, twines and textiles.

# 4.2 Pharmacokinetics and duration of action

This chapter details some of the more important aspects of the pharmacokinetics of $\Delta^9$-tetrahydrocannabinol (THC), the principal active component of cannabis, including the absorption, bioavailability, half-life and metabolic fate.

Readers are directed to a number of review articles and other relevant papers listed in the monograph for THC.[10–13]

## ABSORPTION AND BIOAVAILABILITY

Cannabis is consumed by inhalation by either smoking or using a bong or water pipe, or by ingestion of baked cannabis products. THC and other cannabinoids are absorbed by all of these routes. Eating fresh cannabis leaf will not allow significant absorption of THC, since THC is activated by a heating process by a decarboxylation reaction.

### Oral consumption

The ingestion of cakes or other sweet products, using the seed or the oil of the cannabis plant, is popular in some countries. Ingestion of THC is inefficient. Estimates of the bioavailability after oral absorption are 6%. The peak concentration of THC occurs at 1–5 h after consumption, although 60–90 min is more typical. The peak concentration ranges from 4 to 11 ng/mL THC after a 20 mg cookie.[14]

### Smoking

Smoking cannabis is most popular and produces a much quicker absorption with maximum plasma concentrations occurring within a few minutes of smoking. The amount absorbed is also much higher than with ingestion; studies show a bioavailability of 14–50%.[6,14,15] Clearly the amount absorbed will depend on the technique used to smoke the cigarette and how much is inhaled.

### $\Delta^9$-THC

The smoking of a cigarette containing 1.75% THC (16 mg) gives peak plasma concentrations of ~80 ng/mL, with a range of 50–130 ng/mL, within 15 min of smoking.[16] Correspondingly, higher concentrations are achieved with cigarettes containing a higher THC content. Peak THC concentrations of 200 ng/mL can be achieved with high-THC-content cigarettes.[17]

Once absorption has taken place, THC is rapidly distributed to tissues, concentrations being highest in adipose (fat) tissue due to its low water solubility and high affinity for fatty tissues. This distribution phase results in a rapid decline in blood plasma THC concentrations.

# Cannabis

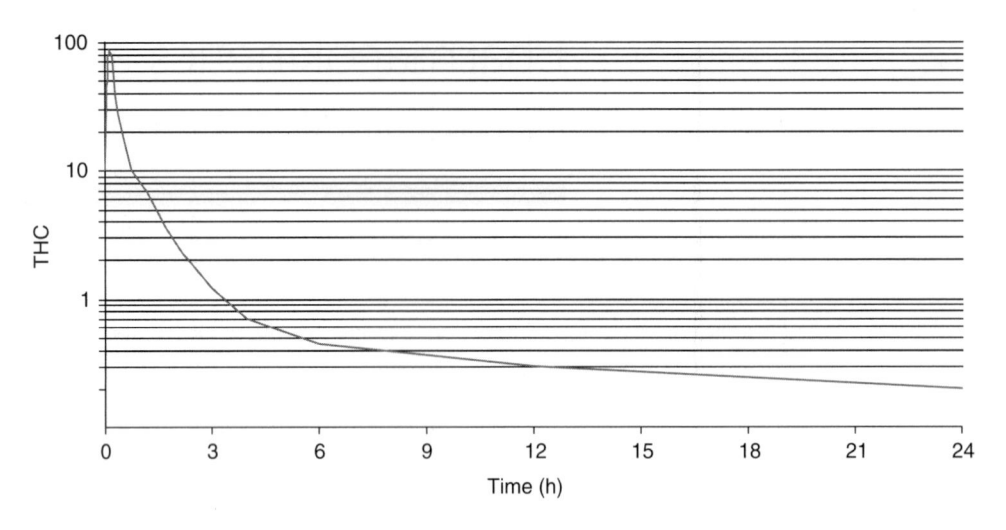

**Fig. 4.3** A typical concentration versus time profile of THC (ng/mL) following a 15 mg cigarette of cannabis on a log concentration scale

THC concentrations greater than 10 ng/mL are uncommon after 1 h even after moderate to high doses of cannabis.[18]

The terminal elimination half-life of THC is reported as 4.3 days, with a range of 3–13 days,[19] although a shorter half-life of about 1 day has also been quoted.[20] At first glance, this relatively long half-life contradicts the well-known short action of cannabis. However, this half-life is calculated after the process of distribution to tissues has taken place and represents the terminal phase of the elimination curve. Figure 4.3 shows a typical plasma concentration versus time profile after one 1.75% cannabis cigarette. A very quick peak level is seen followed by a rapid redistribution phase up to about the end of the first hour and a slower distribution phase beyond 1 h (see normal scale graph). Beyond 6 h there is an even slower elimination phase. This biphasic log-linear decline is typical of many drugs. There is little difference in the pharmacokinetics of THC in men and women.[13]

In high-dose (3.5% cigarette) users of marijuana, concentrations of THC can be detected for up to 24 h after last use (>0.5 ng/mL).[16] In fact it is not uncommon in regular users to detect THC at concentrations >1 ng/mL at 12 h after the last use of cannabis. For this reason a blood concentration less than 2 ng/mL may not suggest recent use and could be carried over from use days earlier. However, behavioural effects of cannabis may not occur at these levels (see Chapter 4.4). While sensitive assays can detect THC down to 0.1 ng/mL, it may not be practicable to measure concentrations less than 2 ng/mL, unless only proof of prior exposure is required.

### 11-Nor-$\Delta^9$-tetrahydrocannabinol-9-carboxylic acid

11-Nor-$\Delta^9$-tetrahydrocannabinol-9-carboxylic acid (carboxy-THC) is one of the main metabolites of THC and is found in the blood of cannabis users. Because of difficulties in measuring THC accurately, laboratories frequently measure this inactive metabolite rather than THC. Plasma concentrations of unconjugated carboxy-THC following a 1.97% THC cannabis cigarette peak at 43 ng/mL (SD 10 ng/mL) at 20 min after smoking. By 6 h plasma concentrations have fallen to 13 ng/mL (SD 2.8 ng/mL).[17]

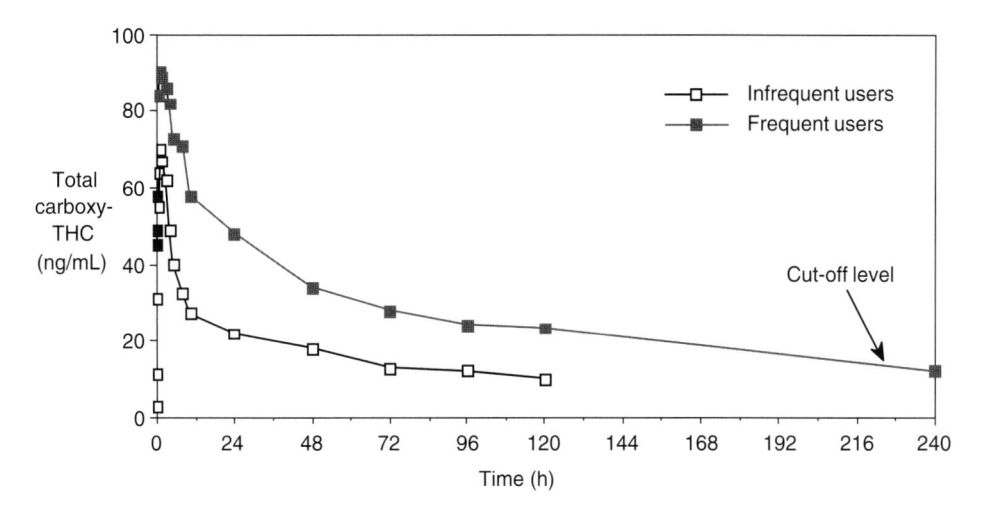

**Fig 4.4** Free and total 11-nor-$\Delta^9$-tetrahydrocannabinol-9-carboxylic acid (carboxy-THC) concentrations in plasma following a standard 5 mg intravenous dose of cannabis (after Kelly and Jones, 1992[21])

Intravenous administration of 5 mg THC (this mimics absorption by smoking of one cigarette reasonably well) gives peak concentrations of 40 ng/mL at 5–45 min in frequent users of marijuana and 44 ng/mL at 20–30 min post-dose in frequent users of marijuana. Pre-dose concentration of carboxy-THC may be significant in frequent users, with studies showing average levels of 18 ng/mL, although these are usually undetectable in infrequent users (<1 ng/mL).[21]

Occasionally total carboxy-THC (free and conjugated carboxy-THC) is measured. The administration of 5 mg THC intravenously gives peak concentrations of carboxy-THC in infrequent marijuana users at 70 ng/mL at 45–180 min post-dose, and 90 ng/mL in frequent users of marijuana. The higher plasma concentration in frequent users is because the pre-dose concentration is already 45 ng/mL.[21] The half-lives of free and total carboxy-THC are similar in the two groups and average about 5 days, although shorter half-lives of about 2 days have been reported.[20] Conjugated carboxy-THC is detectable in plasma for up to 12 days in frequent users, although concentrations fall below 15 ng/mL between 6 and 12 days in the frequent group and 2 and 6 days in the infrequent group.

Any back calculation to estimate amount consumed or time of consumption will need to take into account any baseline concentrations for carboxy-THC and of course individual variations in absorption and handling of the drug once absorbed. In most cases it will not be possible to calculate a likely dose or time of ingestion. Higher doses of THC will give proportionally higher concentrations of all THC species and will allow detection for a longer period of time. In the data above, individual variations in plasma concentrations of ±50% are not unusual and should at least be expected in real life.

### 11-Hydroxy-$\Delta^9$-tetrahydrocannabinol

11-Hydroxy-$\Delta^9$-tetrahydrocannabinol is produced from THC by metabolism and also exhibits THC-like activity. Blood concentrations are rapidly detected following a 1.75% or 3.55% marijuana cigarette within 15–20 min. This metabolite is only detectable in blood for

12–24 h after normal-strength marijuana cigarettes.[16] This metabolite is present in much higher concentrations following ingestion of cannabis products.

## PREDICTION OF TIME OF ADMINISTRATION

### Blood THC and carboxy-THC concentration ratios

Some researchers have investigated blood concentration ratios of THC and THC metabolites in order to predict time of administration. The ratio of free carboxy-THC to conjugated carboxy-THC is greater than two up to 30 min after a intravenous dose of THC.[21] In the same study, the ratio of THC to total carboxy-THC was less than one up to about 45 min after a intravenous dose. It is not clear how robust these ratios are, although it is likely that oral administration will produce more carboxy-THC during the first-pass effect and thereby change these ratios. There is no good relationship between blood THC and either blood or urine carboxy-THC concentrations.[22]

Some researchers have used urinary carboxy-THC concentrations in excess of 80 ng/mL to imply impairment. However, others have found little predictive value in using urinary carboxy-THC concentrations, especially since 24% of users would have blood THC concentrations of less than 1 ng/mL, a concentration that does not normally cause impairment. Many persons with impaired THC concentrations would not be impaired based on urinary carboxy-THC concentrations.[22] The use of lower urinary carboxy-THC concentrations would further increase the error.

A ratio of blood carboxy-THC to THC of less than 4 : 1 has been suggested to imply impairment; however, while this is indicative of recent THC exposure, it is not predictive since cases with a low (non-impairing) THC concentration could also have a ratio of less than 4 : 1.[22]

Algorithms have been used to assess the relationship between blood THC and carboxy-THC concentrations. The use of log-transformed blood concentrations and time has provided a better correlation and predictive potential,[18] although there are still a significant number of outliers, including cases with blood THC concentrations of less than 2.0 ng/mL.

THC concentrations in excess of 2–3 ng/mL and urinary 8β,11-dihydroxy-THC concentrations in excess of 15–20 ng/mL have been suggested as indicative of smoking within 6 h.[23] This relationship has not been confirmed by others, nor has this relationship been tested in chronic heavy users or after other routes of administration.

In conclusion, there are currently no useful predictive concentrations or algorithms of THC and its metabolites in blood or urine that have been shown to be capable of replacing the measurement of blood THC and obviating some form of impairment assessment.

## METABOLISM AND BIOLOGICAL ACTIVITY OF METABOLITES

The metabolism of THC is complex, with over 20 metabolites identified. However, only three are of any significance: the 11-hydroxy, the 9-carboxy and the glucuronide of 9-carboxy-THC (Table 4.1). Other metabolites found in blood are the 8- and 2′-hydroxy-THC metabolites (Fig. 4.5).[24] The 8-hydroxy metabolite exists in both the 8α- and 8β-isomers, of which

## Pharmacokinetics and duration of action

**Table 4.1** Selected pharmacokinetic parameters of THC

| | | |
|---|---|---|
| Absorption (% of intravenous) | Oral | 6% |
| | Smoking | 14–50% |
| Blood concentration (one typical cigarette)[a] | $\Delta^9$-THC | 0–200 ng/mL |
| | 11-Hydroxy-THC | 0–10 ng/mL |
| | 11-Nor-$\Delta^9$-THC-9-carboxylic acid-free | 0–50 ng/mL |
| | 11-Nor-$\Delta^9$-THC-9-carboxylic acid-total[a] | 0–100 ng/mL |
| Volume of distribution | Acute dosing | 9 L/kg |
| | Chronic dosing | 11 L/kg |
| Half-life (distribution) | $\Delta^9$-THC | <1 h |
| Half-life (elimination) | $\Delta^9$-THC | 1–4 days |
| | 11-Nor-$\Delta^9$-THC-9-carboxylic acid | 2–5 days |

| | | Urine | Faeces |
|---|---|---|---|
| Excretion (oral dose) | $\Delta^9$-THC | Trace | 1–6% |
| | 11-Hydroxy-THC | – | 1–4% |
| | 11-Nor-$\Delta^9$-THC-9-carboxylic acid | 3–4% | 1–11% |
| | Polar acids | 6–7% | 1–6% |

[a] Higher concentrations are expected for frequent users.

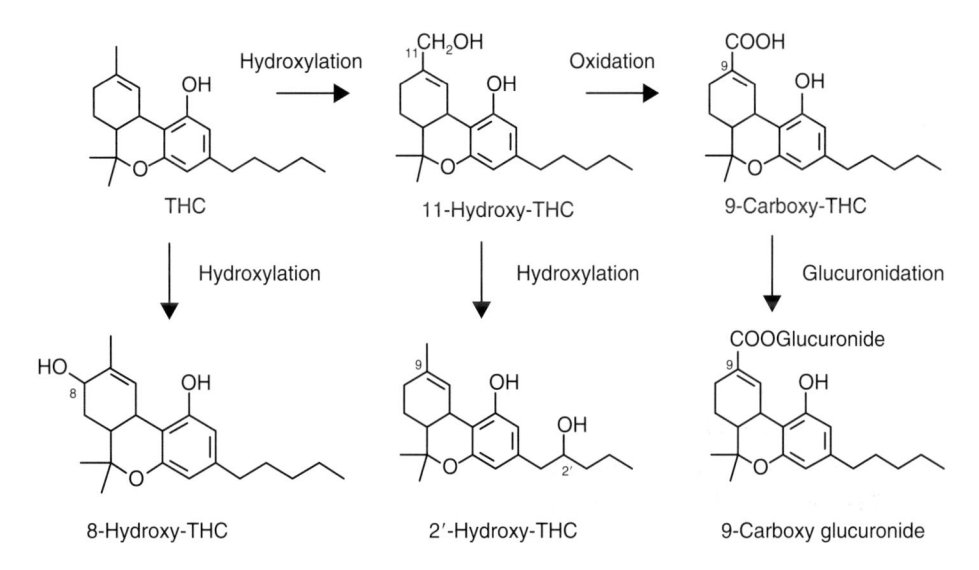

**Fig. 4.5** Metabolic pathways of THC

the β form has the most activity.[12] The hydroxy metabolites possess some THC-like activity, particularly the 11-hydroxy; however, they are not regarded as contributing significantly to the psychoactive effects of cannabis following smoking. Dihydroxy metabolites, other hydroxylated metabolites, and polar metabolites are also known to occur. Oral administration of cannabis will produce larger amounts of these hydroxy metabolites due to the first-pass effect, although it is not clear to what extent they contribute to the biological effects of cannabis.

The 9-carboxy metabolite (also known as 11-carboxy-THC) is extensively conjugated with glucuronic acid and is present in plasma and urine largely as the conjugated form. This is the major metabolite of THC, and is most often targeted in blood and urine analyses.

## EXCRETION

### THC intake by smoking

THC is essentially completely metabolized and excreted as polar hydroxy, carboxy and conjugated forms.[25] Approximately 20% of a dose is excreted in urine, and 40% in faeces. 9-Carboxy-THC is the main metabolite excreted as the glucuronide conjugate, although about 2% is excreted as the 11-hydroxy form.

Urine concentrations of carboxy-THC peak average at 90 and 153 ng/mL within 6 h following the smoking of 1.75% (16 mg) and 3.55% (34 mg) cannabis cigarettes.[26] Similar urinary concentrations are observed after 10 mg smoked[23] and 5 mg intravenous administration.[21] There is a large variation in the amounts excreted between and within studies.

Detectable carboxy-THC (measured as such by GC-MS) persists for up to 12 days following low to moderate doses of cannabis (16–36 mg smoked, or 5 mg intravenous).[21,26,27] Higher doses (56 mg over 2 days) give detection times in urine up to 25 days in regular users of marijuana.[19]

Detection times in urine in light, moderate and high users of marijuana during total abstinence from cannabis can take approximately 29, 63 and 77 days, respectively using a 20 ng/mL cut-off. Higher cut-offs such as 100 ng/mL give considerably shorter detection times, being a maximum of 11, 34 and 45 days, respectively for the three groups.[28]

Figure 4.6 shows an example of the urinary excretion profiles in low (once per month), moderate (once per week) and high users of cannabis (two or three times per week). Low users rapidly excrete carboxy-THC and drop below the 15 ng/mL cut-off within ~5 days, while high-dose users are still over the cut-off level after 12 days. It is of interest that the pre-dose urinary carboxy-THC is positive in regular users since accumulation of metabolite occurs between doses. Daily use of cannabis will produce even higher urine concentrations again. There is little difference in the metabolism and excretion of THC in men and women.[13]

Variation in urine concentrations of cannabinoids occurs for a number of reasons, including variable rates of metabolism, release of THC from fat and tissues, and variations in urine output. Creatinine measurements in urine are used to correct for renal function. A low water output will concentrate any products, compared with a high urine flow. Kidney function will also affect drug excretion. For this reason, if carboxy-THC concentrations in urine are used to produce sanctions or affect employment status, it is recommended to correct urinary cannabinoids for creatinine content.

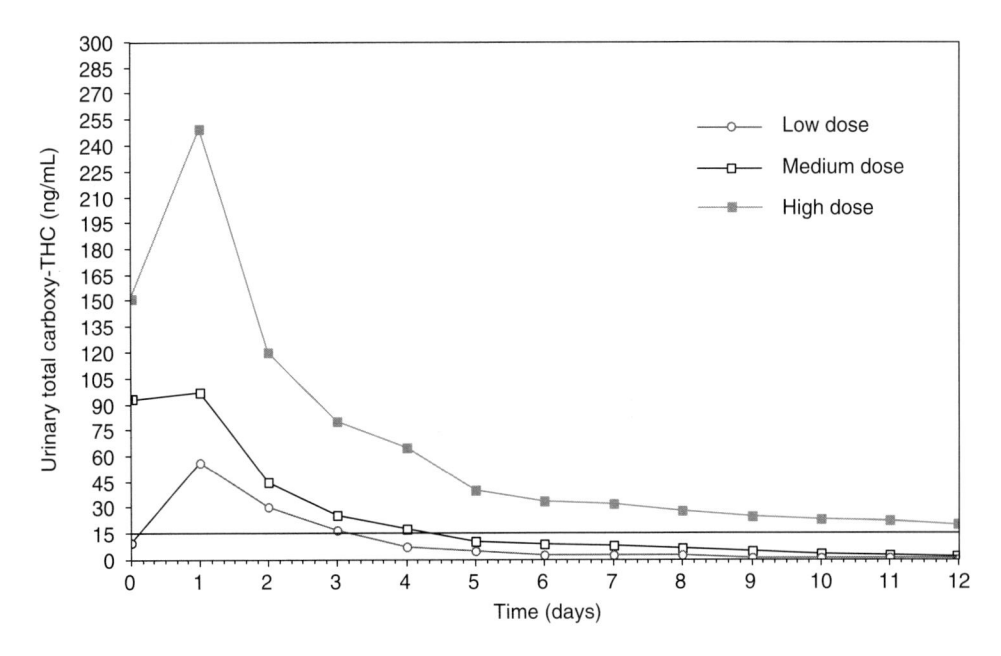

**Fig. 4.6** Urinary excretion of total carboxy-THC in low-, moderate- and high-dose users of cannabis (adapted after Ellis et al., 1985[28])

## THC intake by oral consumption

The oral availability of cannabis is about 6%, which means that only 6% of the ingested THC is absorbed into the blood stream. The remainder is metabolized prior to entry into the blood stream, or is not absorbed. Consumption of marijuana-laced brownies (cookies) containing the equivalent of 1–2 cigarettes produces significant behavioural and physiological changes as well as significant carboxy-THC in the urine. Detection times in urine range up to 12 days using a 20 ng/mL cut-off and 8 days using a 75 ng/mL cut-off.[29]

It is likely that the oral activity is higher than expected from THC concentrations due to a much higher production of 11-hydroxy-THC, which is also biologically active.

## DURATION OF ACTION

The duration of action of cannabis is usually short and more closely follows the blood THC concentrations than the carboxy-THC metabolite. However, the pharmacological and physiological effects (see Chapter 4.4) do not parallel the blood concentrations of THC. The peak effect is experienced about 15–30 min after smoking whereas the peak plasma concentration of THC is achieved within minutes. The pharmacological effects often last for 2–4 h, whereas the THC concentrations rapidly decline after their peak.[14,17,30,31] This lack of relationship of effect with blood concentration is common with other drugs, and should be regarded as expected rather than unexpected.

Occasional users of cannabis show a dose-dependent reduction in ability to perform divided attention tasks (Aluisi battery) and to recall correctly for about 2 h after smoking 2% or 3% THC-containing cigarettes.[32]

Table 4.2  Summary of studies describing blood concentrations of THC

| Reference | Protocol | Intake of THC | THC blood levels, ng/mL | Carboxy-THC blood levels, ng/mL | Comments |
|---|---|---|---|---|---|
| 14 | Eleven males with prior experience – infrequent and frequent exposure to cannabis – given cannabis smoking, oral and intravenous in a cross-over design, 1 week apart | 19 mg smoked<br><br>20 mg oral<br><br>5 mg intravenous | 33–119 ng/mL at 3 min; 18% bioavailability<br>4–11 ng/mL at 1–5 h; 6% bioavailability | | Well designed; psychological effects also measured |
| 30 | Marijuana smoked by 6 regular users, 2 cigarettes spaced 2 h apart | 1% cigarette | 46–188 ng/mL (1st smoke)<br>37–102 ng/mL (2nd smoke) | | Psychological effects and heart rate measured |
| 17 | Six regular male users smoked 3 strengths of cigarette in a randomized cross-over trial | 1.32% cigarette<br>1.97% cigarette<br>2.54% cigarette | 100 ± 10 ng/mL<br>120 ± 11 ng/mL<br>163 ± 19 ng/mL (peak) | Unconjugated<br>34 ± 8 ng/mL<br>43 ± 10 ng/mL<br>50 ± 8 ng/mL | Psychological effects and heart rate measured; kinetics over 6 h |
| 15 | Marijuana (deuterated THC) smoked and given intravenously to 9 men: 5 heavy users and 4 light users | 8.6–9.9 mg smoked; 5 mg intravenous | Mean 16 (10–44) ng/mL at 10 min; 0.5 ng/mL at 6 h; and 0.2 ng/mL at 12 h | | Bioavailability of smoked marijuana was 14% in light and 27% in heavy users; no pharmacokinetic tolerance found |
| 23 | Marijuana smoked in 2 cigarettes over 30 min by 10 regular social users | 10 mg smoked | 85 ng/mL at 5 min; 1 ng/mL at 2 h | Conjugated<br>26 ng/mL at 30 min | |

**Table 4.2** (continued)

| Reference | Protocol | Intake of THC | THC blood levels, ng/mL | Carboxy-THC blood levels, ng/mL | Comments |
|---|---|---|---|---|---|
| 46 | Ten males smoking 1 cigarette daily were given deuterated THC by smoking over 2 days | 56 mg deuterated THC | Half-life THC 4.3 ± 1.6 days (2.6–12.6 days) | | Kinetic data over 28 days for THC; shows long terminal elimination half-life of THC in regular users |
| 47 | Marijuana smoked by 24 regular users | Approximately 20 mg smoked, amount inhaled unknown | 13 ± 10 ng/mL at 40 min | 22 ± 22 ng/mL at 40 min | |
| 16 | Six regular male users smoked 2 strengths of cigarette at weekly intervals | 1.75% (16 mg) 3.55% (34 mg) | 84 (50–129) 162 (76–267) | *Unconjugated carboxy-THC* 24 (15–54) 54 (22–101) | Good kinetic data and graphs; also measured 11-OH metabolite; placebo controlled study |
| 21 | Eight males, 4 frequent and 4 infrequent users, given intravenous THC | 5 mg intravenously | F half-life 117 ± 17 min IF half-life 93 ± 31 min | *Unconjugated carboxy-THC* F half-life 5.2 ± 0.8 days IF half-life 6.2 ± 6.7 *Conjugated carboxy-THC* F half-life 6.8 ± 4.5 IF half-life 3.7 ± 2.0 | Conjugated carboxy-THC seen in plasma for 12 days; ratios of free carboxy-THC to conjugated, or THC/carboxy-THC, ratios only predictive to 30–45 min post-dose |

F: frequent (user); IF: infrequent (user).

Table 4.3 Summary of studies describing urine concentrations of carboxy-THC

| Reference | Protocol | Intake of THC | Peak urine level Mean ± SD and range | Detection time in urine (screen) | Detection time in urine ± SD and range[a] | Half-life ± SD (days) |
|---|---|---|---|---|---|---|
| 26 | Single smoked cigarette in 6 drug-free volunteers | 1.75% THC (16 mg) 3.55% THC (34 mg) | 90 ± 32 (11–234) ng/mL 153 ± 49 (30–318) ng/mL | | 34 ± 9 (8–68) h 89 ± 10 (27–122) h | |
| 27 | Single smoked cigarette in 6 drug-free volunteers | 1.75% THC 3.55% THC | No data | 13 ± 7 h (51 ± 39)[b] 36 ± 13 h (93 ± 36)[b] | 34 ± 22 h 89 ± 23 h | |
| 21 | Single intravenous 5 mg THC in 4 frequent and infrequent users | 5 mg | F 97 ± 65 (50–153) ng/mL IF 56 ± 29 (44–97) ng/mL | F 0–2 (2 to >12)[b] days IF 0 (1–3)[b] days | F 6 to >12 days IF 2–6 days | |
| 19 | Four cannabis cigarettes over 2 days to 13 male regular users, abstinence for 28 days | 56 mg smoked over 2 days | | 3–25 days[c] | 3–25 days[d] | cTHCp 2.6–12.4 days cTHCu 0.8–9.8 days |
| 36 | Passive inhalation of cannabis smoke to drug-free volunteers | 30 min exposure in a car with volume 1650 L, following 2 or 6 cigarettes | 30 ng/mL on day 2 (unhydrolyzed cannabinoids) | 4 days | | |

192

**Table 4.3** (continued)

| Reference | Protocol | Intake of THC | Peak urine level Mean ± SD and range | Detection time in urine (screen) | Detection time in urine ± SD and range[a] | Half-life ± SD (days) |
|---|---|---|---|---|---|---|
| 23 | Marijuana smoked in 2 cigarettes over 30 min by 10 regular social users | 10 mg smoked | 20–107 ng/mL total between 0 and 6 h post-dose | | | |
| 28 | 86 chronic users followed for almost 3 months in a supervized setting | 60% used cannabis at least daily, users of 2–21 years | Light users: 27 days[e]<br>Moderate users: 32 days<br>Heavy users: 34 days<br>All users: 32 days | | Above 20 ng/mL for 46 consecutive days, or 77 days to drop below cut-off for 10 consecutive days | |
| 37 | Passive inhalation in 6 volunteers over 1 h in a closed room | 2.5–2.8% content | Small transient increase over 20 ng/mL cut-off, in only 2 urines | | | |
| 34 | Passive inhalation in 5 volunteers exposed to side-stream smoke of 4 and 16 cigarettes | 2.8% content, 1 h each day for 6 days | Three subjects tested positive to EMIT 100 after exposure to 16 cigarettes | 4 cigarettes: 0–6 h[c]<br>16 cigarettes: 22–141 h[c] | 4 cigarettes: 0–25 h[f]<br>16 cigarettes: 53–218 h[f]<br>Peak level 4 cigarettes: 12 ng/mL<br>Peak level 16 cigarettes: 87 ng/mL | Well-designed study; shows EMIT reactivities over 100, and carboxy-THC levels approaching 100 ng/mL |

[a] 15 ng/mL GC-MS cut-off; [b] 100 ng/mL cut-off and in parentheses 20 ng/mL cut-off using EMIT d.a.u.; [c] 20 ng/mL cut-off EMIT; [d] HPLC using 7 ng/mL cut-off; [e] EMIT d.a.u. measured as extended duration (days from last use to last positive detection); [f] 5 ng/mL cut-off. THC: Δ⁹-tetrahydrocannabinol; cTHC: 11-carboxy-THC; F: frequent (user); IF: infrequent (user); p: plasma; u: urine.

# Cannabis

Oral consumption of marijuana-laced brownies containing the equivalent of one to two cigarettes produces a duration of action of about 8 h.[29] The longer duration is caused by the slower absorption and the greater contribution to the behavioural effects by metabolites (principally 11-hydroxy-THC).

See Chapter 4.5 for more details of behavioural effects of cannabis.

## ALTERNATIVE SOURCES OF CANNABINOIDS

### Passive smoking

Inhalation of side-stream smoke from tobacco smoking is now well established as a risk factor. Cannabis is no different if smoked. Unwitting persons in a confined area, or adjacent to an active smoker of marijuana, will inhale significant amounts of cannabis smoke.[33–37]

Exposure for 30 min in a confined area (motor vehicle with air space of 1650 L and smoking a 1.5% cigarette) produces plasma concentrations of THC of 1.3–6.3 ng/mL, and urine concentrations (over 20 ng/mL EMIT cut-off) are positive in volunteers who have never used cannabis before.[36] Similar results were found in another study after 1 h exposure to 2.8% cigarettes in a larger room (15 500 L).[37] In both studies urine EMIT® results did not exceed the 50 ng/mL cut-off concentration.

Repeated exposure to 16 marijuana cigarettes (2.8% strength) for 1 h for each of six consecutive days in a small unventilated room (12 200 L) produces strong cannabinoid responses in urine, some even exceeding the 100 ng/mL cannabinoid calibrator. GC/MS confirmation of carboxy-THC produces urine concentrations up to 87 ng/mL (fourth day).[33,34]

Passive smoking can clearly produce relatively large exposures in situations of large-scale use of cannabis in confined areas, although exposures producing urinary cannabinoids, or equivalent, of less than 50 ng/mL is more usual.[38]

### Consumption of hemp products

Hemp is a form of *Cannabis sativa* that contains little or no $\Delta^9$-THC (typically <0.5%). Hemp is used to produce long fibres for the textile and paper industries. Hemp seeds and oil derived from the seeds have appeared in cosmetics and health foods.

Consumption of these products can lead to positive cannabinoid levels in urine. Ingestion of Swiss cannabis seed oil has produced peak urine concentrations of carboxy-THC of almost 300 ng/mL and gave detectable concentrations for over 5 days.[39] Analysis of this oil gives THC contents of 3–1500 µg/g (i.e. up to 0.15% content by weight). Legal hemp products that contain a maximum of 50 µg/g THC are unlikely to produce more than a transient positive reaction in urine.

Consumption of 15 mL cold pressed hemp oil as a herbal remedy twice daily for 4 days produces an EMIT 50[i] positive reaction in urine from the end of the first day to at least 2 days after the last dose. Urinary concentrations of carboxy-THC reach a maximum of 68 ng/mL

---

[i] Equal to or greater than a 50-mg/mL carboxy-THC calibrator.

# Pharmacokinetics and duration of action

and remain over the 15 ng/mL cut-off for over 2 days after the last dose.[40] Lower concentrations are also detected using hemp seed oil.[41]

German-sourced food products produced from hemp contain up to 4.4 µg/g THC, while hemp seed oil sourced in Germany contained up to 150 µg/g THC. Consumption of a hemp food bar gave a positive THC concentration in blood (maximum 6 ng/mL).[42] Consumption of hemp seed snack bars may not produce urinary readings above the cut-off level.[43]

## NABILONE: A SYNTHETIC CANNABINOID

Nabilone is a synthetic drug related chemically to THC that is available in a number of countries (see Fig. 4.2). The rapid uptake into tissues and metabolism to a range of related compounds is similar to THC. The half-life in plasma is reported as 2 h, although related compounds are present in blood for at least 20 h. The drug is mainly excreted in faeces rather than urine as polar metabolites.[44] A number of synthetic cannabinoids are known with varying pharmacokinetic properties.[9,45]

## Synopsis

### PHARMACOKINETICS AND DURATION OF ACTION

1 Oral consumption of cannabis leads to an absorption of only about 6% and produces a slow build-up to maximum blood concentrations of THC over 60–90 min. Maximum blood concentrations are 4–11 ng/mL after 20 mg cannabis.
2 The smoking of cannabis leads to only about 14–50% absorption of THC; however, absorption is rapid leading to peak plasma concentrations within a few minutes. Peak concentrations of THC are 50–129 ng/mL after smoking a 16 mg cigarette.
3 THC is rapidly distributed into tissues leading to a rapid fall in blood concentrations after absorption. Plasma concentrations above 10 ng/mL after 1 h are uncommon. The terminal elimination phase has a half-life of 4 days, which means that THC will accumulate in blood in regular users.
4 Blood concentrations of THC under 2 ng/mL are not predictive of recent use due to this carry-over effect.
5 Metabolism of THC is extensive leading to numerous products. Only the 11-hydroxy and a few other hydroxylated substances possess any biological activity. The major metabolite, carboxy-THC, is inactive and is the most measured THC species.
6 The major metabolite, carboxy-THC, is found in blood shortly after use and persists in blood for up to 1 week due to its half-life of 5 days, and with regular use may persist in blood for some weeks.
7 There is no predictive relationship of THC and its metabolites that provides any accurate calculation of timing of administration.
8 Urinalysis allows detection of cannabinoids for up to 11 weeks after use, although in light users carboxy-THC is only detectable for about 2 weeks.
9 The physiological and pharmacological effects of cannabis persist in most users for only 2–4 h after use.

10 Passive smoking can lead to a false detection of cannabis use. Exposure to heavy cannabis use in a confined area, or after several exposures, can lead to cannabinoid positive reactions in urine of 100 ng/mL. Light to moderate exposure is unlikely to exceed urine concentrations of 20 ng/mL.
11 Consumption of hemp food products (products made from the oil or seeds) can also lead to a false positive conclusion of active cannabis use. Unusually high content of THC and/or consumption of significant amounts of material can lead to cannabinoid reactions of over 100 ng/mL. Concentrations of less than 20 ng/mL are more usual.

# 4.3 Mechanisms of action

The active constituents of marijuana act on the central nervous system (CNS) on specific recognition sites termed receptors in the same way as opioids and benzodiazepines act on their receptors. The cannabinoid receptor belongs to a family of receptors known as G-protein coupled receptors, in which their activation inhibits the enzyme adenylate cyclase that then produces an intracellular mediator. THC and the known psychoactive cannabinoids inhibit this enzyme, and it is believed that this mediates most of the effects of cannabis. This receptor also affects movement of calcium through ion channels.

The cannabinoid receptor is localized to specific regions of the brain that are known to be sites of action for THC. These sites include hippocampus and cortex for cognitive effects (memory and learning), and basal ganglia and cerebellum, which control balance and co-ordination. This site is known as $CB_1$, and differs from a peripheral binding site known as $CB_2$, which may play a role in modulating immune response and inflammation. The lack of cannabinoid receptors in the brain stem explain the lack of life-threatening toxicity exhibited by cannabis, since the brain stem regulates breathing and other functions vital for life.

The physiological functions of these receptors are affected by a number of neuronal systems modulated by other drugs of abuse, namely the opioid (morphine), GABA (benzodiazepines), dopamine, serotonin (amphetamines and cocaine) and cholinergic receptors.[48]

The presence of a specific receptor for THC raises questions of the physiological role for this receptor. Endogenous substances have been isolated that appear to mimic the action of THC and may even be the endogenous cannabinoids. These substances include anandamide (after the Sanskrit for bliss), and 2-arachidonyl glycerol (Fig. 4.2). These chemicals are derivatives of arachidonic acid, an essential precursor for the formation of prostaglandins and related substances. Their roles and the question of whether they are the endogenous cannabinoids are yet to be fully determined. However, it seems reasonable to conclude that both substances interact with cannabinoid receptors in both peripheral and central sites to produce a wide range of effects. Administration of these substances to laboratory animals produce effects that are quite similar to those produced by THC.[49] Nevertheless, there are pharmacological differences between the plant-derived THC and the endogenous cannabinoids that could be due to either pharmacodynamic or pharmacokinetic differences.

# 4.4 Pharmacological actions and therapeutics

Cannabis produces a host of behavioural and physiological changes. These are probably best summarized as a pleasant, dreamy state with impairment of cognitive and psychomotor functions.

While these responses are often only short lived, there is a view that cannabis is a relatively harmless drug used domestically or socially. Cannabis has a range of quite important physiological effects, many of which are reviewed elsewhere.[48,50]

## ACUTE PHYSIOLOGICAL EFFECTS

The smoking of cannabis produces measurable increases in heart rate, blood pressure and body temperature. Heart rate acceleration is dose dependent and can be as much as 50% within 30 min of a dose, which declines to the normal rate usually within 2 h.[17] Blood pressures also rise, particularly systolic pressure. A 5-mg dose of THC can raise systolic pressure by 25 mmHg, which then declines to normal over the next few hours.[21] Similarly, body temperature rises in a dose-dependent manner.

Cannabis is also known to lower intraocular pressure, reduce lacrimation, redden the conjunctiva, cause small increases in the size of pupils and diminish reaction to light, causing photophobia.[45] Indeed, cannabis users often show no lacrimation when peeling onions.

All of these physiological changes are associated with behavioural changes that show only a poor relation with plasma concentration of THC. Figure 4.7 illustrates the delay, and the longer duration of cannabis, in self-reported psychological effects compared with the blood THC concentration. The heart rate increases are also delayed but do not endure for as long as the subjective change in mood.

## ACUTE BEHAVIOURAL CHANGES

Psychological changes experienced with smoking cannabis include a transient euphoric effect with associated emotional and cognitive changes that are usually perceived as a 'high'. These effects are subjective experiences that cannot be quantified. Figure 4.7 illustrates the time-course of this 'high' relative to THC plasma concentrations. Blood concentrations of THC in excess of 5 ng/mL are strongly suggestive of recent cannabis use.

In some subjects, particularly naïve users, dysphoria occurs. This manifests as anxiety, paranoia, panic and generally unpleasant feelings. Depersonalization and restlessness also

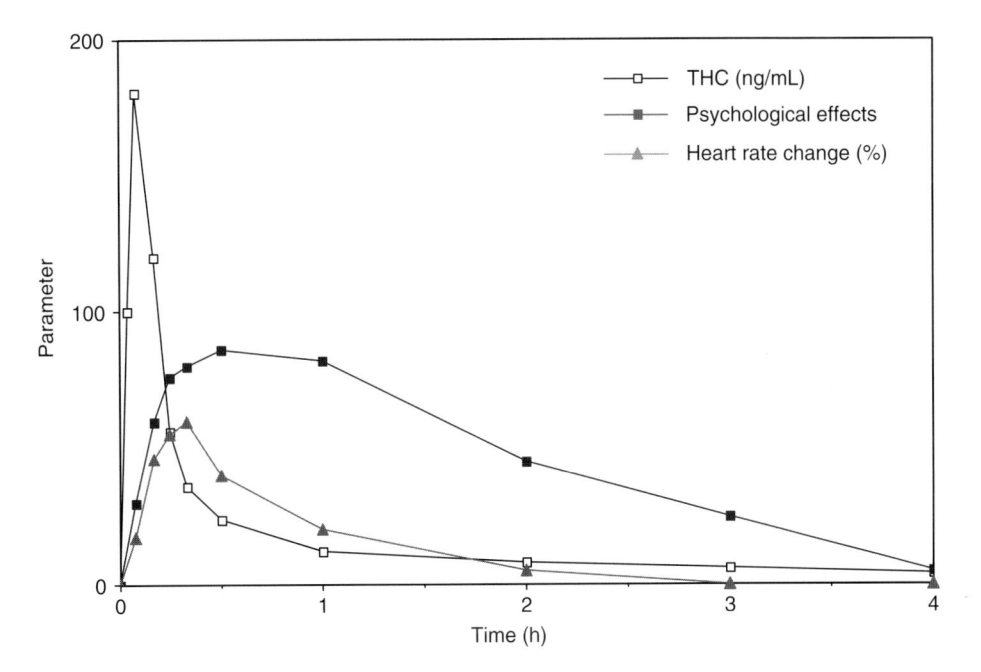

**Fig. 4.7** Simulated time changes for THC blood concentration, self-reported psychological effect and increase in heart rate following a standard dose of cannabis

occur. In some users, flashbacks occur, similar to those experienced with LSD. As with many drug users, there is often a psychological basis for drug reactions.

Cognitive skills, such as correct recall of numbers or facts, simple calculations on demand and perceptual tasks, particularly those requiring sustained vigilance, are significantly impaired by cannabis, even from low-potency cigarettes. Several reviews are available.[11,12,48,51] These cognitive effects are relatively short lived and appear to have a similar time course to other physiological changes.

There is no general increase in aggressiveness observed in persons under the influence of cannabis, rather an increased passivity is more often noted. However, acute paranoid or manic psychoses induced by cannabis intoxication may lead to increased risk of aggression and violent acts.

## Effects on driving skills

Cannabis produces a reduction in performance skills, including reaction times to stimuli, road-tracking performance, divided attention tasks, and hand–eye co-ordination. Simple and complex sensory functions are clearly impaired by normal doses of THC.[52]

The decrements in performance are, generally speaking, not measurable after 4 h, although fine motor skills may be affected for longer.[53] These decrements are unlikely to be measurable clinically unless motor skills have been tested prior to administration of cannabis.

Cannabis decreases speed and risk taking in both open-road and city-driving situations.[54] It is not clear if this is a direct effect of the cannabinoids, or an over-reaction by the driver to perceived impairment.

## CHRONIC AND ADVERSE HEALTH EFFECTS

### Lung disease and cancers

The process of smoking marijuana, like smoking tobacco, forces a large quantity of products into the lungs of the individual, many of which are formed by pyrolysis during the heating stage. In this process inactive cannabinoids rapidly decarboxylate to THC. A number of other cannabinoids are released (possibly over 60), as well as other products, including polycyclic hydrocarbons such as benzpyrene, a known carcinogen also found in tobacco smoke. Like tobacco, carbon monoxide, hydrogen cyanide and carcinogenic nitrosamines are also inhaled by the smoker.

Daily marijuana smoking has been shown to precipitate pulmonary dysfunction such as cough, wheeze and sputum formation, and may lead to chronic obstructive lung diseases. This is usually only present in heavy long-term use, although it may be difficult to distinguish tobacco-related causes of lung disease from tobacco smoking, since most users smoke both types of cigarette.[55]

Standard laboratory tests on cannabis extracts have been found to cause mutations, inhibit DNA and RNA synthesis, and inhibit the immune response. It is therefore of no surprise to find that long-term inhalation of cannabis smoke has caused similar detrimental effects on the lungs as tobacco smoking. Initially, symptoms of airways obstruction and squamous cell hyperplasia (a form of abnormal cell growth) occur, as well as other abnormalities of cells in the epithelium. Squamous cell cancers with lymph node involvement have been recognized in the head and neck of young marijuana or hashish smokers, as well as tongue cancers in heavy users.[56] There is also a 10-fold higher incidence of leukaemia in children of women who have smoked during pregnancy. Behavioural abnormalities and retarded development are also associated with active cannabis use during pregnancy.

### Memory and learning

Long-term cannabis use impairs short-term memory, overall learning and other cognitive processes.[48,50] This impairment will persist for much longer than the presence of THC in body tissues, and may even be permanent. There is, however, little scientific evidence to distinguish these changes from other factors, such as development of mental disease.

### Schizophrenia and other mental disorders

Acute psychotic-like reactions lasting for a few hours are known following cannabis use, particularly heavy use. This consists of paranoid ideation, illusions, hallucinations, delusions, depersonalization, confusion, restlessness and excitement.[57] Long-term cannabis users tend to become withdrawn and indifferent and develop an 'amotivational syndrome'. In this state they are less likely to become confrontational or violent although there is a considerable body of knowledge that links marijuana use to acute psychotic episodes.[56] This link is equivocal since other researchers find little evidence of a psychotic state distinguishable from cannabis intoxication.[57,58]

The incidence of an acute toxic psychotic-like state (known as dagga in South Africa among southern African blacks) is known to be high in a population in which over 60% are users of cannabis. Toxic psychoses are represented by a variety of clinical presentations, including schizophrenia, paranoia, maniform psychoses and organic psychoses.[ii] Unfortunately, the contribution made by cannabis in these people is difficult to establish due to the presence of other confounding factors and their low socioeconomic status.[59]

Epidemiological studies involving large numbers of persons are showing an increased incidence of schizophrenia in cannabis users.[60] People who have used cannabis more than 50 times exhibit a six-fold higher rate of schizophrenia than non-users. It is important to point out that there is also a strong association with diagnosis of other psychiatric diseases. It is possible that persons developing schizophrenia and other forms of psychiatric disease are more likely to use cannabis, or that cannabis triggers physiological changes in the brain that lead to mental disease. These questions are at present unresolved.

## Other effects

Other effects of cannabis include abnormal menstruation and anovulation in women, and decreased serum testosterone, decreased sperm count and impaired sperm motility with abnormal morphology in men.

Cannabis may have adverse effects in surgical patients receiving anaesthetics. This is because cannabis affects the cardiovascular system and may enhance the effects of opioids and other CNS active drugs.

## MEDICAL USES

Despite the illegal nature of the drug and the adverse effects noted above, cannabis, or more particularly THC, has a number of legitimate medical uses. These uses include treatment of nausea and vomiting in persons receiving chemotherapy (approved in the USA and some other counties and prescribed as Marinol capsules) and in patients who do not respond to conventional anti-emetics, and for stimulating appetite in patients with AIDS. Chemotherapy in persons with AIDS has also been approved in some countries, but its use is potentially dangerous in these patients since cannabis is believed to compromise the immune system.[61]

Cannabis is also known to lower the intraocular pressure in glaucoma, although its use for this indication is unlikely given that many other drugs are available for this purpose, and that its efficacy is probably not caused by THC but rather by another constituent in cannabis.[45,62]

Cannabinoids appear to have analgesic properties, and are being investigated for the treatment of chronic pain conditions. Their ability to possess anti-inflammatory and anti-anxiety

---

[ii] In maniform psychosis, patients are agitated and restless, speech is pressured, patients have grandiose thoughts and actions that have no purpose. Schizophreniform psychosis presents as blunting of effects, withdrawal, lack of movement, actions or ideas, and bizarre somatic or other delusions and thought disorders. Organic psychosis presents as clouding or fluctuating consciousness, disorientation, and decrement in thought and intellect. Paranoid psychosis presents as paranoid ideation with an apparent congruent mode.[59]

# Cannabis

properties may assist in the analgesic response. A 20-mg dose of THC may have the same analgesic potency as 120 mg codeine. This effect seems to be at the spinal or supraspinal level and is enhanced by opioids.[63] Its use in pain management is unclear, but it is noteworthy that THC enhances the effects of opioid narcotics and other CNS active drugs. However, more research is required to fully understand the efficacy of THC and other cannabinoids.[48,64]

Other perceived uses that have not been proven medically include its use to treat convulsions, muscle spasticity and bronchial asthma. Synthetic forms of THC are also available, e.g. nabilone and levonantradol.

## Synopsis

### PHARMACOLOGICAL ACTIONS AND THERAPEUTICS

1. Marijuana produces a pleasant, dreamy 'high', with impairment of emotive, cognitive and psychomotor functions.
2. This impairment reduces performance involving complex mental or motor skills, such as those involved in driving motor vehicles and operating fine machinery.
3. These effects are usually short lived, lasting for only a few hours at most.
4. Cannabis also produces measurable increases in heart rate, blood pressure and body temperature, reduces intraocular pressure, reduces lacrimation, induces photophobia and causes eye reddening.
5. Chronic (regular) use may lead to long-term impairment of memory and learning skills, as well as possibly contributing to lung disease and cancers involving the respiratory system, and increases the propensity to develop schizophrenia.
6. High doses may even induce a psychotic-like state.
7. Medical uses of cannabis, or THC, include reduction of nausea following chemotherapy.
8. Cannabis may also be useful for treatment of glaucoma, to increase appetite, and to act as an analgesic. The efficacy and safety of cannabis for these conditions is not proven.

# 4.5 Tolerance and dependence

The phenomena of tolerance and dependence have been discussed elsewhere (see Chapter 1.6). Similarly to other drugs of abuse, cannabis users develop tolerance to the physiological and psychological effects of THC. A number of useful reviews are available that describe the biology and psychological consequences of cannabis use.[48,51,61,65]

## TOLERANCE

Tolerance is now known to occur to many of the behavioural effects of cannabis as well as to the changes in blood pressures and heart rate. Regular use of cannabis results in little if any increase in heart rate or blood pressure; rather users may even experience a decrease in heart rate.[51,65]

Persons using cannabis regularly experience fewer of the dysphoric and nauseating effects and experience less mood-altering activity. The subjective high experienced by cannabis users will also decline in intensity with repeated use.[66] However, tolerance does not develop to the CNS depressants effects of cannabis to the same degree as some of the cardiovascular changes.[67]

However, the development of tolerance shows significant variability between subjects, although naïve or social users will experience greater impairment of psychomotor and cognitive responses than regular users.

There is no evidence that tolerance is caused by altered pharmacokinetics of cannabis. In other words, chronic use of cannabis results in the same blood concentrations of THC as achieved when first used.

Interestingly, cannabis and alcohol produce some degree of cross-tolerance, i.e. regular consumption of alcohol can reduce the effects of cannabis, and vice versa. This interrelation between the two most widely used drugs may also explain why they are frequently used together.

## DEPENDENCE

The ability of cannabis to produce dependence is more controversial and depends more on the terms used to define dependence. Old definitions of dependence included the presence of tolerance and withdrawal, whereas modern definitions, such as that of the American Psychiatric Association,[68] define the syndrome as follows:

> The essential feature of this disorder is a cluster of cognitive, behavioural and physiological symptoms that indicate that a person has impaired control of psychoactive substance use and continuous use of the substance despite adverse consequences.

# Cannabis

A diagnosis of drug dependence is made if any three of nine criteria are met (see Chapter 1.6). These include symptoms of compulsion to use the drug, high value attached to drug use by the individual, and drug-seeking behaviour, as well as symptoms of tolerance and abstinence syndromes. By this definition, cannabis can cause dependence to develop in users.

An abstinence syndrome has been observed in animals and in humans given high doses of THC. This consists of yawning, piloerection (goose pimples), anorexia, anxiety, irritability, sleeplessness, sweating, tremors and photophobia, which are similar to the abstinence symptoms associated with the minor tranquillizers, and are reversed by consumption of THC.[65] The smoking of two to four cigarettes daily for 10 days can produce an abstinence syndrome.[69]

The change in lifestyle caused by compulsion to use the drug and to seek money to fund the habit, and the continual psychotropic effects, while under the influence, are probably the biggest negative factors with cannabis – and indeed all drugs of dependence. It has been estimated that approximately 20% of persons who have used cannabis more than five times become dependent users.[65] Clearly, the risk of dependence increases with the frequency of using the drug. An estimated one in 10 will establish a dependence on the drug. As with many drugs of abuse, the risk of dependence is highest in 18–29-year-old males, and in those with poor academic achievement, deviant adolescent behaviour and poor parental relationships.

Comobidity is associated with dependence on cannabis. This includes major depression and other forms of drug abuse, including alcohol dependence.[70]

The extent of dependence on cannabis and other drugs can be gauged by the absolute numbers attending drug treatment centres. The 1992 National Census of Clients of Australian Treatment Service Agencies listed 6% of over 5000 clients with cannabis as the main drug problem.[71]

It is also important to note that cannabis smokers will often mix their marijuana leaves with tobacco. In this context, it is sometimes difficult to isolate the nicotine-induced dependence from that caused by THC and other cannabinoids.

## Synopsis

### TOLERANCE AND DEPENDENCE

1 Regular use of cannabis produces tolerance to its actions, resulting in less mood-altering activity, fewer effects on heart rate and blood pressure, and less dysphoria, but subjects may not become tolerant to its effects on cognitive and psychomotor activity.
2 Dependence is also exhibited by regular cannabis users within a week or two.
3 Withdrawal from cannabis in dependant users results in an abstinence syndrome characterized by anxiety, dysphoria, irritability, sleeplessness, anorexia, sweating and photophobia.
4 It is estimated that 10% of persons who have ever used cannabis will develop some degree of dependence on the drug.

# 4.6 Toxicology

Cannabis is a unique drug: it causes changes in a number of physiological parameters and produces significant and often profound behavioural changes, yet it has not been linked directly to an acute death. It can cause significant clinically observable impairment, and for this reason its use by motor vehicle drivers is one of most frequent associations in forensic cases.

## PREVALENCE OF THC IN FORENSIC CASES

Drug screening in toxicology laboratories reports cannabinoids, particularly THC or 11-hydroxy-THC and/or carboxy-THC in more cases than probably any other drug apart from alcohol. Statistics show a highest incidence of cannabis use in drug-related deaths, particularly those involving heroin. The reasons for this may relate to the propensity of heroin users to consume other psychoactive substances, or to the fact that it may increase the effects of the opioid.[63] The incidences in other types of medical examiner/coroners cases are shown in Table 4.4.

The prevalence of cannabis use shown in Table 4.4 are likely to reflect the incidence in similar cases in many of the European countries and the USA, which frequently report active use in over 10% of the population. Moreover, a higher proportion of the younger or male population use cannabis than the older population or females.

## CONTRIBUTION OF CANNABIS USE TO DEATH

There is little evidence that death is caused directly by misuse of cannabis. There have been no reported cases of death attributed directly to cannabis. This is surprising given the marked behavioural and cardiovascular changes caused by modest doses of cannabis.

Since ingestion or inhalation of cannabis use can come only from the cannabis plant material, it is likely that an overdose is not possible without suffering from the unpleasant effects

**Table 4.4** Incidence of THC and cannabinoids in various categories of sudden death

| | |
|---|---|
| All coroners' cases | 10.8% |
| Drug-related deaths | 22.0% |
| Heroin-related deaths | 36.0% |
| Homicides | 16.9% |
| Drivers of motor vehicles | 16.7% |
| Suicides (non-drug-related) | 13.2% |
| Natural deaths | 2.2% |

Derived from the Victorian Institute of Forensic Medicine toxicology statistics.

of the consumption or inhalation of too much leaf material. In this respect this is similar to tobacco. Tobacco smoking rarely, if at all, causes sudden death from inhalation of too much nicotine, but consumption of nicotine in a pure form has led to death. (Nicotine has been used as an insecticide, usually in the form of a concentrated solution.)

It is likely that if a pure form of THC is ingested in too high a dose, death can occur. The availability of capsules of THC, and synthetic variations of THC, may allow this to happen. However, THC and other psychoactive drugs do not show appreciable activity on the brain stem, which controls much of the nervous control to the lungs and heart. Respiratory depression, a common toxic effect of many other CNS depressants, does not manifest itself with cannabis. When CNS depression does occur, it is usually from other co-administered drugs, such as alcohol, opioids or the benzodiazepines.

Cannabis does increase the effects of alcohol, opioids and possibly other CNS active drugs, such as benzodiazepines. Consequently, co-consumption of cannabis with other CNS depressant drugs may lead to an increased toxic response. In reality, a contribution by cannabis is difficult to prove in such cases when other CNS active drugs are present.

## CONTRIBUTION TO MOTOR VEHICLE ACCIDENTS

The contribution of cannabis to road traffic accidents is subject to controversy despite the high incidence of THC in drivers involved in accidents. Drivers killed in crashes have had variable prevalences of cannabinoids detected ranging from 2.5% to over 30% (Table 4.5).

Drivers apprehended for driving under the influence of drugs are frequently positive to cannabis, or combinations of drugs with cannabis, particularly alcohol. The incidence of THC in apprehended drivers in Nordic countries ranges from 3% to 15%.[85] Similar prevalences occur elsewhere including the USA and Australia.[86]

Terhune and colleagues examined almost 2000 fatally injured drivers in the USA using a method of responsibility analysis to assess the contribution of drugs to the accidents. The authors found that the responsibility rate for drivers with THC in their blood decreased compared with the drug-free control group. This of course contrasts with alcohol-positive drivers who show significant increases in risk.[87] A similar result was found in another study conducted in the USA[79] and more recently in Australia.[72] Limited conclusions can be drawn from the early Australian study, since only the inactive metabolite carboxy-THC was

Table 4.5 Prevalence of cannabinoids in fatally-injured drivers

| Country | Prevalence (%) | Reference |
|---|---|---|
| Australia | 11–22 | 72, 73 |
| USA | 7–37 | 74–81 |
| Norway | 5 | 82 |
| Canada | 11 | 83 |
| England/Wales | 2.5 | 84 |

measured in most cases. On the other hand, other reports have suggested an increase in culpability for cannabis users involved in crashes.[88,89]

However, THC does impair, as outlined previously. Recent studies in Australia on fatally-injured drivers suggest that drivers with THC concentrations over 2 ng/mL are more likely to be responsible for the crash.[90,91] At lower THC concentrations, or in cases with no measurable THC but with detectable carboxy-THC, there tends to be a slightly lower risk. This latter observation is consistent with observations that cannabis users reduce speed to compensate (at least partly) for their perceived impairment.[54]

It is noteworthy that cannabis impairment produces delayed reaction times, poor road-tracking performance, and decrements in divided attention tasks and hand–eye co-ordination. Inattentiveness is also a recognized sign of cannabis intoxication, leading to lack of perception of change in traffic signals and traffic flows.

The high rate of detection of cannabis-impaired drivers in jurisdictions using the American-style Drug Recognition Expert programme further confirms the problems associated with cannabis use on road safety (see Section 8).

## IMPAIRING BLOOD CONCENTRATIONS OF THC

From the early chapter on pharmacokinetics (Chapter 4.2), blood concentrations of THC above 2 ng/mL is suggestive of recent use. However, inter-individual differences in behavioural response, and the problem of the possible development of tolerance, precludes any definitive blood concentration to be assigned that is predictive of impairment except in extreme cases. Nevertheless, as the previous paragraphs suggest, drivers with significant THC in blood (probably over 2 ng/mL) tend to present as impaired and culpable.

Any evaluation or interpretation of blood concentrations of THC or its metabolites must take into account all available information and establish, if possible, the regularity of cannabis use, how much is normally used, and when the last use occurred. These questions clearly take into account whether tolerance to the behavioural effects is likely, and enable an expert to form a balanced view on the likely exposure to THC.

The measurement of carboxy-THC leads to further assumptions about previous use and possible build-up of blood concentrations, and, because it is inactive pharmacologically, is less able to predict possible behavioural changes than the measurement of THC itself.

## Synopsis

### TOXICOLOGY

1 Cannabinoids present as one of the most common drug types in forensic toxicology laboratories, and are often found in over 10% of all cases.
2 The highest incidences in sudden deaths are in drug-related (22%), homicides (17%), and drivers of motor vehicles (17%).

## Cannabis

3 The incidence in other types of forensic cases is similar, although wide variations exist from one jurisdiction to another.
4 Cannabis is not regarded as a substance capable of causing death, except in the rarest of circumstances, but it may enhance effects of opioids and other CNS active drugs.
5 THC is linked to behavioural changes, particularly those contributing to accidents involving motor vehicles.

# 4.7 Case reports

## CASE REPORT 4.1 PROOF OF CANNABIS USE

This 30-year-old female was under probation by the court and risked losing custody of her child because of drug use.

A urine test was positive for cannabinoids taken 32 days after the court order to abstain from drug use. It gave a result of 29 ng/mL of 11-nor-9-carboxy-THC.

The woman denied using drugs in this period and challenged the court interpretation that she had used cannabis in the last 32 days.

This scenario is unfortunately quite common and predictably leads to a conclusion of drug use by the person concerned. Drug use cannot be proven by this process for two main reasons. Carboxy-THC can be found in urine for up to 11 weeks after last use, and the test cannot necessarily exclude her exposure to passive smoking or other forms of inadvertent ingestion.

The carboxy-THC result of 29 ng/mL is low and would be entirely consistent with either possibility.

Serial collections of urine (monthly or weekly) would be helpful in this type of case (custody, prison testing, probation, workplace testing, etc.) to establish changes in time, although small oscillations (particularly slightly raised levels) can occur due to changing body physiology and urine output. Large increases in urinary cannabinoids will usually mean exposure or ingestion of cannabis. Corrections for urinary creatinine can reduce some of these fluctuations.

It is recommended that tests for sobriety be included with urinalysis (at meetings with officials) to establish any likely degree of intoxication or impairment. Alternatively, blood concentrations of THC can be measured to indicate recent ingestion of cannabis.

## CASE REPORT 4.2 THC BACK CALCULATION

A driver involved in a fatal collision was admitted to hospital for treatment of his injuries.

A routine blood specimen was taken for the purposes of alcohol and drug testing. This specimen was taken 2 h after the collision. Analysis showed THC was present at 0.5 ng/mL. No other drugs were detected.

The police requested a back calculation for the likely THC concentration at the time of the collision.

Such calculations are not useful since a large range of estimates are possible. These are summarized below. The formula used for calculations is based on the estimation of the loss of

# Cannabis

THC by multiplying the half-life expressed as beta (0.693/half-life in hours) by the numbers of hours elapsed. This is added to the natural logarithm of the measured blood concentration.

*Assumption 1.* Driver has not recently used cannabis and was in terminal phase of elimination, hence half-life of THC is 28 h (range 19–96 h). THC concentration is antilog of ($\log_e$ 0.50 + 693 × 2/28) = 0.53 ng/mL.

*Assumption 2.* Driver was smoking shortly before crash and was therefore in distribution phase of THC elimination, hence apparent half-life is 0.5 h (range 0.2–2 h). THC concentration is antilog of ($\log_e$ 0.50 + 0.693 × 2/0.5) = 8.0 ng/mL.

The presence of 8 ng/mL of THC in blood is highly suggestive of impairment being present in the driver, in the absence of other information. Alternatively, a level of 0.5 ng/mL emanating from use at least several hours earlier is not likely to lead to clinically measurable impairment.

Consequently, back calculations for THC are not recommended.

## CASE REPORT 4.3 CANNABIS INTOXICATION WHILE DRIVING – I

A 25-year-old male drove his motor vehicle (A) through a red light of a controlled intersection colliding with another vehicle (B) travelling through the intersection facing a green light. The driver of vehicle B was killed.

Immediately following the accident the driver of vehicle A was in a state of shock and had suffered minor head and limb abrasions that were treated at a local hospital.

Blood taken from the driver (A) 2 h after the accident returned with a carboxy-THC (total) reading of 25 ng/mL. The police subsequently charged him with culpable driving (manslaughter involving a motor vehicle).

There was no evidence to suggest the driver was driving abnormally before the accident. The accident occurred some 10 min after starting his car.

In this case a serious accident has occurred by the actions of a man who had been using marijuana. The toxicological evidence shows a positive concentration of the inactive metabolite of THC. This result demonstrates a likely use of cannabis, but because this metabolite is inactive, and could have come from ingestion several days previously, no conclusion can be made of possible impairment at the time of the accident.

The absence of abnormal driving behaviour before the accident, i.e. dangerous or erratic driving, or previously not obeying traffic signals may suggest that he was not so impaired to be incapable of proper control of a motor vehicle.[iii] A better test would be a clinical assessment of impairment by a trained physician or drug recognition expert. Hospitalization, even for a few hours for minor injuries, unfortunately often prevents any useful timely clinical examination.

---

[iii] Current Australian test for driving under the influence in most jurisdictions.

Short of admission by the driver, the only illegality that can be proven is dangerous or reckless driving and failing to obey a traffic signal. This would not be sufficient to sustain a culpable driving charge. An assessment of his sobriety immediately after the accident (if impaired) and a large positive THC level may enable an expert to conclude very recent use of cannabis associated with significant impairment.

## CASE REPORT 4.4 CANNABIS INTOXICATION WHILE DRIVING – 2

A 28-year-old female was driving her motor vehicle in a built-up area and was observed to be driving slowly and occasionally erratically. She was observed to drive through a stop sign and almost caused an accident. At this stage, she was forced to pull over by the police.

Initial discussions with the driver showed her to be in a dishevelled and 'spaced-out' state suggesting drug use. A breath alcohol returned a blood alcohol concentration of 0.045%. The driver was subsequently taken to the local police station and was examined by a forensic medical officer for possible alcohol or drug use leading to impairment. This examination took place 45 min after she was taken to the station.

The physician confirmed the initial signs by the police officer and concluded, based on a number of tests, that her cognitive and psychomotor functions were impaired with mild signs of horizontal gaze nystagmus with bloodshot eyes. There was no evidence of any medical conditions or injuries.

Blood taken from the driver at 75 min after the intercept returned with a BAC of 0.038%, a carboxy-THC (total) reading of 45 ng/mL, and a $\Delta^9$-THC reading of 5 ng/mL. The police subsequently charged her with driving under the influence of drugs.

In this case a police officer observed driving behaviour that suggested the driver was either unwell or drug affected. The act of entering an uncontrolled intersection without stopping alerted the police officer to stop the driver. Initial observations by the officer suggested drugs were being used by the driver since the slightly positive BAC did not accord with her physical state. These preliminary signs were confirmed by a trained medical practitioner who also ruled out medical conditions that might have caused or contributed to her state. The toxicological evidence of a positive concentration $\Delta^9$-THC and the inactive metabolite of THC confirmed that her medical state was probably caused by a combination of cannabis and alcohol use.

The medical examination, together with evidence of THC being present in concentrations consistent with recent use, and the police observations of driving irregularities, is the best possible scenario to establish a driving under the influence of drugs (DUID) case.

In some cases, there will be less evidence to prove a DUID case. In these situations, a DUID charge can still be proven but generally this must require good evidence of irregular driving behaviour or at least good evidence by a forensic medical officer (or equivalent) of a drug-affected state. If neither of these is available, a DUID case based solely on laboratory evidence of drug use is weak.

# References for Section 4

1. NIDA. *Prevalence of various types of drugs*. NIDA; 1995.
2. Commonwealth Department of Health and Family Services. *National Drug Strategy Household Survey*: Survey Report. Commonwealth Department of Health and Family Services; 1998.
3. Lynskey M, White V, Hill D, Letcher T, Hall W. Prevalence of illicit drug use among youth: results from the Australian School Students' Alcohol and Drugs Survey. *Aust NZ J Public Health* 1999; 23(5): 519–24.
4. Ashton CH, Kamali F. Personality, lifestyles, alcohol and drug consumption in a sample of British medical students. *Med Educ* 1995; 29(3): 187–92.
5. *United Nations World Drug Report*. New York: Oxford University Press; 1997.
6. Von Taeschner K-L. *Das Cannabis Problem*. Cologne: Deutsche Aerzte-Verlag; 1986.
7. Frank M, Rosenthal E. *Marijuana growers guide*. Berkeley, USA: And/or Press; 1978.
8. Turner CE. Marujuana research findings: 1980. Chemistry and metabolism. *NIDA Res Monogr* 1980; 31: 81–97.
9. Pertwee RG. Pharmacology of cannabinoid CB1 and CB2 receptors. *Pharmacol Ther* 1997; 74(2): 129–80.
10. Cone EJ. Marijuana effects and urinalysis after passive inhalation and oral ingestion. In: Chiang CN, Hawks RL, eds. *Research findings on smoking of abused substances*. Maryland: National Institute on Drug Abuse; 1990.
11. Jones RT. Drug of abuse profile: cannabis. *Clin Chem* 1987; 33:72B–81B.
12. Mason AP, McBay AJ. Cannabis: pharmacology and interpretation of effects. *J Forens Sci* 1985; 30(3): 615–31.
13. Wall ME, Sadler BM, Brine D, Taylor H, Perez-Reyes M. Metabolism, disposition, and kinetics of delta-9-tetrahydrocannabinol in men and women. *Clin Pharmacol Therapeut* 1983; 34: 352–63.
14. Ohlsson A, Lindgren JE, Wahlen A, Agurell S, Hollister LE, Gillespie HK. Plasma delta-9 tetrahydrocannabinol concentrations and clinical effects after oral and intravenous administration and smoking. *Clin Pharmacol Ther* 1980; 28(3): 409–16.
15. Ohlsson A, Lindgren J-E, Wahlen A, Agurell S, Hollister LE, Gillespie HK. Single dose kinetics of deuterium labelled delta 1-tetrahydrocannabinol in heavy and light cannabis users. *Biomed Mass Spectrom* 1982; 9: 6–10.
16. Huestis MA, Henningfield JE, Cone EJ. Blood cannabinoids. I. Absorption of THC and formation of 11-OH-THC and THCCOOH during and after smoking marijuana. *J Anal Toxicol* 1992; 16(5): 276–82.

# References

17. Perez-Reyes M, DiGuiseppi S, Davis K, Schindler VH, Cook CE. Comparison of effects of marijuana cigarettes of three different potencies. *Clin Pharmacol Therapeut* 1982; 31: 617–24.
18. Huestis MA, Henningfield JE, Cone EJ. Blood cannabinoids. II. Models for the prediction of time of marijuana exposure from plasma concentrations of delta 9-tetrahydrocannabinol (THC) and 11-nor-9-carboxy-delta 9-tetrahydrocannabinol (THCCOOH). *J Anal Toxicol* 1992; 16(5): 283–90.
19. Johansson EK, Hollister LE, Halldin MM. Urinary elimination half-life of delta-1-tetrahydrocannabinol-7-oic acid in heavy marijuana users after smoking. *NIDA Res Monogr* 1989; 95: 457–8.
20. Hunt CA, Jones RT. Tolerance and disposition of tetrahydrocannabinol in man. *J Pharmacol Exp Therapeut* 1980; 215: 35–44.
21. Kelly P, Jones RT. Metabolism of tetrahydrocannabinol in frequent and infrequent marijuana users. *J Anal Toxicol* 1992; 16(4): 228–35.
22. Moody DE, Monti KM, Crouch DJ. Analysis of forensic specimens for cannabinoids. II. Relationship between blood delta 9-tetrahydrocannabinol and blood and urine 11-nor-delta 9-tetrahydrocannabinol-9-carboxylic acid concentrations. *J Anal Toxicol* 1992; 16(5): 302–6.
23. McBurney LJ, Bobbie BA, Sepp LA. GC/MS and EMIT analyses for tetrahydrocannabinol metabolites in plasma and urine of human subjects. *J Anal Toxicol* 1986; 10: 56–64.
24. Wall ME, Brine DR, Pitt CG, Perez-Reyes M. Identification of delta-9-tetrahydrocannabinol and metabolites in man. *J Am Chem Soc* 1972; 94(24): 8579–81.
25. Kanter SL, Hollister LE. Marihuana metabolites in urine of man. VII. Excretion patterns of acidic metabolites detected by sequential thin layer chromatography. *Res Commun Chem Pathol Pharmacol* 1977; 17(3): 421–31.
26. Huestis MA, Mitchell JM, Cone EJ. Urinary excretion profiles of 11-nor-9-carboxy-delta 9-tetrahydrocannabinol in humans after single smoked doses of marijuana. *J Anal Toxicol* 1996; 20(6): 441–52.
27. Huestis MA, Mitchell JM, Cone EJ. Detection times of marijuana metabolites in urine by immunoassay and GC-MS. *J Anal Toxicol* 1995; 19(6): 443–9.
28. Ellis GM, Mann MA, Judson BA, Schramm NT, Tashchian A. Excretion patterns of cannabinoid metabolites after last use in a group of chronic users. *Clin Pharmacol Therapeut* 1985; 38: 573–8.
29. Cone EJ, Johnson RE, Paul BD, Mell LD, Mitchell J. Marijuana-laced brownies: behavioral effects, physiologic effects, and urinalysis in humans following ingestion. *J Anal Toxicol* 1988; 12(4): 169–75.
30. Perez-Reyes M, Owen M, Di Guiseppi S. The clinical pharmacology and dynamics of marijuana cigarette smoking. *J Clin Pharmacol* 1981; 21: 201S–207S.
31. Reeve VV, Robertson WB, Grant J, Soares JR, Zimmermann EG, Gillespie HK, *et al.* Hemolyzed blood and serum levels of delta-9-THC: effects on the performance of roadside sobriety tests. *J Forens Sci* 1983; 28: 963–71.

32. Kelly TH, Foltin RW, Emurian CS, Fischman MW. Performance-based testing for drugs of abuse: dose and time profiles of marijuana, amphetamine, alcohol, and diazepam. *J Anal Toxicol* 1993; 17(5): 264–72.
33. Cone EJ, Johnson RE. Contact highs and urinary cannabinoid excretion after passive exposure to marijuana smoke. *Clin Pharmacol Therapeut* 1986; 40: 247–56.
34. Cone EJ, Johnson RE, Darwin WD, Yousefnejad D, Mell LD, Paul BD, et al. Passive inhalation of marijuana smoke: urinalysis and room air levels of delta-9-tetrahydrocannabinol. *J Anal Toxicol* 1987; 11(3): 89–96.
35. Law B, Mason PA, Moffat AC, King LJ, Marks V. Passive inhalation of cannabis smoke. *J Pharm Pharmacol* 1984; 36(9): 578–81.
36. Mørland J, Bugge A, Skuterud B, Steen A, Wethe GH, Kjeldsen T. Cannabinoids in blood and urine after passive inhalation of cannabis smoke. *J Forens Sci* 1985; 30(4): 997–1002.
37. Perez-Reyes M, Di Guiseppi S, Mason AP, Davis KH. Passive inhalation of marihuana smoke and urinary excretion of cannabinoids. *Clin Pharmacol Ther* 1983; 34(1): 36–41.
38. Falck R. Passive inhalation of marijuana smoke [letter]. *JAMA* 1983; 250(7): 898.
39. Lehmann T, Sager F, Brenneisen R. Excretion of cannabinoids in urine after ingestion of cannabis seed oil. *J Anal Toxicol* 1997; 21(5): 373–5.
40. Struempler RE, Nelson G, Urry FM. A positive cannabinoids workplace drug test following the ingestion of commercially available hemp seed oil. *J Anal Toxicol* 1997; 21(4): 283–5.
41. Callaway JC, Weeks RA, Raymon LP, Walls HC, Hearn WL. A positive THC urinalysis from hemp (cannabis) seed oil [letter]. *J Anal Toxicol* 1997; 21(4): 319–20.
42. Alt A, Reinhardt G. Positive cannabis results in urine and blood samples after consumption of hemp food products. *J Anal Toxicol* 1998; 22: 80–1.
43. Fortner N, Fogerson R, Lindman D, Iversen T, Armbruster D. Marijuana-positive urine test results from consumption of hemp seeds in food products. *J Anal Toxicol* 1997; 21(6): 476–81.
44. Rubin A, Lemberger L, Warrick P, Crabtree RE, Sullivan H, Rowe H, et al. Physiologic disposition of nabilone, a synthetic cannabinol derivative, in man. *Clin Pharmacol Therapeut* 1977; 22(85–91).
45. Razdan RK, Howes JF. Drugs related to tetrahydrocannabinol. *Med Res Rev* 1983; 3: 119–46.
46. Johansson E, Halldin MM, Agurell S, Hollister LE, Gillespie HK. Terminal elimination plasma half-life of delta 1-tetrahydrocannabinol (delta 1-THC) in heavy users of marijuana. *Eur J Clin Pharmacol* 1989; 37(3): 273–7.
47. Moeller MR, Doerr G, Warth S. Simultaneous quantitation of delta-9-tetrahydrocannabinol (THC) and 11-nor-9-carboxy-delta-9-tetrahydrocannabinol (THC-COOH) in serum by GC/MS using deuterated internal standards and its application to a smoking study and forensic cases. *J Forens Sci* 1992; 37(4): 969–83.
48. Ashton CH. Adverse effects of cannabis and cannabinoids. *Br J Anaesthes* 1999; 83(4): 637–49.

49. Martin BR, Mechoulam R, Razdan RK. Discovery and characterization of endogenous cannabinoids. *Life Sci* 1999; 65(6–7): 573–95.
50. Chait LD, Pierri J. Effects of smoked marijuana on human performance: a critical review. In: Murphy A, Bartke J, eds. *Marijuana/cannabinoids: neurobiology and neurophysiology*. Boca Raton: CRC Press; 1992.
51. Dewey WL. Cannabinoid pharmacology. *Pharmacol Rev* 1986; 38: 151–78.
52. Stark P, Dews PB. Cannabinoids. I. Behavioural effects. *J Pharmacol Exp Therapeut* 1980; 214: 125–30.
53. Yesavage JE, Leirer VO, Denari M, Hollister LE. Carry-over effects of marijuana intoxication on aircraft pilot performance: a preliminary report. *Am J Psychiat* 1985; 142: 1325–9.
54. Robbe HWJ. *Influence of marijuana on driving*. Maastricht: CIP-Data Koninklinik Bibliothek, The Hague; 1994.
55. Van Hoozen BE, Cross CE. Marijuana. Respiratory tract effects. *Clin Rev Allergy Immunol* 1997; 15(3): 243–69.
56. Nahas G, Latour C. The human toxicity of marijuana. *Med J Australia* 1992; 156: 495–7.
57. Mathers DC, Ghodse AH. Cannabis and psychotic illness. *Br J Psychiat* 1992; 161: 648–53.
58. Thomas H. Psychiatric symptoms in cannabis users. *Br J Psychiat* 1993; 163: 141–9.
59. Solomons K, Neppe VM, Kuyl JM. Toxic cannabis psychosis is a valid entity. *South African Med J* 1990; 78: 476–81.
60. Andreasson S, Allebeck P, Engstrom A, Rydberg V. Cannabis and schizophrenia. A longitudinal study of Swedish conscripts. *Lancet* 1987; 2: 1483–5.
61. Abood ME, Martin BR. Neurobiology of marijuana abuse. *Trends Pharmacol Sci* 1992; 13: 201–6.
62. *The pharmacological basis of therapeutics*, latest edn. New York: McGraw Hill.
63. Manzanares J, Corchero J, Romero J, Fernandez-Ruiz JJ, Ramos JA, Fuentes JA. Pharmacological and biochemical interactions between opioids and cannabinoids. *TIPS* 1999; 20: 287–93.
64. Calignano A, La Rana G, Giuffrida A, Piomelli D. Control of pain initiation by endogenous cannabinoids. *Nature* 1998; 394(6690): 277–81.
65. Hall W, Solowij N, Lemon J. *The health and psychological consequences of cannabis use*. Canberra: Australian Government Publishing Service; 1994.
66. Georgotas A, Zeidenberg P. Observations on the effects of four weeks of heavy marijuana smoking on group interaction and individual behaviour. *Comp Psychiat* 1979; 20: 427–32.
67. Compton DR, Dewey WL, Martin BR. Cannabis dependence and tolerance production. *Adv Alcohol Subst Abuse* 1990; 9(1–2): 129–47.
68. Association AP. *Diagnostic and Statistical Manual of Mental Disorders (DSM-III-R)*. 3rd edn, revised. Washington: American Psychiatric Association; 1987.
69. Jones RT, Benowitz NL, Herning RI. Clinical relevance of cannabis tolerance and dependence. *J Clin Pharmacol* 1981; 21(8–9 suppl.): 143S–152S.

70. Grant BF, Pickering R. The relationship between cannabis abuse and DSM-IV cannabis abuse and dependence. *J Substance Abuse* 1999; 10(3): 255–64.
71. Chen R, Mattick RP, Baillie A. *Clients of Treatment Service Agencies*. Canberra: Australian Government Publishing Service; 1993.
72. Drummer OH. Drugs in drivers killed in Australian road traffic accidents. Melbourne: Department of Forensic Medicine, Monash University; March 1994. Report no. 0594.
73. Haworth N, Vulcan P, Bowland L, Pronk N. Fatal single vehicle crashes study. Melbourne: Monash University Accident Research Centre; September 1997. Report no. 122.
74. NHTSA. *The incidence and role of drugs in fatally injured drivers*. National Highway Traffic Safety Administration; December 1993. Traffic Tech, NHTSA Technology Transfer Series, 57.
75. Dishinger PC, Birschbach J. Alcohol and drug use among victims of vehicular crashes admitted to trauma centers. In: Perrine MW, ed. *Alcohol, drugs and traffic safety – T89*. Chicago, Illlinois: National Safety Council; 1990. pp. 586–94.
76. Caplan YH, Levine BS, Goldberger BA. Drugs in driver fatalities: a preliminary study in the State of Maryland. In: Perrine MW, ed. *Alcohol, drugs and traffic safety – T89*. Chicago, Illinois: National Safety Council; 1990. pp. 824–8.
77. Budd RD, Muto JJ, Wong JK. Drugs of abuse found in fatally injured drivers in Los Angeles County. *Drug Alcohol Depend* 1989; 23: 153–8.
78. Fortenberry JC, Brown DB, Shevlin LT. Analysis of drug involvement in traffic fatalities in Alabama. *Am J Drug Alcohol Abuse* 1986; 12: 257–67.
79. Williams AG, Peat MA, Crouch DJ, Wells JK, Finkle BS. Drugs in fatally injured young male drivers. *Public Health Rep* 1985; 100: 19–25.
80. Mason AP, McBay AJ. Ethanol, marijuana, and other drug use in 600 drivers killed in single-vehicle crashes in North Carolina, 1978–1981. *J Forens Sci* 1984; 29: 987–1026.
81. Logan BK, Schwilke EW. Drug and alcohol use in fatally injured drivers in Washington State. *J Forens Sci* 1996; 41(3): 505–10.
82. Gjerde H, Beylich KM, Morland J. Incidence of alcohol and drugs in fatally injured car drivers in Norway. *Accid Anal Prev* 1993; 25(4): 479–83.
83. Cimbura G, Lucas DM, Bennett RC, Donelson AC. Incidence and toxicological aspects of cannabis and ethanol detected in 1394 fatally-injured drivers and pedestrians in Ontario (1982–1984). *J Forens Sci* 1990; 35: 1035–41.
84. Everest JT, Tunbridge RJ. The incidence of drugs in road accident fatalities in Great Britain. In: Perrine MW, ed. *Alcohol, drugs and traffic safety – T89*. Chicago, Illinois: National Safety Council; 1989. pp. 595–601.
85. Christophersen AS, Ceder G, Kristinsson J, Lillsunde P, Steentoft A. Drugged driving in the nordic countries – a comparative study between five countries. *Forens Sci Int* 1999; 106: 173–90.
86. Committee RS. Inquiry into the effects of drugs (other than alcohol) on road safety in Victoria. Melbourne, Australia: Parliament of Victoria; 1996. Final Report.
87. Terhune KW, Ippolito CA, Hendricks DL, Michalovic JG, Bogema SC, Santinga P, *et al*. The incidence and role of drugs in fatally injured drivers. Washington: US

Department of Transportation, National Highway Traffic Safety Administration; 1992 October 30. Report DOT HS 808 065.
88. Simpson HM. Epidemiology of road accidents involving marijuana. *Alcohol, Drugs Driving* 1986; 2(3–4): 15–30.
89. Crouch DJ, Birky MM, Gust SW, Rollins DE, Walsh JM, Moulden JV, *et al*. The prevalence of drugs and alcohol in fatally injured truck drivers. *J Forens Sci* 1993; 38(6): 1342–53.
90. Drummer OH, Gerostamoulos J. The contribution of cannabis to road crashes. In: Australia and New Zealand Forensic Science Society Annual Meeting; Goldcoast, Queensland; 2000.
91. Drummer OH, Batziris H, Gerostamoulos J. Involvement of drugs in accident causation. In: National Road Safety Summit; Canberra, Australia; 1998. pp. 201–6.

# 5 Opioids

| | | |
|---|---|---|
| **Foreword** | | 220 |
| 5.1 | Source and structures | 221 |
| 5.2 | Pharmacokinetics and duration of action | 225 |
| 5.3 | Mechanisms of action | 238 |
| 5.4 | Pharmacological actions and therapeutics | 241 |
| 5.5 | Adverse reactions and dependence | 246 |
| 5.6 | Toxicology | 249 |
| 5.7 | Case reports | 261 |
| **References for Section 5** | | 265 |

# Foreword

The opioids are a large family of drugs that possess pharmacological activities related to morphine, the principal member of the group. Modifications of the morphine molecule include codeine and oxycodone, while synthetic compounds such as pethidine and methadone mimic the narcotic analgesic actions of morphine. By definition, opioids[i] also include the naturally occurring peptides that exhibit analgesic activity: the enkephalins, endorpins and dynorphins.

The opioids are a particularly important class of drugs in medicine due to their ability to relieve pain and reduce suffering; unfortunately, mainly through heroin, they are also one of most abused group of drugs. One-third of all persons treated in Australia for drug dependence (35 000–50 000) are opioid users and in 1995 there were 17 000 persons attending methadone treatment centres for opioid dependence.[1] In Australia alone, over 800 persons die each year from the use of heroin, and an estimated 200 000, or almost 1% of the population, are users of the drug.[1,2] Hospital admission episodes due to opioid overdose have been estimated to exceed 2000 annually.[3] Crime is linked to opioid use. Self-reported criminal activities (breaking, entering and stealing) of heroin users were 100 times those of non-users.[4] A high proportion of heroin users are involved in petty crime, in the selling of drugs, and in prostitution.[1]

While opioids are primarily analgesic drugs, there are other drugs that also act as analgesics that are not covered in this book. These include acetylsalicyclic acid (aspirin), paracetamol (acetaminophen in the USA), the non-steroidal anti-inflammatory drugs (NSAIDs), and a number of other drugs used in the treatment of pain.

This section will not attempt to provide a comprehensive summary of the pharmacology of each opioid member; that would overwhelm readers. Rather, a review of the pharmacological and pharmacokinetic properties of the main members of this family of drugs is presented. A description of their common medical uses and adverse effects, their ability to produce tolerance and dependence, and finally aspects of their toxicology with applications of this information in forensic cases are also included.

---

[i] Another term in common use, opiates, refers to drugs that exhibit morphine-like behaviour.

# 5.1 Source and structures

Opioids are a large family of drugs with well over 30 members in active use throughout the world. Because of the diversity of members, this section will deal predominantly with morphine, heroin, codeine, pethidine (merperidine) and some of the other members with important clinical uses and that find a presence on the street. These include methadone, laevamethadryl acetate and naltrexone, which are used in treatment programmes for opioid-dependent persons.

## SOURCES OF OPIOIDS

Opioids, with the exception of some (e.g. heroin), are available by prescription in a number of formulations: oral (normal and sustained release) tablets, sublingual tablets, solutions for injection, solutions for oral ingestion, suppositories, skin patches for transdermal delivery, and other pharmaceutical formulations. Details of the availabilities of these legal medicines can be obtained from the respective national listing of approved medicines and such references as Martindale.[5] Summaries of most common opioids are found in the monographs in the Appendix.

Heroin is widely available as an illicit drug. Heroin derives from the synthetic acetylation of morphine, or from crude extracts of the exudate from the opium poppy (*Papaver somniferum*). The exudate, or sticky gum, is known as opium and contains many alkaloids; morphine at ~10% content is the most important. Low amounts of codeine (0.5%) are also present in the gum, although the content varies from one sub-species to another and according to country of origin. The opium poppy grows in the tropical highlands of South East Asia (Burma, Laos, Thailand, Vietnam and Yunnan Province of China) and in central and southern Asia (Afghanistan, Pakistan, India), as well as in Mexico and Columbia.[3]

Legal growing of the opium poppy occurs in Australia (Tasmania), France, Spain, Turkey and India. Australia is the leading producer of morphine, supplying 44% of the world market for poppy straw, which is used to extract the morphine alkaloid.[6]

In some countries (e.g. New Zealand) codeine is demethylated in clandestine laboratories to morphine ('homebake' procedure).[7] Acetylation and formation of the hydrochloride salt yields a white crystalline powder. This powder is cut with inert sugars such as glucose and lactose and is sold on the street as heroin. Occasionally, other substances are found laced with the heroin that will modify the pharmacology and toxicology of the drug. These include lignocaine (lidocaine), quinine, strychnine and paracetamol (acetaminophen).[8] Street purities of heroin vary from less than 5% to over 70%.[3] Crude extracts such as 'Mexican black' are also a significant source of heroin. Street names for heroin include smack, skag, H, horse and hammer.

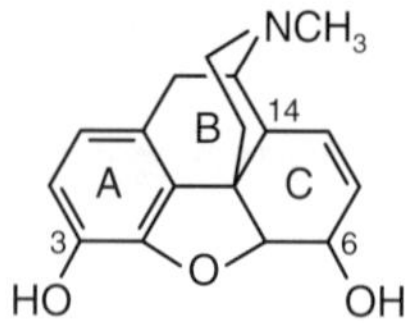

# Opioids

**Fig. 5.1** Structure of morphine

Important carbon positions are numbered, together with three of the ring systems.

## STRUCTURAL FEATURES

The structure of morphine is shown in Fig. 5.1. The main features are the three fused ring systems, labelled A, B and C, the two hydroxy substituents at the 3- and 6-positions, and the N-methyl group. A fourth ring is fused to the B-ring and contains the nitrogen (N). Variations of the morphine molecule involve these hydroxyl groups and variations in the fused ring systems. For example codeine is 3-O-methyl-morphine, and oxycodone has the 6-hydroxy converted to a keto group and contains an additional hydroxy at the 14-position.

A number of synthetic opioids have been developed that resemble morphine when viewed as a 3-D image on the receptor, although at first glance they do appear quite different. These are shown in Fig. 5.2. The relative potencies of these opioids are shown in parentheses alongside the name, i.e. strong, moderate or weak.

### Agonists

The most important opioids are N-ethylmorphine, dihydrocodeine, hydromorphone, hydrocodone, methadone, pethidine (meperidine in the USA), and fentanyl. Other examples of potent opioids also exist, including alfentanil, levorphanol, l-α-acetylmethadol (LAAM), etorphine, and remifentanil.

Designer[ii] opioid drugs exist and are particularly potent and toxic substances. These include the fentanyl derivatives, para-fluorofentanyl, α-methylfentanyl and 3-methylfentanyl. China white is 3-methylfentanyl, which is some 6000 times more potent than morphine and is active from a few micrograms. Designer opioids of pethidine (meperidine) are also known.

### Antagonists

These are a class of opioids that block the actions of morphine, but do not have any activity themselves. They are used, for example, as antidotes to morphine and heroin toxicity, e.g. naloxone. Another antagonist, naltrexone, is also used to treat opioid dependence. Their structures are shown in Fig. 5.3.

### Partial agonists/antagonists

A further type of opioids is drugs that behave like morphine (i.e. act as agonists), but also act as antagonists. These mixed agonist–antagonists are based on the morphine structure and include buprenorphine, butorphanol, and pentazocine (Fig. 5.4).

---

[ii] A designer drug is a drug modified from a legal pharmaceutical substance intended for recreational use.

Source and structures

**Natural and semi-synthetic phenanthrenes (a)**

Morphine (strong)

Ethylmorphine (weak)

Oxycodone (moderate)

Codeine (weak)

Oxymorphone (strong)

Heroin (strong)

**Synthetic phenylheptylamines (b) and phenylpiperidines (c)**

Methadone (strong, b)

Propoxyphene (weak, b)

Alfentanil (strong, c)

Pethidine (meperidine) (moderate, c)

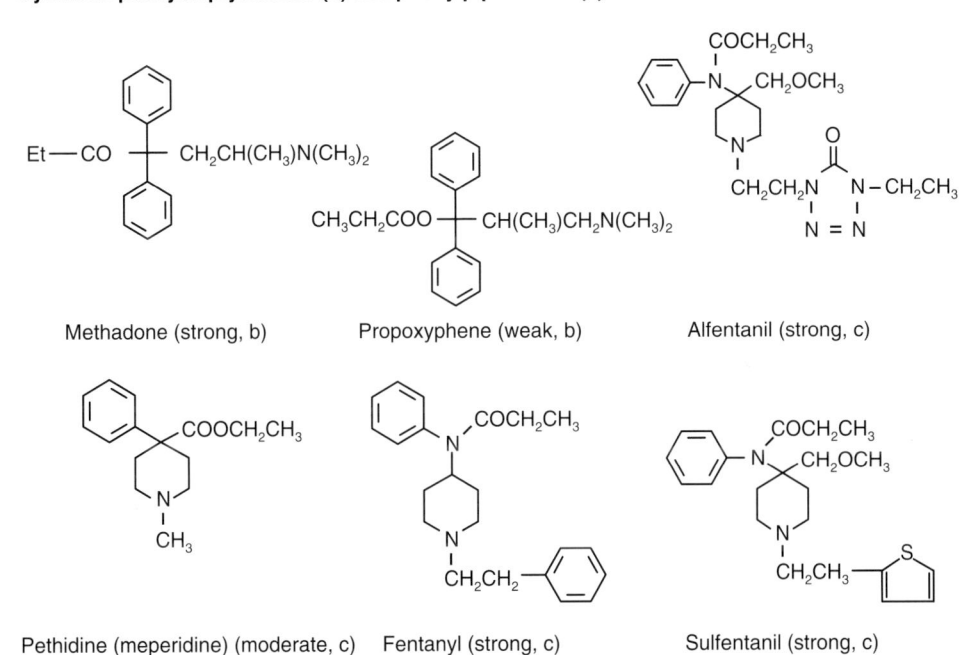

Fentanyl (strong, c)

Sulfentanil (strong, c)

**Fig. 5.2** Structures of opioid agonists

Naloxone

Nalorphine

Naltrexone

**Fig. 5.3** Structures of opioid antagonists

223

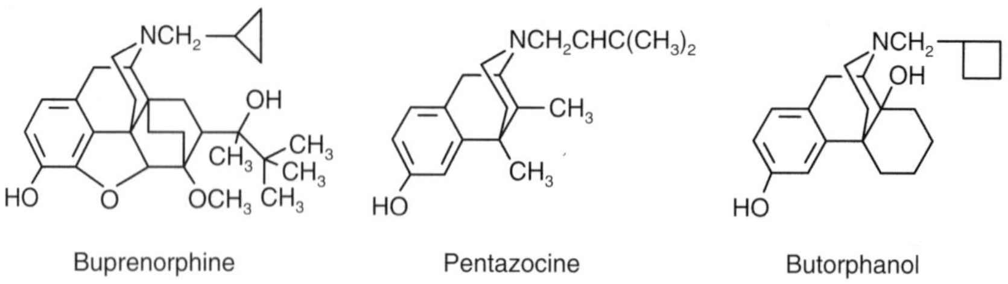

# Opioids

Buprenorphine        Pentazocine        Butorphanol

**Fig. 5.4** Structures of mixed agonist–antagonists

# Synopsis

## SOURCE AND STRUCTURES

1 Opioids (opiates) are a large family of drugs that are either naturally (morphine), derived from morphine by chemical modification (codeine, oxycodone, dihydrocodeine, hydrocodone, hydromorphone, etc.), or obtained synthetically (fentanyl, methadone, pethidine (meperidine), propoxyphene, etc.).

2 Legal opioids are available as oral (normal and sustained release) tablets, oral solutions, parenteral injections, sublingual tablets, skin patches and rectal suppositories.

3 Heroin is produced in clandestine laboratories either from acetylation of morphine derived from the opium poppy or from demethylation of codeine ('homebake'), and often comes as a white powder mixed with inert sugars such as lactose and glucose, or as a black gum known as 'Mexican black'. Occasionally, other active substituents are added, which can substantially increase toxicity. Street purities range from less than 5% to over 70%.

4 Street names for heroin include smack, skag, H, horse and hammer.

5 Morphine is the archetypal structure based on a phenanthrene ring system. Semi-synthetic opioids are based on various modifications of the hydroxyl groups, ring systems, the nitrogen, and the double bond on ring C.

6 Some opioids act as partial agonists, that is they do not exhibit full activity. The best example is buprenorphine.

7 Opioid antagonists such as naloxone and naltrexone block the effects of opioid agonists and find use either as antidotes or to treat opioid dependence.

# 5.2 Pharmacokinetics and duration of action

This chapter details some of the more important aspects of the pharmacokinetics of morphine and other opioids, including their absorption, oral bioavailability, half-lives and metabolic fate.

Readers are directed to a number of texts, as well as review articles and other relevant papers listed in the monographs for each drug (Appendix).[9–14]

## ABSORPTION AND BIOAVAILABILITY

### Oral absorption

The opioids have variable degrees of oral absorption and bioavailability. Heroin is almost totally hydrolysed to morphine before it reaches the systemic circulation, whereas the oral bioavailability of morphine is quite variable and ranges from 15% to 64%, depending on the person, the type of morphine formulation, dose and state of health. Oral bioavailabilities average 20–30%. This means that less than one-third of morphine ingested orally is available. Consequently, a 10 mg intravenous dose is equivalent to approximately 30–50 mg orally. Other opioids such as codeine, oxycodone and pethidine have much higher oral bioavailabilities (see Table 5.1).

Plasma concentrations of morphine correlate poorly with dose, with only 35% of the variation in plasma concentrations explained by the dose.[15] Individual variability in terms of pharmacokinetics, absorption and metabolism is the reason for the remaining variation. There is, however, little evidence of non-linearity of plasma concentrations with morphine dose; even the ratio of concentrations of morphine conjugates to morphine are relatively constant with dose. This means that persons receiving increasing doses of morphine will produce correspondingly higher blood concentrations providing other factors have remained constant.

First-pass metabolism accounts for the large loss of morphine following oral dosing (Fig. 5.5). In Fig. 5.5 the same dose of morphine orally gives rise to lower plasma concentrations (~one-third) than intravenous dosing (note semi-logarithmic plot).

Table 5.1 shows recommended doses, relative potencies to morphine, pharmacokinetic half-lives, and oral bioavailabilities for selected opioids.

### Absorption from other routes

Morphine is absorbed from essentially all routes with the exception of intact skin. This includes oral, sublingual and buccal, rectal, vaginal, spinal, intramuscular, intranasal and transbronchial routes.

## Opioids

**Table 5.1** Doses, relative potencies to morphine, half-lives and bioavailabilities for selected opioids

| Drug | Usual dose (mg)[a] | Relative potency[b] | Half-life (h)[c] | Bioavailability[d] | Usual therapeutic blood concentrations (mg/L) |
|---|---|---|---|---|---|
| Buprenorphine[e] | 0.2–24 | 25–50 | 3–6 | 30 | |
| Codeine | 8–60 | 0.08 | 2–4 | High | 0.01–0.25 |
| Dihydrocodeine | 30–60 | 0.1 | 2–4 | High | |
| Ethylmorphine | 25–50 | 0.1 | 2–3 | N/A | 0.1–0.3 |
| Heroin | >5 | 1.5 | <0.1 | <1% | 0.01–1.0[g] |
| Fentanyl[f] | 0.05–0.2 | 50 | 1–6 | N/A | 0.01–0.05 |
| Methadone | 5–120 | 1.0 | 8–55 | 50% | 0.02–0.5 |
| Naltrexone | 25–100 | N/A | 10 | 20% | 0.002–0.10 |
| Morphine | >10 | 1.0 | 1–8 | 20–30% | 0.01–1.0 |
| Oxycodone | 10–15 | 0.8 | 2–8 | 80% | 0.01–0.2 |
| Pethidine (merperidine) | 5–150 | 0.125 | 2–4 | 50% | 0.1–0.8 |
| Propoxyphene | 192–390 | ~0.03 | 4–24 | 30–70% | 0.1–0.8 |
| Tramadol | 50–100 | 10 | 5–7 | 75% | 0.1–0.6 |

[a] Dose range normally prescribed; [b] relative pharmacological potency to morphine; [c] pharmacokinetic half-life of terminal elimination phase; [d] oral bioavailability, relative to intravenous dose; [e] sublingual dose, very low oral bioavailability; [f] usually given parenterally; [g] as morphine.

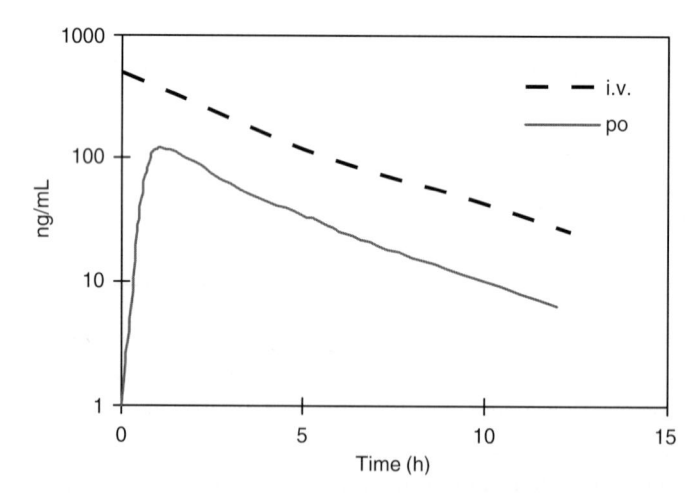

**Fig. 5.5** Stylized plasma concentration versus time plots for morphine after 50 mg intravenous (i.v.) and oral doses (po)

Rectal absorption of morphine appears to be better than oral, since first-pass metabolism in the liver is bypassed. An oxycodone suppository has a bioavailability of 60%, but the absorption is slow and is delayed with peak blood concentrations achieved much later than for oral doses.[16]

Sublingual absorption of opioids is variable. Buprenorphine (55%) and fentanyl (51%) are best absorbed, while methadone (34%) and morphine (18%) are absorbed to a lesser extent. Oxycodone, heroin and laevorphanol appear to be absorbed by this route. Maintaining a slightly basic oral pH increases sublingual absorption since more drug is unionized.[17] Fentanyl can also be absorbed from skin patches.

Morphine can be injected epidurally, intrathecally or intraventrically with good results, although morphine crosses the blood–brain barrier slowly. Morphine can also be given through a nebulizer resulting in a rapid effect, but only 5% of the drug is delivered to the systemic circulation.[18] Intramuscular administration of morphine can also be used to directly inject drug without involving liver first-pass metabolism.

There is little difference in the pharmacokinetics of morphine when given orally, sublingually or buccally. Morphine-6-glucuronide is found in concentrations greater than free morphine after all routes of administration, particularly oral, sublingual and buccal, which give rise to ratios around 6 : 1. The corresponding ratio for morphine-3-glucuronide is 30 : 1.[19]

Intranasal routes, or 'snorting', and smoking ('chasing the dragon' and 'ack ack') are now increasingly common routes for the use of heroin (in the USA), particularly heroin with high purity, and heroin in the non-salt form ('free base'). These routes absorb drug efficiently and quickly and avoid the use of syringes with the concomitant risk of infection. See later in this chapter for the pharmacokinetics of heroin and urinary excretion of heroin after different routes of administration.

The more potent opioids, alfentanil, buprenorphine, fentanyl and sulfentanil, are normally given by non-oral routes.

## Half-life and duration of action

The half-lives for most of the common opioids are relatively short. Morphine has a half-life of only a few hours at most, requiring frequent top-ups for maintenance of analgesia, often in the form of continuous morphine infusions. In contrast, methadone has a long pharmacokinetic half-life, often in excess of 1 day. The duration of action, in most cases, parallels the pharmacological response of opioids. Drugs with short half-lives will not accumulate greatly between doses, unless regular frequent doses are administered or intravenous infusions are used.

In contrast, methadone taken once a day will accumulate substantially over the first week of use reaching blood concentrations many times higher than obtained on the first day. This has significant consequences in clinical practice and in the treatment of opioid-dependent persons (see Chapter 5.6). Similar degrees of accumulation will occur with other relatively long half-life drugs, such as propoxyphene and LAAM (see monographs in the Appendix). See Table 5.1 for a list of half-lives of common opioids.

## Metabolism

Due to the diversity of chemical structures, the metabolism of opioids varies significantly between members. Morphine is essentially completely metabolized by glucuronidation at the 3- and 6-positions, whereas methadone is dealkylated leading to a cyclized product. Dealkylation pathways are also important for the drugs with larger substituents on the

# Opioids

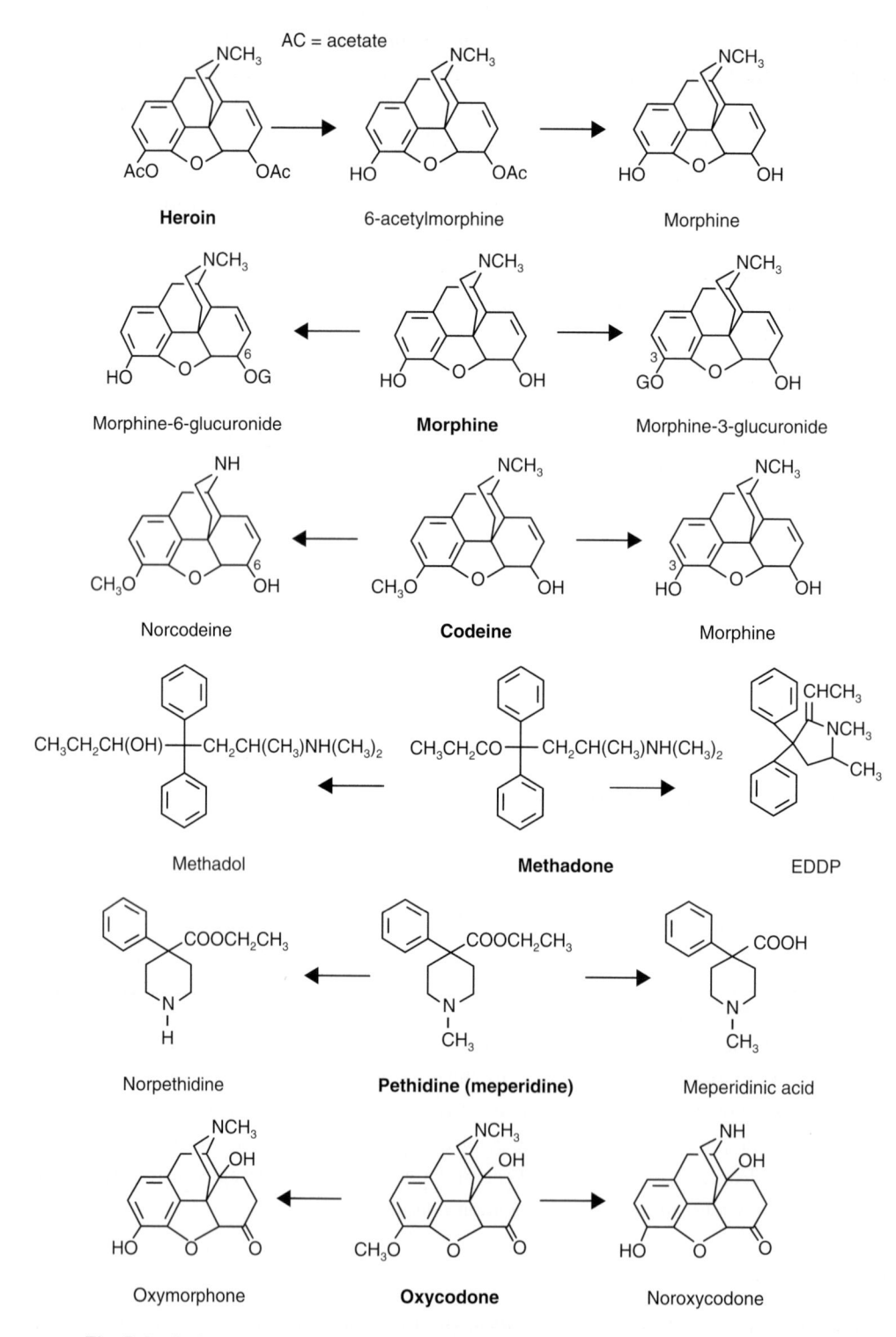

**Fig. 5.6** Pathways of metabolism of selected opioids
The two most common pathways are shown; see monographs (Appendix) for other metabolites.

N-atom, e.g. buprenorphine, butorphanol and pentazocine. Some metabolic pathways are illustrated in Fig. 5.6.

## Genetic differences and metabolic interactions

The pathways used to metabolize opioids involve both phase I and II metabolism. The CYP2D6 isozyme (isoenzyme) is largely responsible for phase I metabolism of O-methylated opioids (see Section 1).

The activity of the CYP2D6 enzyme system is affected by inheritance, as well as other factors. For example, the main metabolic pathway for codeine and ethylmorphine is the bioconversion to morphine through O-dealkylation. Some 7% of Caucasians are deficient in this enzyme and are unable to produce significant amounts of morphine.[20–22] In these people, codeine and ethylmorphine is a far weaker analgesic than in those who are able to produce morphine. The same enzyme is involved in the bioconversion and activation of oxycodone to oxymorphone, hydrocodone to hydromorphone, and the bioconversion to the active norpethidine from pethidine (meperidine), etc. The efficacy and toxicity of these drugs will therefore be affected by this genetic difference.

Methadone metabolism proceeds through at least three CYP450 enzymes, of which the 3A4 is most significant. Methadone metabolism is affected by a number of drugs and it also inhibits the metabolism of drugs proceeding through the 2D6 isozyme (see later in this chapter).

Cimetidine (used in the treatment of gastric and duodenal ulcers) will inhibit metabolism of opioids requiring microsomal cytochrome enzymes. A related drug ranitidine has also been associated with raised morphine concentrations.[15]

## Excretion

Morphine is rapidly excreted in urine as glucuronides by renal excretion, with up to 85% of the dose recovered in urine within 24 h. Only small amounts are excreted unchanged (2–10%). Following intravenous use, larger amounts of unchanged morphine are excreted in urine compared with oral use. Codeine is not produced by the metabolism of morphine.

Heroin, which is rapidly converted to morphine (within minutes), has a similar excretion profile, although small amounts of 6-acetylmorphine (6-AM) are found in the urine of most heroin users. The presence of this metabolite distinguishes heroin use from morphine. Small amounts of codeine are also present in the urine of heroin users as a result of the presence of codeine, or acetylcodeine, in the heroin.

Codeine users excrete from 2% to 23% (mean 10%) of the dose as morphine (and morphine glucuronides). Substantially greater amounts of morphine are formed following ingestion of ethylmorphine than after codeine. Urinary morphine to ethylmorphine concentrations are greater than unity during the 12–24 h period and climb to over 10 after 24 h as the urinary concentrations decrease. There is, however, considerable individual variability in the metabolism and excretion of ethylmorphine.[23]

The glucuronide metabolites of morphine and other opioids such as codeine and oxycodone are excreted into bile together with smaller amounts of parent drug. Estimates for morphine suggest about 10% is excreted into bile. Some of this biliary-excreted drug is likely to be re-absorbed, including the glucuronide conjugates (following hydrolysis in the intestine). This process is known as entero-hepatic recirculation and is responsible for a second absorption peak in the plasma concentration versus time profile of orally administered morphine.

## PHARMACOKINETICS IN VARIOUS PHYSIOLOGICAL STATES

### The elderly

Age-related changes for opioid narcotics are generally similar to those seen with other drugs, although the magnitude of the change will be dependent on the importance of phase II conjugation on the overall metabolic fate.

The clearance of morphine is reduced in the elderly (>65 years). This is associated with a smaller volume of distribution and higher blood or plasma concentrations.[24] Similar changes are likely for codeine and other phenanthrene opioids relying primarily on glucuronidation for metabolism.

More significant changes are likely with opioids metabolized primarily by the liver microsomal P450 system, e.g. pethidine (meperidine) and methadone. Clearance of pethidine (meperidine) and methadone is reduced in the elderly, requiring halving of doses.

### The young

Morphine pharmacokinetics are largely independent of age from 1 to 15 years old.[25] It is likely that under 1 year of age a reduced clearance will occur due to underdevelopment of liver enzymes.[26] Age studies in children showed clearance and half-life correlates with postnatal age. The morphine half-life reduced from 8 h in neonates under 1 week old to 2.6 h in 2–6-month-old infants.[27] The pharmacokinetics of morphine in the young may be more complex since the pharmacokinetics of morphine in neonates (gestational ages 24–41 weeks, postnatal age 4–43 h) using heroin infusions (diamorphine) is not markedly dissimilar to adults.[28]

### Liver disease

The liver has a large reserve of enzymes involved in glucuronidation, hence morphine metabolism is little affected by minor liver dysfunction. However, cirrhosis and other serious liver damage will reduce clearance leading to a longer half-life.[29] Variations in liver blood flow, degree of liver damage and extrahepatic metabolism complicates any prediction on the extent of impairment.[14] Liver disease may also affect the production of plasma proteins, which can also affect the amount of drug available for biological activity.

Clearance of pethidine (meperidine) is markedly reduced in liver disease and acute viral hepatitis, while methadone is less affected. Similar effects are likely with those opioids metabolized by dealkylation pathways.

### Kidney disease

Persons with significant kidney disease are more sensitive to morphine requiring an appropriate dose reduction. Morphine plasma concentrations increase (approximately double), and the glucuronide metabolites increase two- to three-fold.[15] Kidney disease reduces the ability of the glucuronide conjugates of morphine, and other opioids, to be excreted, hence causing an accumulation in blood.[30] The increased pharmacodynamic effect is due to increased morphine-6-glucuronide (which is pharmacologically active), and to haemodynamic changes.

## Cancer sufferers

There does not appear to be any significant change in the pharmacokinetics of morphine in persons receiving morphine for cancer pain or other forms of pain. There is a linear dose–concentration relationship for morphine over the dose range 20 mg to at least 750 mg per day. A change would be expected, however, if the weight of the patient changes dramatically and/or organ failure sets in. There does not appear to be any tolerance to the pharmacokinetic properties of the drug, rather only to the pharmacodynamic properties, i.e. analgesia.

## PHARMACOKINETIC PROFILES OF SELECTED OPIOIDS

### Morphine

Much of the pharmacokinetics of morphine has been described earlier and is covered in the section on heroin later this chapter. Useful references are also cited.[14,15,19,31]

Morphine is removed relatively rapidly by the body with a half-life ranging from 1 to 8 h. Plasma (or blood) concentrations decline with time similar to that described in Fig. 5.7 following intravenous or oral dosing. Morphine has a low oral bioavailability, therefore morphine is far more potent when given by injection (intravenous, intramuscular, intrathecal, epidural, etc.) than by the oral route.

The formation of glucuronide conjugates is also an important feature of the pharmacokinetics and toxicology of morphine. Laboratories will often measure morphine as total

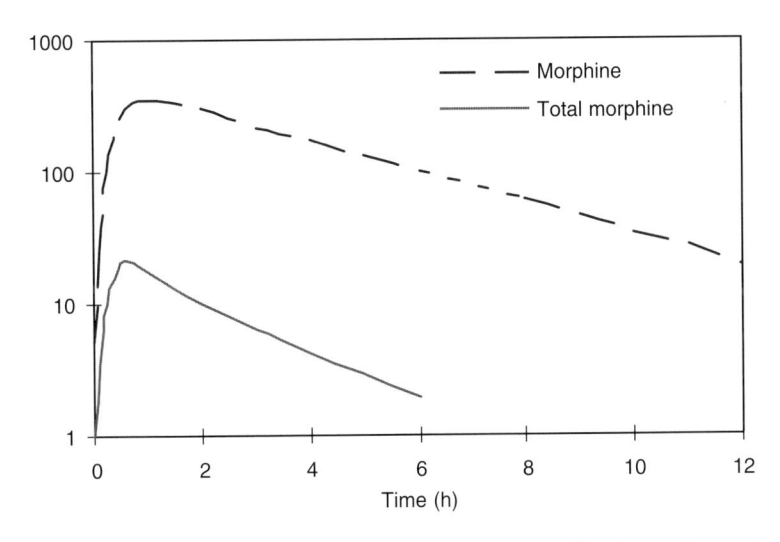

**Fig. 5.7** Stylized graph showing plasma concentration versus time profile of morphine and total morphine following a 10 mg oral dose of morphine

morphine, which includes free morphine and the sum of the two glucuronide conjugates. This total morphine concentration is often far higher than concentration of morphine itself (Fig. 5.7). One of the reasons for the measurement of total morphine is the greater ease associated with measuring these higher concentrations, since morphine levels are often undetectable after several hours. There is also little evidence to suggest that correlations of physiological effect are better if the active free morphine is measured alone. However, measurement of free morphine can provide a better estimate of time of ingestion than total morphine. In some cases, measurement of both free and total morphine may assist in estimating time of use.

There is evidence that morphine 6-glucuronide (M6G) is biologically active and contributes to the effects of morphine.[32] Increasingly, laboratories are measuring these metabolites of morphine to provide an improved ability to interpret the likely effects of morphine.

M6G (and the inactive 3-glucuronide, M3G) is produced in higher amounts following oral administration compared with other routes (intravenous, sublingual, buccal, etc.).[19] Plasma concentrations of M6G are four- to nine-fold those of morphine after oral administration and decline with a half-life of 3–11 h. M3G has a half-life of 2–9 h and is present in concentrations five times that of M6G.

In chronic high-dose situations, such as in morphine-resistant pain, plasma concentrations of morphine and morphine glucuronides can reach very high levels (without incurring a toxic response). In cases with daily doses ranging up to 1 g, mean plasma concentrations of morphine, M6G and M3G are 58, 390 and 2600 ng/mL, respectively. The mean total morphine concentration is ~2.1 mg/L.[31]

## Heroin

Heroin is widely used as an illicit drug, but is also used in some countries to treat neonates for distress (as an intravenous infusion), as a sedative and to synchronize the breathing of infants with a ventilator.[28] Heroin can also be used to treat chronic severe pain.

### Intravenous heroin

This is the most common route of injection and delivers the drug fastest to the brain. The actions are dependent on injection within a vein; missed injections will cause a slower and less complete drug absorption (subcutaneous or intramuscular).

Pharmacokinetic studies of intravenous heroin show peak heroin plasma concentrations are obtained within 2 min of dosing and are not detected after 30 min. Morphine concentrations are detectable at 1 min and peak at 5 min. Miosis (pinpoint pupils) and the behavioural effects persist for 4–6 h. Higher doses will give longer lasting effects, although these effects will depend on the tolerance (or neuroadaptation) developed to heroin. Half-lives for heroin, 6-AM and morphine are approximately 3, 10 and 120 min, respectively.[33]

Urine detection times for morphine following research doses of heroin (6–20 mg) range up to 1–2 days if a 300 ng/mL cut-off concentration is used. 6-AM will only be detectable in urine for 2–8 h following heroin use, although in some subjects no 6-AM will be detectable.[34] Higher doses will prolong the detection time in urine.

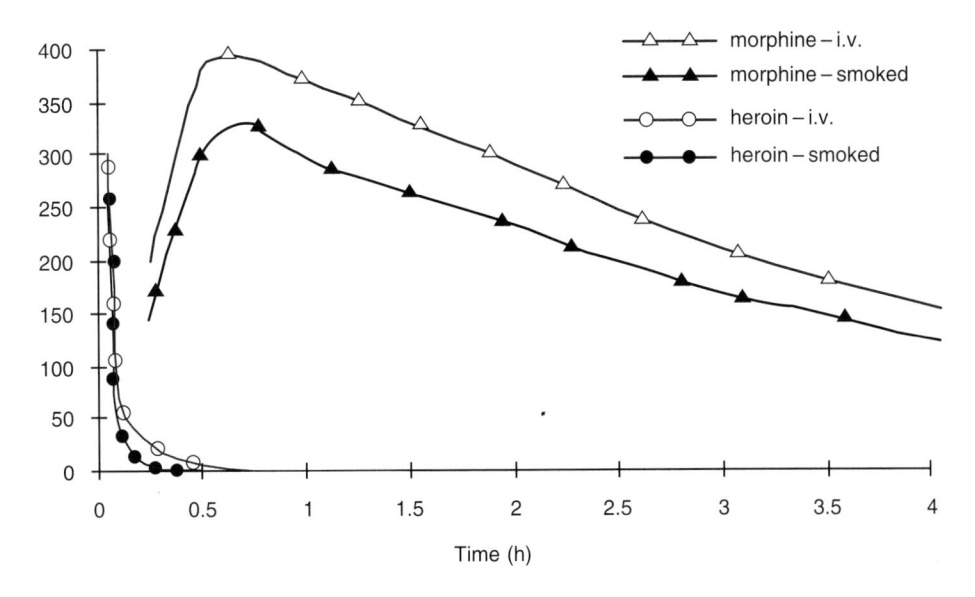

**Fig. 5.8** Plasma concentrations of morphine and heroin following intravenous and smoked administration

Smoked heroin
Smoking heroin has become an increasingly common route of administration by heroin users. Heroin can be smoked straight, in a similar manner to cocaine ('chasing the dragon'), or by adding to, or dipping in, cigarettes ('ack ack'). Freebase heroin gives a greater smoking yield than the use of the hydrochloride salt since less drug is destroyed by the heat. The prevalence of route of administration is very much dependent on changing attitudes and trends, and varies widely from one jurisdiction to another. The prevalence of smoking has been estimated as 40% in New York[35] and even higher in South East Asia (74%).[36] In Australia smoking is not a popular route of administration.

The prevalence is also likely to increase as the purity of street heroin rises and as more heroin users avoid injection by syringe, to reduce the risk of transmission of HIV and other infections, and to reduce scarring of veins.

The smoking of heroin is not as efficient as intravenous use. Estimates suggest that chasing the dragon may be only half as efficient as intravenous use, in terms of absorbed heroin. The 'ack ack' route is half as efficient probably due to a greater pyrolysis (destruction by heat) of the heroin during smoking. These estimates of drug availability will depend on the technique used and particularly how much smoke is actually inhaled. When inhaled, heroin is likely to reach the brain within 20 s.

Pharmacokinetic studies of smoked heroin base show peak heroin plasma concentrations are reached within 1–5 min of smoking and are not detected after 30 min. Morphine concentrations also peak at 1–5 min. The initial distribution half-lives of heroin and morphine are 3 and 19 min, respectively. 6-AM behaves similarly giving a half-life of 5 min. The bioavailability of smoked heroin compared with intravenous heroin ranges from 5% to 45% (as morphine). Miosis (pinpoint pupils) persists for 4 h and the behavioural effects are similar in magnitude and duration as intravenous injections of like doses of heroin.[33] Saliva contains

**Table 5.2** Characteristics of heroin administration by different routes

| Route of administration | Relative bioavailability[a] (%) | Duration of action[b] (h) | Urine detection time[c] (days) |
| --- | --- | --- | --- |
| Intravenous | 100 | 4–8 | 1–2 |
| Intramuscular | 100 | 4–6 | 1–2 |
| Nasal insufflation (snorting) | 80 | 4–8 | 1–2 |
| Smoking | 20–40 | 4 | ~1–2 |

[a] Relative to intravenous injection = 100%; [b] measured by miotic and behavioural effects; [c] using a morphine cut-off of 300 ng/mL. Note these characteristics will depend on a number of factors, including the dose and tolerance.

comparatively high concentrations of heroin (to blood) and retains heroin longer than blood concentrations.[37]

### Snorted heroin

Snorting heroin has also become increasingly used to avoid the danger of intravenous injections and the risk of HIV transmission. As for smoking, the higher the purity of heroin the greater will be the effects.

Heroin concentrations peak in blood within 5 min, while 6-AM and morphine concentrations peak at 5–10 min and within 60 min, respectively following snorting of heroin hydrochloride. Elimination half-lives of heroin, 6-AM and morphine are 5, 10 and 90 min, respectively. Changes in miosis (pupil size) and behavioural changes are similar to those observed after intramuscular administration. Miosis persists for 4–6 h after intranasal administration.[38] In subjects snorting 12 mg heroin, urine concentrations of 6-AM (cut-off limit 10 ng/mL) and morphine (cut-off limit 300 ng/mL)[iii] remain detectable for about 3 and 34 h, respectively. Higher doses will enable longer detection times. The amount absorbed is one-half to one-third of that absorbed by intramuscular injection, although the physiological and behavioural effects are similar.[39]

### Intramuscular heroin

Pharmacokinetic studies of intramuscular heroin give peak heroin plasma concentrations within 5 min of dosing and are not detected after 30–45 min. Morphine concentrations are detectable at 5 min and peak at 10 min. 6-AM plasma concentrations peak within 5 min of dosing and are not detected after 1.5 h. Miosis (pinpoint pupils) persists for 4–6 h and the behavioural effects are similar in magnitude and duration as with intravenous injections of like doses of heroin. Absorption can be highly variable depending on the site of injection, but is slower than intravenous.[38]

---

[iii] Measured as total morphine, i.e. morphine plus glucuronides.

## Fentanyl and its derivatives

Fentanyl is a synthetic opioid some 50–100 times more potent than morphine. It is usually administered by intravenous infusion as a narcotic anaesthetic, but can also be administered sublingually and dermally. It has a short pharmacokinetic half-life (1–6 h), but its actions are terminated by tissue distribution rather than metabolic clearance and excretion. This is similar to THC, thiopentone (barbiturate anaesthetic) and quazepam (benzodiazepine) in which very high fat solubility causes rapid distribution into tissues leading to low blood concentrations and rapid diminution of action. Chronic or repeated use can cause saturation of these tissue sites causing a prolonged narcosis and respiratory depression. Fentanyl is subject to abuse, particularly by the medical profession, which has greater access to it. The effects of fentanyl and its derivatives are generally similar to other opioids.

There are a number of fentanyl derivatives available throughout the world; alfentanil, sulfentanil, lofentanil and carfentanil have been reviewed by Mather.[40] Alfentanil is less distributed into body fat than fentanyl, while the properties of sulfentanil lie between alfentanil and fentanyl. Usual doses of fentanyl for anaesthesia are 0.05–0.2 mg. Plasma concentrations of fentanyl following therapeutic use are typically less than 10 ng/mL, although concentrations over 100 ng/mL are obtained in some surgical procedures.

Since blood concentrations of fentanyl are low it is best measured by GC-MS techniques, although specific radioimmunoassays are available for screening and quantitation analyses. The greatest concentrations of fentanyl occur in lung, kidney, spleen and fat. In contrast, alfentanil shows affinity for stomach compared with other tissues, hence its presence in gastric contents should not necessarily imply oral consumption.

## Codeine

Codeine is one of the most widely used opioids. It is freely available in some countries as low-dose over-the-counter preparations with other drugs such as aspirin and paracetamol. Codeine is a weak analgesic whose narcotic properties are likely to be substantially mediated by the minor metabolite, morphine. It is of interest that ~7% of the population are poor metabolizers of codeine to morphine due to their deficiency in the CYP2D6 isozyme. These people are less likely to respond to codeine use as an analgesic.

Blood concentrations of codeine in all subjects (poor metabolizers and normal metabolizers) following a 50 mg oral dose range from 0.05 to 0.15 mg/L (mean 0.09 mg/L). This peak concentration occurs at 0.3–1.5 h (mean 1 h). The elimination half-life of codeine is 2.5 h. The concentration of codeine glucuronide are approximately 15 times higher than codeine itself and decline with a half-life of ~2 h. Morphine concentrations are often only a fraction of codeine concentrations in plasma (~2%) in normal metabolizers and are undetectable in poor metabolizers.[41]

Urinary excretion shows a number of metabolites, including codeine glucuronide (~70%), codeine (~3.5%), traces of morphine 3- and 6-glucuronides, and morphine. Morphine excretion in normal metabolizers is 6%, but only 0.3% in poor metabolizers.

As discussed previously, the ratio of urinary codeine and morphine concentrations is >1 until about 22–36 h when it becomes less than unity.[42] The change in urinary codeine morphine ratios is due to the longer half-life of morphine. Urinalysis can detect codeine use for 1–2 days, depending on the dose used and methods employed.[43]

## Methadone

Methadone differs from morphine since its oral activity is similar to its intravenous potency and because it has a long terminal elimination half-life. Half-lives of 1 day are often quoted, but the half-life can vary at least five-fold with a range of 8.5–58 h.[44] The half-life is complicated by two apparent elimination half-lives (mean 14 and 55 h).[45] Once-daily dosing will cause an accumulation of blood and tissue levels for at least 1 week of dosing, even without dose adjustment, resulting in a three- to eight-fold increase in blood concentrations of methadone.[45]

Blood concentrations of methadone following a single dose of 15 mg peak at 0.075 mg/L. Chronic dosing will produce blood concentrations of 0.1–0.5 mg/L. Higher doses produce correspondingly higher blood concentrations after steady state has been reached at 1 week, although there is wide individual variability.

The pharmacokinetics of methadone are further complicated by the variation in half-life with urinary pH. Subjects with acidic urine have half the elimination half-life of those with basic urine (20 versus 43 h). This is also associated with a corresponding change in body clearance. The oral bioavailability of methadone is also variable, varying from 40% to over 90%.[44]

Changes in the pharmacokinetics and metabolism of methadone from acute to chronic treatment in maintenance treatment are also known. The urinary and faecal excretion of methadone and its monomethylated metabolite increased from 22% to 62% and the urinary metabolite to methadone ratio triples during chronic therapy.[45] Lower urinary pH and increases in renal clearance in the first month of treatment have also been observed.[46]

Methadone metabolism and therefore its excretion are affected by a number of drugs, all of which affect the activity of P450 enzymes. Antiviral drugs used to treat HIV infection, such as ritanovir, decrease blood concentrations of methadone by increasing the activity of the enzymes.[47,48] Similar effects are seen with barbiturates and some anticonvulsants, such as phenytoin,[49] and with the antifungal drug fluconazole.[50]

Serotonin re-uptake antidepressants such as fluvoxamine increase blood concentrations of methadone and predispose the patient to an increased risk of toxicity.[49,51]

Methadone can be injected intravenously, particularly if solid methadone is available. The kinetics of this route will be similar to other drugs administered intravenously. Very high blood concentrations are obtained within minutes followed by a rapid distribution phase and a much slower elimination phase, which is identical to oral administration.

Methadone is found in low concentrations in breast milk of mothers, but the dose presented to suckling babies is minimal and unlikely to provide a significant problem to the neonate.[52,53]

## Naltrexone

Naltrexone is an antagonist of the opioid receptor and is used in the treatment of opioid dependence. Peak concentrations of naltrexone following an oral dose of 100 mg are 44 ng/mL at 1 h, although there is a wide range in plasma concentrations. The elimination half-life is ~10 h resulting in significant plasma concentrations at 24 h (2 ng/mL). There is little accumulation of naltrexone during chronic administration. One dose of 100 mg naltrexone blocks the effects of 25 mg morphine for up to 48 h.[54]

The major metabolite, β-naltrexol, is also active and reaches higher plasma concentrations than naltrexone, and the half-life is slightly longer than the parent drug.

## Synopsis

**PHARMACOKINETICS AND DURATION OF ACTION**

1. Opioids have variable oral absorption; essentially no heroin reaches the blood after oral use, and some 20–30% of morphine is bioavailable, while the synthetic opioids such as methadone and pethidine (meperidine) show good oral bioavailability.
2. Most of the potent opioids are designed not for oral use, but for parenteral injections (intramuscular, intravenous, epidural, intrathecal) for specialist medical use. Skin patches exist for fentanyl, sublingual tablets exist for buprenorphine, and rectal suppositories for oxycodone are available, as well as numerous sustained-release formulations.
3. Heroin can be taken by nasal insufflation (snorting), by inhalation of vapours or by smoking, as well as by the usual intravenous injection.
4. Half-lives of opioids are generally short (morphine has a half-life of 2–3 h); however, drugs such as methadone with a half-life exceeding 1 day must be used quite differently to prevent undue accumulation of drug and risk of toxicity.
5. Opioids are metabolized both by conjugation (phase I) metabolism (e.g. morphine, codeine, etc.), as well as oxidative phase II processes (codeine, methadone, pethidine (meperidine), etc.) and show genetic variability leading to a small group of persons with an inability to produce some metabolites (i.e. morphine from codeine).
6. Most opioids are excreted into urine substantially as metabolites. Morphine-like drugs will show similarity in urine excretion products and require careful evaluation to prevent false conclusions of heroin or morphine use in codeine users, or heroin use in morphine users.
7. Age and disease states affect the pharmacokinetics (and response) to opioid drugs. Liver disease mostly affects those drugs metabolized by phase II processes, kidney disease affects all opioids, while advanced age tends to cause a gradual decline of all metabolic and excretory processes. Children, with the exception of neonates, show little difference to adults in the pharmacokinetics of morphine.
8. Pharmacokinetic profiles of morphine, heroin (various routes of administration), codeine, fentanyl, methadone, and naltrexone are provided.

# 5.3 Mechanisms of action

Opioids, like the benzodiazepines, interact with specific binding sites in the CNS. It is this interaction that results in most, if not all, of the pharmacological effects of morphine and its analogues. The receptors are located mainly in the brain and spinal cord regions, although there are receptors in peripheral tissues such as the gastrointestinal system.

Opioids are believed to mimic the actions of endogenous substances that are natural analgesics. These endogenous substances termed 'endogenous opioid peptides' include β-endorphin, leu-enkephalin and met-enkephalin as well as dynorphins (A and B) and neoendorphins (α and β). These peptides are present at brain sites containing the specific opioid receptors and are released by the body to modulate pain.

When opioids bind to specific receptors in the spinal cord (nerves that transmit pain) they inhibit the release of excitatory neurotransmitters. Opioids also inhibit the release of neurotransmitters in primary afferent nerve fibres that relay pain signals to nerves in the spinal cord. The net result is a powerful analgesic effect. The actual biochemical mechanism for these processes is complex and are not completely understood. However, they involve changes in the coupling of a G-protein to the regulatory enzyme adenylate cyclase. This produces an intracellular mediator and facilitates the opening of $K^+$ ion channels, and inhibits opening of $Ca^{++}$ channels.[55]

There are three main types of receptors based on their location and function; these are called μ (mu), δ (delta) and κ (kappa), and each has sub-types. The receptor classification of opioids is based on the relative affinity of opioids to these receptor types and to their effects.

The following references are recommended reading on the mechanisms of opioid action and classification of opioid receptor sub-types.[11,55,56]

## MU-OPIOID RECEPTOR

Morphine acts mainly on the μ-receptor, which is primarily responsible for the analgesic actions of opioids. Most of the common opioids are full agonists (produce maximum positive response) at the μ-receptor. This receptor is also responsible for the often unwanted effects of opioids, such as respiratory depression, constriction of pupils (miosis), reduction in motility of the gastrointestinal system, as well as the euphoric effects, sedation and physiological dependence.

The selectivity of actions of certain opioids is shown in Table 5.3. This shows that the most common opioids act on the μ-receptor. Some opioids show activity at the other receptor types. The receptor antagonists naloxone and naltrexone block the effects of agonist opioids at these μ-sites as well as the other receptor types. More selective agents have now been identified that show less activity at the other receptor types.[55]

## DELTA-OPIOID RECEPTOR

This opioid receptor occurs at different locations within the brain to the μ-receptor but also mediates analgesia, respiratory depression, euphoria and dependence. The functional

# Mechanisms of action

**Table 5.3** Receptor selectivities for some opioids[a]

| Opioid | μ (mu) | δ (delta) | κ (kappa) |
|---|---|---|---|
| **Full agonists** | | | |
| Codeine | + | + | − |
| Etorphine | +++ | +++ | +++ |
| Fentanyl | +++ | + | − |
| Methadone | +++ | + | + |
| Morphine | +++ | + | + |
| Pethidine (meperidine) | +++ | + | + |
| Sulfentanil | +++ | + | − |
| **Partial agonists** | | | |
| Buprenorphine | +++[a] | − | Antagonist |
| Pentazocine | Antagonist | + | ++ |
| **Antagonists** | | | |
| Naloxone | Antagonist | Antagonist | Antagonist |
| Naltrexone | Antagonist | Antagonist | Antagonist |

[a] Partial receptor agonist at this receptor; number of + indicates relative agonist activity; − no activity.

significance of this receptor is less clear but seems to be involved more with peripheral pain control. The classical opioids have only weak activity at this receptor. Etorphine is the best agonist.

## KAPPA-OPIOID RECEPTOR

This receptor occurs in the spinal cord and mediates spinal analgesia and sedation, and supports only low physical dependence. Pentazocine and etorphine are the best opioid drugs at this site.

## OTHER ACTIONS

There are other recognition sites such as the sigma receptor, which is not selective for opioids and appears to account for the hallucinogenic and dysphoric properties of opioids, and the hallucinogens phencyclidine and ketamine.

# Synopsis

## MECHANISMS OF ACTION

1 Opioids interact with specific recognition sites, or receptors, in the brain and other parts of the body.
2 These sites are regulated by endogenous opioids, such as the enkephalins, endorphins and dynorphins.

## Opioids

3 Opioids act on these receptors to inhibit excitatory neurotransmitters in the brain and inhibit transmission of pain signals to the spinal cord.
4 There are three main sub-types of opioid receptors that have been characterized: μ (mu), δ (delta) and κ (kappa).
5 The mu-opioid receptor is the main opioid receptor site and is responsible for the principal analgesic action of morphine and other related opioids.
6 The delta-opioid receptor occurs at different locations in the brain to mu-opioid receptors and is involved more with peripheral pain control. Etorphine is the best opioid acting on this receptor sub-type.
7 The kappa-opioid receptor occurs in the spinal cord and mediates spinal analgesia. Pentazocine is the most effective drug at this opioid receptor subtype.
8 The opioid-receptor antagonists (naloxone etc.) block the actions of opioids at all opioid receptor sub-types.

# 5.4 Pharmacological actions and therapeutics

The main pharmacological uses of opioids are for the relief of pain, both acute and chronic. The definition of pain is too complex to easily detail here. Readers are referred elsewhere.[12,56,57] Nociception is a term used by pharmacologists to refer to the mechanism by which the body responds to noxious peripheral stimuli. Pain is a subjective response to a variety of situations including those deriving from noxious stimuli, e.g. tissue damage, and is not always associated with nociception. Chronic pain is usually defined as pain that outlasts the precipitating tissue injury.

This chapter reviews the pharmacological effects of opioids and their clinical uses. A number of reviews or texts are recommended reading.[56,58,59]

## USES OF OPIOIDS

### Analgesia and euphoria

Morphine and the other opioids are effective in most types of acute and chronic pain, although pain of neuropathic origin, such as phantom limb, trigeminal neuralgia, etc., is less well controlled. Importantly, morphine and its derivatives also reduce the affective component of pain, i.e. the emotional or psychological component. This is important in chronic pain states where emotional distress can be severely debilitating. The use of morphine will therefore reduce suffering.

The euphoric effects are an important component of reducing distress in persons and are likened to a sudden elevation of mood, even an orgasm, particularly if used intravenously. Euphoria is not always present and depends on the circumstances. Distressed patients will usually achieve an euphoric state, while long-term sufferers of chronic pain may even feel dysphoric.

The euphoric state is clearly one of the main reasons for the recreational use of heroin and other opioids.

Euphoria is mediated through the μ-opioid receptor, although weak opioids acting on this sub-type, such as codeine, dihydrocodeine and ethylmorphine, do not exhibit this effect.

### Acute pulmonary oedema and respiratory distress

Morphine is used intravenously to treat pulmonary oedema due to left ventricular failure and in neonates to treat respiratory distress.

## Diarrhoea

Opioid narcotics are well known to produce constipation. This effect is used to treat diarrhoea. Those designed to minimize CNS side effects are preferred. These include diphenoxylate and codeine.

## Anaesthesia

Opioids are frequently used as pre-medicant drugs before anaesthesia and surgery, and are used in operations as adjuncts to other anaesthetics, or as primary anaesthetics in cardiovascular surgery to minimize cardiovascular depression. Because of their direct action on the spinal cord, opioids are used as regional analgesics by administration into the epidural or subarachnoid spaces of the spinal column. For example, doses of epidural morphine are only 3–5 mg. Fentanyl is often used in surgical procedures as an anaesthetic, as are related opioids such as alfentanil and sulfentanil.

## Suppression of cough reflex

The weaker opioids show antitussive activity and are used to suppress cough. Codeine at low doses acts as an antitussive. Other drugs used as antitussives exhibit little if any analgesic activity and are unlikely to produce dependence. These include pholcodine, dihydrocodeine, ethylmorphine and dextromethorphan.

One of the important adverse reactions in abusers of opioids such as heroin, or in patients on methadone programmes, is the suppression of the cough reflex, which can lead to respiratory difficulties.

# SIDE EFFECTS OF OPIOIDS

## Respiratory depression

All opioids produce depression of the respiratory centres with normal analgesic doses. The response is exhibited by a decrease in rate and depth of breathing. The depressant effect is associated with a decrease in the sensitivity of the respiratory centre to carbon dioxide. Opioids produce this effect without causing depression of the brain regions (medulla) that control cardiovascular function. Other drugs that act as CNS depressants usually exhibit non-specific depression of the medullary centres, e.g. barbiturates, alcohol, etc., and if present, will exacerbate the opioid effects on respiration.

Patients with respiratory disease such as emphysema, kyphoscoliosis, cor pulmonale and asthma are also more likely to develop adverse respiratory reactions to opioids.

## Nausea and vomiting

Almost half of patients using opioids experience nausea and vomiting, but this effect usually declines in severity with repeated dosing, i.e. tolerance develops. Drugs can be used to minimize these side effects, such as metoclopramide (Maxolon and others).

## Gastrointestinal tract and genito-urinary system

One of the better-known effects of morphine is constipation; this is a significant side effect caused by reduction in motility and an increase in tone of the gastrointestinal system. These effects may worsen existing bowel complaints, cause biliary spasm, and cause pancreatitis. Its effect on the genito-urinary system may provide difficulty in passing urine. This also leads to a reduced rate of gastric emptying and will retard the absorption process of other co-administered drugs.

## Pupillary constriction

Miosis is caused by direct action of opioids on the $\mu$- and $\kappa$-opioid receptors and can be diagnostic of opioid use. Tolerance does not develop to any significant degree with repeated dosing; hence, heroin-dependent persons will normally exhibit some degree of miosis. Drugs can be used to mask miosis, in particular atropine and related alkaloids found in deadly nightshade (*Atropa belladonna*) and in many of the Solanaceae family including *Datura* species. Coma and hypoxia will also cause pupillary dilatation.

## Cardiovascular changes

Morphine and related opioids produce little direct effect on blood pressure and heart function. However, they inhibit baroreceptor reflexes, which can lead to sudden orthostatic hypotension and fainting in a person who suddenly sits or stands from a supine position. High doses may even precipitate bradycardia and hypotension directly.

Different opioids can have specific effects on the cardiovascular system. Morphine and pethidine (meperidine), but not fentanyl, also release histamine, which can lead to hypotension. Pethidine (meperidine) can cause an atropine-like effect causing a high heart rate, while fentanyl and sulfentanil can cause a profound lowering of heart rate at higher doses.

Opioids in combination with other drugs particularly the phenothiazines (thioridazine etc.) can cause hypotension. Opioid overdose following a sudden intravenous injection of heroin will of course exacerbate these effects and may lead to cardiovascular collapse due to a reduction in peripheral resistance and hypotension.

Opioids also cause bronchoconstriction leading to asthma-like symptoms and are therefore not advised in asthmatics.

## Effect on the central nervous system and on cognitive functions

Opioids affect both the sensory and affective components of pain, providing pain is present. Opioids can also produce sedation and narcosis. Drowsiness leading to sleep is one of the typical effects of a person using heroin or morphine, although the sleep is not usually deep. Conscious state is often clouded leading to a diminution of mental state. Apathy, reduced visual acuity, reduced physical activity and lethargy are also common. The user is more likely to be in a 'drugged' or 'stoned' state, although there is a component of paradoxical excitement.

Respiratory depression is a major side effect and can occur at low doses unless tolerance has developed. This respiratory depression is affected by the conscious state. Persons awake and in pain are less likely to develop respiratory depression than those asleep. In fact most deaths of methadone users occur during the night.[60–62] Factors that affect respiratory function include respiratory disease, pneumonia and emphysema. Other CNS depressant drugs will exacerbate this effect.

Miosis (pinpoint pupils) is a readily observable symptom of opioid use and is a tell-tale sign of opioid overdose. Interestingly, significant tolerance does not develop to this effect, although drugs such as atropine and the belladonna alkaloids can reverse the miotic effects of opioids.

These side effects are important to consider in the overall profile of a heroin addict because they contrast with drug effects seen with the amphetamine-like stimulants and cocaine. Sedation and reduced cognition are also important in situations involving monotonous activity such as car driving, where inattention and fatigue are more likely to operate.

### Opioids and the effect on food and water intake

Opioids are known to increase alcohol drinking, which is blocked by the opioid antagonist naltrexone. It is therefore not surprising that many heroin users also drink alcohol. In fact over 30% of all heroin deaths have consumed significant amounts of alcohol prior to death.[63,64] This assumes more importance since alcohol will also substantially contribute to any toxic effect of opioids.

Benzodiazepines also increase thirst. Opioid antagonists block the thirst and increased food consumption induced by benzodiazepines. Biochemical links have also been established in which benzodiazepines release enkephalin from brain regions such as the striatum. This suggests a link between endogenous opioids (enkephalin etc.) and the benzodiazepine sites of action probably by interconnecting neural pathways.[65] This link is supported by the high prevalence of benzodiazepines in heroin users.[64,66]

### Effects on behavioural aggression

There is no particular aggressive reaction attributed to opioids, although opioids may modify the behavioural reactions to other drugs such as alcohol, amphetamines and benzodiazepines. See individual sections on these drugs for more details.

## NON-MEDICAL USES OF OPIOIDS

Clearly opioids have a large non-medical use, although this should best be referred to as abuse. Heroin is the main abused opioid, although most other opioids are also abused. These are either obtained by prescription under false pretences, obtained from burglaries of medical and pharmaceutical premises, or, in the case of heroin, produced in clandestine laboratories.

The reasons for their use are multifactorial but usually stem from social and/or psychological needs. The neurobiology of opioid abuse is reviewed.[55]

## THERAPEUTICS

Therapeutic concentrations of opioids vary widely depending on their potency (and consequently dose), protein binding, volume of distribution and rate of metabolism, and as the next section details, the degree of tolerance. Since persons using opioids can develop tolerance to doses well over a factor of 50, plasma concentrations of drug do not relate to an effect unless tolerance can be quantified. In practice, tolerance cannot be properly quantified. While plasma concentrations of morphine and pethidine (meperidine) have been defined for minimum analgesia in acute use, there is no safe therapeutic concentration for opioids. Blood concentrations of opioids, which can produce a therapeutic response (i.e. analgesia), can equally well cause respiratory depression.

Therefore therapeutic concentrations of opioids overlap completely with toxic (fatal) concentrations. Table 5.1 provides an indication of blood plasma concentrations expected for the various opioids.

The additional use of sedatives such as benzodiazepines can result in enhanced sedation and drowsiness. Mixing opioids with alcohol or other drugs will also exacerbate the effects.

## Synopsis

**PHARMACOLOGICAL ACTIONS AND THERAPEUTICS**

1 The main pharmacological uses of opioids are:
   (a) to relieve mild to moderate pain (codeine, propoxyphene);
   (b) to relieve moderate to severe pain (morphine, methadone, oxycodone, pethidine (meperidine));
   (c) to treat pulmonary oedema and respiratory distress (morphine, heroin);
   (d) to treat diarrhoea (diphenoxylate, codeine);
   (e) to supplement other anaesthetics or act as anaesthetics (fentanyl derivatives);
   (f) to relieve coughing (weak opioids with antitussive action, pholcodine, dextromethorphan, dihydrocodeine).

2 Side effects of opioids include:
   (a) respiratory depression, which can occur at therapeutic doses;
   (b) nausea and vomiting;
   (c) constipation, increase in biliary pressure, difficulty in micturition, pancreatitis;
   (d) pupillary constriction (miosis);
   (e) cardiovascular changes: hypotension, low heart rate;
   (f) bronchoconstriction and asthma-like symptoms;
   (g) respiratory depression, or arrest of respiration;
   (h) clouding of conscious state, lethargy, reduced visual acuity;
   (i) increased thirst, leading to increased alcohol consumption.

3 Therapeutic concentrations of moderate to strong opioids overlap completely with toxic concentrations.

4 Other CNS active drugs increase potential for toxic response when used with opioids (see Chapter 5.6).

# 5.5 Adverse reactions and dependence

The opioids are probably better known for their side effects and adverse reactions than most other classes of drugs. Tolerance, dependence and even addiction characterize these drugs. Other important adverse reactions are also a feature of opioids. This chapter reviews these features for the main members of the family. Cited texts are recommended reading.[58,59]

## DEPENDENCE AND TOLERANCE

Heroin, morphine and many of the other opioids are well known to produce tolerance and dependence with repeated use. This applies particularly with those opioids with μ-activity such as heroin, morphine, pethidine (meperidine), fentanyl and methadone. Tolerance develops rapidly to the analgesic, euphoriant, sedative and respiratory depressant effects of opioids, but not to the miotic and constipating effects.

The mechanism for the development of tolerance and drug dependence is complex and not fully understood but is believed to involve a reduction in the number of μ-receptors and a reduction in the efficiency in coupling of the receptor to its biochemical responses, which include calcium ($Ca^{++}$) flux into cells, inhibition of adenylate cyclase and protein phosphorylation.

The tolerance developed to opioids can be substantial. A 20-mg dose of morphine (intravenously) can kill an opiate-naïve person, whereas daily doses of over 2000 mg (2 g) can be tolerated in a person accustomed to the drug. This tolerance can develop quite rapidly, even within hours in patients receiving morphine by continuous intravenous infusion. In practice, illicit drug users tend to use heroin sporadically resulting in high and low blood concentrations with relatively long intervals between doses. In this situation drug tolerance and physiological dependence are unlikely to develop to any significant degree.

On the other hand, oral administration of morphine or another orally active opioid, such as methadone, oxycodone, pethidine (meperidine), etc., can lead to a longer period of action because of the delayed and sustained nature of oral absorption. Persons using drugs with long half-lives such as methadone are particularly prone to developing tolerance since substantial accumulation will occur from one dose to another.

Cross-tolerance occurs with opioids, as it does for the benzodiazepines. This means that a person tolerant to morphine will also be tolerant to other opioids acting on the μ-opioid receptor.

## WITHDRAWAL SYMPTOMS

Abstinence symptoms in tolerant persons abstaining from opioids are characteristic, and include anxiety, chills, diarrhoea, gooseflesh, hostility, hyperthermia, muscular aches, rhinorrhoea,

# Adverse reactions and dependence

**Table 5.4** Symptoms associated with abstinence and opioid toxicity

| Symptoms of abstinence[a] | Symptoms of toxicity |
|---|---|
| Anxiety | Bradycardia (low heart rate) |
| Chills | Difficulty with urination |
| Diarrhoea | Headache |
| Gooseflesh | Noisy breathing when sleeping |
| Hostility | Pinpoint pupils |
| Hyperthermia | Reduced respiratory rate |
| Muscular aches | Sleepy and narcosed |
| Rhinorrhoea (runny nose) | Unrousable sleep |
| Sweating | Unsteady gait |
| Tachycardia (high heart rate) | Vomiting |
| Tachopnoea | |
| Vomiting | |

[a] Assuming person has become physiologically dependent to opioids. Symptoms are organized alphabetically in each column.

sweating and vomiting. These are distinguishable from signs of toxicity (Table 5.4). As with all drug withdrawal symptoms, the time of onset, and the intensity and duration of symptoms will depend on numerous variables not least of which are the type of opioid used and the frequency of administration.

In general, withdrawal from opioids with short half-lives, e.g. heroin and morphine, will produce a rapid onset of symptoms compared with methadone. Heroin users will exhibit abstinence symptoms within 6–10 h, which become maximal at about 36–48 h. Symptoms gradually subside over 1 week. Methadone users will require much longer (several days) to reach maximum abstinence symptoms.

There appears to be a significant component of psychological dependence in heroin users, (see Section 1) which is related to the euphoric sensation achieved with the intravenous injection and a range of social pressures that led to drug use in the first place. This should not be confused with physical (chemical) dependence, which has a physiological basis.

The opioid receptor antagonists (naloxone, nalbuphine, naltrexone), or mixed agonist/antagonists (pentazocine) will often produce abstinence symptoms in opioid-dependent persons. These symptoms can be severe if a person has developed a significant tolerance. The use of these agents is not recommended unless an overdose to an opioid is suspected. Many must also be used intravenously due to their low oral bioavailability.

## IMPORTANT DRUG INTERACTIONS

Benzodiazepines can interact with potent opioids causing a reduction in blood pressure and an enhanced pharmacological response. This phenomenon has been reported for sulfentanil, fentanyl and morphine. In addition, combining a benzodiazepine such as midazolam with morphine or fentanyl increases anaesthesia and the depression of the CNS. In fact, midazolam and fentanyl are commonly combined in minor surgical procedures. Diazepam (and probably other benzodiazepines) boosts the effects of methadone in maintenance subjects.[66]

A second well-known drug interaction is combining an opioid with a neuroleptic drug (antipsychotic drug). For example, fentanyl and droperidol are used to induce a neuroleptanalgesic state in which the patient is in a trance; i.e. calm and indifferent to the surroundings. Other neuroleptics such as thioridazine or chlorpromazine are also used to enhance analgesic potency of morphine; they enhance the possibility of low blood pressure.

Since some opioids are metabolized by the microsomal enzyme system, enzyme inhibitors will reduce clearance, increase the intensity of effect, and increase the duration of action. This phenomenon has been seen with the antibiotic erythromycin, which reduces the half-life of alfentanil, and with quinidine, which increases the half-life of codeine. Other interactions of this type are possible since a number of drugs inhibit this enzyme system. Drugs most likely to be affected are pethidine (meperidine), methadone, propoxyphene and the fentanyl analogues since these are subject to dealkylative metabolism mediated by the microsomal enzymes.

## Synopsis

**DEPENDENCE AND TOLERANCE**

1. Opioids cause a rapid development of tolerance, within hours in some circumstances.
2. Tolerance develops to the analgesia, euphoriant, sedative and respiratory depressant actions of opioids.
3. Tolerance dose not develop to miosis (pinpoint pupils) or constipation.
4. Tolerance to morphine can result in 50-fold higher doses being required to achieve the same pharmacological effect.
5. Cross-tolerance develops to all opioids.
6. On abstinence from opioids in tolerant persons, withdrawal effects develop.
7. Symptoms of withdrawal include anxiety, gooseflesh, diarrhoea, hostility, hyperthermia, muscular aches, vomiting and sweating.
8. Opioids with short pharmacokinetic half-lives produce more severe abstinence symptoms earlier than longer acting drugs. Symptoms for morphine develop within 6–10 h.
9. There is a significant psychological basis to opioid dependence that should not be confused with physiological (or chemical) dependence.
10. Important drug interactions with opioids include:
    (a) benzodiazepines, which potentiate analgesic activity and cause a lowering of blood pressure;
    (b) drugs that inhibit microsomal metabolism;
    (c) neuroleptics, which enhance analgesia and may even induce a trance-like state.

# 5.6 Toxicology

Concentrations of drugs in blood and other specimens are normally used to interpret possible time frames of ingestion or exposure and assist in establishing likely pharmacological effects. Unfortunately, the therapeutic and toxic concentrations of most opioids overlap completely. Hence blood and tissue concentrations alone can provide no useful guide to potential toxicity, unless concentrations are clearly well in excess of those normally experienced in therapeutic use and the tolerance to opioids is known. Therefore, these limitations place real restrictions on the toxicological interpretation of cases involving opioids.

This chapter reviews the toxicology of opioids and discusses factors that can affect the interpretation of toxicological data.

## HEROIN AND MORPHINE

Toxic reactions to the use of opioids leading to unconsciousness are common. Over 70% of heroin users have witnessed a non-fatal adverse reaction to heroin[iv] and at least 25% have witnessed a fatal adverse reaction to heroin.[67,68] In addition, most heroin users experience adverse reactions to heroin. Almost all long-term users (>12 years) have had such an experience.

As expected, heroin users have a high mortality compared with the rest of the community. Estimates of risk of death vary widely, but range from 15 to 30 per thousand per year and may be as high as 50 per thousand per year for American and British addicts discharged from detoxification.[69] The mortality rate for people regularly using heroin is more than 13 times that of the general community.[70] The greater part of this high risk is death from an adverse reaction to heroin, or from suicide or trauma.

### Hospital admissions

Subjects presenting to hospital accident and emergency units following an adverse reaction to opioids are usually unconscious and show signs of respiratory distress. If opioid use is suspected, then treatment with positive-pressure oxygen and naloxone (or another opioid antagonist) will rapidly reverse the effects of the opioid, providing the brain has not had hypoxic damage. Constriction of pupils is a tell-tale sign of opioid toxicity, unless hypoxia has occurred, in which case pupillary dilatation will occur and mask signs of opioid toxicity.

Following arousal of the patient, the use of supportive care to maintain adequate breathing and to maintain adequate blood pressure and heart rate are normally all that is required. Further treatment with naloxone may be needed if the effects of the opioid persist. Naloxone

---

[iv] The term overdose is deliberately avoided here since overdose may imply a deliberate ingestion of an excess of drug; in most cases the adverse reaction to heroin is caused by polydrug use.

has only a short pharmacokinetic half-life (duration of action 1–2 h). Suspected cases of drug toxicity to long-acting opioids (e.g. methadone) will require regular dosing with naloxone.

In many cases presentations to hospital are the result of mixed drug ingestions with CNS depressant drugs such as alcohol, benzodiazepines, antipsychotic drugs and the tricyclic antidepressants. Since these other drugs will also depress the CNS, they may add significantly to the toxic effects of opioids. Patients not responding immediately, or only responding partially to the effects of naloxone (or any other opioid receptor antagonist), may be under the influence of other drugs. For this reason drug screens are useful to establish what other drugs may have been co-ingested. From an acute management point of view drug screens based on blood testing are often far more useful, providing they can be conducted rapidly.

## Death associated with heroin use

Deaths due to heroin are one of the most common causes of sudden and unexpected death. Incidences in Australia are about three deaths per 100 000 population per year. Estimates of yearly mortality rates vary from 1% to 3% of heroin users per year, which is 6–20 times those expected for non-drug users of the same age and gender. It is of interest that the average age of a heroin-related death is the late twenties, which is usually several years after initiation to heroin. While this high mortality is in part due to viral (HIV and hepatitis) infections, earlier onset of natural disease and increased incidence of violent outcomes, the leading cause of death is opioid toxicity.[71]

Heroin deaths are most often classified by the circumstances; i.e. knowledge of deceased being a heroin user, indications of recent heroin use including analysis of seized drug paraphernalia, and of course anatomical signs of drug death. Anatomical signs include pulmonary oedema and congestion of lungs, needle puncture marks perhaps with subcutaneous and perivenular haemorrhages, and presence of antibodies to hepatitis C and others. However, none of these are specific to heroin, nor do they necessarily indicate the cause behind the death. For this reason toxicology testing must be conducted to establish the nature of the poison, if present.

In most deaths attributed to heroin use, other drugs have also been used (often in as many as 90% of cases), many of which are CNS depressant drugs in concentrations likely to contribute to opioid toxicity. The most significant drug is ethanol (alcohol), which is present in over one-third of cases, with an average BAC in excess of 0.1%. Studies have shown that lower morphine concentrations are required to cause death in the presence of significant amounts of alcohol.[72] The benzodiazepines are present in more cases, although relatively few cases show overt misuse of these drugs. Amphetamine and cannabis use is widespread, as is the use of antidepressants and antipsychotics. A summary of blood concentrations and drugs detected in heroin-associated deaths is shown in Table 5.5.

In some countries (e.g. the USA) cocaine is a significant problem and contributes substantially to heroin mortality (see Section 2).

Recently, cannabis is believed to play a role in reinforcing some of the actions of morphine, including antinociception, sedation, hypotension and inhibition of bowel motility.[73]

The mean blood concentrations of morphine and other morphine species are no different to those subjects receiving legitimate morphine for analgesia, nor are they different in occasional

**Table 5.5** Demographic and toxicological profiles of typical heroin deaths[a]

| Demographics | | | |
|---|---|---|---|
| Age | Median 28–30 years | | |
| Gender | 80% male | | |
| **Morphine species** | **Median (mg/L)** | **Range (mg/L)** | |
| Morphine | 0.25 | 0–0.8 | |
| Normorphine | 0.15 | 0–0.26 | |
| Morphine-3-glucuronide | 0.4 | 0.1–2.2 | |
| Morphine-6-glucuronide | 0.1 | 0.01–0.5 | |
| Total morphine | 0.6 | 0.05–2.5 | |
| **Other drugs** | **Mean (%)** | **Range** | **Prevalence (%)** |
| Ethanol | 0.13 | 0.01–0.33 | 30–40 |
| Benzodiazepines | | | 40–60 |
| Cannabis | | | 30–40 |
| Antidepressants | | | 5–20 |
| Amphetamines | | | 5–10 |
| Methadone | | | 5 |
| Antipsychotics | | | 5 |
| Cocaine | | | <1 |

[a] Based on heroin-related deaths in Victoria.

versus long-term users of heroin.[74] Morphine concentrations in blood are not significantly affected by postmortem artefacts such as redistribution or metabolism.[74,75] Since blood morphine concentrations are largely uninterpretable (as a cause of death), there is little value in just measuring concentrations of morphine in blood. This is further reinforced by the variable morphine concentrations depending on the route of administration. This comment applies to both morphine and to total measures of circulating morphine (total morphine).[v] There may be some value in measuring morphine metabolites and in measuring morphine content in other specimens.

Urine concentrations can provide some information in heroin deaths. The absence of morphine in urine, or the presence of low concentrations (<1 mg/L), will strongly suggest death occurred shortly after a heroin dose but, more importantly, indicates lack of physiological opioid dependence (see Table 5.6). An opioid-dependent person is very likely to use the opioid at least once per day ensuring measurable concentrations of morphine species in urine at all times. The lack of significant opioid dependence will increase the risk of an acute death due to heroin.

Morphine, morphine conjugates (M3G, M6G) and the heroin metabolite 6-AM are relatively stable in urine for the first 1–2 days of death, or after collection, although high ambient

---

[v] Many laboratories measure total morphine (morphine plus morphine 3- and 6-glucuronide conjugates), rather than free morphine itself.

Table 5.6  Toxicological indicators in heroin deaths

| Type of heroin death | Indicators |
| --- | --- |
| Immediate death | High blood free morphine levels (>0.5 mg/L) |
| | Low blood concentrations of conjugates |
| | Absence of morphine in urine (<300 ng/mL) |
| Sub-acute death (death in less than 3 h)[a] | Free morphine levels in blood under 0.5 mg/L |
| | Free morphine to conjugated morphine[b] >1.0 |
| | Free morphine+M6G to M3G ratio >1.0 |
| | Total morphine levels under 1 mg/L |
| Delayed death (death after 3 h)[a] | Low concentrations of morphine in blood |
| | Free morphine to conjugated morphine[b] ≤1.0 |
| | Urinary total morphine levels (>5 mg/L) |

[a] In delayed death; [b] sum of M3G and M6G concentrations.

conditions and extended exposure can cause hydrolysis of 6-AM to morphine.[74,76] Heroin and 6-AM are spontaneously converted to morphine in blood and other tissues by the action of esterases. Consequently, morphine concentrations will elevate in the first few hours after death as all remaining heroin and 6-AM is consumed.

There is some uncertainty as to whether morphine glucuronides are stable postmortem. Recent studies have shown that M3G and M6G are stable in postmortem blood (and urine) at 4°C and 23°C over 4 weeks, but at 37°C a 15–30% loss occurs.[74] Extended exposure over 12 months can lead to substantial, or even complete, loss of morphine glucuronides in urine.[77] Morphine glucuronides are apparently stable in plasma stored at −20°C for 101 weeks.[78]

Bile concentrations of morphine are usually very high due to biliary excretion and are often several-fold higher than blood. This allows re-absorption of morphine and morphine conjugates to occur in the bowel. This is called entero-hepatic recirculation and causes a flat or double-humped blood concentration versus time profile for morphine or heroin. Biliary total morphine concentrations are significantly higher in delayed deaths, persons using very high doses and in persons using heroin regularly.[vi] There are, however, few data in the literature to support any strong conclusions made from biliary concentrations of morphine and its metabolites.

Morphine-6-glucuronide is biologically active (see Chapter 5.4) and, arguably, contributes to the pharmacological and toxicological effects of morphine and heroin. Morphine-6-glucuronide concentration in blood in combination with morphine has been shown to be significantly higher in persons dying from a delayed death (>3 h after use) (Table 5.6). In time, other measurements may also prove useful to assist in the interpretation of a heroin-related death.

There seems to be no relation to the quality of heroin on the streets (i.e. purity) and the mortality rate.[79] The variety of other factors associated with heroin toxicity, such as tolerance and use of other drugs, probably play the dominant role in the mortality to heroin.

---

[vi] A regular user in this context implies at least daily use.

Table 5.7  Pathological findings in heroin deaths[a]

**Frequent findings**

Antibodies to hepatitis C and chronic inflammation of liver

Aspiration of vomit

Frothing in mouth and nose (a manifestation of pulmonary oedema)

Pulmonary oedema and congestion

Tissue scarring, bruising and needle track marks with perivenular and subcutaneous haemorrhages

**Less frequent findings**

Cardiomegaly

Coronary heart disease

Cutaneous foreign body granulomas

Petechial haemorrhages

Pulmonary foreign body granulomas

Splenomegaly

[a] In alphabetical order.

## Mechanisms of heroin deaths

The principle mechanism of death in heroin-related cases is respiratory depression. All moderate to strong opioids produce depression of the respiratory centres even with normal analgesic doses.

Opioid toxicity following a sudden intravenous injection of heroin can lead to cardiovascular collapse due to a reduction in peripheral resistance and hypotension. Opioids also cause bronchoconstriction leading to asthma-like symptoms, which will exacerbate any respiratory depression. It is not surprising, therefore, that pulmonary oedema (heavy lungs) and bronchopneumonia are common pathological findings in heroin deaths, particularly those in which some delay has occurred to death. These are essentially a manifestation of respiratory depression. Table 5.7 summarizes the important pathological findings in deaths caused by use of heroin. While these findings are associated with heroin deaths, not all will be necessarily present at postmortem.

Impurities in heroin, or the injection of particulate matter into the veins, can lead to death, although there is little information to suggest that this is an issue in such deaths.

## OTHER OPIOIDS

The characteristics of some selected opioids are described below, together with some toxicological data. As for most heroin-related deaths, multiple drug use is common in cases of opioid abuse. Alcohol, the benzodiazepines, cocaine and the amphetamines are the most frequent drugs co-abused. In most cases, fatal concentrations of the opioid will be lowered due to their combined effects on the CNS.

## Buprenorphine

This partial agonist is perceived as far safer than heroin and is widely used in some countries for substitution treatment. Buprenorphine has a low oral bioavailability, but due to its high potency and high lipid solubility it can be delivered sublingually with adequate bioavailability. The duration of action lasts some 72 h depending on the dose. Typical doses range to 8 mg daily, although higher doses are possible.

Abuse of the drug through intravenous injection and the concomitant use of benzodiazepines may predispose to a much greater risk of death.[80,81] Blood concentrations of fatalities attributed to this combination have ranged from 1.1 to 29 ng/mL.

## Codeine

Death from codeine alone occurs rarely, but has been reported. Fatalities involving codeine have been reported in cases with total concentrations as low as 0.1 mg/L, although it is more usual for concentrations to exceed 1.0 mg/L.[13,82–84] In a review of over 100 fatalities, codeine concentrations have been at least 0.4 mg/L and total codeine[vii] concentrations have been at least 2 mg/L.[85] In most cases involving codeine, other drugs are also detected which are usually more toxic than codeine itself.[85] The presence of morphine in the blood of cases is also more likely to contribute to a toxic response, since morphine is the more active form of codeine. In the 7% of individuals who are incapable of producing significant amounts of morphine (see Chapter 4.2), codeine overdose is less likely to cause death.

The ratio of free to total codeine concentrations in fatalities attributed to codeine alone or to a combination of drugs is often about 1 : 3, although individual variations will occur.[85] Particularly high ratios (greater than 1 : 2) would suggest very recent exposure, probably within 1 h.

Codeine is often associated with heroin deaths, principally due to the presence of codeine (as acetylcodeine) in the heroin itself. The opium poppy produces small amounts of codeine, in addition to the morphine and other alkaloids. When this occurs, the morphine concentration in urine (and other tissues) is much higher than the codeine concentration (~10 : 1 ratio). Urinary ratios of codeine to morphine greater than 0.2 will strongly suggest additional codeine consumption. In some cases of heroin use, no codeine is detectable in urine. Codeine is not produced from the metabolism of morphine.[86]

## Dextromoramide

This is a relatively little used narcotic analgesic, although it was favoured as an injectable opioid in the 1980s when it was more freely available. A number of fatalities have been reported that describe fatal blood concentrations of 0.3 mg/L and higher, although claims are made of fatal concentrations in excess of 0.04 mg/L. The toxicity potential is clearly dependent on a number of factors, including route of injection and presence of other drugs.[87]

Dextromoramide is present in bile in significant concentrations, and in urine, kidney and lung.[88]

---

[vii] Codeine plus codeine-6-glucuronide concentration measured following hydrolysis of conjugate.

## Dihydrocodeine

This mild analgesic and antitussive drug has many similarities to codeine, in terms of its potency, toxicity and routes of metabolism. Deaths attributed to dihydrocodeine range from 0.8 mg/L.[89] Symptoms are similar to those experienced with morphine and codeine.

## Fentanyl

Fentanyl has a potency some 50–100 times that of morphine. Designer variations, such as 3-methylfentanyl, are more potent again. Consequently, the risk of death in an abuse setting is far higher than for the more commonly used opioids. In the USA, hundreds of deaths have been attributed to fentanyl or one of its analogues, largely through intravenous use.[90] Elsewhere, abuse tends to be restricted to health professionals with access to the drug.

Fentanyl and its modern counterparts in anaesthesia, alfentanil, remifentanil, sulfentanil, etc., show rapid tissue distribution into deep tissue sites. In normal doses this distribution terminates, or limits, their biological activities. Their solubility is so high in tissues that transdermal patches can be used to control delivery of small but effective doses through the skin.[91]

The fentanyls exhibit essentially the same profile of adverse effects as morphine. For example, respiratory depression is exhibited at therapeutic doses. Blood concentrations of fentanyl usually range up to 3 ng/mL, while fatal blood concentrations of fentanyl range from 0.2 ng/ml, with a mean of 3 ng/mL.[92] Slightly higher concentrations are observed in deaths in anaesthetized patients (5–45 ng/mL).[93] Liver concentrations of fentanyl are higher than blood in liver ($\times 10$) and brain ($\times 5$).

## Hydrocodone

This opioid is largely used as an antitussive (cough medicine) and is usually available as a syrup combined with other drugs. Fatal toxicity can develop at blood concentrations as low as 0.2 mg/L.[94] Signs of toxicity are similar to those seen with morphine. The main active metabolite is hydromorphone, which is present in bile in particularly high concentrations.[95]

## Methadone

Methadone is used primarily to treat opioid-dependent people – largely heroin users. Methadone maintenance programmes (MMPs) are used worldwide to substitute opioid use with a long-acting, orally available opioid. These programmes have been quite successful with varying estimates of their success.[96,97] Epidemiological studies have shown that the relative risk of death of an opioid user is 3–4 times less on MMPs, but is still much higher than the average person.[96,98] Daily doses of approximately 80 mg are needed for methadone to substantially compete with the actions of co-administered heroin. When this occurs, the risk of heroin toxicity in persons choosing to continue abuse of heroin is minimized. At this stage plasma concentrations of methadone are at least 100 ng/mL.[99]

However, reports have commented on the increased risk of death in the early stages of MMPs.[60,61,100,101] In these cases, death usually occurs at home during sleep, many hours after

Table 5.8 Blood concentrations of methadone in various types of methadone-associated death[a]

| | | |
|---|---|---|
| Methadone death | First stage of MMP (<14 days), n=20 | 0.44±0.27 (0.1–1.1) |
| | Following illicit use of methadone, n=22 | 0.48±0.39 (0.15–1.8) |
| Polydrug death | Subjects on long-term MMP, n=20 | 0.82±0.69 (0.1–2.8) |
| Non-drug death | Death caused by non-drug suicide, car accidents, etc. | 0.42±0.37 (0.05–1.6) |

[a] A review of 89 methadone-associated deaths occurring in Victoria from 1994 to 1996;[105] all concentrations in mg/L and are in femoral blood.

the peak pharmacokinetic blood concentration has occurred. This increased death rate is recognized as being largely due to the difficulty in assessing the opioid dependence of new clients. Most people claiming to be heroin addicts either are occasional users or are opioid naïve. Occasional use of heroin will not produce chemical dependence, and if started on a programme at doses in excess of their established tolerance, can lead to fatal consequences. Oral doses of methadone as low as 20 mg can be fatal, particularly after a few days of treatment, due to accumulation of drug in blood and tissues.[viii]

A further difficulty is the diversion of some legally prescribed methadone to unsuspecting persons.[100,102,103] Uncontrolled or inappropriate use of methadone is therefore more dangerous than heroin because of this long half-life. The risk of death at the start of an MMP has been calculated as seven-fold higher than the risk prior to entering the programme.[100] This risk reduces substantially after stabilization on the MMP.

Toxicologically, the blood concentrations of persons on MMPs are the same as those who have died from the toxic effects of methadone, although they tend to be elevated somewhat from postmortem redistribution (Table 5.8).[104] These usually range from about 0.1 to 1.0 mg/L. This lack of separation of therapeutic and toxic concentrations is similar to morphine. Consequently, the assessment of the death can only be made on the circumstances, i.e. lack of clearly defined history of physiological dependence to opioids in a setting of starting an MMP. Of course, other factors seen with heroin deaths, such as polydrug use and presence of natural disease, may contribute. In a few cases direct abuse of methadone will occur from diverted legal supplies of methadone syrup or an overdose of tablets prescribed for pain.[100]

Pathological signs of toxicity to methadone are similar to other opioids, notably signs of respiratory depression and associated hypoxia. There is a high rate of hepatitis C serology and bronchopneumonia in methadone-related deaths.[61] Measurements of methadone concentrations in other specimens such as liver probably offer no advantage over peripheral blood alone.[61] However, analysis of gastric contents is always useful to establish, or refute, recent ingestion.

---

[viii] Methadone has a half-life of 1 day or longer and will reach much higher blood concentrations during the first week of treatment.

## Pentazocine

Pentazocine has had a history of abuse, particularly in the USA in the 1970s–1980s when the combination of Talwin (pentazocine) and tripelennamine (Pyribenzamine) were used by injection of the crushed tablets. Numerous deaths were reported with fatal blood concentrations ranging from 0.2 mg/L.[106,107] A common pathological finding in these subjects was diffuse pulmonary granulomatosis with adjacent arteriolar and capillary thrombosis. Identifiable foreign bodies within the vessel walls and lumena were often noted with birefrigent crystals of talc-like material within the foreign body cells. This was caused by the injection of the excipients in the crushed tablets.

Overdose to pentazocine alone has been reported.[108] In these subjects, the classic signs of narcotic overdose are not present (i.e. respiratory depression and miosis) since pentazocine is active at kappa- and sigma-opioid receptors. Symptoms of overdose include seizures, high blood pressure, hypotonia, dysphoria, hallucinations, delusions and agitation. Naloxone, effective in treating heroin toxicity, is only effective in much higher doses in subjects suffering from pentazocine toxicity.[108]

The addition of naloxone to pentazocine tablets has largely prevented abuse of this opioid by blocking its effects if used intravenously. Oral administration inactivates naloxone, while preserving pentazocine activity.

## Propoxyphene

Propoxyphene is a close analogue of methadone chemically, although it is a much weaker narcotic drug and is usually regarded as an analgesic. However, it has had widespread use as an analgesic for mild to moderate pain, often in combination with other non-narcotic analgesics such as paracetamol (acetaminophen) and aspirin. Unfortunately, it has been subject to much abuse and has caused the death of a large number of people in Australia, Europe and the USA.[109] Its toxicity stems from a combination of respiratory depression and its potent membrane stabilizing activity, which leads to heart conduction defects and cardiac arrhythmias.

Propoxyphene is rapidly metabolized to norpropoxyphene, which is also active and toxic. In most cases blood and tissue concentrations of norpropoxyphene exceed those of the parent. The relatively long half-life (up to 24 h) of the parent and metabolite leads to accumulation with chronic use, substantially increasing the risk of a toxic reaction. This risk is increased in the elderly and in those with impaired liver function, due to a reduced metabolic clearance.

Propoxyphene undergoes substantial postmortem redistribution. Blood concentrations in cardiac blood have been shown to increase over 10-fold.[110] Smaller increases are observed in peripheral (femoral) blood. For this reason blood concentrations of propoxyphene are even less reliable than for other opioids. Where doubt exists over a cause of death, it is recommended to also measure liver and gastric contents for propoxyphene and norpropoxyphene. Fatal liver concentrations range from ~20 mg/kg for parent and metabolite.

Because of the ease of metabolism of propoxyphene and postmortem artefacts, propoxyphene and norpropoxyphene concentration ratios should be treated with caution. The ratio is also likely to change during putrefaction, although there are few hard data to quantify these changes.

## Tramadol

Tramadol is not a typical opioid analgesic and has only a low affinity for μ-opioid receptors. It has central analgesic activity and is used for the treatment of moderate to severe pain. The drug inhibits serotonin and noradrenaline re-uptake, which is significant in blocking nociceptive impulses at the spinal level. The O-desmethyl metabolite (often known as M-1) is twice as active as an analgesic and binds with greater affinity to mu-opioid receptors.

The drug produces little respiratory depression by virtue of its weak opioid activity but it does produce seizures in cases involving misuse of the drug. It has low lipid solubility, hence it is unlikely to show significant postmortem redistribution. A number of cases involving fatalities are reported, usually involving significant amounts of other CNS active drugs.[111–114]

## TOXIC CONCENTRATIONS OF OPIOIDS

A summary of toxic opioid blood concentrations is shown in Table 5.9. These should only be used as a guide since other factors discussed throughout this chapter will affect the toxic response.

## DISTINGUISHING SOURCE OF OPIOID FROM URINE PROFILE

The principal opioids that are of concern with regard to their possible source are heroin, codeine and morphine. Metabolically (see Fig. 5.6) they are closely linked; heroin is metabolized to

Table 5.9  Toxic blood concentrations of opioids

| Drug | Minimum toxic concentration in blood (mg/L) |
|---|---|
| Codeine[a] | >0.4 |
| Dextromoramide | >0.3 |
| Dextropropoxyphene[b] | >1.0 |
| Dihydrocodeine | >0.8 |
| Fentanyl | >0.0002 |
| Hydrocodone | >0.2 |
| Morphine[a] | >0.01 |
| Oxycodone | >0.2 |
| Pethidine (merperidine) | >1.0 |
| Pentazocine | >0.2 |
| Methadone | >0.1 |
| Tramadol | >2 |

[a] Free drug concentrations; [b] norpropoxyphene concentrations often exceed 2 mg/L, but in some situations fatal concentrations of propoxyphene may be lower than 1.0 mg/L.

**Table 5.10** Criteria for distinguishing heroin, codeine and morphine use[a]

- Presence of 6-AM in urine confirms heroin use
- Presence of small amounts of codeine (<10%) relative to morphine suggests, but does not confirm, heroin use
- Presence of relatively large amounts of codeine relative to morphine suggests, but does not confirm, use of codeine
- Presence of low concentrations of codeine and morphine (both <2 mg/L) does not distinguish between codeine and heroin use
- Presence of morphine (and no codeine) in urine does not distinguish morphine from heroin use unless other criteria are established
- Urinary total morphine concentrations greater than 5 mg/L and total codeine to total morphine ratio less than 0.125 indicates heroin use[b]

[a] Species measured as total drug and glucuronide conjugates; [b] after Fuller, 1997.[115]

morphine, as is codeine. Furthermore, heroin usually contains small amounts of codeine, which means that urine of heroin users contains both codeine and morphine leading to a possible confusion with codeine users. Morphine consumption (by any route) does not produce 6-AM or codeine in urine, while 6-AM presence in urine confirms heroin use.

Urine profiles can be used to distinguish these drugs providing the following criteria in Table 5.10 are adhered to.

## INGESTION OF POPPY SEEDS AND MORPHINE EXCRETION

The presence of morphine in urine during random or targeted drugs of abuse testing can result from the ingestion of poppy seeds. Poppy seeds are used in curry sauces in Asian cooking and in many forms of baking such as bread rolls, bagels and speciality cakes. Poppy seeds contain morphine, although the content varies widely from country to country. In Australia, poppy seeds have contained ~100 µg/g seed. The contents of seeds from other sources are: Spanish 251 µg/g, Dutch 4 µg/g and Turkish 5–27 µg/g.[116–119]

The ingestion of amounts of poppy seeds consistent with normal eating behaviour will lead to morphine excretion in urine, and will, in some instances, exceed the normal urinary 300 ng/mL cut-off applied to drugs of abuse testing. Urine morphine concentrations can easily exceed 1000 ng/mL if poppy seeds contain an appreciable content of morphine. For example, consumption of 2 g of poppy seeds will produce ~0.2 mg morphine.

Codeine is usually also present but will hardly ever exceed 300 ng/mL. Morphine will be detectable in urine for about 24 h.[116,117,119] Ingestion of poppy seed Danish or streusel has given urine concentrations of morphine in excess of 5000 ng/mL.[118] 6-AM is not present in the urine of poppy seed consumers. However, only the presence of this metabolite can differentiate heroin use from other sources of morphine.

Abuse of, and addiction to, poppy seeds and poppy seed extracts has been reported.[13,120,121]

## Synopsis

### TOXICOLOGY

1. Heroin deaths are by far the most frequent of opioid-related deaths and occur in opioid-dependent persons at a rate of 1–2% per year. The mortality from heroin use is some 6- to 20-fold that of the average person and occurs most frequently in males aged in their late twenties or thirties who are often also using other drugs.
2. Heroin is used intravenously, but is also smoked and snorted. Smoking and snorting provide rapid effects with similar duration of actions as intravenous use.
3. Heroin deaths are characterized by the sudden nature of the death, presence of drug paraphernalia at scene, presence of needle puncture marks, presence of hepatitis C antibodies, presence of heavy lungs and congestion of organs, and petechial haemorrhages.
4. Blood and urine testing for morphine can confirm recent use of opioid, and other drugs that have contributed. Toxicology can assist in reconstructing the relevant background to the death, and assist in distinguishing acute versus chronic use, and delayed versus rapid death. Urine testing may confirm use of heroin by presence of 6-AM.
5. Ingestion of poppy seeds can lead to false conclusion of heroin use.
6. Consumption of codeine will also lead to excretion of morphine in urine. Only 93% of the population is capable of producing significant morphine from codeine.
7. Methadone is a more toxic drug than heroin if misused due to its long pharmacokinetic half-life, potent narcotic effects, and high relative oral bioavailability. Use of low starting doses (20 mg) is recommended in persons starting methadone maintenance programmes to avoid accumulation over the next days to toxic levels.
8. Fentanyl and other potent lipid-soluble opioids such as alfentanil and sulfentanil can produce the same dependence and toxicity as heroin and morphine and may have the advantage of being absorbed sublingually and dermally as well as the usual routes.

# 5.7 Case reports

## CASE REPORT 5.1 OCCUPATIONAL DRUG TESTING

This 35-year-old person was a regular employee of a large firm producing high-tech electronic equipment. The company had a policy of workplace testing to guard against the use of drugs affecting the skills of their workforce and thereby endangering the lives of colleagues.

A routine urine test by a reputable laboratory gave a positive test to morphine at a concentration of 400 ng/mL. No codeine was detected.

In this case, a number of possibilities exist. The employee may have used morphine, an antitussive producing morphine other than codeine (e.g. ethylmorphine), poppy seeds, or heroin.

The subject's use of drugs should clearly be questioned and legal drugs eliminated from the list of possibilities, including morphine use for pain control. If ethylmorphine has been used (and is legally available in the country), then analysts will also detect ethylmorphine in urine. The same comments apply to codeine use. Consumption of poppy seeds can lead to transient urinary morphine concentrations above the cut-off level of 300 ng/mL.

Heroin use is the remaining possibility. The detection of 6-acetylmorphine (6-AM) is unequivocal proof of heroin use, but may not always be present in urine, or may only be present in low concentrations. The use of highly sensitive GC-MS techniques to detect 6-AM down to at least 0.01 mg/L is strongly recommended in these cases.

## CASE REPORT 5.2 ACUTE HEROIN DEATH

This 25-year-old male was a known drug user, mainly heroin and speed, since the age of 16. He had recently been released from prison after serving 6 months for assault and robbery. Two days after his release he was found dead, lying in a public park. An empty syringe was located near the body. According to the forensic pathologist, death had occurred at least several hours earlier.

External examination was unremarkable. Internal examination showed some mild inflammatory changes in the liver consistent with his hepatitis C positivity and pulmonary oedema of the lungs. Otherwise, the autopsy was unremarkable. Tissues including femoral blood, liver, gastric contents, bile, vitreous humour and urine were taken for routine toxicology. Toxicology showed:

# Opioids

| | | |
|---|---|---|
| Morphine, free | Blood | 0.09 mg/L |
| Morphine, total | Blood | 0.19 mg/L |
| 6-AM | Urine | 0.1 mg/L |
| Morphine, total | Urine | 0.1 mg/L |
| Ethanol (alcohol) | Blood | 0.11 g/100 mL |
| Diazepam | Blood | 0.2 mg/L |
| Nordiazepam | Blood | 0.2 mg/L |

Analysis of the syringe contents detected heroin, 6-acetylmorphine and morphine. The pathologist concluded death was due to 'mixed drug toxicity'.

In this case the pathologist excluded natural disease processes and injuries and attributed the cause of death as drug-related based on the circumstance of a known heroin user dying suddenly. The analysis of the syringe strongly suggests recent heroin use. The toxicology confirms recent heroin use by the detection of 6-AM in urine and the presence of significant morphine in blood. The presence of a trace of morphine in urine (rather than much larger amounts) suggests lack of opioid dependence and a rapid death after injection (within 15 min).

The period of incarceration and recent release from prison further suggests likely recent heroin use and lack of tolerance to opioids. Alcohol was present in significant amounts that would also contribute to the sudden death. The contribution of the low concentrations of diazepam to the death is uncertain, but is likely to be small.

## CASE REPORT 5.3 DELAYED HEROIN DEATH

This 32-year-old female was a known regular user of heroin. She had appeared stuporous for a few hours before going to sleep on the couch. She was found dead the following morning. Death had probably occurred earlier in the night.

External examination revealed chronic inflammatory changes in the front of the left elbow consistent with chronic intravenous drug abuse. Internal examination showed congestion of the liver and spleen and mild fatty changes in the liver, pulmonary oedema of the lungs, early-stage bronchopneumonia and petechial haemorrhages. Otherwise, the autopsy was unremarkable. Toxicology showed:

| | | |
|---|---|---|
| Morphine, free | Blood | 0.30 mg/L |
| Morphine, total | Blood | 1.5 mg/L |
| 6-AM | Urine | Not detected (<0.01 mg/L) |
| Morphine, total | Urine | 40 mg/L |
| Morphine, total | Bile | 80 mg/L |
| Codeine, total | Urine | 2 mg/L |
| Temazepam | Blood | 2.3 mg/L |
| Oxazepam | Blood | 0.2 mg/L |

The pathologist concluded death was due to 'mixed drug toxicity'. In this case the pathologist concluded that tissue congestion, the petechial haemorrhages and lung changes were secondary to respiratory depression induced by heroin and other drugs. The toxicology testing showed significant free and total morphine concentrations in blood. The presence of high concentrations of morphine in bile and urine suggested either a delayed death and/or chronic use of heroin. Note urine concentrations are far higher than in Case 5.2. The absence of 6-AM in urine does not exclude heroin use, but does not prove it either. Codeine in urine is often associated with heroin, although it can derive from codeine use.

Interestingly, a very high concentration of the benzodiazepine temazepam was detected. This will contribute to the CNS depressant effect of heroin/morphine and would be consistent with her persistent stuporous state. Death during sleep is characteristic of deaths occurring from respiratory depression associated with mixed drug toxicity. In such cases, bronchopneumonia is often seen together with other anoxic and agonal changes (pulmonary oedema etc.). Oxazepam is a known active metabolite of temazepam.

In this case, death was due to the accumulated respiratory depressant effects of heroin/morphine while using high doses of a benzodiazepine.

## CASE REPORT 5.4 METHADONE DEATH

This 33-year-old male was found dead in his bed at around 0800 h. He had gone to bed complaining of tiredness and headaches and been observed to be sleeping soundly with loud snoring at 2200 h the previous night. He had commenced a methadone maintenance programme some 3 days earlier at a dose of 40 mg after being advised to seek help for his heroin dependency. This was taken daily as syrup from the local pharmacist. He had been a sporadic user of heroin for over 12 years.

Pathological examination revealed congestion of liver, spleen and pulmonary oedema in the lungs. Antibodies to hepatitis C were detected on serology testing and chronic persistent hepatitis was noted.

Toxicology showed the presence of methadone in femoral blood (0.3 mg/L) and liver (0.4 mg/kg), but no methadone was detected in gastric contents. A small amount of temazepam was also detected in blood (0.1 mg/L).

The cause of death was given as methadone toxicity in a man recently starting a methadone maintenance programme.

Methadone is a long-acting opioid that will accumulate in body tissues over the first week of regular dosing.[60,100] Consequently, a 40 mg single dose on day 1 will assume a much greater effect over the next few days. Persons who do not have an opioid dependency when starting a programme will be most at risk to toxicity. Sporadic or occasional users are unlikely to exhibit significant opioid-dependency and need close monitoring in the early stages of a methadone programme. The use of starting doses of 20–30 mg is recommended. Dose adjustment may take place after the first week, if required.

## Opioids

Tiredness, lethargy, unsteady gait, drowsiness, and headaches are often seen in persons suffering from excessive methadone. Deep unrousable sleep with snoring are characteristic of a drug-induced state associated with a high risk of death. Positive serology results and liver pathology are commonly seen in drug users. Congestion of organs, oedema of lungs, and occasionally bronchopneumonia and petechial haemorrhages are the result of compromised respiratory function. The methadone blood concentration is rarely of value in interpreting likely toxic reactions to methadone.

# References for Section 5

1. *United Nations World Drug Report.* New York: Oxford University Press; 1997.
2. Commonwealth Department of Health and Family Services. *Statistics on Drug Abuse in Australia 1994.* Canberra: Commonwealth Department of Health and Family Services; 1994.
3. ABCI. *Australian Illicit Drug Report 1998–99.* Canberra: Australian Bureau of Criminal Intelligence; March 2000.
4. Fox R, Matthews I. *Drugs policy: fact, fiction and the future.* Sydney: Federation Press; 1992.
5. Martindale W. *Martindale's: the complete drug reference*, 32nd edn. London: Pharmaceutical Press; 1999.
6. United Nations. *International Narcotics Drug Control Board Annual Report.* Vienna: United Nations; 1997.
7. Bedford KR, Nolan SL, Ohrusy R, Siegers JD. The illicit preparation of morphine and heroin from pharmaceutical products containing codeine: 'homebake' laboratories in New Zealand. *Forens Sci Internat* 1987; 34: 197–204.
8. Shesser R, Jotte R, Olskhaker J. The contribution of impurities to the acute morbidity of illegal drug use. *Am J Emerg Med* 1991; 9: 336–42.
9. Boerner U. The metabolism of morphine and heroin in man. *Drug Metab Rev* 1975; 4: 39–73.
10. *Physician's Desk Reference.* Montvale, NJ: Medical Economics Company; 1998.
11. *Goodman and Gilman's the pharmacological basis of therapeutics*, latest edn. New York: McGraw Hill; 1996.
12. Rang HP, Dale MM, Ritter JM. *Pharmacology*, 3rd edn. London: Churchill Livingstone; 1995.
13. Baselt RC, Cravey RH. *Disposition of toxic drugs and chemicals in man,* 3rd and later edns. Foster City, CA: Year Book Medical Publishers; 1990.
14. Glare PA, Walsh TD. Clinical pharmacokinetics of morphine: a review. *Therapeut Drug Monit* 1991; 13: 1–23.
15. McQuay HJ, Carroll D, Faura CC, Cavaghan DJ, Hand CW. Oral morphine in cancer pain: influences on morphine and metabolite concentration. *Clin Pharmacol Therapeut* 1990; 48: 236–44.
16. Leow KP, Cramond T, Smith MT. Pharmacokinetics and pharmacodynamics of oxycodone when given intravenously and rectally to adult patients with cancer pain. *Anaesthet Analges* 1995; 80: 296–302.

17. Weinberg DS, Inturissi CE, Reidenberg B, Moulion DE, Nip TJ, Wallenstein S, et al. Sublingual absorption of selected opioid analgesics. *Clin Pharmacol Therapeut* 1988; 44: 335–42.
18. Masood AR, Thomas SHL. Systemic absorption of nebulised morphine compared with oral morphine in healthy adults. *Br J Clin Pharmacol* 1996; 41: 250–2.
19. Osborne R, Joel S, Trew D, Slevin M. Morphine and metabolite behaviour after different routes of administration: demonstration of the importance of the active metabolite morphine 6-glucuronide. *Clin Pharmacol Therapeut* 1990; 47: 12–19.
20. Liu Z, Mortimer O, Smith CAD, Wolf CR, Rane A. Evidence for a role of cytochrome P450 2D6 and 3A4 in ethylmorphine metabolism. *Br J Clin Pharmacol* 1992; 39: 77–80.
21. Chen ZR, Somogyi AA, Bochner F. Polymorphic O-demethylation of codeine. *Lancet* 1988; ii: 914–15.
22. Yue QY, Svensson JO, Alm C, Sjoqvist F, Sawe J. Codeine O-demethylation cosegregates with polymorphic debrisoquine hydroxylation. *Br J Clin Pharmacol* 1989; 28: 629–45.
23. Popa C, Beck O, Brodin K. Morphine formation from ethylmorphine: implications for drugs-of-abuse testing in urine. *J Anal Toxicol* 1998; 22: 142–7.
24. Baillie SP. Age and the pharmacokinetics of morphine. *Age Aging* 1989; 18: 258–62.
25. Dahlstrom B, Bolme P, Feychting H, Noack G, Paalzow L. Morphine kinetics in children. *Clin Pharmacol Therapeut* 1979; 26: 354–65.
26. Coffey B, Shader RI, Greenblatt DJ. Pharmacokinetics of benzodiazepines and psychostimulants in children. *J Clin Psychopharmacol* 1983; 3(4): 217–25.
27. Pokela ML, Olkkola KT, Seppala T, Koivisto M. Age-related morphine kinetics in infants. *Develop Pharmacol Therapeut* 1993; 20: 26–34.
28. Barrett DA, Barker DP, Rutter N, Pawula M, Shaw PN. Morphine, morphine-6-glucuronide and morphine-3-glucuronide pharmacokinetics in newborn infants receiving diamorphine infusions. *Br J Clin Pharmacol* 1996; 41(6): 531–7.
29. Hasselstrom J, Eriksson S, Persson A, Rane A, Svensson JO, Sawe J. The metabolism and bioavailability of morphine in patients with severe liver cirrhosis. *Br J Clin Pharmacol* 1990; 29: 289–97.
30. Woolner DF, Winter D, Frendin TJ, Begg EJ, Lynn KL, Wright GJ. Renal failure does not impair the metabolism of morphine. *Br J Clin Pharmacol* 1986; 22: 55–9.
31. Goucke CR, Hackett LP, Ilett KF. Concentrations of morphine, morphine-6-glucuronide and morphine-3-glucuronide in serum and cerebrospinal fluid following morphine administration to patients with morphine-resistant pain. *Pain* 1994; 56: 145–9.
32. Paul D, Standifer KM, Inturisi CE, Pasternak GW. Pharmacological characterisation of morphine-6β-glucuronide, a very potent morphine metabolite. *J Pharmacol Exp Therapeut* 1989; 251: 477–83.
33. Jenkins AJ, Keenan RM, Henningfield JE, Cone EJ. Pharmacokinetics and pharmacodynamics of smoked heroin. *J Anal Toxicol* 1994; 18(6): 317–30.
34. Cone EJ, Welch P, Mitchell JM, Paul BD. Forensic drug testing for opiates: I. Detection of 6-acetylmorphine in urine as an indicator of recent heroin exposure; drug and assay considerations and detection times. *J Anal Toxicol* 1991; 15(1): 1–7.

35. Kramer TH, Fine J, Bahari B, Ottomanelli G. Chasing the dragon: the smoking of heroin and cocaine. *J Substance Abuse Treat* 1990; 7: 65.
36. Mohan D, Adityanjee, Saxena S, Lal S. Changing trends in heroin abuse in India. *Bull Narcot* 1985; 37: 19–24.
37. Jenkins AJ, Oyler JM, Cone EJ. Comparison of heroin and cocaine concentrations in saliva with concentrations in blood and plasma. *J Anal Toxicol* 1995; 19(6): 359–74.
38. Cone EJ, Holicky BA, Grant TM, Darwin WD, Goldberger BA. Pharmacokinetics and pharmacodynamics of intranasal 'snorted' heroin. *J Anal Toxicol* 1993; 17(6): 327–37.
39. Cone EJ, Jufer R, Darwin WD, Needleman SB. Forensic drug testing for opiates. VII. Urinary excretion profile of intranasal (snorted) heroin. *J Anal Toxicol* 1996; 20(6): 379–92.
40. Mather LE. Clinical pharmacokinetics of fentanyl and its derivatives. *Clin Pharmacokinet* 1983; 8: 422–46.
41. Yue QY, Hasselstrom J, Svensson JO, Sawe J. Pharmacokinetics of codeine and its metabolites in caucasian healthy volunteers: comparisons between extensive and poor metabolisers of debrisoquine. *Br J Clin Pharmacol* 1991; 31: 635–42.
42. Lafolie P, Beck O, Lin Z, Albertioni F, Boreus L. Urine and plasma pharmacokinetics of codeine in healthy volunteers: implications for drugs-of-abuse testing. *J Anal Toxicol* 1996; 20: 541–6.
43. Cone EJ, Welch P, Paul BD, Mitchell JM. Forensic drug testing for opiates, III. Urinary excretion rates of morphine and codeine following codeine administration. *J Anal Toxicol* 1991; 15(4): 161–6.
44. Meresaar U, Nilsson MI, Holmstrand J, Anggard E. Single dose pharmacokinetics and bioavailability of methadone in man studied with a stable isotope method. *Eur J Clin Pharmacol* 1981; 20(6): 473–8.
45. Verebely K, Volavka J, Mule S, Resnick R. Methadone in man: pharmacokinetic and excretion studies in acute and chronic treatment. *Clin Pharmacol Therapeut* 1975; 18(2): 180–90.
46. Nilsson MI, Widerlov E, Meresaar U, Anggard E. Effect of urinary pH on the disposition of methadone in man. *Eur J Clin Pharmacol* 1982; 22(4): 337–42.
47. Geletko SM, Erickson AD. Decreased methadone effect after ritonavir initiation. *Pharmacotherapy* 2000; 20(1): 93–4.
48. Hsu A, Granneman GR, Bertz RJ. Ritonavir. Clinical pharmacokinetics and interactions with other anti-HIV agents. *Clin Pharmacokinet* 1998; 35(4): 275–91. [Published erratum appears in *Clin Pharmacokinet* 1998; 35(6): 473.]
49. Schlatter J, Madras JL, Saulnier JL, Poujade F. Drug interactions with methadone. *Presse Med* 1999; 28(25): 1381–4.
50. Cobb MN, Desai J, Brown LS, Jr., Zannikos PN, Rainey PM. The effect of fluconazole on the clinical pharmacokinetics of methadone. *Clin Pharmacol Ther* 1998; 63(6): 655–62.
51. DeMaria PA, Jr., Serota RD. A therapeutic use of the methadone fluvoxamine drug interaction. *J Addict Dis* 1999; 18(4): 5–12.
52. Wojnar-Horton RE, Kristensen JH, Yapp P, Ilett KF, Dusci LJ, Hackett LP. Methadone distribution and excretion into breast milk of clients in a methadone maintenance programme. *Br J Clin Pharmacol* 1997; 44(6): 543–7.

53. Geraghty B, Graham EA, Logan B, Weiss EL. Methadone levels in breast milk. *J Hum Lact* 1997; 13(3): 227–30.
54. Verebey K, Volavka J, Mule SJ, Resnick RB. Naltrexone: disposition, metabolism, and effects after acute and chronic dosing. *Clin Pharmacol Therapeut* 1974; 20: 315–28.
55. Di Chiara G, North RA. Neurobiology of opiate abuse. *Trends Pharmacol Sci* 1992; 13(5): 185–93.
56. Way WL, Fields HL, Way EL. Opioid analgesics and antagonists. In: Katzung BG, ed. *Basic and clinical pharmacology*, 7th edn. New Jersey: Prentice Hall International; 1998. pp. 496–515.
57. Fields HL, Basbaum AI. *Endogenous pain control mechanisms*. Edinburgh: Churchill Livingstone; 1989.
58. Ellenhorn MJ. *Medical toxicology*. Baltimore: Williams Wilkins; 1996.
59. *Goodman and Gilman's the pharmacological basis of therapeutics*, various edns. Basingstoke: Macmillan; 1998.
60. Drummer OH, Syrjanen M, Opeskin K, Cordner S. Deaths of heroin addicts starting on a methadone maintenance programme. *Lancet* 1990; 335(8681): 108.
61. Drummer OH, Opeskin K, Syrjanen M, Cordner SM. Methadone toxicity causing death in ten subjects starting on a methadone maintenance program. *Am J Forens Med Pathol* 1992; 13(4): 346–50.
62. Caplehorn JR, Drummer OH. Mortality associated with New South Wales methadone programs in 1994: lives lost and saved. *Med J Aust* 1999; 170(3): 104–9.
63. Zador D, Sunjic S, Darke S. Heroin-related deaths in New South Wales, 1992: toxicological findings and circumstances. *Med J Aust* 1996; 164: 204–7.
64. Tracqui A, Kintz P, Ludes B. Narcotic-related deaths in Strasbourg, France: five year survey (1991–95) and recent trends. In: American Academy of Forensic Sciences; 1998. San Francisco, CA.
65. Cooper SJ. Benzodiazepine-opiate antagonist interactions in relation to feeding and drinking behaviour. *Life Sci* 1983; 32: 1043–51.
66. Stitzer ML, Griffiths RR, McLellan AT, Grabowski J, Hawthorne JW. Diazepam use among methadone maintenance patients: patterns and dosages. *Drug Alcohol Depend* 1981; 8: 189–99.
67. Loxley W, Carruthers S, Bevan J. Overdose among injecting drug users: findings from the Australian study of HIV and injecting drug use (ASHIDU). In: Hall W, ed. International Opioid Overdose Symposium. Sydney: National Drug and Alcohol Research Centre, NSW; 1997. pp. 49–61.
68. Powis B, Strang J, Griffiths P, Taylor C, Williamson S, Fountain J, *et al.* Self-reported overdose among injecting drug users in London: extent and nature of the problem. *Addiction* 1999; 94(4): 471–8.
69. Caplehorn JR, Dalton MS, Haldar F, Petrenas AM, Nisbet JG. Methadone maintenance and addicts' risk of fatal heroin overdose. *Subst Use Misuse* 1996; 31(2): 177–96.
70. Hulse GK, English DR, Milne E, Holman CD. The quantification of mortality resulting from the regular use of illicit opiates. *Addiction* 1999; 94(2): 221–9.

71. Darke S, Zador D. Fatal heroin 'overdose': a review. *Addiction* 1996; 91(12): 1765–72.
72. Ruttenber AJ, Kalter KD, Santinga P. The role of ethanol abuse in the etiology of heroin-related death. *J Forens Sci* 1990; 35: 891–900.
73. Manzanares J, Corchero J, Romero J, Fernandez-Ruiz JJ, Ramos JA, Fuentes JA. Pharmacological and biochemical interactions between opioids and cannabinoids. *TIPS* 1999; 20: 287–93.
74. Gerostamoulos J. The toxicological interpretation of heroin deaths. Melbourne: Monash University; 1998.
75. Logan BK, Snirnow D. Postmortem distribution and redistribution of morphine in man. *J Forens Sci* 1996; 41: 37–46.
76. O'Neal CL, Poklis A. Simultaneous determination of acetylcodeine, monoacetylmorphine, and other opiates in urine by GC-MS. *J Anal Toxicol* 1997; 216: 427–32.
77. Liu Z, Lafolie P, Beck O. Evaluation of analytical procedures for urinary codeine and morphine measurements. *J Anal Toxicol* 1994; 18: 129–33.
78. Milne RW, Nation RL, Reynolds GD, Somogyi AA, van Crugten JT. High-performance liquid chromatographic determination of morphine and its 3- and 6-glucuronide metabolites: improvements to the method and application to stability studies. *J Chromatogr* 1991; 565: 457–64.
79. Risser D, Uhl A, Stichenwirth M, Hoeningschabel S, Hirz W, Schneider B, *et al*. Quality of heroin and heroin-related deaths from 1987 to 1995 in Vienna, Austria. *Addiction* 2000; 95(3): 375–82.
80. Reynaud M, Petit G, Potard D, Couty P. Six deaths linked to concomitant use of buprenorphine and benzodiazepines. *Addiction* 1998; 93(9): 1385–92.
81. Tracqui A, Ludes B. Buprenorphine-related deaths among drug addicts in France: a report on 20 fatalities. *J Anal Toxicol* 1998; 22: 430–4.
82. Nakamura GR, Griesemer EC, Noguchi TT. Antemortem conversion of codeine to morphine in man. *J Forens Sci* 1976; 21: 518–24.
83. Wright JA, Baselt RC, Hine CH. Blood codeine concentrations in fatalities associated with codeine. *Clin Toxicol* 1975; 8: 457–63.
84. Kintz P, Tracqui A, Mangin P. Codeine concentrations in human samples in a case of fatal ingestion. *Int J Legal Med* 1991; 104(3): 177–8.
85. Gerostamoulos J, Burke MP, Drummer OH. Involvement of codeine in drug-related deaths. *Am J Forensic Med Pathol* 1996; 17(4): 327–35.
86. Mitchell JM, Paul BD, Welch P, Cone EJ. Forensic drug testing for opiates. II. Metabolism and excretion rate of morphine in humans after morphine administration. *J Anal Toxicol* 1991; 15(2): 49–53.
87. *Clarke's isolation and identification of drugs,* 2nd edn. London: Pharmaceutical Press; 1986.
88. Kintz P, Tracqui A, Mangin P, Lugnier AA, Chaumont AJ. Fatal intoxication by dextromoramide: a report on two cases. *J Anal Toxicol* 1989; 13(4): 238–9.
89. Peat MA, Sengupta A. Toxicological investigations of cases of death involving codeine and dihydrocodeine. *Forens Sci Internat* 1977; 9: 21–32.

90. Allen A, Cooper D, Kram T. 'China White': alpha-methylfentanyl. *Microgram* 1981; 14(3): 26–32.
91. Calis K, Kohler D, Corso D. Transdermally-administered fentanyl for pain management. *Clin Pharm* 1992; 11: 22–36.
92. Henderson G. Fentanyl-related deaths: demographics, circumstances, and toxicology of 112 cases. *J Forens Sci* 1991; 236: 422–33.
93. McGee M, Marker E, Jovic M, Stajic M. Fentanyl related deaths in New York city. In: Annual Meeting of the American Academy of Forensic Science. New Orleans, LA; 1992.
94. Morrow PL, Faris EC. Death associated with inadvertant hydrocodone overdose in a child with a respiratory tract infection. *Am J Forens Med Pathol* 1987; 8(1): 60–3.
95. Park JI, Nakamura GR, Griesemer EC, Noguchi TT. Hydromorphone detected in bile following hydrocodone ingestion. *J Forens Sci* 1982; 27(1): 223–4.
96. Farrell M, Ward J, Mattick R, Hall W, Stimson V, Des Jarlais D, et al. Methadone maintenance treatment in opiate dependence: a review. *Br Med J* 1994; 309: 997–1001.
97. Proceedings of Expert Workshop on the Induction and Stabilisation of Patients onto Methadone. Canberra: National Drug Strategy; 2000. Monograph Series no. 39.
98. Caplehorn JR, Dalton MS, Cluff MC, Petrenas AM. Retention in methadone maintenance and heroin addicts' risk of death. *Addiction* 1994; 89(2): 203–9.
99. Lorimer N, Schmid R. The use of plasma levels to optimise methadone maintenance treatment. *Drug Alcohol Depend* 1994; 30: 241–6.
100. Caplehorn J, Drummer OH. Mortality and NSW methadone programs: lives lost and saved. *Med J Australia* 1999; 170: 104–9.
101. Clark JC, Milroy CM, Forrest ARW. Deaths from methadone use. *J Clin Forens Med* 1995; 2: 143–4.
102. Williamson PA, Foreman KJ, White JM, Anderson G. Methadone-related overdose deaths in South Australia, 1984–94. *Med J Aust* 1997; 166: 302–5.
103. Cairns A, Roberts ISD, Benbow EW. Characteristics of fatal methadone overdose in Manchester, 1985–94. *Br Med J* 1996; 313: 264–5.
104. Milroy CM, Forrest ARW. Methadone deaths: a toxicological analysis. *J Clin Pathol* 2000; 53: 277–81.
105. Drummer OH. The toxicology of methadone and its involvement in sudden death. In: Tedeschi L, ed. The International Association of Forensic Toxicologists Annual Conference. Padua, Italy; 1997.
106. Monforte JR, Gault R, Smialek J, Goodin T. Toxicological and pathological findings in fatalities involving pentazocine and tripelennamine. *J Forens Sci* 1983; 28(1): 90–101.
107. Polklis A, Mackell MA. Pentazocine and tripelennamine (T's and Blues) abuse: toxicological findings in 39 cases. *J Anal Toxicol* 1982; 6: 109–14.
108. Challoner KR, McCarron MM, Newton EJ. Pentazocine (Talwin) intoxication: report of 57 cases. *J Emerg Med* 1990; 8(1): 67–74.
109. Somerai S, Avorn J, Gortmaker S, Hawley S. Effect of Government and commercial warnings on reducing prescription misuse: the case of propoxyphene. *Am J Public Health* 1987; 77: 1518–23.

110. Yonemitsu K, Pounder D. Postmortem toxico-kinetics of co-proximol. *Internat J Legal Med* 1992; 104: 347–53.
111. Moore KA, Cina SJ, Jones R, Selby DM, Levine B, Smith ML. Tissue distribution of tramadol and metabolites in an overdose fatality. *Am J Forens Med Pathol* 1999; 20(1): 98–100.
112. Levine B, Ramcharitar V, Smialek JE. Tramadol distribution in four postmortem cases. *Forens Sci Internat* 1997; 86(1–2): 43–8.
113. Michaud K, Augsburger M, Romain N, Giroud C, Mangin P. Fatal overdose of tramadol and alprazolam. *Forens Sci Internat* 1999; 105: 185–9.
114. Goeringer KE, Logan GD, Christian GD. Identification of tramadol and its metabolites in blood from drug-related deaths and drug-impaired drivers. *J Anal Toxicol* 1997; 21: 529–37.
115. Fuller DC. A statistical approach to the prediction of verifiable heroin use from total codeine and total morphine concentrations in urine. *J Forens Sci* 1997; 42(4): 685–9.
116. El Sohly HN, El Sohly MA, Stanford DF. Poppy seed ingestion and opiate urinalysis: A closer look. *J Anal Toxicol* 1990; 14: 308–10.
117. Pelders MG, Ros JJW. Poppy seed: differences in morphine and codeine content and variation in inter- and intra-individual excretion. *J Forens Sci* 1996; 41(2): 209–12.
118. Selavka CM. Poppy seed ingestion as a contributing factor to opiate-positive urinalysis results: the pacific perspective. *J Forens Sci* 1991; 36(3): 685–96.
119. Lo DST, Chua TH. Poppy seeds: implications of consumption. *Med Sci Law* 1992; 32(4): 296–302.
120. King MA, McDonough MA, Drummer OH, Berkovic SF. Poppy tea and the baker's first seizure [letter]. *Lancet* 1997; 350(9079): 716.
121. Struempler RE. Excretion of morphine following the ingestion of poppy seeds. *Milit Med* 1988; 153: 468–70.

# 6 Ethanol

| | | |
|---|---|---|
| **Foreword** | | 274 |
| 6.1 | Types and sources of alcohol | 275 |
| 6.2 | Pharmacokinetics, metabolism and duration of action | 278 |
| 6.3 | Mechanisms of action | 290 |
| 6.4 | Pharmacological actions and therapeutics | 292 |
| 6.5 | Adverse reactions, tolerance and dependence | 297 |
| 6.6 | Toxicology | 300 |
| 6.7 | Case reports | 309 |
| **References for Section 6** | | 313 |

# Foreword

Alcohol is the common word for the simple chemical ethanol.[i] There is in fact a large family of chemicals that belong to this generic term. Some of these alcohols surface from time to time in forensic cases, particularly methanol and the propanols, but predominantly the main alcohol of interest in forensic science is ethanol. Ethanol will be the subject of this section and, except for a passing reference, other alcohols will not be discussed.

Ethanol is a product of fermentation by the action of certain yeasts on the sugars in fruits and cereals and is probably the oldest drug known to humans. This natural series of chemical reactions has led to a huge variety of drinks and beverages and foods for consumption. The free availability of alcohol-containing beverages has not surprisingly led to abuse. Alcohol is the most widely used drug in Western and many other societies and is second to tobacco in terms of health costs to the community. Estimates suggest that ~10% of those drinking alcohol have alcohol-related problems that adversely affect their lives and those of their families.[1] This is a serious problem since the great majority (>85%) of most Western communities consume this drug. The mortality rate of those persons drinking six or more drinks daily is 50% higher than non-drinkers,[2] and alcohol is linked to acts and crimes of violence such as in suicide, accidental deaths, homicides and child abuse.[3] Alcohol is at least a part cause of death in approximately one-third of all drug-related deaths.

Despite its simple chemical nature, ethanol has complex pharmacology and pharmacokinetics, and despite many thousands of research articles covering all conceivable aspects of its actions, there is still much unknown concerning the actions of ethanol.

This section provides an overview of the source and availability, pharmacology, pharmacokinetics and toxicology of ethanol, and includes case reports to illustrate some important concepts and their relevance to forensic cases.

---

[i] This section will refer to alcohol and ethanol, or ethyl alcohol, as though they are one drug. When other alcohols are mentioned, they will be specifically named.

# 6.1 Types and sources of alcohol

Ethanol (or ethyl alcohol) is one of a number of alcohols, which are characterized by the presence of a hydroxyl group (OH) on the molecule. While this definition covers many chemicals and drugs, the definition is best restricted to those simple molecules that possess a hydrocarbon chain as the backbone and contain a hydroxyl group at one of the positions.

Compounds that possess two adjacent hydroxyl groups are known as diols, or glycols. An important example of this is ethylene glycol (an antifreeze). Glycerol contains three adjacent hydroxyl groups.

This chapter provides an overview of the range of alcohols and details their sources and physical properties.

## STRUCTURES OF ALCOHOLS

The structures of ethanol and related simple alcohols are shown in Fig. 6.1. Propanol and isopropanol are isomers, i.e. they contain the same number and type of atoms, but are arranged in different ways. Propanol is also called 1-propanol, or propan-1-ol. Isopropanol is also named 2-propanol or propan-2-ol.

## PHYSICAL PROPERTIES OF ALCOHOLS

Simple alcohols such as those listed in Fig. 6.1 are volatile liquids at room temperatures and are good solvents. Ethanol has a wide use industrially and domestically as a solvent for a variety of goods including paints, perfumes, domestic cleaning preparations, and in liquid pharmaceuticals such as elixirs. The distillation of alcohol in the presence of water will produce an azeotrope (distils at 78.1°C) that contains 95.6% ethanol and 4.4% water. This is normally used to fortify beverages and as a solvent, unless dehydrated ethanol is required. This is then produced by a special distillation process to remove the water.

| $CH_3OH$ | $CH_3CH_2OH$ | $CH_3CH_2CH_2OH$ | $CH_3CHCH_3$ with OH |
|---|---|---|---|
| Methanol | Ethanol | Propanol | Isopropanol |
| b.p. 64.7°C | b.p. 78.4°C | b.p. 97–98°C | b.p. 82.5°C |

**Fig. 6.1** Structures of common simple alcohols
b.p.: boiling point at 1 atmosphere pressure.

# Ethanol

Isopropanol is also used in swabs to cleanse and disinfect skin before injections or venipuncture for the collection of blood.

## HISTORICAL ASPECTS AND SOURCE

Ethanol as an alcoholic beverage has been recognized by humans from c. 4200 BC when early scenes on pottery from Mesopotamia depicted the fermentation process. Brandy has been known since about 100 AD and the Scottish and Irish have distilled whisky since the 15th century. The North Americans banned the sale and use of alcohol products in the 1920s (prohibition) but were forced to repeal the Act in 1933 because of widespread illegal production and consumption.

For many communities alcohol is an important social drink and is often consumed with a meal, or simply consumed for pleasure. Aside from restrictions for the sale to underaged persons, alcohol products in most Western communities are available without restriction. Ethanol is produced by the fermentation of fruits, grains and other food products, particularly rye, barley, malt and grapes.

Fermentation of such food occurs by the presence of suitable bacteria in the mixture. These can be natural yeasts or from yeasts added to facilitate the fermentation process. The most common bacteria used are *Saccharomyces rose*, *S. carlsbergensis*, *S. cerevisiae*, and *S. ellipsoideus*. Fermentation will usually stop at alcohol concentrations of 10–12%. Alcoholic beverages with greater than this concentration are produced by fortification with pure alcohol obtained by distillation. Industrial-grade ethanol is normally produced synthetically from petroleum and from ethylene.

## ALCOHOLIC CONTENT OF BEVERAGES

The alcoholic content of beverages varies from less than 1% for some ultra-light or dealcoholized drinks to ~50% for some spirits. The typical contents of common alcoholic beverages are summarized in Table 6.1 together with an estimate of the number of standard

Table 6.1 Alcoholic strengths of common beverages

| Beverage | Strength (% v/v) | Standard measure[a] |
|---|---|---|
| Beer | | |
|    Normal strength | 4–6 | 3.75 |
|    Light beer | 2–3 | 1.9 |
| Table wines (red, white, champagnes) | 8–12 | 8.2 |
| Fortified wines (sherry, vermouth, port) | 14–22 | 13.5 |
| Liqueurs | 15–40 | 20 |
| Spirits (whisky, rum, brandy) | 35–45 | 30 |

[a] Standard measure is defined here as 10 g ethanol in a normal measure sold at a licensed premise; calculation is based on a 750-mL bottle at the mid-point alcohol concentration of each type of beverage.

# Types and sources of alcohol

**Table 6.2** Alcoholic strengths of common products

| Product | Strength (% v/v) |
|---|---|
| Aftershaves | 15–80 |
| Colognes | 40–60 |
| Cough and anti-histamine syrup/mixture/elixir | 2–25 |
| Gasohol (fuel for cars) | 10 |
| Methylated spirit | 80–95 |
| Mouthwashes | 10–25 |
| Perfumes | 25–95 |

measures per 750-mL bottle. This latter measure provides a guide to the number of drinks per type of alcoholic beverage.

It is common practice to sell alcohol as a standard measure, hence one standard drink will contain approximately 10 g of ethanol. A common exception is light beer,[ii] which contains approximately half this amount of alcohol in a 200-mL glass.

## ALCOHOLIC CONTENT OF COMMERCIAL PRODUCTS

Ethanol is present in a large range of pharmaceutical mixtures (syrups and elixirs) as well as a host of other industrial and domestic products, including perfumes, mouthwashes and after-shaves. Methylated spirit is essentially pure ethanol with some water and a chemical added to impart a smell and an unpleasant taste (Table 6.2).[iii]

## Synopsis

### TYPES AND SOURCES OF ALCOHOL

1. Ethanol (or ethyl alcohol) is one of a number of alcohols, which are characterized by the presence of a hydroxyl group (OH) on the molecule.
2. Ethanol is a water-soluble molecule with a boiling point of 78°C produced by fermentation of fruits and grains, or from catalytic action on ethylene derived from petroleum.
3. Ethanol is used widely as an industrial solvent, as well as in perfumes and colognes, mouthwashes and pharmaceutical elixirs and mixtures.
4. Alcoholic beverages contain variable amounts of ethanol: beers 2–6%, wines 8–12%, fortified wines 14–22%, spirits 35–45% and liqueurs 15–40%.
5. Other simple alcohols of interest are methanol, propanol and isopropanol.

---

[ii] In some countries 'light' may refer to the colour or body of the beer, rather than the alcohol concentration.

[iii] An unpleasant tasting chemical is added to methylated spirit to prevent oral consumption.

# 6.2 Pharmacokinetics, metabolism and duration of action

The pharmacokinetics, metabolism and excretion of alcohol are unique among drugs. The volatility of alcohol and the rate-limiting metabolism of alcohol in the liver places this drug in an unusual position relative to other drugs, in that the usual rules of half-life and other pharmacokinetic factors are different to those for other drugs. Many forensic practitioners have often simplified the pharmacokinetics of ethanol to extrapolate blood concentrations to earlier time points or to estimate dose. Unfortunately, the pharmacokinetics of ethanol are complex and a number of factors influence the rate of absorption and elimination of ethanol.

This chapter reviews the pharmacokinetics and metabolism of ethanol and how this affects our ability to measure and interpret the presence of ethanol. A number of key scientific papers or reviews are useful reading on this subject.[4-6]

## ABSORPTION

### Oral absorption and blood concentrations

Ethanol is rapidly absorbed when any one of the vast varieties of alcohol-containing beverages, cocktails or other liquid products is consumed. Absorption occurs in the stomach, although most ethanol is absorbed in the lower intestine, as for most other drugs. Peak blood concentrations of ethanol occur at about 30 min, although the time to peak concentration ($T_{max}$) may not occur until 2 h, if large doses are consumed or gastric emptying is delayed. Gastric emptying is important since it governs the rate the access of drug to the main absorptive surfaces in the lower intestine (see review by Holford, 1987[5]). The consumption of large doses in relatively short periods of time (>4 drinks in 1 h) retards the $T_{max}$ since the rate of ethanol absorption is rate limiting, i.e. the body has a finite absorption rate, and therefore a longer time is required to absorb all the ingested ethanol. This has implications in back calculations since the drug may still be absorbing 2 h after the last drink.

The consumption of light beers is becoming an increasing trend, particularly in those countries with a relatively low legal driving limit, e.g. Australia (0.05%) and Sweden (0.02%). Consumption of one 330-mL bottle of 1.8% w/v beer over 5 min produced an average blood alcohol concentration (BAC) of 0.008% (range 0.002–0.011% in four men and four women). Consumption of 660 mL beer of 3.0% w/v strength gives blood levels of 0.032% (range 0.026–0.044%) (see Fig. 6.2).[7]

The variability in absorption times in social drinkers is further highlighted by Winek et al.[8]

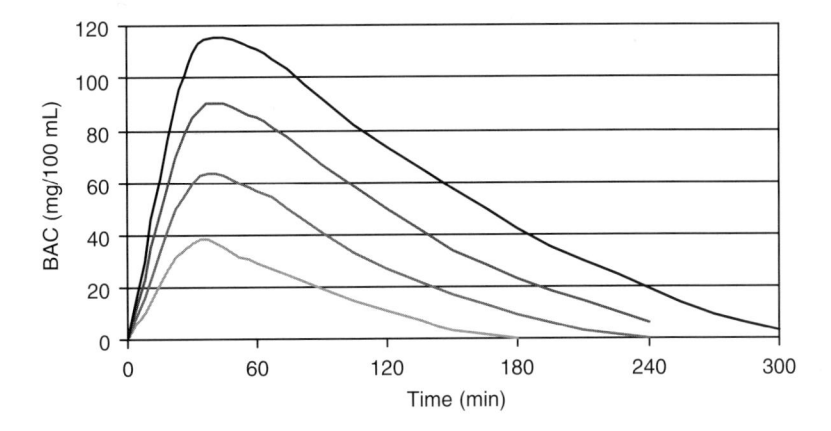

**Fig. 6.2** Effect of increasing alcohol dose and blood concentrations

The bioavailability of normal doses (<4 drinks per hour) of ethanol is about 80%, that is 80% of the ethanol ingested is available to the body after oral absorption. This bioavailability increases with increasing doses and becomes almost 100% with large doses, as the metabolic losses become insignificant with increasing dose.

A simple relationship is known that relates an oral dose of ethanol to a peak ethanol concentration in subjects who have been fasting:[9]

$$C_{max}\ (g/100\ mL^{iv}) = 0.002 \times \text{dose (g per 70 kg body weight)} \qquad (1)$$

With this relationship, a 30 g dose of ethanol (three glasses of full-strength beer consumed quickly) would produce a peak BAC of 0.06% (g/100 mL) on an empty stomach. While this relationship does not include a number of possible variables it may be used as a guide to predicting peak BACs.

Clearly persons with a lower body weight produce a higher BAC, and those with a higher body weight would produce correspondingly lower peak BACs. For example, a person with a body weight of 50 kg would produce a peak BAC of 0.084%, while a person with a body weight of 120 kg would produce a peak BAC of 0.035%.

### Widmark formula

The Widmark equation allows the dose of ethanol consumed after a certain time to be calculated from a BAC.[10] This formula is shown below:

$$A = r \times \rho \times (C_t + (\beta \times t)) \qquad (2)$$

where: A = dose of ethanol in grams; r = is a constant (0.68 men, 0.55 women); ρ = body weight; $C_t$ = BAC at time t; and β = zero-order elimination rate constant.

This formula can provide a reasonable estimate of dose in some people, but it is limited in that there is variability in r between subjects, and β can vary substantially between

---

iv Units of g/100 mL is the same as % (strictly gram per cent).

# Ethanol

subjects. Friel et al.[11] have suggested revision of the constants for men and women to 0.71 and 0.65, respectively.

If breath alcohol concentrations are used,[v] multiplication by 2300 gives an estimate of the BAC, but again this is subject to variation.[11] Modern breath analysis instruments automatically correct for this factor depending on the legally approved factor. Mean calculated ethanol doses using the Widmark formula are lower than actual doses up to 125 min after drinking. Mean underestimates ranged from 12 to 14 mL of 100 proof vodka. Calculated doses overestimate actual doses in some subjects. At the 95% confidence level, the calculated dose could underestimate it by as much as 30 mL (~15 g ethanol) vodka.

A number of factors affect ethanol absorption. These include intake of food, other drugs and disease states.

## Effect of food

The consumption of food during or before ingestion of ethanol has a marked effect on the absorption and bioavailability of ethanol. The peak blood concentration ($C_{max}$) may be halved following a standard meal (Fig. 6.3).[12] This effect is dependent on the type of food ingested. Carbohydrate-rich foods seem to a have a larger effect than fatty meals, although both affect alcohol absorption.[13] The reduced BAC following food appears to be a combination of delayed absorption leading to a reduced rate of absorption and a reduced absorption of ethanol.[14] Food also affects the elimination (clearance) when ethanol is given by intravenous infusion, suggesting that food has a direct effect on enzyme oxidation systems.[15]

Consumption of 660 mL beer of 3.0% w/v strength with food gave blood levels of 0.024% (range 0.020–0.029%). This compares with levels of 0.032% (range 0.026–0.044%) observed while fasting.[7]

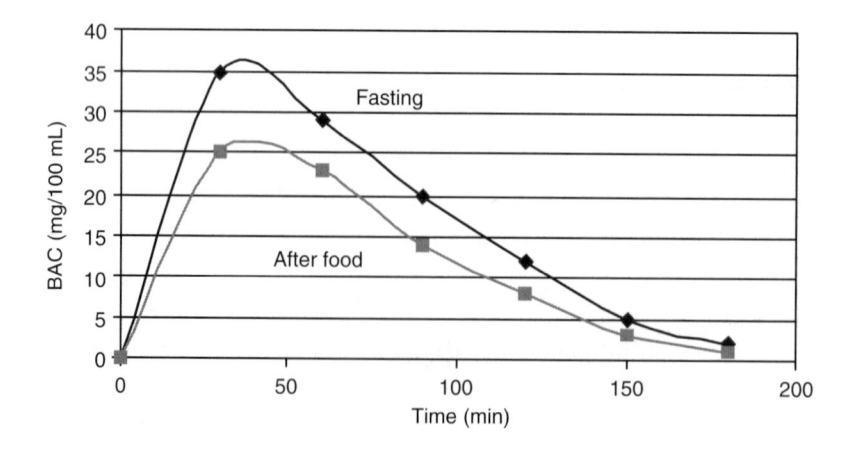

**Fig. 6.3** Effect of food on the absorption of alcohol

---

[v] Alcohol is found in breath, but at much lower concentrations than blood.

## Other routes of absorption

Since ethanol is such a simple molecule with a high fat solubility, it is likely to be absorbed by all of the usual routes. In practice, ethanol is almost always taken orally. Ethanol is absorbed in the pulmonary circulation (if inhaled from vapour etc.), but the breath concentrations are so low that no practical amount of ethanol would be absorbed.[5]

## METABOLISM

The metabolism of ethanol is largely mediated through the enzyme alcohol dehydrogenase (ADH) in the liver. This enzyme converts ethanol to acetaldehyde, which in turn is metabolized by aldehyde dehydrogenase to acetate (at physiological pH), and eventually also to carbon dioxide (see Fig. 6.4). Both enzymes utilize the cofactor nicotinamide adenine dinucleotide (NAD). This cofactor must be present in sufficient concentrations for the enzymes to function, and is the rate-limiting factor.

There are other enzymes capable of oxidizing ethanol. These include catalase, which uses hydrogen peroxide as cofactor, and a microsomal P450 enzyme called CYP2E1, or simply microsomal oxidizing system (MEOS). Catalase is unlikely to be a significant enzyme since tissue concentrations of hydrogen peroxide are very low; however, the MEOS is considered a potentially important enzyme system in some situations.[16] Evidence suggests that the MEOS may be induced by regular ethanol consumption (such as in alcoholics[vi]). If this occurs, then the MEOS system will play a larger role in the metabolism of ethanol in chronic users compared with social drinkers.

Another enzyme, UDP-glucuronyltransferase, forms the minor metabolite ethyl glucuconide.[17] This metabolite may be a marker of heavy alcohol consumers.[18]

## Elimination of ethanol

Ethanol is eliminated by a number of mechanisms, although the predominant process is metabolism in the liver. Other processes include expiration in breath, urine excretion and transpiration (sweating), and possibly some metabolism in other tissues including the stomach.

Gastric ethanol metabolism accounts for only 0.2% of the dose, and ethanol elimination by the lung and kidney accounts for 1.3–1.7% of the dose.[19]

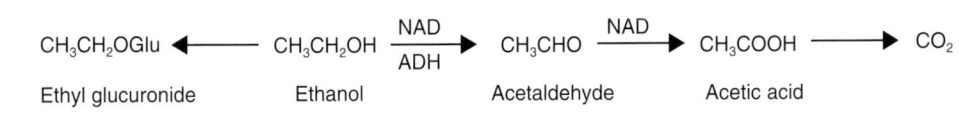

$$CH_3CH_2OGlu \leftarrow CH_3CH_2OH \xrightarrow[ADH]{NAD} CH_3CHO \xrightarrow{NAD} CH_3COOH \rightarrow CO_2$$

Ethyl glucuronide    Ethanol    Acetaldehyde    Acetic acid

Fig. 6.4   Metabolic pathways of ethanol

---

[vi] There are varying definitions used for alcoholics in the literature, including those persons who consume more than 80 g ethanol per day constantly, and show signs of alcohol-seeking behaviour and signs of dependence.

# Ethanol

This elimination assumes a zero-order process[vii] with a constant rate of loss of ethanol and is the basis of the Widmark formula (see earlier). While this has been convenient to back calculate a BAC from a single BAC, it has been known for some time that this is an oversimplification. Ethanol is actually eliminated with Michaelis–Menten kinetics by virtue of its metabolism by ADH:

$$-\frac{dC}{dT} = \frac{V_m C}{K_m + C} \qquad (3)$$

where: dC/dT = rate of elimination; $V_m$ = maximal enzyme rate (velocity); C = concentration at time T; and $K_m$ = Michaelis constant.

The elimination of alcohol is dependent on dose, but since BACs above 0.02% saturate the enzyme, the elimination of ethanol at BACs above 0.02% is almost a linear decline (pseudolinear).[20] However, only relatively small increases in elimination rate are observed with increasing steady-state BAC.[21]

The rate of elimination of ethanol from blood is often taken as 0.015%/h, although a number of studies have shown rates varying from 0.012 to 0.027%/h[5] and 0.009 to 0.036%/h.[22] A study of over 2000 drivers in whom paired blood samples were taken, spaced at least 60 min apart, showed a range from 0.01 to 0.06%/h.[23]

Ethanol elimination is dose dependent with higher doses showing a faster elimination rate.[24] Studies in drinking drivers have shown only a small dose-dependent increase in the rate of elimination with BAC.[25]

Alcoholics also show an enhanced elimination rate compared with social drinkers. For subjects classified as non-drinkers (consume less than 170 g of ethanol/month), the mean ethanol elimination rate is 0.012%/h. For subjects classified as social drinkers (consume more than 170 g but less than 840 g of ethanol/month), the mean ethanol elimination rate is 0.015%/h. For alcoholics, the mean ethanol elimination rate is 0.030%/h.[26] While these data show discrete variations in ethanol elimination depending on the amount of ethanol consumed, there is approximately a 30% variability between groups (Fig. 6.5).

Not all persons classified as alcoholics have enhanced elimination rates.[22] Since some alcoholics have rates similar to social drinkers it raises the question of whether disease states or conditions such as liver disease, congestive heart failure and other conditions reduce the elimination of ethanol in these cases.

There is evidence that in some people (~20%) a rapid increase in alcohol metabolism occurs following even a single dose of alcohol.[27] Elimination rates increasing by more than 40% are observed in these persons. This physiological response, possibly caused by an increase in the regeneration of NADH to NAD, may offer protective effects in these individuals to the development of alcoholism.

There is a small difference in ethanol blood concentrations between arterial and venous blood during the absorptive and distribution phases (<0.01%), but not in the elimination phase.[28]

---

[vii] Zero-order elimination refers to a constant rate of elimination irrespective of dose (or BAC), as distinct from first-order elimination, which is exponentially dependent on blood concentration.

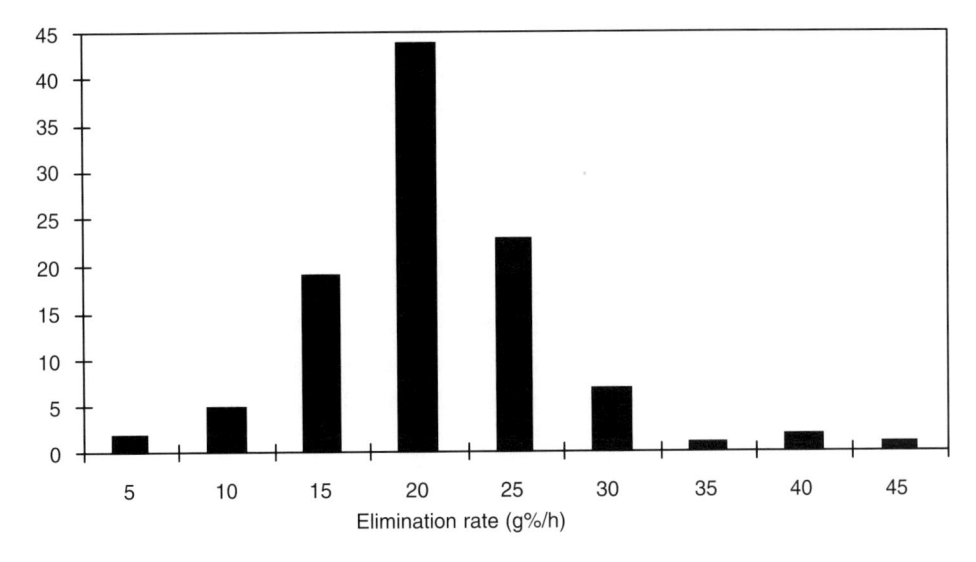

**Fig. 6.5** Frequency distribution of the rate of elimination of ethanol (adapted from Jones, 1993[22])

### Effect of age and gender

In a study of the ethanol elimination of 1090 DUI[viii] suspects the mean elimination rate for females (0.0214%/h) was significantly higher than males (0.0189%/h).[25] In contrast, Friel *et al.* (1995) found no difference in the elimination rate for 97 men and 77 women.[11] There is some unsubstantiated evidence that women eliminate alcohol more rapidly in the mid-luteal phase of the menstrual cycle.[29] On balance there appears to be little difference in elimination of alcohol between sexes providing an appropriate adjustment is made for differences in body weight. The elimination rate may be affected by the person's age.[30,31]

### Effect of race

Polymorphism of genes expressing the enzyme ADH and aldehyde dehydrogenase are known.[32] Different alleles encode subunits of the enzymes that differ in the rate they metabolize ethanol (isozymes). The Han, Mongolian, Korean and Elunchun populations in Northern China differ in allele frequencies, with the Elunchun having a much lower frequency of ADH2*2 alleles, and the Mongolian and Elunchun having a much lower frequency of ALDH2*2 alleles. Within each population, alleles at one or more of these three loci are protective against alcoholism, although the populations differ in which loci play significant roles. The protective allele at each locus (ALDH2*2, ADH2*2, and ADH3*1) encodes a subunit that either metabolizes ethanol to acetaldehyde more rapidly or slows the conversion of acetaldehyde to acetate. These data demonstrate that genetic differences in the enzymes that metabolize alcohol can substantially affect the risk for alcoholism. Variations in ADH isozymes also exist among other racial groups.

---

[viii] DUI: driving under the influence (of alcohol).

Compared with Caucasians, the Japanese have a low sigma-ADH activity, which reduces first-pass metabolism of ethanol at low but not high alcohol concentrations. However, blood alcohol levels are similar because of the higher elimination rates in Japanese due to the hepatic β2-ADH variant.[33]

Ethanol elimination is significantly higher in the normal ALDH Japanese men than those with this deficiency and the ethanol elimination rate in normal ALDH subjects is greater than that in Caucasians.[34]

The mean elimination rate of African Americans having beta 3-containing ADH isozymes is significantly faster than those with only β1β1-ADH isozymes. Within each of these groups, men have marginally lower ethanol disappearance rates than women.[35] For men, the elimination rate ranged from 0.0106%/h (β1β1) to 0.0125%/h (β3β3), whilst for women the rates are 0.0121%/h and 0.0137%/h, respectively.

The black American population has a significantly higher maximum blood ethanol concentration and area under the blood ethanol concentration versus time curve than the other populations studied, when either a single dose or multiple doses of ethanol are ingested. These increases are due to the presence of a considerable amount of the β3β3-ADH isoenzyme, with a Michaelis constant ($K_m$) of 34 mM in the black American population.[19]

The alcohol-flush reaction occurs in Asians who inherit the mutant ALDH2*2 allele, which produces an inactive aldehyde dehydrogenase enzyme. In these individuals, high blood acetaldehyde levels are believed to be the cause of the unpleasant symptoms that follow drinking. The ADH2*2 and ADH3*1, alleles that encode the high-activity forms of alcohol dehydrogenase, as well as the mutant ALDH2*2 allele, are less frequent in alcoholics than in controls. The presence of ALDH2*2 is associated with slower alcohol metabolism and the most intense flushing. In those homozygous for ALDH2*1, the presence of two ADH2*2 alleles correlates with slightly faster alcohol metabolism and more intense flushing, although a great deal of variability occurs.[36]

Despite these findings there appears to be no correlation between rate of ethanol clearance and race, sex, age, or time of day in intoxicated patients arriving at hospital emergency centres.[37] This suggests that body weight, overall health and alcohol-induced tolerance are the major factors affecting alcohol clearance rates.

## EXCRETION AND DETECTION TIMES

Most of the ethanol consumed (>95%) is metabolized to acetaldehyde and ethyl glucuronide. Acetaldehyde is in turn metabolized to acetate and carbon dioxide. Consequently the urinary excretion of ethanol is very small (~0.3% of dose).

Other processes include expiration in breath (0.7% of dose) and transpiration (sweat ~0.1%). There is evidence of ADH in the stomach walls, although there is little evidence that ethanol metabolism in the stomach accounts for anything other than trace amounts.

There will be some reduction in the elimination rate at low BAC because of the Michaelis–Menton kinetics. However, the detection time of alcohol in urine is roughly proportional to the dose consumed. Four measures of alcohol would be eliminated in approximately 5 h allowing for 1 h absorption time. Twelve measures of alcohol would take approximately 13 h.

In practice, high-dose consumers will have a higher elimination rate that can reduce the detection time by up to a factor of two. The retention of alcohol in the bladder is likely to increase detection time for a few hours.

## DRUGS AFFECTING ABSORPTION AND ELIMINATION

A number of drugs are known to affect ethanol pharmacokinetics causing changes in the BAC and duration of action of the drug. It is important to note that any effect by co-consumed drugs has little or no medico-legal significance, that is, it is no defence if the clearance of alcohol is reduced by other drugs consumed.

### Enzyme inhibitors

Disulfiram (Antabuse) is a drug used to treat alcohol dependence and acts to inhibit aldehyde dehydrogenase, the enzyme responsible for the deactivation of acetaldehyde produced by the action of ADH on ethanol (see Fig. 6.4). This inhibition has the consequence of building up tissue levels of the toxic acetaldehyde and causing flushing, hyperventilation, high heart rate, and considerable distress and unpleasant effects, and usually has the effect of dissuading the user from further alcohol consumption.[38]

Calcium carbimide (cyanamide) also inhibits aldehyde dehydrogenase.[39] The orally active antidiabetic drug chlorpropamide, and to a lesser extent tolbutamide, the antibacterial drugs metronidazole and tinidazole, and the cephalosporin antibiotics cephamandole and latamoxef cause flushing.[40–42] Women who use metronidazole pessaries for the local treatment of vaginal infection are at risk of adverse effects if co-consuming alcohol. A life-threatening interaction between the antifungal drug griseofulvin and alcohol has been reported.[43]

### Other drug interactions

The fruit sugar fructose has been touted as being able to increase the metabolism of ethanol (and therefore reduce the possibility of being caught drink driving). The basis for this is to increase liver levels of NAD and thereby accelerate the action of ADH. Data tend to suggest that consumption of high doses of fructose leads to an acceleration of up to 40% in the metabolism of ethanol (review, Ref. 4), although there is great variability between subjects.[44] In practice, the amount of fructose that must be consumed to cause an effect is very high and is likely to lead to other side effects.

Nutritional status is an important factor. Low nutritional status resulting from chronic alcohol abuse inevitably leads to reductions in vitamin intake. NAD is produced from nicotinic acid, one of the B-group of vitamins,[ix] and must be regenerated from NADH or replaced from the diet to maintain adequate supplies for ADH and aldehyde dehydrogenase. The vitamin thiamine is also affected by poor nutrition and is often added to bread and other foods as supplements. Vitamin supplements are used in the treatment of alcoholics.

---

[ix] Deficiency in nicotinic acid (known as niacin) and other B-group vitamins leads to the disease known as pellegra characterized by dermatitis of the skin exposed to sunlight, stomatitis, sores, magenta tongue, inability to digest foods, and diarrhoea.

# Ethanol

Ingestion of large doses of ethanol (BAC >0.3%) will retard gastric emptying and absorption in the lower intestine. Drugs such as the antibiotic erythromycin, the prokinetic agent cisapride and the antinausea drug metoclopramide increase gastrointestinal motility and accelerate absorption, while morphine and the other opioids decrease motility (see Section 5) and reduce the rate of absorption.

Drugs such as cimetidine and ranitidine, which are used to treat duodenal ulcers and reduce acid secretion, have no effect on ethanol pharmacokinetics.[5] However, smoking increases the rate of disappearance of ethanol by up to 20%, due presumably to induction of liver enzymes. Alcohol reduces the clearance of benzodiazepines metabolized not only by N-demethylation and oxidation pathways,[45] but also apparently to lorazepam which is conjugated.[46] Oxazepam is not affected. These changes may in part be related to the alterations in tissue NAD/NADH cofactor concentrations. This phenomenon may also apply to opioids and the barbiturates. In liver disease, these changes will be greater.

Acute consumption of excessive alcohol inhibits formation of the toxic metabolite N-acetyl-para-benzoquinone following overdose with paracetamol (acetaminophen), but not in alcoholics who show induction of enzymes that increase the formation of this toxic metabolite.[47] Doxycycline (antibiotic), pentobarbital (sedative) and tolbutamide (antidiabetic) show similar phenomena.

Drugs such as propranolol[x] reduce the BAC, presumably because of the effects on blood flow to the liver.[48] Other drugs affecting liver blood flow will affect the clearance of ethanol.

Reviews on the pharmacokinetic interactions between alcohol and drugs are worthwhile reading.[38,45,47]

Disease states such as congestive heart failure will lower liver blood flow and affect liver clearance. Liver disease is the most important condition affecting ethanol clearance, although advanced liver disease such as cirrhosis is required before any significant reduction in clearance occurs. Renal failure does not markedly affect elimination of ethanol.[49]

## MARKERS OF ALCOHOL CONSUMPTION

### Ethyl glucuronide

Ethyl glucuronide serum concentrations are higher in regular drinkers suspected of driving under the influence, compared with naïve or social drinkers. A serum ethyl glucuronide of greater than 5 mg/L when the BAC is less than 0.10% has been suggested as representing alcohol misuse.[18] The half-life of this metabolite is estimated at 2–3 h, hence it will be present some time after ethanol has been removed from blood.

### Methanol

Methanol is the simplest alcohol and is known to be present as a normal endogenous substance at serum concentrations of ~0.3–0.9 mg/L (or 0.0001%). Methanol is metabolized by

---

[x] Propranolol belongs to the beta-blocker class of antihypertensive drugs, and reduces blood pressure by dilating blood vessels (reducing peripheral resistance) and lowering heart rate.

the same enzymes that metabolize ethanol. These produce formaldehyde and carbon dioxide as successive metabolites, but only when ethanol is not present in a person. Ethanol competes with methanol for these enzymes and is preferentially metabolized.[50] Chronic heavy alcohol consumption is known to cause a build-up of methanol over time to concentrations that are not only detectable by laboratories performing analysing for ethanol,[xi] but also begin to exert a toxic effect. This is exacerbated by the presence of methanol in alcoholic beverages. Methanol concentrations are highest in brandy (200–300 mg/L) and whisky (80–200 mg/L), with lesser amounts in red wine (60–100 mg/L), white wine (20–40 mg/L), vodka (1–100 mg/L), and beer (1–10 mg/L).[51]

The critical ethanol concentration above which no methanol is eliminated is 0.02%. The half-life of methanol is 1.4–3.3 h.[50]

In forensic cases the presence of methanol in alcoholics above 10 mg/kg is unusual and strongly implies chronic alcoholism, an embalmed body, or ingestion of methanol. Methanol poisonings in Western countries are uncommon since alcohol-based solvents including methylated spirits contain only ethanol. Some embalming fluids contain methanol, as well as other chemicals (formaldehyde, volatile fragrant oils, etc.).

## Biochemical markers

Biochemical markers for alcoholism include γ-glutamyltransferase (GGT) and carbohydrate-deficient transferrin (CDT). CDT appears to show promise as a postmortem marker of alcoholism.[52] The CDT quotient (to transferrin) of greater than 10% is regarded as being abnormal.

# DURATION OF ACTION

The duration of action of ethanol is primarily affected by the clearance of ethanol from the body. While there are differences in sensitivity to ethanol from one person to another, and variations exist in the rate of elimination, persons consuming low to moderate amounts of alcohol will be affected by alcohol for a shorter period than those consuming a large amount of alcohol.

As a rule of thumb, humans eliminate approximately one measure of alcohol per hour.[xii] Persons who have consumed four glasses of normal strength beer (200 mL at 5% v/v), or four glasses of wine (100 mL at 10% v/v), would have a detectable BAC for approximately 4 h. Persons consuming 12 measures would be affected for the most part of 12 h.

# EFFECTS OF ALCOHOL ON DRUG PHARMACOKINETICS

Ethanol is known to affect the pharmacokinetics of a large number of drugs. This can occur by an effect on the absorption process, or by an alteration in clearance, probably related to

---

[xi] Only those laboratories using gas chromatographic analysis.
[xii] This rule makes many approximations, but can provide a rough guide to the clearance and duration of action of alcohol when accuracy is not necessary.

**Table 6.3** Selected pharmacokinetic studies for alcohol

| Reference | Cases/gender | Age (years)[a] | Dose | $T_{max}$[b] (min) | $C_{max}$[c] (g%) | $\beta$[d] (%/h) | Comments |
|---|---|---|---|---|---|---|---|
| 54 | 48M | 20–60 | 0.68 g/kg (55 g) neat whisky, fasting | 54 (30–120) | 0.092 (0.061–0.123) | 0.0126 (0.0097–0.0147) | Ranges in 95% confidence limits |
| 7 | 4M, 4F | 27, 28 | 330 mL 1.8% beer in 5 min | — | 0.002–0.011 | 0.015 | Two light beer strengths under various conditions |
|  | 9M | 53 | 660 mL 3.0%, fasting, or after food | 30–50 | 0.026–0.044 | 0.012 |  |
|  |  |  | 660 mL 3.6%, fasting, or after food | 30–50 | 0.023–0.054 | 0.014 |  |
|  |  |  |  | 30–70 | 0.020–0.029 |  |  |
|  |  |  |  | 30–50 | 0.020–0.039 | 0.011 |  |
| 31 | 50M | 21–81 | Intravenous ethanol 0.57 g/kg over 1 h (46 g) | 60 | Y 0.11–0.21 | 0.034 | No significant age effect when corrected for body mass |
|  |  |  |  | 60 | O 0.14–0.20 | 0.029 |  |
| 12 | 24M | 19–27 | 0.3 mg/kg (21 g) before food and after food | 27 | 0.040 | 0.017 | Significant food effect |
|  |  |  |  | 37 | 0.021 | 0.009 |  |
| 22 | 150 | 20–60 | Three doses of alcohol given on an empty stomach, 0.51, 0.68 and 0.85 g/kg, respectively (41, 54 and 68 g) | — | 0.075 | 0.090–0.013 | Shows dose-dependent increase in BAC, and little change in elimination rate |
|  |  |  |  | — | 0.091 | 0.010–0.017 |  |
|  |  |  |  | — | 0.146 | 0.012–0.016 |  |
| 49 | 4M, 3F | 65 | Two doses of 0.4 g/kg before (B) and after (A) haemodialysis and food | — | B 0.088±0.013 | 0.0157 | Little effect on pharmacokinetics caused by dialysis |
|  |  |  |  | — | A 0.092±0.013 | 0.0185 |  |

[a] Average age, or range; [b] time to peak blood/serum concentration; [c] peak blood/serum concentration; [d] elimination rate; F: female; M: male; Y: young group, 21–56 years; O: old group, 57–81 years.

an effect on the drug metabolizing systems. See Lane *et al.* (1985) for an excellent review on this topic.[47]

The drugs of abuse discussed in this book are affected by alcohol. The clearance of the benzodiazepines diazepam, chlordiazepoxide, clobazam, lorazepam and triazolam, and pentobarbitone are reduced during short-term administration of ethanol. However, for many of these drugs it is uncertain what changes take place under long-term alcohol usage. The solubility of benzodiazepines will be increased with any significant co-consumption of alcohol. This may facilitate the rate of absorption of benzodiazepines. In the presence of ethanol, cocaine is metabolized to cocaethylene, an active and toxic form of cocaine.

Methadone has been shown to increase brain and liver concentrations, reduce biliary concentrations, and reduce N-demethylation after short-term alcohol administration in rats.[53]

## Synopsis

### PHARMACOKINETICS, METABOLISM AND DURATION OF ACTION

1 Ethanol is absorbed orally; peak blood concentrations occur between 0.5 and 2 h.
2 Peak BAC for a small 330-mL bottle of 1.8% light beer is 0.008% in men and women. Peak BAC for two small 330-mL bottles of 3.0% beer is 0.032%.
3 Two measures of alcohol (~20 g) give a peak BAC of 0.04% in adult males on an empty stomach, but only 0.02% with a meal.
4 Ethanol is metabolized to acetaldehyde by the enzyme ADH; acetaldehyde is metabolized to acetate by aldehyde dehydrogenase. Both enzymes require NAD, which is produced from the vitamin niacin. Ethanol, in high concentrations or in alcoholics, is also metabolized by a microsomal enzyme oxidizing system (MEOS).
5 Ethanol is primarily eliminated by metabolism. The rate of decline in plasma is essentially zero order above BAC 0.02% and ranges from 0.01 to 0.04%/h. The mean elimination rate in novice or social drinkers is 0.015%/h, but this increases in regular consumers and alcoholics.
6 There is little difference in the elimination rate between males and females and with advancing age providing adjustments for body weight are made.
7 There are some differences in the pharmacokinetics of ethanol between racial groups with Japanese and African Americans showing slightly higher elimination rates.
8 Urinary excretion of ethanol accounts for ~0.3% of the absorbed dose, while breath and sweat account for 0.7% and 0.1%, respectively.
9 Disulfiram, metronidazole and some other drugs inhibit metabolism of aldehyde dehydrogenase, resulting in the accumulation of the highly toxic acetaldehyde.
10 Other drugs such as erythromycin, cisapride, metoclopramide and propranolol can affect gastrointestinal motility or liver blood flow and affect absorption of ethanol.
11 Ethyl glucuronide, methanol and carbohydrate-deficient transferrin may be useful markers of alcoholism, both clinically and postmortem.

# 6.3 Mechanisms of action

Ethanol has an exceedingly complex pharmacology for such a simple molecule. This chapter provides a review of some of more significant mechanisms of action of this drug and provides an introduction to later chapters that describe the effects associated with alcohol ingestion and alcohol abuse.

Readers are advised to refer to other texts and to a review article for a more detailed account of the mechanisms of action of ethanol.[55,56]

## CNS MECHANISMS

Ethanol is a central nervous system (CNS) depressant and acts to increasingly depress various functions in the brain and the nervous system generally. It also acts to depress organ function generally and its actions in many ways resemble those of the volatile anaesthetics such as chloroform, ether and the modern halogenated anaesthetics. The increase in disorder and fluidity of membranes in nerves and cells explains many of the effects of ethanol.

Despite the often non-specific depression of nerve and cellular function, it is now recognized that ethanol does have specific functions that help to explain its psychoactive actions. Ethanol is now known to affect a number of excitatory and inhibitory amino acid transmitters as well as dopamine and serotonin (5-HT).[55]

One of the mechanisms is enhancement of GABA-mediated inhibition, which is akin to the mechanism of action of benzodiazepines and barbiturates. Ethanol has less specific and consistent effects on this receptor system than the benzodiazepines. The benzodiazepine antagonist flumazenil has been used to treat alcohol dependence[57] as has the opioid antagonist naltrexone. The fact that both of these receptor antagonists have some effect illustrates the effect of ethanol on the GABA system and the connection of the GABAergic neurons[xiii] with opioid receptors in the brain. This also explains why benzodiazepines (and barbiturates) enhance the actions of ethanol, and vice versa (see Chapter 6.7).

Ethanol also enhances the actions of serotonin at the 5-HT$_3$ receptor (significant receptor system involved in behaviour) and the nicotinic acetylcholine receptor in the CNS. Both receptors are excitatory, whereas most of the actions of ethanol are to augment inhibitory systems (such as GABA) or inhibit excitatory systems, such as inhibiting the opening of voltage-sensitive Ca$^{++}$ channels affected by glutamate. Glutamate acts on receptors (NMDA type) that are involved in learning and the acquisition of memory.

These varied effects on excitatory and inhibitory nerve processes in the CNS account for the complex pharmacology of alcohol and the variable responses observed in persons using the drug. It also accounts for the serious and irreversible changes caused by chronic alcohol abuse.

---

[xiii] Neurons that utilize GABA as neurotransmitter.

Pharmacodynamic tolerance develops to chronic alcohol use and is thought to involve adaptive changes in membranes, receptors systems in the brain together with their associated ion channels, and intracellular messengers that are involved in expressing receptor- or ion-mediated signals.[58]

## PERIPHERAL MECHANISMS

At high enough concentrations, ethanol blocks nerve conduction in peripheral nerves and in the CNS by affecting sodium and potassium conduction through ion channels. This accounts for the serious toxic effects evident at high ethanol concentrations. Chronic heavy use may also be associated with a peripheral neuropathy leading to sensory loss in the hands and feet.

Ethanol also affects cardiovascular function by depressing cellular activity in part due to its inhibitory effect in the CNS. Cardiac arrhythmias such as atrial fibrillation and elevation of the QT-interval[xiv] can cause serious problems, including sudden death. Ethanol also produces vasodilatation, which is the cause of the flushed appearance of some alcohol users. Effects on platelet function and lipoproteins (increase in HDL concentration) may lead to initial protection against atherosclerosis (clogging of arteries) and formation of thrombi (clots in blood vessels).

There is also a range of other haematological changes secondary to liver disease. Ethanol also produces a number of endocrine effects including increased output of adrenal steroid hormones, increased secretion of ACTH and increased plasma hydrocortisone. An increased urine output (diuresis) caused by ethanol is well known and may lead to dehydration. Liver damage caused by excessive alcohol intake is most well known (see later, p. 293).

## Synopsis

**MECHANISMS OF ACTION**

1 Ethanol acts to increasingly depress various functions in the brain (CNS) and the nervous system generally.
2 Ethanol depresses nerve transmission generally, including those nerves supplying vital organs and the vascular system.
3 Ethanol affects a number of excitatory and inhibitory transmitter systems in the CNS, including acetylcholine, GABA, serotonin, dopamine and glutamate receptors.
4 Enhancement of GABA mediation inhibition is similar to that caused by the benzodiazepines and probably explains the additivity of effects of ethanol and benzodiazepines in humans.
5 The effect on various CNS transmission systems explains the variable responses, both excitatory and inhibitory, in persons using ethanol.
6 Effects on peripheral systems include heart, lungs and kidneys, as well as endocrine and numerous biochemical functions.

---

[xiv] This is one of the important indicators of heart function seen in the electrocardiogram.

# 6.4 Pharmacological actions and therapeutics

Ethanol has been used in a huge variety of social drinks and herbal or medicinal tonics for thousands of years. Its social use as a recreational drug, and its use as a serious drug of abuse, is arguably more blurred than for any other drug. As the previous chapter introduced, the pharmacology of ethanol is varied and complex.

The functions of ethanol can be separated into those affecting the CNS, the cardiovascular system, the liver and gastrointestinal system, effects on other systems and its biochemical actions.

## CNS EFFECTS

The effects on CNS function are probably the most significant. Ethanol at blood concentrations (BAC) in excess of ~0.02% produces decrements in motor co-ordination (e.g. ability to perform hand–eye co-ordination), speech articulation, intellectual performance, judgement and sensory discrimination. Slurred speech and unsteadiness on the feet are tell-tale signs of alcohol intoxication. There is no clear threshold at which intoxication begins to manifest, but overt intoxication usually only becomes clearly evident clinically at BACs above 0.1%.

The actual impairment at a given BAC is often higher as the ethanol concentration rises rather than when it falls. This may be more of a pharmacokinetic phenomenon associated with the actual brain concentration, but also may be related to a degree of tolerance established to the effects of ethanol. Hang-over effects the morning after too much alcohol consumption are well known.

Alcohol also produces a sense of euphoria, although this is less pronounced than for heroin and cocaine, but more importantly produces disinhibition and increased self-confidence. These latter effects result in gregarious behaviour, and other actions that may normally be suppressed. This can manifest itself as aggression, with loud and outrageous behaviour. The reduced judgement that accompanies alcohol intoxication can lead to serious behavioural changes in persons when confronted by others, or an increased argumentativeness that again may lead to aggressive and violent outcomes.

The change in mood caused by alcohol is not always predictable. Some people react as presented in the previous paragraph, while others may become sleepy, introverted or even depressed.

Whatever behaviour emanates from alcohol use, cognitive actions (memory and judgement) are impaired together with the psychomotor actions. These effects are best illustrated

## Pharmacological actions and therapeutics

in driving tests and driving behaviour in alcohol-affected persons. The risk of being involved in an accident is measurable between 0.05% and 0.08% (BAC) and increases exponentially as the BAC rises.[59,60] Of interest in drivers using alcohol are their delayed and impaired reactions to driving situations caused by the depression of psychomotor and cognitive functions, but also their increased risk taking and increased speed.

The CNS effects become increasingly greater with rising BAC. At very high BAC (>0.2%) serious toxicity becomes apparent and by 0.3% coma is increasingly likely. Depression of respiration is the most serious toxic CNS effect at high BAC. Death can occur from respiratory failure at 0.4% BAC, although other complications capable of causing death can occur at lower concentrations (see Chapter 6.6).

Chronic abuse often leads to permanent brain damage.[61] Loss of memory and dementia are common. Blackouts (episodes of amnesia) associated with chronic ethanol abuse result from a disorder of central serotonergic neurotransmission, as well as general loss of brain functions. Memory function can be improved by the treatment with a serotonin re-uptake inhibitor zimeldine.[62]

Neuropsychiatric disturbances or brain diseases such as Wernicke's encephalopathy, Korsakoff's psychosis, central pontine myelinolysis and general cerebellar degeneration are known.[58] Alcoholics also have a higher incidence of peripheral nerve disorders, particularly polyneuropathies (general irreversible loss of nerve function). Nicotinic acid deficiency (due to chronic depletion of NAD used in its metabolism) and general nutritional and vitamin deficiency (particularly thiamine) appear to be major causes for these conditions.[56,63] As for other drugs of abuse, maintenance of proper nutrition reduces harm associated with chronic use. Abrupt withdrawal may also be associated with a range of problems, including fitting (see later, p. 298).

## CARDIOVASCULAR SYSTEM

Small to moderate doses of alcohol have few direct effects on blood pressure and heart rate. However, vasodilation of blood vessels in the skin causing 'flushing' is common. Vasodilation in larger vessels such as the coronary arteries also occurs. Importantly, moderate consumption of alcohol does lead to a reduced incidence of atherosclerosis.

Contrary to popular opinion, alcohol causes increased heat loss by dilation of skin capillaries and through increased sweating. Lowering of core body temperature is therefore a real possibility when exposed to the elements without sufficient protection.

Chronic excessive use leads to changes (usually increases) in cardiac output and importantly can predispose to cardiomyopathy, heart conduction changes, congestive heart failure and cardiac arrhythmias. Myopathy of other muscle groups, such as skeletal muscle, can also occur. Indeed, chronic excessive use is also a risk factor for the development of high blood pressure and stroke.

## LIVER AND GASTROINTESTINAL SYSTEM

Alcohol causes mobilization of fat from peripheral tissue resulting in its accumulation in the liver. This is particularly common in regular users of alcohol and in binge drinking. Increased fat content of liver leads to chronic inflammation of the liver (hepatitis) and a condition known as 'fatty liver' (steatosis), and may be observable temporarily after even low doses of alcohol. The inhibition of secretion of protein from liver cells also results in accumulation of protein. Both the accumulation of fat and protein, while reversible initially, can lead to irreversible changes and cirrhosis. Malnutrition and vitamin deficiency contributes significantly to this process.

Cirrhosis and associated conditions such as ascites and congestive heart failure are serious, life-threatening diseases.

Alcohol is an irritant to the stomach and increases the release of gastrin, with irritation increasing with the amount ingested and the concentration of alcohol in the stomach itself. Alcohol abuse produces a high incidence of erosive gastritis (inflammation of stomach) and ulceration with subsequent blood loss. Pancreatitis, both acute and chronic, is also associated with regular alcohol consumers due to release of secretin and obstruction of the pancreatic duct.

## OTHER EFFECTS

### Kidney

Consumption of alcohol induces a diuretic effect on the kidney by a decrease in renal tubular reabsorption of water. This leads to a preferential loss of water and dehydration by inhibiting secretion of the antidiuretic hormone. This effect is worse for high-alcohol-content beverages. The use of low-alcohol beverages or the concomitant consumption of water is recommended to reduce dehydration.

### Biochemical and endocrine abnormalities

A number of hormonal and biochemical changes are caused by alcohol consumption.[64] Alcohol is likely to affect most if not all endocrine functions, including adrenals, pituitary, hypothalamus, gonads and thyroid glands. Some of these have been briefly mentioned earlier.

Alcohol affects glucose metabolism. Hypoglycaemia is not an uncommon occurrence, together with diabetic ketoacidosis, in which acetone bodies are present in tissues, particularly on alcohol withdrawal.

The ability of alcohol to raise high-density lipoproteins (HDL) and to inhibit platelet aggregation at BAC levels under 0.10% is the likely reason for a mild protecting effect against the development of ischaemic heart disease and atherosclerosis. Much higher consumption of alcohol has the reverse effect and leads to premature ischaemic heart disease, arrhythmias and associated vascular abnormalities.

Perhaps one of the most significant effects of excessive alcohol consumption is the interference in a number of critical biochemical cycles by the utilization of large amounts of the cofactor NAD (see Chapter 6.2). Since chronic abuse or binge drinking involves the consumption of 100 g or more of ethanol in a session, enormous quantities of NAD are consumed. The resultant production of NADH causes unphysiological production of lactate, fatty acids with possible adverse effects on the citric acid cycle, and fatty acid oxidation. The net result is depletion of NAD and AMP.[xv] At the same time large quantities of acetate (acetic acid) is produced.

## Cancers

Alcoholics show an increased incidence of mouth, pharynx, larynx, oesophagus, liver and lung cancers compared with the normal population.

## Fetal alcohol syndrome

Alcohol consumption during pregnancy results in a higher risk of adverse fetal development. Fetal alcohol syndrome (FAS) normally manifests in moderate to heavy drinkers (>4 drinks per day) or binge drinkers, and results in varying levels of mental retardation and behavioural abnormalities. In extreme cases, retarded growth, abnormal facial and cranial development, and congenital heart problems and other malformations occur. These effects result from the teratogenic effects of ethanol and the metabolite acetaldehyde, by inhibiting embryonic cellular proliferation. These children also have impaired immune systems and are more susceptible to diseases.

# THERAPEUTIC USES OF ETHANOL

Many people will argue that a glass or two of wine or a few glasses of beer are therapeutic. There are now published studies that support the lowering of risk of atherosclerotic disease of arteries in persons using less than four measures of alcohol per day. Despite this effect, any alcohol above BAC 0.02% will cause some impairment of psychomotor and cognitive functions. At BAC 0.05% this impairment becomes significant in most people. Those consumers who have developed some tolerance to the drug, without necessarily becoming alcoholics, may require slightly higher BACs to record a measurable loss of performance.

Alcohol has had a variety of other uses. Alcohol in small quantities improves digestion and acts as a hypnotic. Its ability to cause drowsiness is useful when sleep is desired or when recovering from a minor head cold.

Alcohol is an excellent solvent for pharmaceuticals, and for the preparation of disinfectants, liniments and rubbing agents. Alcohol is used to reduce skin ulceration in bedridden persons. Alcohol when applied to the skin increases sweating and aids the loss of body heat during fever.

Ethanol is also used to treat methanol poisoning. Ethanol competes with ADH and is preferentially metabolized, reducing the formation of toxic formaldehyde and formic acid metabolites of methanol.

---

[xv] AMP (adenosine monophosphate) is used to produce ATP, the key energy source in cells. ATP is produced enzymatically using NADH as an energy source.

# Ethanol

## Synopsis

**PHARMACOLOGICAL ACTIONS AND THERAPEUTICS**

1. Alcohol causes decrements in cognitive and psychomotor skills at BACs >0.02%.
2. Alcohol produces disinhibition and increased self-confidence, and in many people loud and outrageous behaviour leading to aggression and violence. In others, it may lead to introversion and depression.
3. Clinical signs of alcohol intoxication are usually only evident at BACs >0.1%. Serious depression of vital functions occurs at >0.2%.
4. Alcohol produces skin flushing caused by vasodilation associated with increased loss of body heat, diuresis and dehydration, and in some cases gastritis and ulcerations of the stomach, pancreatitis and gall stones.
5. Chronic use leads to a high incidence of brain damage presenting as memory loss, dementia and psychoses, which often are exacerbated by nutritional deficiencies.
6. Liver cirrhosis is the result of chronic fatty liver and hepatitis caused by chronic high-dose alcohol consumption.
7. Alcoholics present with a greater incidence of heart disease, atherosclerosis, oral, lung and liver cancers, cardiac and skeletal muscle myopathies, and stroke.
8. Alcohol abuse during pregnancy increases the risk of a range of fetal malformations, including fetal alcohol syndrome.
9. Biochemical abnormalities are common and are due to excessive production of NADH and ATP, resulting in increased fatty production and interferences in key biochemical metabolic cycles including glucose metabolism.
10. Endocrine abnormalities are also common, caused by the release of steroids and interferences of other hormones from the adrenals, gonads, hypothalamus, thyroid and pituitary.
11. Therapeutic uses of low doses of alcohol include improving digestion, reducing fever, and use as a disinfectant and as a mild hypnotic.

# 6.5 Adverse reactions, tolerance and dependence

The previous two chapters have detailed the mechanisms and effects caused by alcohol and in particular excessive alcohol consumption. This chapter details the abuse potential of alcohol, and the potential for alcohol users to become dependent and elicit tolerance. Despite its legal status, alcohol is a more abused drug than all of the other illegal drugs put together.

## ABUSE POTENTIAL

Ethanol is regarded as a drug with moderate to high abuse potential. This means that regular users will have a reasonable chance of becoming dependent on ethanol, and by definition, exhibit many or all of the criteria associated with dependence as defined by the American Medical Association and other health bodies (see Chapter 1.6).

The likelihood of developing alcohol-related illnesses increases substantially beyond about four drinks per day in men, and two to three drinks for women. A high risk for developing a dependence on alcohol starts at more than eight drinks per day for men, and more than five drinks per day for women (heavy drinkers). Estimates of the prevalence of alcoholics in the community vary up to 10% of the drinking population,[1] and in those drinking six or more alcoholic drinks daily the increase in mortality is 50%.[2]

Children of alcohol-dependent persons have a four-fold higher risk of becoming alcohol-dependent themselves.[65]

## ADVERSE REACTIONS

The best indication for alcohol-related dependence is frequent intoxication (probably daily) and the onset of illnesses classically related to alcohol abuse or alcoholism. These include upset stomachs (gastritis), ulcers, flushed face, loss of memory, sleep disturbances, increased blood pressure and weight gain.

Additionally, there are a range of social markers that although not specific for alcoholism may initiate further investigation. These include behavioural changes, absenteeism, etc. Long-term changes late in alcoholism include dementia, psychoses, and liver disease leading to cirrhosis. General nutritional and vitamin deficiency occurs early in the abuse stage. See the previous section for details of these illnesses.

## TOLERANCE

Both pharmacokinetic and pharmacodynamic tolerance occur to the effects of chronic alcohol use. Pharmacokinetic tolerance results in an increased ability to eliminate ethanol. The rate per hour increases from an average of 0.012–0.015%/h to 0.02–0.03%/h. This is believed to be caused by induction of the microsomal enzyme oxidizing system (MEOS) but also may be due to improved recycling of the NADH produced from alcohol metabolism. Consequently, even larger daily doses of alcohol are required to maintain a defined BAC.

Chronic alcohol consumers develop tolerance to the effects of alcohol (pharmacodynamic tolerance). Whereas visual recognition of intoxication is frequently evident at BACs of 0.1% in social drinkers, alcoholics may require much higher levels to attain this level of apparent intoxication. A study on 110 alcoholics admitted to a detoxification programme showed that 80% were positive to alcohol and 64% had BACs >0.2%, the highest being 0.44%.[66] Clinical examination of these subjects on entry showed most had no clinical signs of intoxication (speech, gait, vision, verbal comprehension, pupil size and co-ordination) and five of the ten individuals with BACs >0.35% showed normal speech. A varying response to other signs was noted, but not all individuals failed all other tests.

Anecdotal reports in the literature show many examples of extreme BAC readings well over 0.4%. Survival after a BAC of 1.5% with only signs of agitation, abdominal pains and slight confusion has been published.[67]

However, it is a misnomer to suggest that alcoholics are not impaired at 0.1% (or even lower concentrations). Their general cognitive and psychomotor skills are impaired, but their visual appearance to outsiders may not suggest overt intoxication. Late-stage alcoholics will have suffered permanent loss of brain function, which will further reduce their reaction times and cognitive performance.

## DEPENDENCE AND ABSTINENCE

Withdrawal symptoms of persons with alcohol dependence are well characterized. These include anxiety, irritability, tremor and insomnia in the early stages, leading to fever, sweating, disorientation, hallucinations and delirium tremens.[68] This process may take from 1 to 2 weeks. Alcoholic seizures are well known in withdrawing alcoholics. These develop within 2 days of withdrawal and are generalized rather than localized to one region of the brain. Diabetic ketoacidosis is also common and leads to a build-up of α-ketoacids and acetone with associated glucose abnormalities. Untreated, there is a significant morbidity and mortality associated with these conditions.

Drugs used to treat withdrawal include clonidine (0.2 mg several times daily for a few days), benzodiazepines (oral or intravenous) and chlormethiazole (oral or intravenous). The sedative chlormethiazole (Hemineurin M etc.) is commonly used in loading doses of 400–800 mg with additional drug to maintain sedation.

# Adverse reactions, tolerance and dependence

## Synopsis

### ADVERSE REACTIONS, TOLERANCE AND DEPENDENCE

1. Alcohol has a moderate to high abuse potential with up to 10% of users becoming dependent and developing into alcoholics.
2. The likelihood of developing an alcohol-related illness starts at >4 drinks per day for men and >2 drinks per day for women (moderate to heavy drinkers).
3. A high risk for developing a dependence on alcohol starts at >8 drinks per day for men and >5 drinks per day for women (heavy drinkers).
4. The best indication for alcohol-related dependence is frequent intoxication and the onset of vitamin or nutritional deficiency. Long-term changes include dementia, psychoses, encephalopathies, polyneuropathies, ischaemic heart disease, biochemical abnormalities and liver cirrhosis.
5. Pharmacokinetic tolerance develops with chronic abuse, causing an increased elimination rate often over 0.02%/h.
6. Pharmacodynamic tolerance reduces visual evidence of intoxication at BACs normally associated with intoxication in social or naïve consumers. BACs much greater than 0.1% are tolerated.
7. Withdrawal symptoms of persons with alcohol dependence are well characterized and include excessive anxiety, irritability, tremor and insomnia, leading to fever, sweating, disorientation, hallucinations, convulsions and delirium tremens.
8. Clonidine, chlormethiazole and benzodiazepines are used to treat alcohol withdrawal.

# 6.6 Toxicology

Alcohol is present in more forensic cases than probably any other drug and is a contributing agent in many traffic accidents, acts of violence and drug-related deaths. While evidence for its involvement in a adverse or toxic response at marginal blood concentrations (BAC <0.1%) is weak, the drug clearly shows an increase in toxicity at higher BACs. This chapter reviews the toxicology of ethanol and its involvement in forensic cases.

## PREVALENCE IN FORENSIC CASES

Ethanol is a factor in a large proportion of deaths reported to coroners. Statistics on the incidences of alcohol in various types of coroners cases are shown in Table 6.4.

The median BAC in drug-related deaths, drivers, homicides and suicides is often greater than 0.15%, indicating that most of those cases positive for ethanol are likely to be substantially affected by the presence of ethanol at the time of their death. Many jurisdictions in other parts of the world have shown high incidences of alcohol in unnatural deaths, including car accidents, suicides, drug deaths and homicides, with rates in these groups often exceeding 50%.[69–84]

While only the drug-related cases have causes of death attributed to drug toxicity, the presence of alcohol in the other cases will have led to impairment of cognitive and psychomotor skills. Contribution to motor vehicle accidents by alcohol is high and increases exponentially with rising BAC.[59,60,85] The relative risk at a BAC 0.05% is approximately double that for drug-free drivers. At a BAC 0.1% the risk is between 5- and 10-fold, which then increases to 25-fold at BAC 0.15%.

There is also a strong association between violence and alcohol use.[86] Heavy drinking and verbal arguments usually precede violent acts, and the victim is as likely as the offender to

**Table 6.4** Incidences of ethanol in various categories of sudden death

| Type of case | Incidence (%) | (BAC), g% |
|---|---|---|
| All coroners' cases ($n = 2121$) | 25 | To 0.63 |
| Drug-related deaths ($n = 350$) | 38 | To 0.63 |
| Homicides ($n = 71$) | 41 | To 0.40 |
| Drivers of motor vehicles ($n = 216$) | 28 | To 0.30 |
| Suicides (non-drug-related) ($n = 515$) | 33 | To 0.41 |
| Natural deaths ($n = 595$) | 13 | To 0.33 |
| Accidents (not MVAs) ($n = 161$) | 24 | To 0.48 |

MVA: motor vehicle accident.
Taken from the Victorian Institute of Forensic Medicine Toxicology database.

initiate an altercation. However, it is the precipitator of the altercation who is more likely to be intoxicated.[87] The BAC in the persons involved in the altercation are likely to well exceed 0.1%, indicating a high likelihood of alcoholic intoxication at the time of many violent criminal offences, including theft and white-collar crime. In a follow-up study of over 1000 alcoholics after several years after treatment, 4% had died by violent means. Suicide and homicide were the leading causes of violent death, with deaths in fires, and pedestrian and other accidents also occurring with some frequency.[88]

Alcohol is also a significant factor in homicide–suicides for both the assailant and the victim.[89]

## FERMENTATION

Putrefaction in bodies will in most cases lead to formation of ethanol in tissues. The rate of formation is variable and will depend on the amount of glucose (sugar) in the blood and tissues, the temperature, the flora of bacteria capable of producing ethanol, and of course the period from death to sampling.

Mannitol is a sugar that is used in emergency medicine to lower intracranial pressure when an intracranial haemorrhage occurs. If a subject dies with this substance present in blood there is a likelihood of accelerated postmortem fermentation leading to the formation of significant amounts of ethanol.

In two reported case studies, the BACs were 0.05% and 0.064% (12-h and 6-day intervals from death to autopsy).[90] In these cases alcohol was absent in the urine, which alerted to the possibility of an artefact.

Alcohol is rarely produced in urine from putrefaction or fermentation processes, unless glucose is present (in diabetics) and the microorganism *Candida albicans* is present.

## COLLECTION ARTEFACTS

There have been some discussions in the literature concerning possible artefacts caused by skin swabbing prior to venipuncture falsely elevating BAC. Skin swabbing, used to disinfect the skin prior to skin puncture, has involved use of ethanol, although commercial swabs are usually based on isopropanol. Small differences have been noted when ethanol has been used to swab skin,[91] but it is likely that this difference is too small to be significant even if ethanol swabs are used, unless gross carelessness is involved.[92,93]

## REDISTRIBUTION AND DIFFUSION

Since ethanol is a simple non-ionizable molecule soluble in water, the distribution of ethanol in cadavers is relatively uniform throughout the body and equilibrates with the aqueous component of tissues and fluids. Postmortem changes do occur from one site to another, although they tend to be minor (compared with many drugs). In one study, a variation of 0.15–0.22% occurred through 13 collection sites, giving a standard deviation of 0.017%.[94]

Unfortunately, there are exceptions. Postmortem diffusion from stomach and bowel contents to neighbouring sites is known to affect blood taken from the abdominal and thoracic areas. Artificial instillation of alcohol-containing solutions into the stomach of alcohol-free cadavers led to positive readings for alcohol in blood. Highest concentrations were found in the pericardial fluid, left pulmonary vein and aorta, and lowest were found in the femoral vein. This diffusion was temperature and time dependent.[95] In practice there is little diffusion if putrefaction has not yet set in, or if heart chamber blood is used.[96]

Similar diffusion of ethanol is found when alcohol-containing vomitus is present in the trachea. Significant amounts of alcohol, and indeed other drugs, are found in pulmonary vessels, aortic blood and the superior vena cava after 48 h at room temperature.[97]

The case report of a 48-year-old male alcoholic found dead lying face down on the carpet raises an interesting problem. In this case, there was evidence of gastric aspiration at autopsy and histologic examination. The distribution of ethanol was very unusual: femoral blood, 0.26% and 0.27% (two samples); heart blood, 0.64%; vitreous humour, 0.76%; urine, 0.08%; bile, 0.62%; liver, 0.25%; and gastric contents, 2.5 g. In addition, this man ingested isopropanol, and according to the history, may also have ingested acetone in the form of nail polish remover. The distribution of both isopropanol and acetone was as expected, which was approximately in proportion to the aqueous content of the respective tissues. It was proposed that agonal or postmortem aspiration of the ethanol-rich vomitus and postmortem fermentation could account for the apparently elevated concentrations of ethanol in heart blood and bile. The elevated vitreous ethanol was explained if ethanol diffusion occurred across the eye in the agonal phase or at postmortem from gastric aspirate in the carpet.[98]

## TISSUE CONCENTRATIONS

A host of specimens have been analysed for alcohol content. In contrast to most drugs, the ethanol concentration varies little between tissues, since ethanol equilibrates to the aqueous component of cells. Individual tissues do have certain advantages and disadvantages. These are briefly discussed below.

### Blood or plasma

Blood, plasma or even serum are most often used to determine the presence of alcohol. The concentrations between blood and plasma (serum) are slightly different due to the different water content. On average plasma concentrations are higher than blood concentrations by a factor of 1.12–1.18.[99]

Heart blood concentrations tend to be very similar to femoral blood concentrations in cadavers provided proper sampling procedures are adopted to avoid contamination and extensive putrefaction has not occurred.[100]

Blood loss with replacements with blood substitutes usually following major trauma has the potential to reduce the BAC. One study failed to find any significant difference after infusion of a blood substitute.[101] This can be explained by the relatively small volume substituted relative to the total aqueous volume of alcohol in the body. In a 70-kg person, the volume of distribution of alcohol is ~30 L; loss of 1 L of blood and its replacement would therefore lead to loss of ~3% of alcohol, assuming equilibrium had been obtained and no further absorption had taken place.

## Bile

Bile alcohol concentrations and BAC are excellently correlated with an average ratio of 0.99 in 89 paired specimens and a correlation coefficient of 0.92.[102] A similar ratio was found in another study of almost 200 cases, although the ratios ranged from 0.32 to 2.91.[103] The mean blood/bile ratio and standard deviation was 1.03 ± 0.32. There was little change to this ratio when corrected for fat content. A ratio of 0.92 was found in another study of 78 post-mortem blood and bile alcohol results covering the full range of BACs.[104]

Bile is subject to bacterial and visceral contamination, hence care should be exercised in its collection and storage.

## Bone marrow

The bone marrow has also been used to measure for alcohol, particularly in cases of decomposition, and has been found to contain concentrations comparable to those in blood. The average blood:bone marrow ratio was 1.26 in a study of cases when the fat content of rib marrow was taken into consideration.[105] Human femur marrow alcohol concentrations are 12–44% (not corrected for fat content) of the corresponding BAC.[106]

## Breath analysis

Breath analysis for ethanol is one of the main tools for the rapid detection of alcohol use.[107] Most police forces around the world use breath-testing devices. These devices rely on the simple principle that ethanol in the pulmonary circulation equilibrates rapidly with alveolar air such that the concentration of ethanol in expired breath is proportional to the BAC.

Depending on the device and procedures used, a blood:breath ratio of 2000–2400 is used by various enforcement agencies to estimate a BAC from the breath result. Whatever factor is used it is important to recognize that humans vary in their blood:breath ratios. Under controlled conditions this ratio can vary from ~2000 to 2800.[108] Consequently, if a breath result is 0.25 mg/L, calibration at 2300 would produce a BAC of 0.058%. If the true blood:breath ratio was 2000 or 2800, then the BACs would be 0.05% and 0.07%, respectively.

This creates a possible dilemma for police forces and the criminal justice system generally if evidential breath analysis is used to prosecute a person for driving under the influence, especially for persons close to the legal limit and persons who have impaired pulmonary function, which can lower the blood:breath ratio to 1200.[109] In some jurisdictions, the breath concentration has legal limits, which reduces the problem of assuming a constant breath:blood ratio.

## Cerebrospinal fluid

There is a good correlation between cerebrospinal fluid (CSF) and blood alcohol concentrations. An average ratio of 1.03 has been obtained.[102]

## Synovial fluid

Synovial fluid (knee joint fluid) is isolated and protected by the bursa sac and the surrounding bone and tissue structures, and consequently is relatively preserved from bacterial attack. No alcohol dehydrogenase is present in synovial fluid.

Studies have found less strong relationships between the BAC and synovial ethanol concentrations. The synovial fluid and BAC ratios range from 0.60 to 0.94, with an average of 0.74.[110] This average has been reported as 0.98 in another study.[111]

## Urine analysis

Urine is sometimes used to assess possible prior consumption of alcohol. As a previous section indicated, the amount of ethanol actually excreted unchanged in urine is only a fraction of 1%. Despite this limited excretion, urine concentrations are generally similar or only slightly higher than those in blood. Urine concentrations tend to be slightly lower in the early stages of absorption since urine in the bladder has a zero or low concentration of alcohol, and tend to be slightly higher during the elimination phase for the converse reason.

Urine:blood concentration ratios in the literature have ranged from $1.33:1$[112] to $1.28:1$[113] and 1.57,[114] although the theoretical ratio (based on water content) is $1.23:1$.[115] Estimates of urine:blood concentration ratio vary from 0.7 to 21 in a study of 5000 forensic cases with a positive alcohol result.[114] A wide range was also observed by Kaye and Cordona.[113] These data suggest that urine should not be used to predict a BAC without incurring a large error.[115]

Correction of urine concentration for creatinine content does not appear to offer any advantages over uncorrected urine volumes.[115]

Urine is less subject to fermentation in the early stages of decomposition depending on bacterial flora and pH of urine. However, persons with urinary tract infections or those with glucose in urine (diabetics) are more likely to produce ethanol in urine.

## Vitreous humour

The vitreous humour is a useful tissue to collect postmortem since it is least likely to be contaminated from visceral fluids and tends to be relatively preserved from bacterial attack. Blood specimens taken from putrefying bodies may have much higher concentrations than those found in the vitreous because of bacterial formation postmortem. In the absence of significant putrefaction the vitreous humour ethanol concentration is similar to the peripheral blood concentration.

Several postmortem studies have compared the blood and vitreous alcohol concentrations.[102,105,116–118] The ratio of blood to vitreous concentrations in these studies and others[116] has given values of 0.57–0.96. A value of 0.85 is the best estimate with a regression coefficient better than 0.8; however, the 95% confidence interval is usually large if one concentration is used to predict the other.[116]

Vitreous humour is most often used to supplement BAC and should be considered as another measure of alcohol content. Where the two values differ, putrefactive formation of ethanol or postmortem artefacts in blood need to be excluded.

## Solid tissues

Ethanol is present in all solid tissues in concentrations proportional to the water content of each tissue. The most common tissues analysed for ethanol are liver (tissue:blood ratio 0.56), muscle (0.93) and brain (ratio 0.65–0.94).[102,118–120]

## TOXICOLOGY AND PATHOLOGY OF ETHANOL

Ethanol can cause death from a combination of respiratory, cerebral and cardiac depression. This usually occurs at BAC >0.4%, although fatalities are known at approximately 0.2%. These lower fatal concentrations of ethanol tend to occur either in persons with already compromised cardio-respiratory function, those in whom aspiration of vomitus occurs, or those whose posture has obstructed their airways (if sleeping or unconscious).

A fatal dose of alcohol in an otherwise healthy person is approximately one bottle of 750 mL whisky or other spirit, six 750-mL bottles of full-strength beer, or 2.5 L of wine. Clearly the duration of drinking, the baseline BAC and the physiological factors mentioned in the previous paragraph will affect the minimum fatal dose.

Persons have survived enormous BACs. Survival after a BAC of 1.127%[121] and 1.51%[122] is known. This illustrates individual variability and their significant tolerance that occurs with regular ethanol consumption.

Young children are at risk from accidental poisoning. Ingestion of 75 mL mouthwash (12.35%) has been reported to have caused hypoglycaemia, coma and tonic seizures in a 2-year-old child.[123] This represents a dose of ethanol of ~9 g.

## Contribution by other drugs and natural disease

The pathological findings associated with chronic alcohol abuse have been described in Chapter 6.5. The presence of encephalopathies and other cerebral disorders, pancreatitis, ischaemic heart disease, atherosclerosis, hepatitis, liver cirrhosis, and diabetic ketoacidosis will all contribute to the toxic effects elicited by a whole range of CNS or cardiodepressant drugs. These drugs are likely to be sedatives, such as the benzodiazepines, barbiturates, tranquillizers, opioids and antidepressants, although the stimulant drugs such as amphetamines and cocaine also interact adversely with alcohol.

### Benzodiazepines

In general, benzodiazepines appear to have little effect on the fatal concentration of alcohol at therapeutic concentrations. Alcohol-related deaths in which no other drug was detected give a mean BAC of 0.36 ± 0.08% ($n = 30$),[xvi] whereas alcohol-related deaths in which diazepam was also detected gave a mean BAC of 0.35 ± 0.04% ($n = 13$). The diazepam concentrations in these cases ranged from 0.1 to 0.7 mg/L (mean 0.3 mg/L), which is consistent with therapeutic use. It is likely that much higher concentrations of diazepam or another benzodiazepine may lower the fatal concentration of alcohol.

---

[xvi] Six years of cases at the Victorian Institute of Forensic Medicine.

# Ethanol

Peripheral blood concentrations in drug-related deaths involving flunitrazepam in the absence of alcohol (mean concentration 0.47 mg/L, $n = 4$) were higher than those in the presence of alcohol (mean concentration 0.18 mg/L, BAC 0.16%, $n = 4$).[124] All of these cases involved the abuse of flunitrazepam since therapeutic flunitrazepam concentrations range up to ~0.02 mg/L.

There is therefore some evidence of the involvement of benzodiazepines, particularly when used to excess.

## Opioids

Combination of opioid drug deaths with alcohol have shown that the minimum fatal concentration of morphine (and presumably dose) is reduced in those subjects in whom alcohol was present at concentrations in excess of 0.2%. In these cases the concentration of morphine and total morphine were halved.[125] The contribution of alcohol in heroin deaths has also been confirmed by other studies. Levine et al.[126] concluded that the use of even small amounts of ethanol with heroin is a risk factor in deaths due to heroin, and this risk increases with rising BAC, particularly above 0.30%. Ruttenber et al.[127] concluded in a study of 505 heroin-related deaths that alcohol at concentrations above 0.10% enhances the toxicity of heroin.

See Case Report 5.2 (p. 261) for effects of alcohol on a heroin-related death.

### Amphetamines

Amphetamine deaths are frequently associated with alcohol use. In San Diego, 34% of amphetamine-associated deaths also involve alcohol.[128] A rate of 34% was reported for Japanese methamphetamine users,[129] and the American Drug Abuse Warning Network (DAWN) report a strong association between methamphetamine-associated deaths and alcohol use.

In Victoria, a review of amphetamine-associated deaths found alcohol to be co-involved in 24%.[130]

Methamphetamine (30 mg intravenously) co-administered to persons using alcohol (1 g/kg) increases heart rate and rate pressure product (heart output and myocardial oxygen consumption) compared with methamphetamine alone. The subjective effects of methamphetamine are not blunted by use of alcohol, although the subjective effects of alcohol are diminished. Alcohol use is not associated with a change in the pharmacokinetics of methamphetamine.[131]

### Cocaine

Alcohol enhances the magnitude and prolongs the euphoric effect of cocaine[132] by reducing the metabolism of cocaine to benzoylecgonine.[133] Cocaethylene, a metabolite of cocaine formed in the presence of ethanol, is as pharmacologically active as cocaine. The concomitant use of alcohol with cocaine is very common, and has been reported to occur in up to 90% of cocaine users.[134] It is of no surprise that the inherent toxicity of their combined use is greater than when either drug is used alone.[132,135] However, the enhancement of cocaine toxicity by alcohol may not be evident when BACs are relatively low.[136]

## Minimum fatal concentrations

Table 6.5 provides a summary of minimum fatal BACs under various conditions. These concentrations reflect the generally higher toxicity of ethanol than often perceived, but they

# Toxicology

**Table 6.5** Minimum fatal blood alcohol concentrations under various conditions

| | |
|---|---|
| Ethanol alone | >0.3% |
| Ethanol plus aspiration | >0.2% |
| Ethanol plus benzodiazepine (low to moderate) | >0.2% |
| Ethanol plus benzodiazepine (high) | >0.1% |
| Ethanol plus heroin (or other opioid) | >0.1% |

Approximations based on a review of over 1000 drug-related cases. Minimum concentrations depend very much on the extent of other drug use, presence of aspiration, position of body and presence of significant natural disease.

should only be used as a guide. Clearly chronic use will lead to tolerance and allow higher blood concentrations to be achieved before developing fatal toxicity. Significant natural disease, particularly cardio-respiratory and liver disease, will also produce lower fatal concentrations.

A minimum of 0.1% BAC has been chosen to elicit significant (measurable) toxicity in cases of mixed drug poisonings. It is at this concentration that clinical signs of intoxication may be evident. Of course lower BAC concentrations will also contribute (to a lower degree), but at this concentration the contribution is often marginal and rarely significant enough to be proven.

## ADVERSE DRUG INTERACTIONS

Disulfiram (Antabuse) (see Chapter 6.2) will inhibit metabolism of acetaldehyde, which causes liver toxicity and cardiac arrhythmias. While disulfiram is used to dissuade consumption of alcohol, it will cause death at much lower alcohol concentrations than simple alcohol poisoning.[137] In these cases acetaldehyde blood concentrations are ~40 mg/L (0.04%).

Metronidazole, a commonly used antibacterial agent, can produce a similar reaction to disulfiram when used in persons consuming alcohol. Metronidazole, like disulfiram, results in the accumulation of acetaldehyde. Blood concentrations of ethanol, acetaldehyde and metronidazole in a death attributed to the accidental coingestion of alcohol and metronidazole were 0.16%, 46 mg/L and 0.4 mg/L, respectively.[138]

Other drugs capable of causing this adverse interaction include the cephalosprorin antibiotics, chloral hydrate and possibly the antidiabetic chlorpropamide, although these drugs are less predictable in their effect on alcohol metabolism.

## Synopsis

### TOXICOLOGY

1 Alcohol (ethanol) is a factor in a large range of deaths, as a contributor to the cause of death in drug-related deaths, by impairing co-ordination and cognitive skills in accidents, by disinhibiting in cases of suicide, or by disinhibiting and provoking violence in homicides.

## Ethanol

2. The median BAC in suicides, homicides, drug-related deaths and motor vehicle accidents is usually over 0.15%.
3. Interpretation of alcohol concentration in specimens is complicated by postmortem artefacts – diffusion from stomach contents and aspiration fluids, and fermentation.
4. Alcohol is found in all tissues at concentrations that mimic their water content.
5. Specimens most preserved from postmortem artefacts are vitreous humour, synovial fluid, urine and bone marrow.
6. Death from alcohol intoxication alone can occur at concentrations as low as BAC 0.2% if aspiration of vomitus or obstruction of airways occurs.
7. Presence of potentially toxic concentrations of another CNS depressant drug or stimulants will contribute to any toxic effect of alcohol (usually >0.10%).
8. Alcoholic liver, heart or cerebral disease will also contribute to a death process initiated by alcohol intoxication.
9. Adverse drug interactions causing an accumulation of the toxic acetaldehyde are known and are caused by disulfiram, metronidazole, the cephalosporins, chloral hydrate and possibly chlorpropamide.

# 6.7 Case reports

## CASE REPORT 6.1 ALCOHOL READ-BACK I

A 20-year-old male (weight 75 kg) has had a blood alcohol measurement taken approximately 5 h after an alleged assault at a night club. He had claimed to have drunk four to five glasses of beer (full strength) and two to three glasses of wine over a period of 4 h. He was not a regular drinker but would occasionally have a binge on the weekend. The BAC was 0.12 g/100 mL.

The prosecution required a back calculation to establish the BAC at the time of the offence and queried the accuracy of the number of drinks consumed.

The back calculation of the BAC some 5 h before the collection of blood involves the process of assuming a certain average elimination rate over this time and making an assumption of when drinking actually finished.

Since alcohol will continue to be absorbed after the last drink, the actual elimination phase may not be evident until about 1 h (range 0–2 h) after the last drink. An elimination rate ($\beta$) of 0.015%/h can be assumed to apply in most social drinkers, with a possible range of 0.01–0.02%/h. For the estimation of dose, the Widmark equation can be used (see Chapter 6.2) substituting the elimination rates used above together with the duration of drinking (4 + 5 h) and the body weight and constant (0.68) for a male.

The table below summarizes the calculations and provides the range of estimates. The back-calculated BAC ranges from 0.16% to 0.22%, and dose consumed from 11 to 15 glasses. These calculations suggest that the accused's account of drinking was probably underestimated.

Consumption of food will raise the best estimate of dose consumed by 0–50%.

| Assumption | Back-calculated BAC[a] (%) | Estimated dose (g) |
|---|---|---|
| $\beta = 0.015$, $t_\beta = 4$ | 0.180 | 122 (12 glasses) |
| $\beta = 0.015$, $t_\beta = 5$ | 0.195 | 130 (13 glasses) |
| $\beta = 0.01$, $t_\beta = 4$ | 0.160 | 107 (11 glasses) |
| $\beta = 0.02$, $t_\beta = 5$ | 0.220 | 153 (15 glasses) |

[a] Assuming elimination time $t_\beta = 4$ or 5 h, and elimination rate = 0.015, 0.010 and 0.020%/h.

# Ethanol

## CASE REPORT 6.2 ALCOHOL READ-BACK 2

In some traffic law jurisdictions, BAC measurements taken more than a certain time after driving are not accepted as the value at the time of driving. Read-back calculations are often requested in these cases to attempt to establish the BAC at the time of a collision. A calculation based on Widmark theory is easily performed.

In this case, drinking began at 1715 h and continued until 2010 h. A collision occurred at 2230 h and the BAC measured by breath analysis at midnight was 0.125%. A read-back calculation gives a possible BAC at the time of the collision between 0.140% and 0.155%. This graph (Fig. 6.6) shows the piecewise linear model of alcohol pharmacokinetics used for basic read-back calculations.

The two cases shown correspond to a 'best case' where absorption is delayed by 2 h and metabolism proceeds at 0.01% per hour, and a 'worst case' where absorption is complete within 30 min and absorption proceeds at 0.02% per hour. Because the exact parameters for any given subject are not known, the best that can be said is that the graphs represent an envelope of possibilities. In cases where the time in question lies in the absorption part of the curve, the BAC cannot be estimated with as much accuracy.

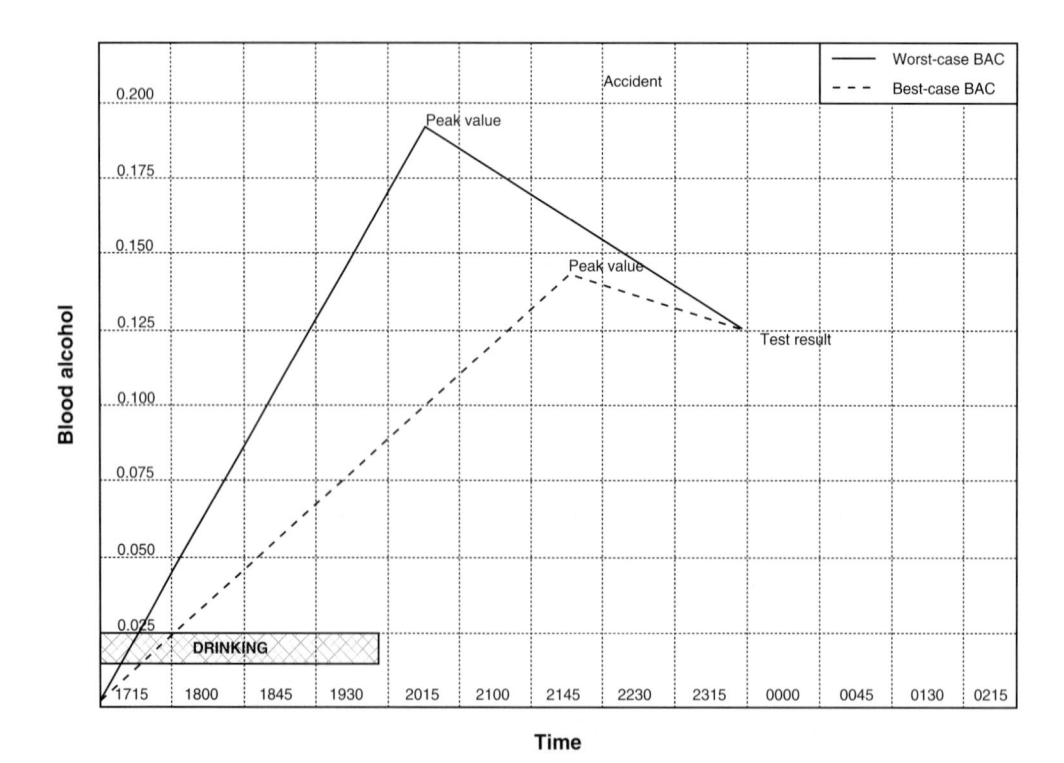

Fig. 6.6 Graphical representation of a read-back of blood alcohol concentration

## CASE REPORT 6.3 ALCOHOL AND HOMICIDE

A case involved the stabbing death of an elderly man (~70 years) by his wife. The accused alleged her husband had continually abused her and refused to believe she had a chronic illness. An argument ensued at which stage the accused stabbed the male. He died some hours later from his injuries.

Toxicology results of the deceased gave a BAC of 0.10%. There was no evidence of alcohol use by the accused.

This is a not too unfamiliar scenario in which a domestic argument has led to a fatal outcome, although in this case the accused has possibly been driven to retaliation by long-standing verbal and violent abuse. Alcohol is more often than not a factor in domestic homicide, or homicide involving known associates, although often both parties are consuming excess alcohol.

Alcohol has the effect of reducing inhibitions and in many cases provoking violent and irrational behaviour. Behavioural changes are often predictable in the one person, and in this case his violent and irrational behaviour was usually associated with excessive consumption of alcohol. Alcoholic intoxication is also associated with partial loss of memory of events occurring during inebriation and subjects may not be perfectly aware of their actions the morning after. In this case, the counsel for the accused could argue self-defence against attack from an irrational and violent person while under the influence of alcohol, in a background of continuing verbal and violent abuse.

The BAC of 0.10% at death some 5 h after his last drink would translate to a BAC of 0.14–0.20% (see Cases 6.1 and 6.2 for calculations). This amounts to ~8–12 glasses of beer, assuming drinking over at least a 3 h period in a 65-kg male.

## CASE REPORT 6.4 ALCOHOL AND PUTREFACTION

A deceased 60-year-old male was found alone lying face-down on the floor of his apartment. The deceased was badly decomposed. There were no obvious signs of struggle or violence.

He had not been seen for approximately 5 days by his neighbours. The ambient temperatures ranged from 18°C to 22°C over this time.

The cause of death was equivocal. There was some evidence of moderate atherosclerosis, but due to the decomposition, any definitive conclusion was ruled out. A full toxicology investigation was conducted to exclude drug involvement.

Toxicology showed a heart blood alcohol of 0.29%, a vitreous alcohol concentration of 0.10% and an urine alcohol concentration of 0.14%.

This is a typical scenario of a death occurring at home alone with some days elapsing before discovery of a body. The circumstances of the case and the observations made by uniformed police attending the scene suggested a natural death, or perhaps a drug-related death.

The heart blood alcohol was much higher than either the vitreous or urine alcohol. Heart blood is more likely to be elevated because of bacterial-mediated fermentation, or postmortem diffusion from stomach contents. In this case, stomach contents were not analysed. The vitreous result was similar to urine, and both specimens were relatively preserved from fermentation processes. It is therefore likely that the true BAC at death was less than 0.14%, and possibly closer to 0.10%. A small formation of ethanol in vitreous is still possible, but less likely in this case.

The analysis of stomach contents for alcohol would have been helpful to establish recent consumption of alcohol. Bone marrow and synovial fluid are also specimens relatively preserved from the fermentation processes.

# References for Section 6

1. Eckhardt MJ, Harford TC, Kaelber CT, et al. Health hazards associated with alcohol consumption. *J Am Med Assoc* 1981; 246: 648–66.
2. Klatsky AL, Armstrong MA, Friedman GD. Alcohol and mortality. *Ann Intern Med* 1992; 117: 646–54.
3. West LJ, Cohen S. Provisions for dependency disorders. In: Holland WW, Detels R, Knox G, eds. *Textbook of public health*. New York: Oxford University Press; 1985. Chapter 9.
4. Baselt RC. Disposition of alcohol in man. In: Garriott JC, ed. *Medicolegal aspects of alcohol*, 3rd edn. Tucson, Arizona: Lawyers and Judges Publishing; 1996. pp. 65–84.
5. Holford NH. Clinical pharmacokinetics of ethanol. *Clin Pharmacokinet* 1987; 13(5): 273–92.
6. Wedel M, Pieters JE, Pikaar NA, Ockhuizen T. Application of a three-compartment model to a study of the effects of sex, alcohol dose and concentration, exercise and food consumption on the pharmacokinetics of ethanol in healthy volunteers. *Alcohol Alcoholism* 1991; 26: 329–36.
7. Jones AW. Concentration–time profiles of ethanol in capillary blood after ingestion of beer. *J Forens Sci Soc* 1991; 31: 429–39.
8. Winek CL, Wahba WW, Dowdell JL. Determination of absorption time of ethanol in social drinkers. *Forens Sci Internat* 1996; 77(3): 169–77.
9. Wilkinson PK, Sedman AJ, Sakmar E, Kay DR, Wagner JG. Pharmacokinetics of ethanol after oral administration in the fasting state. *J Pharmacokinet Biopharm* 1977; 5: 207–24.
10. Widmark EMP. *Principles and applications of medicolegal alcohol determination*. Davis, California: Biomedical Publications; 1981.
11. Friel PN, Baer JS, Logan BK. Variability of ethanol absorption and breath concentrations during a large-scale alcohol administration study. *Alcohol Clin Exp Res* 1995; 19(4): 1055–60.
12. Fraser AG, Rosalki SB, Gamble GD, Pounder RE. Inter-individual and intra-individual variability of ethanol concentration–time profiles: comparison of ethanol ingestion before or after an evening meal. *Br J Clin Pharmacol* 1995; 40(4): 387–92.
13. Sedman AJ, Wilkinson PK, Sakmar E, Weidler DJ, Wagner JG. Food affects on absorption and elimination of alcohol. *J Stud Alcohol* 1976; 37: 1197–214.
14. Lin YJ, Weidler DJ, Carg DC, Wagner JG. Effects of solid food on blood levels of alcohol in man. *Res Commun Chem Pathol Pharmacol* 1976; 13: 713–22.
15. Hahn RG, Norberg A, Gabrielsson J, Danielsson A, Jones AW. Eating a meal increases the clearance of ethanol given by intravenous infusion. *Alcohol Alcoholism* 1994; 29(6): 673–7.

16. Gordon E, Pikkarainen P, Matsuzaki S, Lieber CS. The effect of chronic ethanol consumption on pathways of ethanol metabolism. *Adv Exp Med Biol* 1980; 132: 475–80.
17. Jaakonmaki PI, Knox KL, Horning EC, Horning MG. The characterization by gas–liquid chromatography of ethyl B-D-glucosiduronic acid as a metabolite of ethanol in rat and man. *Eur J Pharmacol* 1967; 1: 63–70.
18. Schmitt G, Droenner P, Skopp G, Aderjan R. Ethyl glucuronide concentration in serum of human volunteers, teetotalers, and suspected drinking drivers. *J Forens Sci* 1997; 42(6): 1099–102.
19. Derr RF. Simulation studies on ethanol metabolism in different human populations with a physiological pharmacokinetic model. *J Pharm Sci* 1993; 82(7): 677–82.
20. Wilkinson PK. Pharmacokinetics of ethanol: a review. *Alcohol Clin Exp Res* 1980; 4(1): 6–21.
21. Wehner HD, Schieffer MC, Krauss S, Hubig M. Concentration dependent ethanol metabolism in steady-state. *Blutalkohol* 1996; 33(1): 17–22.
22. Jones AW. Disappearance rate of ethanol from the blood of human subjects: implications in forensic toxicology. *J Forens Sci* 1993; 38(1): 104–18. [Published erratum appears in *J Forens Sci* 1994; 39(2): 591.]
23. Neuteboom W, Jones AW. Disappearance rate of alcohol from the blood of drunk drivers calculated from two consecutive samples; what do results really mean? *Forens Sci Internat* 1990; 45: 107–15.
24. Wilkinson PK, Reynolds G, Holmes OD, Yang S, Wilkin LO. Nonlinear pharmacokinetics of ethanol: the disproportionate AUC–dose relationship. *Alcohol Clin Exp Res* 1980; 4(4): 384–90.
25. Jones AW, Andersson L. Influence of age, gender, and blood-alcohol concentration on the disappearance rate of alcohol from blood in drinking drivers. *J Forens Sci* 1996; 41(6): 922–6.
26. Winek CL, Murphy KL. The rate and kinetic order of ethanol elimination. *Forens Sci Internat* 1984; 25(3): 159–66.
27. Thurman RG, Cheren I, Forman D, Ewing JA, Glassman E. Swift increase in alcohol metabolism in humans. *Alcohol Clin Exp Res* 1989; 13: 572–6.
28. Jones AW, Norberg Å, Hahn RG. Concentration–time profiles of ethanol in arterial and venous blood and end-expired breath during and after intravenous infusion. *J Forens Sci* 1997; 42(6): 1088–94.
29. Gill J. Women, alcohol and the menstrual cycle. *Alcohol Alcoholism* 1997; 32(4): 435–41.
30. Lucey MR, Hill EM, Young JP, Demo-Dananberg L, Beresford TP. The influences of age and gender on blood ethanol concentrations in healthy humans. *J Stud Alcohol* 1999; 60(1): 103–10.
31. Vestal RE, McGuire EA, Tobin JD, Andres R, Norris AH, Mezey E. Aging and ethanol metabolism. *Clin Pharmacol Ther* 1977; 21(3): 343–54.
32. Shen YC, Fan JH, Edenberg HJ, Li TK, Cui YH, Wang YF, et al. Polymorphism of ADH and ALDH genes among four ethnic groups in China and effects upon the risk for alcoholism. *Alcohol Clin Exp Res* 1997; 21(7): 1272–7.

33. Dohmen K, Baraona E, Ishibashi H, Pozzato G, Moretti M, Matsunaga C, et al. Ethnic differences in gastric sigma-alcohol dehydrogenase activity and ethanol first-pass metabolism. *Alcohol Clin Exp Res* 1996; 20(9): 1569–76.
34. Mizoi Y, Adachi J, Fukunaga T, Kogame M, Ueno Y, Nojo Y, et al. Individual and ethnic differences in ethanol elimination. *Alcohol Alcoholism* 1987; suppl. 1: 389–94.
35. Thomasson HR, Beard JD, Li TK. ADH2 gene polymorphisms are determinants of alcohol pharmacokinetics. *Alcohol Clin Exp Res* 1995; 19(6): 1494–9.
36. Thomasson HR, Crabb DW, Edenberg HJ, Li TK. Alcohol and aldehyde dehydrogenase polymorphisms and alcoholism. *Behav Genet* 1993; 23(2): 131–6.
37. Gershman H, Steeper J. Rate of clearance of ethanol from the blood of intoxicated patients in the emergency department. *J Emerg Med* 1991; 9(5): 307–11.
38. Ferner RE. Interactions between alcohol and drugs. *Adverse Drug Bull* 1998; 189: 719–22.
39. Peachey JE, Brien JF, Roach CA, Loonis CW. A comparative review of the pharmacological and toxicological properties of disulfiram and calcium carbimide. *J Clin Psychopharmacol* 1981; 1: 21–6.
40. Penick SB, Carrier RN, Sheldon JR. Metronidazole in the treatment of alcoholism. *Am J Psychiat* 1969; 125: 1063–6.
41. Porteir H, Chapolin JM, Freysz M, Tanter Y. Interactions between cephalosporins and alcohol. *Lancet* 1980; ii: 263.
42. Groop L, Eriksson CJP, Huupponen R, Ylikahri R, Pelkonen R. Roles of chlorpropamide, alcohol and acetaldehyde in determining the chlorpropamide-alcohol flush. *Diabetologica* 1984; 26: 34–8.
43. Fett DL, Vukov LF. An unusual case of severe griseofulvin–alcohol interaction. *Ann Emerg Med* 1994; 24: 95–7.
44. Brown SS, Forrest JAH, Roscoe P. A controlled trial of fructose in the treatment of acute alcoholic intoxication. *Lancet* 1972(October 28): 898–900.
45. Fraser AG. Pharmacokinetic interactions between alcohol and other drugs. *Clin Pharmacokinet* 1997; 33(2): 79–90.
46. Hoyumpa Jr AH. Alcohol interactions with benzodiazepines and cocaine. *Adv Alcohol Subst Abuse* 1984; 3: 21–34.
47. Lane EA, Guthrie S, Linnoila M. Effects of ethanol on drug and metabolite pharmacokinetics. *Clin Pharmacokinet* 1985; 10(3): 228–47.
48. Wagner JG, Weidler DJ, Lin YJ. New method for detecting and quantitating drug–drug interactions applied to ethanol–propranolol. *Res Commun Chem Pathol Pharmacol* 1976; 13: 9–18.
49. Jones AW, Hahn RG. Pharmacokinetics of ethanol in patients with renal failure before and after hemodialysis. *Res Commun Chem Pathol Pharmacol* 1997; 90(3): 175–83.
50. Haffner HT, Banger M, Graw M, Besserer K, Brink T. The kinetics of methanol elimination in alcoholics and the influence of ethanol. *Forens Sci Internat* 1997; 89(1–2): 129–36.
51. Iffland R, Berghaus G. Experiences with volatile alcoholism indicators (methanol, acetone, isopropanol) in DWI car drivers. In: Berghaus G, ed. International Conference on Alcohol and Traffic Safety. Cologne, Germany; 1993. pp. 63–7.

52. Sadler DW, Girela E, Pounder DJ. Post mortem markers of chronic alcoholism. *Forens Sci Internat* 1996; 82: 153–63.
53. Borowsky SA, Lieber CS. Interaction of methadone and ethanol metabolism. *J Pharmacol Exp Therapeut* 1978; 207: 123–9.
54. Jones AW. Interindividual variations in the disposition and metabolism of ethanol in healthy men. *Alcohol* 1984; 1: 385–91.
55. Samson HH, Harris RA. Neurobiology of alcohol abuse. *Trends Pharmacol Sci* 1992; 13: 206–11.
56. *Goodman and Gilman's the pharmacological basis of therapeutics,* various edns. Basingstoke: Macmillan; 1998.
57. Martens F, Koppel C, Ibe K, Wagemann A, Tenczer J. Clinical experience with the benzodiazepine antagonist flumazenil in suspected benzodiazepine or ethanol poisoning. *J Toxicol Clin Toxicol* 1990; 28: 341–56.
58. Charness M, Simon RP, Greenberg DA. Ethanol and the nervous system. *New Engl J Med* 1989; 17: 442–54.
59. Borkenstein FR, Crowther RF, Shumate RP, Zeil WB, Zylman R. The role of the drinking driver in traffic accidents. *Blutalkohol* 1974; 11(suppl. 1): 1–131.
60. Mounce NH, Pendleton OJ. The relationship between blood alcohol concentration and crash responsibility for fatally injured drivers. *Accid Anal Prev* 1992; 24(2): 201–10.
61. Thomson AD, Pratt OE, Jeyasingham M, Shaw GK. Alcohol and brain damage. *Hum Toxicol* 1988; 7(5): 455–63.
62. Weingartner H, Buchsbaum MS, Linnoila M. Zimelidine effects on memory impairments produced by ethanol. *Life Sci* 1983; 33: 2159–63.
63. The social, medical and legal aspects of alcohol. In: Pluechhahn VD, Cordner SM, eds. *Ethics, legal medicine and forensic pathology,* 2nd edn. Melbourne: Melbourne University Press; 1991.
64. Lands WE. A review of alcohol clearance in humans. *Alcohol* 1998; 15(2): 147–60.
65. Schuckit MA. Genetics and the risk for alcoholism. *J Am Med Assoc* 1985; 254: 2614–17.
66. Perper JA, Twerski A, Wienand JW. Tolerance at high blood alcohol concentrations: a study of 110 cases and review of the literature. *J Forens Sci* 1986; 31: 212–21.
67. Johnson PR. BAC 1.51%! survival. *Lancet* 1982(Dec 18): 1394.
68. Freedland ES, McMicken DB. Alcohol related seizures. II. Clinical presentation and management. *J Emerg Med* 1993; 11: 605–18.
69. Abel EL, Zeidenberg P. Age, alcohol and violent death: a postmortem study. *J Stud Alcohol* 1985; 46(3): 228–31.
70. Holinger PC. Violent deaths as a leading cause of mortality: an epidemiologic study of suicide, homicide, and accidents. *Am J Psychiat* 1980; 137(4): 472–6.
71. Riddick L, Luke JL. Alcohol-associated deaths in the District of Columbia – a postmortem study. *J Forens Sci* 1978; 23(3): 493–502.
72. Hain JR, Ryan DM, Spitz WU. Fatal accidents and blood ethanol levels in adolescents and adults. The Wayne County experience, 1978–1988. *Am J Forens Med Pathol* 1989; 10(3): 187–92.

73. Michaud PA. Violent deaths among adolescents in Switzerland. From epidemiology to prevention. *Pediatrician* 1983; 12(1): 28–36.
74. Haberman PW. Alcohol and alcoholism in traffic and other accidental deaths. *Am J Drug Alcohol Abuse* 1987; 13(4): 475–84.
75. Holinger PC, Klemen EH. Violent deaths in the United States, 1900–1975. Relationships between suicide, homicide and accidental deaths. *Soc Sci Med* 1982; 16(22): 1929–38.
76. Kubo S, Dankwarth G, Puschel K. Blood alcohol concentrations of sudden unexpected deaths and non natural deaths. *Forens Sci Internat* 1991; 52(1): 77–84.
77. Christoffel KK, Anzinger NK, Merrill DA. Age-related patterns of violent death, Cook County, Illinois, 1977 through 1982. *Am J Dis Child* 1989; 143(12): 1403–9.
78. Foster GR, Dunbar JA, Whittet D, Fernando GC. Contribution of alcohol to deaths in road traffic accidents in Tayside 1982–6. *Br Med J (Clin Res Ed)* 1988; 296(6634): 1430–2.
79. Loftus IA, Dada MA. A retrospective analysis of alcohol in medicolegal postmortems over a period of five years. *Am J Forens Med Pathol* 1992; 13(3): 248–52.
80. Smith SM, Goodman RA, Thacker SB, Burton AH, Parsons JE, Hudson P. Alcohol and fatal injuries: temporal patterns. *Am J Prev Med* 1989; 5(5): 296–302.
81. Sinha SN, Sengupta SK, Purohit RC. A five year review of deaths following trauma. *P N G Med J* 1981; 24(4): 222–8.
82. Nashold RD, Naor EM. Alcohol-related deaths in Wisconsin: the impact of alcohol on mortality. *Am J Public Health* 1981; 71(11): 1237–41.
83. Budd RD. The incidence of alcohol use in Los Angeles County homicide victims. *Am J Drug Alcohol Abuse* 1982; 9(1): 105–11.
84. Bastos ML, Galante L. Toxicological findings in victims of traumatic deaths. *J Forens Sci* 1976; 21(1): 176–86.
85. Drummer OH. Drugs in drivers killed in Australian road traffic accidents. Melbourne: Department of Forensic Medicine, Monash University; March 1994. Report no. 0594.
86. Collins JJ, Schlenger WE. Acute and chronic effects of alcohol use on violence. *J Stud Alcohol* 1988; 49(6): 516–21.
87. Murdoch D, Pihl RO, Ross D. Alcohol and crimes of violence: present issues. *Int J Addict* 1990; 25(9): 1065–81.
88. Combs-Orme T, Taylor JR, Scott EB, Holmes SJ. Violent deaths among alcoholics. A descriptive study. *J Stud Alcohol* 1983; 44(6): 938–49.
89. Milroy CM, Dratsas M, Ranson DL. Homicide–suicide in Victoria, Australia. *Am J Forens Med Pathol* 1997; 18: 369–73.
90. Jones AW, Andsersson R, Sakshaug J, Mørland J. Possible formation of ethanol in post-mortem blood specimens after antemortem treatment with mannitol. *J Anal Toxicol* 1991; 15: 157–8.
91. Ryder KW, Glick MR. The effect of skin cleansing agents on ethanol results measured with the Du Pont automatic clinical analyser. *J Forens Sci* 1986; 31: 574–9.
92. Goldfinger TM, Schaber D. A comparison of blood alcohol concentration using non-alcohol and alcohol-containing skin antiseptics. *Ann Emerg Med* 1982; 11: 665–7.

93. Ogden EJD, Gerstner-Stevens J, Burke J, et al. Venous blood alcohol sampling and the alcohol swab. *Police Surg* 1992; 42: 4–5.
94. Jones GR, Pounder DJ. Site dependence of drug concentrations in postmortem blood – a case study. *J Anal Toxicol* 1987; 11: 186–90.
95. Pounder DJ, Smith DR. Postmortem diffusion of alcohol from the stomach. *Am J Forens Med Pathol* 1995; 16: 89–96.
96. Plueckhahn VD. The evaluation of autopsy blood alcohol levels. *Med Sci Law* 1968; 8: 168–76.
97. Pounder DJ, Yonemitsu K. Postmortem absorption of drugs and ethanol from aspirated vomitus – an experimental study. *Forens Sci Internat* 1991; 51: 189–95.
98. Singer PP, Jones GR. Very unusual ethanol distribution in a fatality. *J Anal Toxicol* 1997; 21(6): 506–8.
99. Tagliaro F, Lubli G, Ghielmi S, Franchi D, Marigo M. Chromatographic methods for blood alcohol determination. *J Chromatogr* B 1992; 580: 161–90.
100. Prouty RW, Anderson WH. A comparison of postmortem heart blood and femoral blood ethyl alcohol concentrations. *J Anal Toxicol* 1987; 11: 191–7.
101. Ditt J, Schulze G. The time course of the blood alcohol curve in men after blood loss and infusion of a blood substitute. *Acta Med Legale Soc (Liege)* 1963; 16: 71–6.
102. Backer RC, Pisano RV, Sopher IM. The comparison of alcohol concentrations in postmortem fluids and tissues. *J Forens Sci* 1980; 25: 327–31.
103. Winek CL, Henry D, Kirkpatrick L. The influence of physical properties and lipid content of bile on the blood/bile ethanol ratio. *Forens Sci Internat* 1983; 22: 171–8.
104. Stone BE, Rooney PA. A study using body fluids to determine blood alcohol. *J Anal Toxicol* 1984; 8: 95–6.
105. Winek CL, Esposito FM. Comparative study of ethanol levels in blood versus bone marrow, vitreous humour, bile and urine. *Forens Sci Internat* 1981; 17: 27–36.
106. Isokoski M, Alba A, Laiko K. Bone marrow alcohol content in cadavers. *J Forens Med* 1968; 15: 9–11.
107. Mason MF, Dubowski KM. Breath-alcohol analysis: uses, methods, and some forensic problems – review and opinion. *J Forens Sci* 1976; 21: 9–41.
108. Jones AW, Andersson L. Variability of the blood/breath alcohol ratio in drinking drivers. *J Forens Sci* 1996; 41(6): 916–21.
109. Labianca DA, Simpson G. Medicolegal alcohol determination: variability of the blood-to breath-alcohol ratio and its effect on reported breath:alcohol concentrations. *Eur J Clin Chem Clin Biochem* 1995; 33: 919–25.
110. Ohshima T, Kondo T, Sato Y, Takayasu T. Postmortem alcohol analysis of the synovial fluid and its availability in medico-legal practices. *Forens Sci Internat* 1997; 90: 131–8.
111. Winek CL, Bauer J, Wahba WW, Collom WD. Blood versus synovial fluid ethanol concentrations in humans. *J Anal Toxicol* 1993; 17: 233–5.
112. Heise H. Concentrations of alcohol in samples of blood and urine taken at the same time. *J Forens Sci* 1967; 12: 454–62.
113. Kaye S, Cardona E. Errors of converting a urine alcohol value into a blood alcohol level. *Am J Clin Pathol* 1969; 52(5).

114. Winek CL, Murphy KL, Winek TA. The unreliability of using a urine ethanol concentration to predict a blood ethanol concentration. *Forens Sci Internat* 1984; 25(4): 277–81.
115. Jones AW. Lack of association between urinary creatinine and ethanol concentrations and urine/blood ratio of ethanol in two successive voids from drinking drivers. *J Anal Toxicol* 1998; 22: 184–90.
116. Pounder DJ, Kuroda N. Vitreous alcohol is of limited value in predicting blood alcohol. *Forens Sci Internat* 1994; 65: 73–80.
117. Coe JI, Sherman RE. Comparative study of postmortem vitreous humour and blood alcohol. *J Forens Sci* 1970; 15: 185–90.
118. Felby S, Olsen J. Comparative studies of postmortem ethyl alcohol in vitreous humour, blood, and muscle. *J Forens Sci* 1969; 14: 93–101.
119. Jenkins AJ, Levine BS, Smialek JE. Distribution of ethanol in postmortem liver. *J Forens Sci* 1995; 40: 611–13.
120. Baselt RC, Cravey RH. *Disposition of toxic drugs and chemicals in man*, 3rd edn. Foster City, CA: Year Book Medical Publishers; 1990.
121. Gerild D, Hasselbalch H. Survival after a blood alcohol of 1127 mg/dl. *Lancet* 1981; 15: 363.
122. Johnson RA, Noll EC, Rodney WM. Survival after a serum ethanol concentration of $1\frac{1}{2}$%. *Lancet* 1982; 2: 1394.
123. Hornfeldt CS. A report of acute ethanol poisoning in a child: mouthwash versus cologne, perfume and after-shave. *J Toxicol Clin Toxicol* 1992; 30: 115–21.
124. Drummer OH, Syrjanen ML, Cordner SM. Deaths involving the benzodiazepine flunitrazepam. *Am J Forens Med Pathol* 1993; 14(3): 238–43.
125. Gerostamoulos J. The toxicological interpretation of heroin deaths. Melbourne: Monash University; 1998.
126. Levine B, Green D, Smialek JE. The role of ethanol in heroin deaths. *J Forens Sci* 1995; 40: 808–10.
127. Ruttenber AJ, Kalter KD, Santinga P. The role of ethanol abuse in the etiology of heroin-related death. *J Forens Sci* 1990; 35: 891–900.
128. Bailey DN, Shaw RF. Cocaine- and methamphetamine-related deaths in San Diego County (1987): homicides and accidental overdoses. *J Forens Sci* 1989; 34(2): 407–22.
129. Yamamura T, Hisida S, Hatake K. Alcohol addiction of methamphetamine users in Japan. *J Forens Sci* 1991; 36: 754–64.
130. Bowden M. Report into amphetamine-associated deaths in Victoria for the Victorian Institute of Forensic Medicine. Melbourne: University of Melbourne; 1996.
131. Mendelson J, Jones RT, Upton R, Jacob III P. Methamphetamine and ethanol interactions in humans. *Clin Pharmacol Therapeut* 1998; 57: 559–68.
132. Farre M, de la Torre R, Llorente M, Lamas X, Ugena B, Segura J, et al. Alcohol and cocaine interactions in humans. *J Pharmacol Exp Therapeut* 1993; 266: 1364–73.
133. Parker RB, Williams CL, Laizure SC, Mandrell TD, LaBranche GS, Lima JJ. Effects of ethanol and cocaethylene on cocaine pharmacokinetics in conscious dogs. *Drug Metab Dispos* 1996; 24(8): 850–3.

134. Grant BF, Harford TC. Concurrent and simultaneous use of alcohol and cocaine: results of a national survey. *Drug Alcohol Depend* 1990; 25: 97–104.
135. McCance-Katz EF, Price LH, McDougle CJ, Kosten TR, Black JE, Jatlow PI. Concurrent cocaine–ethanol ingestion in humans: pharmacology, physiology, behavior, and the role of cocaethylene. *Psychopharmacology* 1993; 111: 39–46.
136. Karch SB, Stephens BG, Tseng A. Does ethanol enhance cocaine toxicity? *J Clin Forens Med* 1999; 6: 19–23.
137. Heath MJ, Pachar JV, Perez Martinez AL, Toseland PA. An exceptional case of lethal disulfiram–alcohol reaction. *Forens Sci Internat* 1992; 56: 45–50.
138. Cina SJ, Russell RA, Conradi SE. Sudden death due to metronidazole/ethanol interaction. *Am J Forens Med Pathol* 1996; 17: 343–6.

# 7 Other drugs of abuse

| | | |
|---|---|---|
| **Foreword** | | 322 |
| **7.1** | **LSD** | 323 |
| **7.2** | **Phencyclidine and related hallucinogens** | 326 |
| **7.3** | **Gamma-hydroxy butyrate** | 329 |
| **7.4** | **Volatile substances** | 331 |
| **7.5** | **Case reports** | 334 |
| **References for Section 7** | | 336 |

# Foreword

A number of chemical substances are also abused, although they tend not to be as frequently associated in court proceedings as the drugs covered previously. These include the hallucinogens PCP, LSD and other related chemicals, the night club and date rape substance GHB, and numerous volatile substances.

Their use throughout the world is much more localized than the five main drugs of abuse classes, yet they are capable of causing profound pharmacological and physiological changes in persons exposed to these substances.

This section provides a short summary of the pharmacology, pharmacokinetics and toxicology of these substances relevant to a forensic context.

# 7.1 LSD

## SOURCE AND STRUCTURES

LSD is the abbreviation for lysergic acid diethylamide. It is a chemical derivative of lysergic acid, an ergot alkaloid, which is found in the fungus *Claviceps purpurea* growing on cereal rye and other grains. A number of clinically useful substances are prepared from ergot alkaloids, including ergotamine, dihydroergotamine, ergometrine, ergonovine, methylergonovine, methylergometrine, bromocriptine, ergocornine, ergocryptine, terguride, 2-bromolisuride, lergotrile and methysergide. These are used in obstetrics and gynaecology and endocrinology, and as anti-migraine drugs.

LSD was first discovered in 1943 as a highly potent hallucinogen. Lysergic acid derivatives are also found in morning glory seeds, the Hawaiian baby wood rose and fungus-infected perennial rye grass *Stipa robusta* found in South West USA.

Exposure to ergot alkaloids can lead to prolonged painful vasospasm, drowsiness, nausea, vomiting, diarrhoea, abortion of fetus resulting from stimulation of uterine muscle, and a variety of effects on the CNS including hallucinations.

LSD has been widely abused since the 1960s, particularly by teenagers in various areas of the world, including Europe and the USA. Its popularity is partly due to its wide availability and its relatively low cost (often as low as $5–25 per dosage unit). A street dose normally contains between 25 and 100 μg of LSD, although consumed doses may exceed 300 μg.

Street forms of the drug are usually as 'tabs' or 'tickets' – drug impregnated into small coloured pieces of blotter paper or postage stamps – or less commonly drug impregnated into sugar cubes, tablets, powders, or gelatin squares. Common street names for LSD include acid, trip, mellow, tabs, blotters, dots, tickets, microdots, and jelly beans. Reported usage of LSD in some countries is second to cannabis among the illicit drugs.[1]

## TISSUE CONCENTRATIONS, METABOLISM AND EXCRETION

Peak blood concentrations of LSD are typically less than 10 ng/mL. Maximum plasma concentrations following ~70 μg dose (1 μg/kg) range up to ~2 ng/mL, while doses of 140 μg (2 μg/kg) have given peak concentrations of 5–9 ng/mL.[2,3]

The maximum blood levels occur around 30–90 min, but psychedelic effects of the drug occur within 5–10 min. The elimination half-life is estimated at 3–6 h. Blood concentrations of drug are therefore quite low by 8 h post-dose – often less than 1 ng/mL. The duration of action of LSD parallels approximately the blood concentrations, with 'trips' lasting from a few to several hours depending on the dose used.

LSD is rapidly metabolized with only about 1–3% of an oral dose excreted in the urine as unchanged LSD. The major metabolites in urine are N-desmethyl-LSD (nor-LSD) and

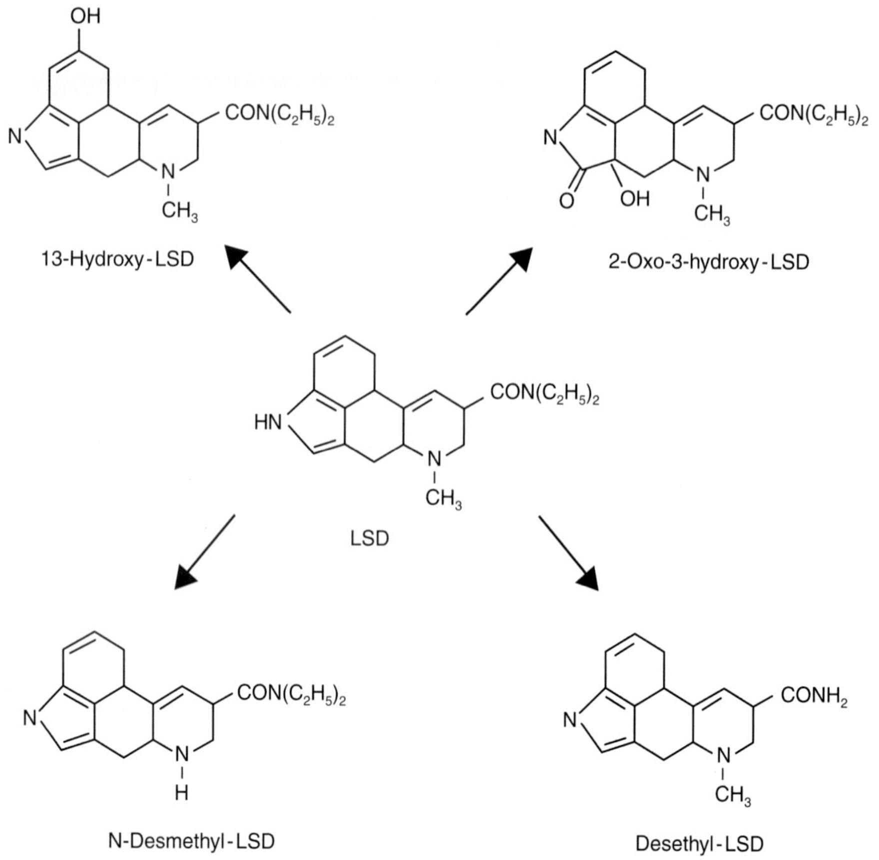

# Other drugs of abuse

**Fig. 7.1** Structures of LSD and some key metabolites

2-oxo-3-hydroxy-LSD (Fig. 7.1). In addition, glucuronide conjugates of 13- and 14-hydroxy-LSD are also present.

Because of the low blood concentrations, LSD is most often measured in urine. Peak urine concentrations following oral ingestion of a typical street dose are normally less than 10 ng/mL and drop below 1 ng/mL within 12–24 h. Therefore, extremely sensitive analytical methods are required to detect LSD use for more than 1 day after ingestion of the drug. 2-Oxo-3-hydroxy-LSD and the glucuronide conjugate of 13-hydroxy-LSD can be detected in urine up to 96 h after administration, whereas LSD can only be detected for 12–24 h post-administration.[4]

Iso-LSD (an inactive isomer at C-8) is often also found in urine, but this is a contaminant of LSD itself.

## MECHANISM OF ACTION

LSD acts as an antagonist of peripheral 5-HT receptors, but acts as an agonist at central (CNS) 5-HT receptors, particularly the subtypes 5-HT$_{1A}$, 5-HT$_{1C}$, and 5-HT$_2$. The 5-HT neuronal system (serotonin system) regulates emotions and thought processes and is affected by amphetamines, cocaine and a range of drugs used to treat affective disorders, e.g. antidepressants.

## PHARMACOLOGICAL ACTIONS AND ADVERSE REACTIONS

The main effect of LSD consumption is altering of perception leading to distorted sounds, smells and visual images. Hallucinations are a manifestation of this effect. Alteration in thought processes occur, hence confusion and illogical actions are common. Occasionally bad trips occur, leading to frightening and dangerous experiences that may result in bizarre behaviour and paranoid delusions, and can produce homicidal and suicidal acts.

LSD was used clinically for the treatment of alcoholism, opioid addiction and psychiatric conditions. It is not regarded now as clinically appropriate or even useful for these conditions. Tolerance develops after 3–6 days of continuous use, but disappears after a short period of abstinence (4–6 days). Discontinuing use of LSD does not result in significant withdrawal symptoms.

## TOXICITY

LSD causes profound hallucinations and disordered thought, but is rarely fatal. Death has been reported from LSD.[5] In this case, serum concentrations were 14 ng/mL. Nevertheless, LSD is considered a highly dangerous drug due to its tendency to produce panic, delirium and bizarre behaviour, sometimes resulting in irrational and injurious acts. These acts can occur with usual doses, even in an experienced LSD user.

It is possible that this drug will be more dangerous when other drugs acting on the serotonin system are used concomitantly, e.g. serotonin re-uptake antidepressants and neuroleptic drugs. Users of LSD are known to also consume alcohol, cannabis and amphetamines.

One of the well-known side effects of LSD is the occurrence of flashbacks. These are repeat hallucinatory and other perceptual experiences occurring after the initial LSD experience has subsided. They may last for minutes to hours, and may occur up to several years after last LSD use. The mechanism is unknown, but is thought to be the result of some permanent serotonergic neuronal damage that shows up later as flashbacks upon a particular stimulation of the serotonergic system. Flashbacks occur in approximately half of the users, regardless of whether they have used LSD regularly.

# 7.2 Phencyclidine and related hallucinogens

Phencyclidine (Fig. 7.2), or PCP, is a synthetic drug that possesses anaesthetic activity but patients in recovery also produced an altered conscious state leading to hallucinations and symptoms of dissociation. PCP was discontinued as an anaesthetic in humans in 1963, but was used in veterinary medicine until 1979.

Another related hallucinogen is ketamine (Fig. 7.2), which is still used as an anaesthetic in humans as well as in animals. PCP analogues prepared in a similar manner to PCP include thienylcyclohexylpiperidine (TCP), phenylcyclohexylpyrrolidine (PHP), phenylcyclopentylpiperidine (PCPP) and phenylcyclohexamine (PCE).

The availability of PCP has largely been restricted to regions of the USA particularly Los Angeles, San Francisco, and the north-eastern corridor. PCP is sold as the powder 'angel dust', as flakes or as a liquid often impregnated in tobacco or cannabis cigarettes, or leaf material. Street doses of PCP range from 1 to 10 mg. Street names for PCP include angel dust, busy bee, cadillac, CJ, crystal, elephant tranquillizer, hog, PeaCe Pill, peace, snorts, and T.

Street names for ketamine include Special K, KitKat, vitamin K, K and ket. It is available for clinical use as Ketalar, and for veterinary use as Ketaset, Ketapex and Ketamil. It comes as solutions for injection, pills, powder or tab form. Ketamine is also commonly cut with cocaine, amphetamine and heroin. LSD tabs are also known to have had ketamine added.[1] Doses are much greater than PCP, often reaching 200–500 mg.

## MECHANISM OF ACTION

The mode of action for PCP and related substances was mentioned earlier. It is believed to interact with a number of brain systems, including blocking the N-methyl-D-aspartate (NMDA) receptor in the cortex and limbic regions, the sigma-opioid receptor, and the dopaminergic system. The dopamine system is possibly responsible for PCP's effect on behaviour, while the sigma-opioid system is responsible for its dysphoria and other unpleasant

Phencyclidine          Ketamine

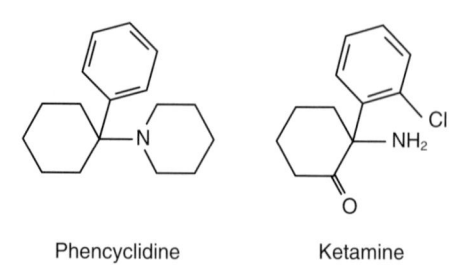

**Fig. 7.2** Structures of phencyclidine and ketamine

effects. The alpha-adrenergic system is activated by PCP causing an elevation in blood pressure. In addition, PCP weakly blocks the cholinergic system resulting in atropine-like effects.

## PHARMACOLOGICAL ACTIONS AND ADVERSE REACTIONS

PCP has actions similar in many ways to those of LSD. It causes distortion of visual and other sensory signals, and produces analgesia similar to opioids, and stereotyped behaviour similar to amphetamines and cocaine. Its ability to produce dysphoria, numbness, nystagmus (horizontal and vertical), miosis, sweating, high heart rate and elevated blood pressures is unwanted and tends to reduce its continued use.

PCP is particularly prone to producing acute psychotic episodes leading to reckless and dangerous actions. In this respect, it is a drug associated with violence and dissociated behaviour. PCP-impaired persons, such as in traffic cases, will typically present with nystagmus, miosis and impaired gait.

Ketamine is used in date rape for its ability to render a victim incapable of defence and to cause amnesia. In this regard it can be compared to flunitrazepam and GHB.

## TISSUE CONCENTRATIONS, METABOLISM AND EXCRETION

Peak plasma concentrations range up to about 2–3 ng/mL following 1 mg oral dose.[6] This occurs within 2–3 h. In subjects examined by drug recognition experts for drug-induced impairment, blood concentrations ranging from 12 to 118 ng/mL have been found.[7] Blood concentrations in casual users have ranged up to 800 ng/mL.[8]

PCP is quickly absorbed by inhalation of smoke or snorting, with psychoactive effects present within minutes. Peak blood concentrations following smoking a parsley cigarette containing 100 µg PCP are 0.15 mg/L.[9] Smoking produces a significant amount of a pyrolysis product, 1-phenylcyclohexene, which can be measured to prove smoking of PCP.

Significant amounts of unchanged drug are excreted into urine (~10%), hence urinalysis is a convenient method to determine exposure to PCP. The drug has a relatively long pharmacokinetic half-life with estimates ranging from 7 to 46 h. The elimination of drug, and of course its duration of action, will depend on the pH of urine, rather like that for the amphetamines.

Blood concentrations of ketamine are substantially higher than those of PCP. Anaesthetic doses produce peak levels of over 6 mg/L, but blood concentrations are likely to be less than 1 mg/L in conscious persons. The metabolite norketamine is present in blood in concentrations similar to ketamine itself. The terminal pharmacokinetic half-life of ketamine is about 2–4 h.

Ketamine is absorbed by the nasal mucosa. Plasma concentrations peak within 20 min, and the norketamine metabolite peaks at 2 h. Norketamine appears in higher concentrations following rectal administration.[10] This is also likely for oral administration, due to its metabolism in the first pass through the liver.

Metabolites of ketamine also include hydroxylated substances. These are conjugated and will form a significant part of the excreted dose. Hydrolysis of these conjugates will allow detection of one or more of the hydroxylated metabolites for longer periods than the parent drug.

## TOXICITY

PCP can cause severe behavioural toxicity leading to violent death, e.g. from jumping from buildings, drowning, stabbing or from collisions with moving vehicles. Indeed, this appears to be the common mode of death in PCP users.[11–13] In these cases blood concentrations range from 0.02 to over 2 mg/L.

PCP can induce high body temperatures leading to rhabdomyolysis, respiratory depression, and seizures with associated multiple organ failure. Pathological findings in deaths also include congestion, bronchopneumonia, alveolar macrophages, pulmonary oedema and aspiration of gastric contents.

Blood concentrations in PCP fatalities range from 0.3 mg/L. Liver concentrations are usually similar to or slightly higher than blood (range 3–12 times blood).[11] Large amounts of PCP are excreted through bile, hence bile is a useful specimen. Because of biliary excretion, the drug will also be present in gastric contents.[14] There is little correlation with blood concentration and clinical symptoms. The concomitant use of other CNS active drugs will further complicate the toxicological interpretation of these cases.[11,15–19]

There have been reports of a contaminant present as a precursor in the synthesis of PCP, namely 1-piperidinocyclohexanecarbonitrile, this being more toxic than PCP itself, possibly through release of cyanide.

# 7.3 Gamma-hydroxy butyrate

Gamma-hydroxy butyrate, or GHB, is a simple molecule prepared from one of a number of precursors, including γ-butyrolactone (GBL), γ-aminobutyric acid, and 1,4-butanediol (BD). The drug was used as an anaesthetic, but the presence of myoclonic seizures and vomiting on withdrawal prevented its further use. It has been sold in health food shops as a weight-reducing agent, as a hypnotic and for stimulating muscle growth. The drug appears to have a limited use to treat narcolepsy and is under investigation for the treatment of alcohol withdrawal syndrome. The substance may also be useful for the treatment of fibromyalgia. The drug is increasingly subject to abuse, particularly in the nightclub scene.

GHB is usually a colourless, odourless, slightly salty tasting liquid freely soluble in water. Because of its solubility and lack of strong taste, it is added to drinks at dances and parties. Consequently, GHB is used in date rape to induce a compliant and amnesic state in women. It is also available as a white powder and in capsule form.

Street names include easy lay, fantasy, georgia home boy, grievous bodily harm, growth hormone boost, G-Riffick, liquid ecstasy, liquid X, liquid E, nature's quaalude, scoop, and thunder nectar (for BD).

## TISSUE CONCENTRATIONS, METABOLISM AND EXCRETION

GHB is rapidly absorbed orally with effects noticeable within 5–15 min. Following oral ingestion, peak blood concentrations occur within 30–45 min. GHB is rapidly eliminated with a blood half-life of less than 1 h (range 0.3–1.0).

Single doses of GHB (25 mg/kg) produce peak serum concentrations of 24–102 mg/L. Doses of 50 mg/kg produce peak concentrations of 48–125 mg/L.[20–22] Non-linear kinetics have been observed with GHB.

Blood concentrations following recreational use range up to 100 mg/L, although higher levels will be seen in some cases, particularly those involving some form of intoxication.

GHB is extensively metabolized with less than 5% appearing unchanged in urine. Urine concentrations can easily exceed 100 mg/L following exposure to psychoactive doses.

Inhibitors of P450 enzymes, particularly the HIV-1 protease inhibitors ritonavir and saquinavir, dramatically reduce clearance of GHB leading to likelihood of a toxic reaction to otherwise non-toxic doses.[23]

## PHARMACOLOGICAL ACTIONS AND ADVERSE REACTIONS

The effects of GHB are similar to alcohol, with which it is commonly associated. Effects include disinhibition, amnesia, confusion, dizziness, and loss of peripheral vision. Higher doses will lead to hypothermia, bradycardia, hypotension, acidosis, hallucinations, somnolence and ultimately loss of conscious state.[24] GHB toxicity can be at least partly reversed with neostigmine or physotigmine.[25,26] Neither flumazenil nor naloxone has been useful in reversing GHB intoxication. It is of interest that persons waking from a GHB-induced coma often show few hang-over effects (see Case Report 7.4).

Relatively low doses of GHB (to 25 mg/kg body weight) do not produce significant impairment of psychomotor functions, but higher doses, or doses combined with known psychoactive drugs, e.g. alcohol and benzodiazepines, will have significant effects on driving performance.[27]

## MECHANISM OF ACTION

GHB is an endogenous substance produced in the amino acid metabolic pathway from the amino, glutamic and aspartic acids. It has been touted to be a neurotransmitter involved in critical brain functions, and appears to inhibit presynaptic uptake of dopamine and act as a weak agonist at the GABA receptor.

## TOXICITY

GHB is a substance produced naturally in humans, although in low amounts, hence caution is advised in interpreting low levels. This is further complicated by significant formation of GHB in postmortem periods, particularly in blood. Reports suggest that over 100 mg/L may be produced in the postmortem period.[28–30] This occurs both before collection of postmortem specimens, as well as during storage, particularly in tubes not properly refrigerated or not containing fluoride as preservative.[30] It should be noted that precursors such as GHL and BD will also be converted to GHB in the body.

GHB is a relatively toxic substance, although doses required to cause death are quite high. A number of deaths have been reported, as well as many more reports of adverse reactions to GHB or its precursors.[25,31–33] In most people, one teaspoonful, which contains ~2.5 g of GHB, is not likely to cause significant adverse effects; larger doses are likely to cause significant toxicity.

A review of a large number of GHB overdoses produced a variety of symptoms, characterized by a Glasgow Coma Scale (GCS) score of less than 13, often as low as 3, bradycardia (<55 bpm), low body temperatures (<35°C), emesis and mild acute respiratory acidosis. Some subjects had low systolic blood pressure, but these had also used alcohol or another drug. The mean time to regain consciousness ranged from 16 to 389 min, the mean being 146 min.[24]

Agitation and extreme combativeness has been seen with subjects admitted to hospital with GHB overdoses requiring physical restraint to protect themselves and health care professionals.[33]

Reports of heart rhythm abnormalities have been reported, particularly first-degree block, right bundle branch block and ventricular ectopy. Some subjects had 'U' waves present.[33]

Fatalities attributed to GHB (or to one of its precursors) alone range from less than 50 mg/L to several hundred. This range is attributed to the fast elimination and breakdown of GHB and its variable toxicity. Given the formation of GHB in postmortem blood, it is preferable to collect urine and vitreous humour to exclude postmortem production.

# 7.4 Volatile substances

Solvents from contact adhesives, notably toluene, petrol (gasoline), halogenated solvents, volatile hydrocarbons such as those found in cigarette lighter refills, aerosol propellants, halocarbon fire extinguishers, and volatile anesthetics form the main constituents of this large group of chemical substances.

Volatile substance abuse (VSA) is a term used to define glue sniffing, inhalant abuse and solvent abuse. The deliberate inhalation of volatile substances in order to achieve some form of intoxication often occurs in adolescents, as well as those persons living in marginal or remote communities. Occupational exposure to volatile substances also occurs and can give rise to acute effects as well as an increased incidence of certain diseases with repeated exposure to significant amounts of substance. This latter subject is not discussed in any detail here.

## TYPES OF VOLATILE SUBSTANCES

The community has access to a large range of volatile substances. The most common volatile substance is ethanol (alcohol) and other low-molecular-weight alcohols, which are covered elsewhere in this text. A selected list of substances is shown in Table 7.1.

The more common abused substances are gasoline (petrol), and the gaseous hydrocarbons, such as liquefied petroleum gas (LPG which is largely propane) and butane, which is found in lighter fluid and aerosol containers, adhesives and fire extinguisher contents.[37,38]

A review of almost 20 000 deaths reported to the coroner of Victoria during an 8-year period to 1997 showed 16 cases related to the use of lower hydrocarbons methane, propane and butane, and four other cases involving exposure to complex hydrocarbons (shellite), methanol, methyl isobutyl ketone and cleaning fluid.

Table 7.1  Common volatile substances

| Chemical group | Volatile substance |
| --- | --- |
| Aliphatic hydrocarbons | Methane, butane, LPG[a], gasoline[b], diesel[b], kerosene[b], aviation gas[b] |
| Aromatic hydrocarbons | Benzene, toluene, xylenes |
| Halogenated hydrocarbons | Chloroform, carbon tetrachloride, dichloromethane, halothane, trichloroethylene |
| Alcohols | Methanol, ethanol |
| Esters | Ethyl acetate, butyl acetate |
| Ethers | Diethyl ether, diisopropyl ether |
| Others | Nitrous oxide, acetone, amyl and butyl nitrites |

[a] Liquefied petroleum gas; [b] contains aromatic hydrocarbon additives such as toluene and xylenes.

It is noteworthy that many of the halogenated hydrocarbons such as chlorofluorohydrocarbons (CFCs) have now been replaced by aliphatic hydrocarbons. While these hydrocarbons are less ozone depleting, they can still have profound effects on the central nervous system.

## TISSUE CONCENTRATION, METABOLISM AND EXCRETION

Inhalation of volatile substances expectably results in rapid absorption, and consequently rapid effects. Responses manifest within seconds. Tissue distribution will lead to a rapid diminution of blood concentrations after the rapid absorption surge, providing there is no continued exposure. These volatile substances are usually lipid soluble and rapidly reach significant concentrations in the brain, and indeed all other organs.

The volatility of these substances will lead to a relatively rapid removal by the body by a combination of expiration of breath and the usual processes of metabolism and excretion. The diverse chemical structures lead to a varying degree of metabolism. However, with few exceptions, the parent substance is responsible for the immediate effects of VSA and is usually the target chemical for forensic toxicologists.

Methanol is metabolized by the same enzyme that metabolizes ethanol, alcohol dehydrogenase (ADH), although at a slower rate. The metabolism of methanol to the toxic formaldehyde is competitively inhibited by the presence of any ethanol. Ethanol can therefore be used to reduce the metabolism and toxicity of methanol.

Toluene is metabolized to hippuric acid, which can be used as a marker for exposure in urine. Benzene is metabolized to hydroxylated metabolites, phenol, catechol and hydroquinone, all of which are eliminated as sulphate or glucuronide conjugates.

## MECHANISM AND FREQUENCY OF USE

Glue sniffing, 'bagging', 'huffing' or 'chroming' are common terms associated with inhalation of products containing volatile substances. Persons can inhale these products directly or by placing material in a plastic bag and inhaling the vaporized contents ('bagging' or 'chroming'). Huffing refers to inhalation of vapours from solvents applied to a rag. Butane lighter fluid is often inhaled by gripping the spray nozzle between the teeth and spraying into the throat directly. Butane 'firebreathing' is also known in which exhaled vapours are set alight.

The highest-risk groups to abuse of volatile substances are children and adolescents. The median age of deaths associated with VSA is 17 years and 79% are under age 20.[38] Most deaths occur alone, at home. In about 41% of cases, death appeared to be only indirectly associated with VSA (trauma 8%, plastic bag over head 19%, and inhalation of stomach contents 14%).[38]

## PHARMACOLOGICAL ACTIONS AND ADVERSE EFFECTS

VSA gives rise to dose-related effects similar to those of other CNS depressants.[39–41] Small doses can rapidly lead to euphoria and other disturbances of behaviour similar to those caused by ethanol (alcohol). Drunken behaviour, unexplained listlessness, anorexia and moodiness are frequent effects resulting from VSA. Auditory and visual hallucinations may also occur. Less obvious effects associated with past use include nausea, abdominal pain, tinnitus, headache, lethargy, unproductive cough, runny nose, sore throat and bloodshot eyes.

Serious impairment of skills required for safe driving of motor vehicles occurs with abuse of all volatile substances. These effects are often initially difficult to distinguish from excessive alcohol consumption due to profound depression of the CNS. Classical effects of CNS depressant drugs are evident, including horizontal gaze nystagmus.

Irreversible damage to the central and peripheral nervous systems is well known after repeated exposure to VSA. This leads to neuropathies and other signs of damage to the nervous systems. Adverse effects on lung function are likely to occur, including irritation and pneumonitis. Hypoxaemia is common. In addition, cardiac arrhythmias and cardiac depression may occur from acute and chronic exposure. When this occurs, risk of death is high. VSA may ultimately produce convulsions and coma.

Death may ensue indirectly, for example after inhalation of vomit, or from direct cardiac, pulmonary or central nervous system toxicity. In some cases, direct effects on the vagal nerve can lead to cardiorespiratory arrest. Situations that lead to increased stress on the cardiovascular system will increase the risk of sudden death; this includes sudden exercise such as running and use of other stimulants or depressant drugs.

Toxicology can rarely be of use in discerning the mechanism of death; rather it provides a means of identifying possible exposed chemicals.

# 7.5 Case reports

### CASE REPORT 7.1 PCP AND VIOLENT BEHAVIOUR LEADING TO DEATH

This 30-year-old man had shown on consecutive days to exhibit bizarre, violent and abnormal behaviour. He was treated for a possible mental disorder with thorazine (an antipsychotic drug). Despite treatment with a major tranquilliser he became violent again and broke furniture. He was eventually restrained with handcuffs and leg restraints but on the way to the hospital he lost consciousness. Despite intensive care, he died 6 days later. He showed strong evidence of rhabdomyolysis with associated renal failure.

At autopsy he also exhibited old needle track marks in the cubital fossa, and numerous petechial haemorrhages were found in the bulbar conjunctiva and eyelids. Abrasions and contusions were found on several parts of the body, a subgaleal haemorrhage was found in the frontal region, lungs were heavy and oedematous, and a focal subepicardial haemorrhage was found in the left ventricle of the heart.

His behaviour and ultimate fate were attributed to injection of PCP.[19]

### CASE REPORT 7.2 DRIVING WHILE INTOXICATED WITH GHB

A 33-year-old male was assessed for sobriety after a crash in which he was at fault. He was found to be disorientated and slow to respond, and had slurred speech and ataxia. His eyes were bloodshot, BP was 124/58 mmHg, pulse was 88–108 bpm, and body temperature was 37.2°C. The subject had horizontal gaze nystagmus and performed poorly on the Romberg test. His pupils were normal size with slow reaction to light. The subject had a bottle of butanediol (BD) in his possession. His blood and urine GHB concentrations were 33 and 714 mg/L. No other drugs were detected in toxicological analysis (after Couper and Logan, 2000[34]).

This case illustrates the substantial impairment capable of being caused by GHB and its precursors consistent with symptoms of CNS depression.

### CASE REPORT 7.3 GHB WITHDRAWAL

A patient admitted to substantial GHB abuse on a daily basis for 2.5 years. Previous attempts at cessation reportedly resulted in diaphoresis, tremors and agitation. The patient's symptoms, negative polypharmacy history, and negative urine and blood toxicological analysis for alcohol, benzodiazepines, sedative-hypnotics, or other substances suggested the diagnosis of GHB withdrawal. Later analysis of a patient drug sample confirmed the presence of GHB. The patient required 507 mg of lorazepam and 120 mg of diazepam over 90 h to control agitation.[35]

This illustrates the possible dangers of regular use of GHB and the development of tolerance and dependence to this drug.

## CASE REPORT 7.4 GHB INTOXICATION

A 23-year-old woman lost consciousness after consuming a considerable amount of alcohol, smoking a few joints and consuming a small amount of GHB about 20 min before her collapse.

On presentation to the emergency department she had a Glascow Coma Scale of 6, a slow heart rate (56 bpm) and slow respiratory rate (8/min), and a low serum potassium (3.22 mM).

Toxicology testing showed alcohol at 0.134 g% and GHB at 125 mg/L.

Forty-five minutes after presentation to hospital she woke up as if she snapped out of a dream. She was nauseated and dizzy, and vomited a few times, and had problems writing her name.

Case report after Louagie et al, 1997.[36]

# References for Section 7

1. ABCI. *Australian Illicit Drug Report 1998–99*. Canberra: Australian Bureau of Criminal Intelligence; 2000 March.
2. Upsall DG, Wailling DG. The determination of LSD in human plasma following oral administration. *Clin Chim Acta* 1972; 36: 67–73.
3. Aghajanian GK, Bing OHL. Persistance of lysergic acid diethylamide in the plasma of human subjects. *Clin Pharm Ther* 1964; 5: 611–14.
4. Reuschel SA, Foltz RL, Percey SE, Liiu S, Eades D. Quantitative determination of LSD and a major metabolite, 2-oxo-3-hydroxy-LSD, in human urine by solid phase extraction and gas chromatography/tandem mass spectromtery. In: Spiehler V, ed. SOFT/TIAFT Annual Scientific Meeting. Albuquerque, NM; 1998. pp. 538–49.
5. Fysh RR, Oon MC, Robinson KN, Smith RN, White PC, Whitehouse MJ. A fatal poisoning with LSD. *Forens Sci Internat* 1985; 28(2): 109–13.
6. Cook CE, Brine DR, Jeffcoat AR, Hill JM, Wall ME. Phencyclidine disposition after intravenous and oral doses. *Clin Pharmacol Ther* 1982; 31: 625–34.
7. Kunsman GW, Levine B, Costantino A, Smith ML. Phencyclidine blood concentrations in DRE cases. *J Anal Toxicol* 1997; 21(6): 498–502.
8. Bailey DN, Shaw RF, Guba JJ. Phencyclidine abuse: plasma levels and clinical findings in casual users and in phencyclidine-related deaths. *J Anal Toxicol* 1978; 2: 233–8.
9. Cook CE, Brine DR, Quin GD, Perez-Reyes M, DiGuiseppi SR. Phencyclidine and phenylcyclohexene disposition after smoking phencyclidine. *Clin Pharmacol Ther* 1982; 31: 635–41.
10. Malinovsky JM, Servin F, Cozian A, Lepage JY, Pinaud M. Ketamine and norketamine plasma concentrations after i.v., nasal and rectal administration in children. *Br J Anaesth* 1996; 77(2): 203–7.
11. Burns RS, Lerner SE. Causes of phencyclidine-related deaths. *Clin Toxicol* 1978; 12: 463–81.
12. Budd RD, Liu Y. Phencyclidine concentrations in postmortem body fluids and tissues. *J Toxicol Clin Toxicol* 1982; 19(8): 843–50.
13. Caplan YH, Orloff KG, Thompson BC, Fisher RC. Detection of phencyclidine in medical examiner's cases. *J Anal Toxicol* 1979; 3: 47–52.
14. Done AK, Aronow R, Miceli JN. The pharmacokinetics of phencyclidine in overdosage and its treatment. *NIDA Res Monogr* 1978; 21: 210–17.
15. Licata M, Pierini G, Popoli G. A fatal ketamine poisoning. *J Forens Sci* 1994; 39(5): 1314–20.

16. Moore KA, Kilbane EM, Jones R, Kunsman GW, Levine B, Smith M. Tissue distribution of ketamine in a mixed drug fatality. *J Forens Sci* 1997; 42(6): 1183–5.
17. Peyton SH, Couch AT, Bost RO. Tissue distribution of ketamine: two case reports. *J Anal Toxicol* 1988; 12(5): 268–9.
18. Kintz P, Sengler C, Mangin P. Fatal anesthesia accident following ketamine in a 6 week old baby. *Bull Internat Ass Forens Toxicol* 1996; 26(3).
19. Reddy SK, Kornblum RN. Rhabdomyolysis following violent behavior and coma. *J Forens Sci* 1987; 32(2): 550–3.
20. Palatini P, Tedeschi L, Frison G, Galimberti L, Gessa GL, Ferrara SD. Dose-dependent absorption and elimination of gamma-hydroxybutyric acid in healthy volunteers. *Eur J Clin Pharmacol* 1993; 45: 353–6.
21. Ferrara SD, Zotti S, Tedeschi L, Frison G, Castagna F, Galimberti L, et al. Pharmacokinetics of gamma-hydroxybutyric acid in alcohol dependent patients after single and repeated oral doses. *Br J Clin Pharmacol* 1992; 34(3): 231–5.
22. Scharf MB, Lai AA, Branigan B, Stover R, Berkowitz DB. Pharmacokinetics of gamma-hydroxybutyrate (GHB) in narcoleptic patients. *Sleep* 1998; 21(5): 507–14.
23. Harrington RD, Woodward JA, Hooton TM, Horn JR. Life-threatening interactions between HIV-1 protease inhibitors and the illicit drugs MDMA and gamma-hydroxybutyrate. *Arch Intern Med* 1999; 159(18): 2221–4.
24. Chin RL, Sporer KA, Cullison B, Dyer JE, Wu TD. Clinical course of gamma-hydroxybutyrate overdose. *Ann Emerg Med* 1998; 31(6): 716–22.
25. Viera AJ, Yates SW. Toxic ingestion of gamma-hydroxybutyric acid. *South Med J* 1999; 92(4): 404–5.
26. Hunderup MC, Jorgensen AJ. Poisoning with gamma-hydroxybutyrate. Cases reported in connection with 'cultural festivals' in August 1999 in Kolding. *Ugeskr Laeger* 1999; 161(50): 6939–40.
27. Ferrara SD, Giorgetti R, Zancaner S, Orlando R, Tagliabracci A, Cavarzeran F, et al. Effects of single dose of gamma-hydroxybutyric acid and lorazepam on psychomotor performance and subjective feelings in healthy volunteers. *Eur J Clin Pharmacol* 1999; 54(11): 821–7.
28. Anderson DT, Kuwahara T. Endogenous gamma-hydroxybutyrate (GHB) levels in postmortem specimens. In: California Association of Toxicologists quarterly meeting. Las Vegas, NV; 1997.
29. Fieler EL, Coleman DE, Baselt RC. Gamma-hydroxybuytrate concentrations in pre- and postmortem blood and urine. *Clin Chem* 1998; 44: 692.
30. Stephens BG, Coleman DE. *In vitro* stability of endogenous gamma-hydroxybutyrate in postmortem blood. *J Forens Sci* 1998: 231.
31. McCutcheon JR, Hall BJ, Schroeder PM, Peacock EA, Baynardo RJ. Fatal intoxication following recreational ingestion of 1,4-butanediol. In: American Academy of Forensic Science Annual Meeting. Reno, NA; 2000. p. 274.
32. Marinetti LJ, Isenschmidt DS, Hepler BR, Schmidt CJ, Somerset JS, Kanluen S. Two gamma-hydroxybutyric acid (GHB) fatalities. In: American Academy of Forensic Science Annual Meeting; Reno, NA; 2000. pp. 274–5.

33. Li J, Stokes SA, Woeckener A. A tale of novel intoxication: a review of the effects of gamma-hydroxybutyric acid with recommendations for management. *Ann Emerg Med* 1998; 31(6): 729–36.
34. Couper FJ, Logan BK. Determination of gamma-hydroxybutyrate (GHB) in biological specimens by gas chromatography-mass spectrometry. *J Anal Toxicol* 2000; 24(1): 1–7.
35. Craig K, Gomez HF, McManus JL, Bania TC. Severe gamma-hydroxybutyrate withdrawal: a case report and literature review. *J Emerg Med* 2000; 18(1): 65–70.
36. Louagie HK, Verstraete AG, De Soete CJ, Baetens DG, Calle PA. A sudden awakening from a near coma after combined intake of gamma-hydroxybutyric acid (GHB) and ethanol. *J Toxicol Clin Toxicol* 1997; 35(6): 591–4.
37. Taylor JC, Norman CL, Bland JM, Ramsey JD, Anderson HR. VSA deaths 1971–1995. *TIAFT Bulletin* 1997; 27(3): 12–18.
38. Anderson HR, Dick B, Macnair RS, Palmer JC, Ramsey JD. An investigation of 140 deaths associated with volatile substance abuse in the United Kingdom (1971–1981). *Hum Toxicol* 1982; 1(3): 207–21.
39. Linden CH. Volatile substances of abuse. *Emerg Med Clin North Am* 1990; 8(3): 559–78.
40. Flanagan RJ, Ruprah M, Meredith TJ, Ramsey JD. An introduction to the clinical toxicology of volatile substances. *Drug Saf* 1990; 5(5): 359–83.
41. Al-Alousi LM. Pathology of volatile substance abuse: a case report and a literature review. *Med Sci Law* 1989; 29(3): 189–208.

# 8  Clinical forensic aspects of drug use

| | | |
|---|---|---|
| **Foreword** | | 340 |
| 8.1 | **Reasons for a forensic medical examination** | 341 |
| 8.2 | **Health status of drug users** | 344 |
| 8.3 | **Principles of an examination scheme for drug-affected persons** | 345 |
| 8.4 | **Clinical forensic opinions** | 348 |
| 8.5 | **Common drug effects seen in clinical medicine** | 349 |
| 8.6 | **Case reports** | 360 |
| **References for Section 8** | | 365 |

# Foreword

This section of the text will discuss aspects of clinical forensic medical practice that relate to the management of drug-impaired persons. While the main emphasis will be on the classes of drugs discussed in this book, there is an enormous number of substances that may be used as drugs and many of them will not easily fit into the broad categories discussed here.

'Classical' effects of drugs may be masked by many phenomena, including injuries, physiological effects such as fatigue, coexisting disease states both physical and psychiatric, and as co-administration of other drugs. Drug use may produce unpredictable or idiosyncratic interactions. In addition, many illicit drugs are actually a mixture of several psychoactive substances that may alter the clinical picture of intoxication. As accurate historical details are notoriously difficult to obtain in many clinical forensic cases, it is important that the examiner has a clear understanding of possible drug effects when called upon to see such patients.

There are very many situations where clinical forensic practitioners come into contact with drug-affected individuals. These range from acute management and treatment of patients[1] to the provision of expert opinions regarding drug effects and appearances as witnesses in court regarding any aspects of the subject. Drug use that has forensic implications may be licit or illicit and the reasons for forensic medical involvement may occur for any possible involvement of the drug-affected person in the legal system. All aspects of such medical involvement may be subject to legal scrutiny and it is very important that observations and actions by medical personnel are adequately documented.

General aspects of forensic practice are outside the scope of this book and are well covered in the relevant literature.[2]

# 8.1 Reasons for a forensic medical examination

Many people detained by law enforcement officers or involved in the legal or custodial systems may have recently consumed one or more drugs and there may be many reasons for medical involvement. These are listed in Table 8.1.

An important part of clinical forensic practice is knowledge of the clinical signs associated with different drug types and interpretation of these in individual cases. This extends to knowledge of withdrawal syndromes that may exhibit clinical signs completely different from the direct effect of the drug.

An important application is the assessment of drug-affected drivers. In this area, attempts have been made to establish systematic examination procedures known as the Standardized Field Sobriety Test (SFST),[4,5] which can be interpreted by non-medical personnel to determine the presence of intoxication and sometimes estimate which classes of drugs may be present (see Table 8.5 on p. 347).[6] This test involves observations and simple psychomotor tests, which are administered in a standardized fashion by specially trained personnel. Each step of administration and observation is performed according to a reproducible protocol. Standard clues are sought and points are allocated to determine a score. Scoring criteria are then used to determine whether impairment exists. The SFST allows evidence to be gathered by police officers, usually for the prosecution of traffic offenders, and medical personnel may not be directly involved. However, knowledge of this procedure is important for forensic medical practitioners who may be required to produce opinions or give evidence based on the findings of an examining officer. In particular, there may be a need to correlate signs of impairment found on SFST with results of toxicological analysis.

Table 8.1  Reasons for a forensic medical examination

- Assessment and treatment of acute intoxication or withdrawal
- Assessment and treatment of medical conditions associated with drug use
- Differentiation of legitimate from illicit drug use
- Examination for evidence of drug effect including withdrawal
- Collection of biological specimens to determine the presence of drugs
- Determination of intoxication in the assessment of fitness to drive a motor vehicle
- Determination of drug effects on *mens rea* or the capacity to form criminal intent
- Determination of drug issues in defences of automatism[3]
- Determination of fitness to be interviewed or to testify in court
- Determination of the appropriateness of custody of an intoxicated person
- Provision of opinions and expert evidence on drug effects after consideration of physical evidence and the results of chemical tests

An important issue in the acute forensic encounter is the question of whether the subject requires medical treatment for their drug-affected state. This may be either for alleviation of acute drug effects or for the treatment of complications or withdrawal syndromes. Many drug users seen in custodial forensic practice will see the medical consultation as an opportunity to obtain drugs and may engage in manipulative or deceptive behaviour in order to convince a practitioner to prescribe sedatives or analgesics. The prescription of psychoactive drugs to detainees is a specialized field that should be undertaken only after appropriate training and experience.[7] In most cases, the custodial setting is not one where optimum medical care for the seriously ill can be provided, especially if there is a requirement for observation of the patient. Any medical conditions that require careful monitoring should be treated in an appropriate health care facility such as a hospital. Particular examples of this are acute alcohol withdrawal, patients with depressed conscious states due to narcotic or sedative (including alcohol) use, and patients with acute excited states who may require monitored seclusion or treatment with sedatives.[8]

The question of whether addicted or drug-affected detainees can be rendered fit for interview by means of drug treatment by forensic medical personnel remains an extremely controversial one.[9] It is certainly possible to reverse intoxication caused by benzodiazepines and opioids by means of the appropriate agent (see individual drug sections). It is also possible to treat withdrawal syndromes due to various drug groups in a manner that greatly increases the comfort of the patient. In general, such treatment should strictly be regarded as symptomatic relief or emergency treatment of a dangerous condition. There is no guarantee that the mental state of the patient after treatment will be at an adequate level to deal with the rigours of an interview that may lead to charges being laid. There are also ethical considerations binding most medical professionals, which makes this a questionable practice in most western societies.[i]

In overdose cases where emergency treatment is needed for life-threatening drug effects, it is wise to arrange transfer to a monitored situation as soon as practicable after the patient has been resuscitated. The possibility of delayed absorption and interactions is ever present, especially in situations where the nature of the drug(s) that have been taken is unknown. This is an important consideration when dealing with individuals who may have concealed drugs in body cavities ('body packers').[10] Absorption in these cases is uncertain and ranges from minimal to massive with unpredictable results. In cases where an ingested container ruptures, there will be a massive dose of the drug delivered rapidly into the bloodstream with immediate effects. If the drug is a stimulant such as cocaine, there will be a rapid onset of confusion, hypertension, hyperthermia, seizures and cardiac arrest. If the drug is an opioid, such as heroin, there will be a rapid onset of extreme sedation, coma, respiratory depression and death. Such cases are medical emergencies and highlight the necessity of dealing with suspected body packers and the like in facilities with access to emergency medical care and hospitalization.

---

[i] Some of these ethical issues are discussed in Amnesty International's 'Declaration on the role of health professionals in the exposure of torture and ill-treatment' (1996). This contains references to the Declaration of Tokyo of the World Medical Association (1975).

A less obvious situation, but one that may have disastrous consequences, is the drug user or dealer who swallows a quantity of drugs when confronted by the authorities. Such persons may appear normal for a period immediately following their arrest but will deteriorate rapidly as the drugs begin to be absorbed. When assessing recent detainees for fitness for interview for drug offences, it is very important to exclude this situation as it may result in a medical emergency or death in custody.

# 8.2 Health status of drug users

Many drug users seen by clinical forensic practitioners will be suffering from medical conditions associated with their lifestyle. While a full discussion of the socioeconomic aspects of drug abuse is beyond the scope of this book, it is important for the practitioner to be aware of the types of medical conditions that may coexist in drug-affected patients. Intravenous drug users in particular may suffer from conditions associated with poverty, poor hygiene and nutrition, and blood-borne infections passed on by needle sharing and sexually transmitted diseases. There is a high incidence of psychiatric morbidity that may coexist in drug abusers. This may make the choice of therapeutic options very difficult. Sometimes the stigmata of acute or chronic drug use will help in immediate clinical assessment, and in some cases they will contribute to the assessment of the chronicity of the problem. There are also significant issues relating to safety both during medical procedures and in the custodial setting, especially when serious infections such as tuberculosis, hepatitis or HIV are involved. Even less serious infections or infestations such as lice or scabies can present a potential problem in the confined conditions of cellblocks.

As with all medical encounters, it is important to obtain as accurate a history as possible when dealing with drug-affected persons in the forensic setting. This is often quite difficult, as there are many confounding factors that may be involved. These are summarized in Table 8.2.

Other sources of information, such as family, friends, medical staff, police and social workers, can be useful sources of information in this respect. Forensic practitioners also need to be familiar with local slang terms and other features of language used on the streets and in the local drug scene. Detainees will often use these terms when giving a history and may not even recognize more formal language used in other areas of society, especially medical terms.

**Table 8.2** Factors that confound an accurate history

- Manipulative behaviour by the subject
- Deliberate untruthfulness
- Conscious states affected by drugs or injury
- Exaggeration of symptoms in an attempt to obtain treatment
- Intellectual disability
- Psychiatric illness

# 8.3 Principles of an examination scheme for drug-affected persons

## OBTAINING A HISTORY

As much history as possible should be obtained from the subject and attending police or other persons. Important data to be sought in the history include those listed in Table 8.3, but a comprehensive history is rarely available.

General medical and/or psychiatric history should include details of drug treatment and medical conditions that may mimic drug effects.[11] Some of these are listed in Table 8.3. There are many drugs used in legitimate medical practice that may affect observations made in clinical forensic examinations. A non-exhaustive list is given in Table 8.4.

An enormous number of medical conditions may produce signs similar to those due to the effects of drugs. It is impossible to give an exhaustive list. However, a knowledge of general medicine will usually help in differentiating the two. When in doubt a medical opinion should always be sought. See also the monographs in the Appendix.

## THE EXAMINATION

The general appearance of the person may give clues as to drug effects. Alcohol intoxication will produce the characteristic smell of alcohol on the breath, and this may be confirmed by breath testing. Users of sedative drugs will appear drowsy or even unconscious. Unconscious or unresponsive patients should not remain in custody particularly if there has been a rapid reduction in conscious state since apprehension. Users of stimulants will be active and agitated, and may show other signs of stimulant effect as described above.

**Table 8.3** Components of an accurate history

- Drugs taken
- Doses
- Timing of drug consumption
- History of recent activities, including sleep and nutrition, or injuries particularly to the head
- A description of the person's state and behaviour at the time of arrest/apprehension
- A description of the person's subsequent behaviour while in custody

# Clinical forensic aspects of drug use

**Table 8.4** Common drug types and their clinical effects

| Drug type | Effect |
| --- | --- |
| Tranquillizers, including benzodiazepines and antipsychotics | Sedation, tremor, other effects of sedatives as described above |
| Anticonvulsants | Sedation, incoordination |
| Analgesics (containing codeine) | Sedation, pinpoint pupils |
| Anorectics and stimulants | Stimulant effects, aggression, etc. |
| Topical ophthalmic medication | Effects on pupil size, may also have systemic effects |
| Antidepressants | Anti-cholinergic effects, hypomania, interactions with other drugs (MAO inhibitors and SSRIs) |
| Methadone | Opioid effects |
| Antimicrobials | May interact to potentiate other psychoactive drugs |
| Anti-parkinsonian drugs | Anti-cholinergic, psychotic reactions |
| Anti-histamines | Sedation, anti-cholinergic effects |
| Non-prescription cough mixtures and similar drugs | Sedation, usually due to anti-histamines, dextromethorphan or codeine; anti-cholinergic or sympathomimetic effects |

Physical examination should include an assessment of the state of consciousness and awareness. Check for orientation, concentration, speech, reflexes, sweating, tremors and muscle tone. Signs of past drug use may include needle track marks, nasal septum changes, evidence of poor hygiene and malnutrition, and signs of systemic diseases such as hepatitis or tuberculosis.

A feature of the SFST is checking pulse and blood pressure and an eye examination. Certain signs may be characteristic of acute drug effects (see Table 8.5).

In cases where withdrawal is occurring, the signs in Table 8.5 may be absent or even reversed, and additional signs may be present as described in the text.

Divided attention and psychomotor tests are features of the SFST that may give clues as to impairment. The information derived from these tests is validated and interpreted purely as an indication of impairment. However, under some circumstances it may be possible to attribute certain observations to specific drugs, e.g. distortion of time perception caused by cannabis or amphetamines. The tests consist of detailed procedures, the extent of which are systematically defined from the first steps of instructing the subject, through observation and scoring of clues. An important part of these tests is the giving of detailed instructions prior to the actual test so that the subject's ability to assimilate and retain instructions is also being assessed. The tests include:

- **The walk and turn test** – subjects are instructed to take nine heel-to-toe steps with their arms by their sides, along a line on the floor, to turn, and then walk back again. Steps are

Table 8.5  Key observations relating to the Standardized Field Sobriety Test

| Drug class | Pulse | Blood pressure | Pupils | Nystagmus | Eye movements | Miscellaneous |
|---|---|---|---|---|---|---|
| CNS stimulants | +/− | Raised | Dilated | Absent | Jerky | 'Speeding' |
| CNS depressants | − | − | Usually normal | Present | Slow | Drowsy |
| Cannabis | + | + | Usually normal | Absent | May be slow | Reddened eyes, tremors |
| Opioids | − | − | Small | Absent | Slow | 'On the nod' |
| Alcohol | +/− | +/− | Normal | Present | Slow/jerky | Alcohol on breath |

to be counted out loud. Clue points are scored for various defined deviations from the procedure, such as stopping, miscounting, losing balance, taking the wrong number of steps, etc.

- **The one leg stand test** – subjects are instructed to stand on one foot with their arms by their sides, with the other held out 15 cm above the ground with the toes pointed. While standing in this position the subject is instructed to estimate 30 s by counting 'one-thousand-and-one, one-thousand-and-two, ..., etc.' Clue points are scored for swaying, putting the foot down, hopping or raising the arms for balance.

# 8.4 Clinical forensic opinions

Clinical forensic practitioners may be requested to provide opinions regarding dosages and effects of drugs, based on observations made by others. The information provided is usually less than optimal and the opinion requested is often more than can be inferred from what is available. Opinions may be sought on a number of possible issues, including those shown in Table 8.6.

In some cases it may be easy to come to an opinion based on apparently obvious information; however, there are many confounding factors that make giving reputable opinions quite difficult. Dose–response characteristics for many drugs of forensic interest are modified by the effects of tolerance as well as by uncertainties of dosage and metabolism.

In the case of alcohol (see below), estimations of blood alcohol concentrations can be made with reasonable accuracy. Unfortunately, the relative ease of providing such opinions has raised a certain expectation that similar opinions can be provided for other drugs. It is rarely possible to give as precise an opinion for other drugs however detailed the knowledge of the pharmacokinetics and effects of the drug in question. Whatever the situation, any opinions must contain a full discussion of the limitations inherent in the process. This maintains the reputation for impartiality and probity that is so important in clinical forensic practice.

In some cases the mere presence of a drug will be a significant finding especially for those drugs whose presence is absolutely forbidden or illegal. In other cases it may only be possible to form an opinion that a particular drug was taken within a limited time if the substance has known pharmacokinetics. If the substance or its metabolites are long lived, such an interpretation is prone to much uncertainty. For some drugs such as alcohol, a mathematical model may be available that allows 'read-back' or in some cases 'read-forward' calculations to predict blood levels and, by inference, effects at certain times.

**Table 8.6** Reasons for requesting clinical forensic opinions

- Estimation of dosages
- Levels of drugs in body fluids and their significance
- Presence or absence of drug effects based on clinical observations
- Physical effects of drugs on the body
- Effects on the capacity to perform complex tasks such as driving
- Effects on capacity to consent to or perform activities including sexual activity
- Effects on fitness to be interviewed or to give evidence in court
- Effects on fitness for custody
- Readback calculations of levels and/or effects at a given time
- Interactions between drugs

# 8.5 Common drug effects seen in clinical medicine

## STIMULANTS

This group of drugs includes amphetamines, other stimulant drugs such as methylphenidate, and amphetamine derivatives such as MDMA (ecstasy). There is a large illicit market for these drugs in many Western societies because of their effects on alertness and reducing the need for sleep. Amphetamines are likely to be abused by people in situations where they are prone to fatigue, such as long-distance truck drivers or students studying for examinations. Stimulant drugs have been used to alleviate fatigue and increase alertness in military personnel, but it is important to distinguish this controlled use with known dosages and opportunities to recover from illicit use where none of these controls apply. Amphetamine derivatives such as MDMA are said to have an enormous consumer market among nightclub patrons and people at dance parties and 'raves', where the drug is used to increase energy and enhance enjoyment of the environment.

Legitimate medical indications for stimulant drugs are few and are usually restricted to specialist practitioners in the relevant fields. In some jurisdictions they are available for treatment of conditions where the patient is pathologically somnolent, such as narcolepsy and sleep apnoea. Stimulants such as dexamphetamine and methylphenidate are also used in the treatment of childhood attention deficit hyperactivity disorder where they have a paradoxical effect of increasing concentration and reducing hyperactivity. The existence of an adult form of this condition and its treatment with stimulants is controversial.[12] The medical use of these drugs may come to forensic attention in situations including assessment of suitability to drive, acute excited states in custody and considerations of drug effect on the ability to form criminal intent.

With the exception of the legitimately prescribed stimulants mentioned above, all other sources of these drugs in most societies are from illegal or clandestine manufacture. These preparations are subject to wide variations in potency and composition and the resulting clinical effects on consumers are likewise variable. In cases where the drugs are taken by injection, are the associated problems of intravenous drug users will be present.

When used in an uncontrolled fashion to alleviate fatigue, users are subject to rebound sedation when drug use is discontinued. This needs to be kept in mind when considering the effects of stimulants on driving ability. When amphetamines have been used to alleviate fatigue, the subject may exhibit rebound signs of depression, exhaustion and fatigue rather than the direct stimulant effect of the drugs. These signs may mimic the effects of sedatives on clinical assessment. The use of preparations of variable effectiveness and in combination with other drugs results in a very dangerous situation in subjects such as long-distance drivers who may suddenly succumb to fatigue with disastrous consequences.

Although stimulants in low doses may have a beneficial effect on the psychomotor skills required for carrying out complex tasks such as driving, in practice this is hardly ever the case. Amphetamines are abused by long-distance truck drivers and others and the result is usually a diminution of driving skills due to the uncontrolled nature of drug use. Undesirable effects such as aggression, lack of judgement, build-up of fatigue and psychotic complications make the use of amphetamines while driving a dangerous practice.

The clinical signs of the acutely intoxicated state are largely those of an excess of sympathetic activity. These include dilated pupils, tachycardia and other arrhythmias, hypertension (which may result in cerebral bleeding), hyperthermia, hyperreflexia, tremors, teeth grinding, restlessness, garrulousness, loss of appetite, dry mouth, urinary retention, diarrhoea, renal failure and seizures. Psychological phenomena include anxiety, agitation, euphoria, hypomania, aggression, hallucinations and paranoia. A psychotic state indistinguishable from schizophrenia can occur. Physical signs of drug use, such as a congested or runny nose, septal damage (inhalation) and venous track marks, may be visible.

Intoxication with cocaine produces more variable and less potent signs of sympathomimetic effects than amphetamines. Sudden death due to acute arrhythmias or acute infarction induced by coronary vasoconstriction may occur and there may also be rapid respiratory depression. Seizures occur prior to death in 50% of fatal cases.[13,14]

In the Standardized Field Sobriety Test, some or all of the above signs are sought. In addition, the eyes are examined for signs consistent with stimulant use. These include mydriasis with a slow pupillary reaction, and the absence of nystagmus.

While the more severe manifestations of stimulant use will result in hospital admission, it is common in some jurisdictions for drug-affected persons to be apprehended by police and kept in custody. In this setting the potential exists for problems to arise because of the detainee's intoxicated state.

Violence and aggression may be a major problem. Stimulant users may not be responsive to verbal commands or attempts to negotiate or reason. The risk of physical injury is high as a result of violent behaviour or physical methods of restraint. The detainee may be affected by chemical agents such as capsicum spray and/or have sustained injuries that are usually exacerbated by attempts to escape or resist. In these situations, it is extremely unwise for forensic medical practitioners to attempt sedation or chemical restraint, especially in the environment of a police cell or arrest scene. Management options for these patients are restricted to physical restraint, sedation or seclusion, all of which require careful monitoring.

Complications of stimulant use that may arise include positional asphyxia and sudden death associated with an acute excited state.[15,16] This arises when a person intoxicated with these drugs is immobilized in a position where respiratory movements are compromised. Because of the increased metabolic demands and energy expenditure in this condition, ventilation is inadequate and death results from hypoxia.

A characteristic withdrawal syndrome does not occur with stimulants such as amphetamine. However, the patient may appear somnolent as a result of the rebound effect and may be depressed. Residual psychotic symptoms may still be present after the acute intoxication phase has passed.

Treatment of stimulant overdoses or acute excited states is best carried out in a hospital emergency department[17] or where resuscitation facilities are available. Treatment follows the general procedures for poisoning cases – where the drug has recently been taken orally, charcoal can be used to prevent further absorption; however, this is of no use when the drug has been inhaled or injected. Specific treatments will depend on the manifestations of the drug and may include tranquillizers such as haloperidol, anti-hypertensives, fluid replacement, beta-blockers, and measures to control seizures and elevated temperatures.[18]

Psychiatric assessments are important in stimulant users as the drugs may produce a very wide range of psychiatric symptoms under various circumstances, including depression, apparent sedation due to fatigue, agitation mimicking manic states, and psychosis. These conditions will have a profound effect on a person's fitness for interview or custody and may change rapidly. This variability makes forensic assessment notoriously difficult (and sometimes dangerous) and highlights the need for careful observation and a low threshold for hospitalizing persons suspected of taking high doses of these drugs.

Expert opinions regarding the effects of stimulants may be sought with respect to psychiatric issues as well as with regard to the interpretation of blood or urine test results and correlation with clinical effects. Because of the wide range of behaviour that may be produced by these drugs, formulating such opinions can be difficult. There is no constant dose–response characteristic for most stimulant drugs. In most cases the interpretation of toxicology tests can only be taken as far as evidence of recent ingestion (within the known pharmacokinetics of the compound) and any opinions of effect from a given dose or level can only be speculative in an individual case.

## BENZODIAZEPINES

Drugs from the benzodiazepine family are very frequently abused and it is therefore common for their effects to be encountered in clinical forensic medicine. Because of the declining availability of sedatives from other groups such as barbiturates, benzodiazepines represent the most commonly encountered non-narcotic sedatives in clinical forensic practice. Benzodiazepines are commonly used as recognized medical treatment for anxiety and other psychiatric disorders, insomnia and epilepsy. They are easily available and it is possible for large amounts of these drugs to be bought legally by obtaining multiple prescriptions; tablets may also be sold on the street.

In the forensic setting, benzodiazepines may be encountered in detainees who have used them in addition to, or as a substitute for, other drugs, such as heroin. This is particularly so in the case of flunitrazepam, which has a reputation as a particularly intoxicating compared with other benzodiazepines and which may be used as self-medication for various perceived psychological problems.[19,20] Enormous amounts of drugs such as diazepam or oxazepam may be taken daily by patients who have developed a tolerance (20–50 tablets or more per day). It is known for intravenous drug users to inject solutions made from tablets, or the liquid contents of temazepam gel-capsules where these are still available. These patients present a management problem in custody as well as for opinions regarding fitness for interview or, in some cases, for court appearance.

Benzodiazepines, particularly flunitrazepam, may have been used as a date rape drug in order to render a victim susceptible to sexual abuse or assault.[21] When taken before driving, the drugs may affect driving skills and the driver may need to be assessed following a collision, or an opinion may be required based on toxicological analyses and observations of behaviour. There are also a large number of people being legitimately treated with benzodiazepines who may come under forensic scrutiny and need psychiatric or other evaluations prior to becoming involved in the legal system. Large doses of benzodiazepines may also be taken in suicide attempts.

The clinical signs of benzodiazepine ingestion are variable, reflecting differences in tolerance, dosage, interactions with other drugs and individual sensitivity. In general the drugs are sedatives and induce a depressed mental state with ataxia, nystagmus, slurred speech, ptosis, hypoventilation, hypo-reflexia and hypotension. Higher doses may lead to unconsciousness and coma. Death may result from respiratory depression, especially in combination with other depressants such as alcohol and in patients with respiratory disease. Psychoactive effects include sedation, amnesia, confusion and fatigue.

Paradoxical reactions may occur with benzodiazepines, including disinhibition, agitation, aggression, delusions and acute rage. These effects are thought to be due to the suppression of inhibitory pathways and are sometimes seen in overdose cases. Any of these effects may be exacerbated by other co-administered drugs, especially alcohol.

In the Standardized Field Sobriety Test the above signs are sought and emphasis placed on eye signs, including horizontal gaze nystagmus, vertical nystagmus (with high doses) and lack of convergence. Pupillary size is usually unaffected. Subjects may be sedated and fail to follow directions adequately. Tests of balance, reflexes and coordination will be impaired.

While habitual users and addicts may maintain a semblance of normality while taking large amounts of benzodiazepine drugs, the question of whether a person may be fit for interview or to represent themselves adequately in legal proceedings is often a difficult one. The drugs all have the potential to seriously disrupt cognitive functions and have an adverse effect on memory and judgement. It is always preferable that people have the benefit of an intact sensorium under difficult circumstances such as police interviews. In general, it is preferable that acutely affected persons have the opportunity to recover prior to being interviewed but final assessment is best made on an individual basis. A patient accustomed to taking benzodiazepines chronically may be less fit for interview in a state of withdrawal than while taking their medication.

Benzodiazepines have the potential to interact with a great many other drugs. In general, there is potentiation of the effects of many sedatives, including alcohol. This extends to the respiratory depressant action of these drugs and makes the combination of alcohol and benzodiazepines a dangerous one in overdose. Because many benzodiazepines such as diazepam have long-lived pharmacologically active metabolic products, there may still be a risk of interactions even after initial effect of the drug has apparently passed off.

The benzodiazepine antagonist flumazenil has a place in the hospital treatment of confirmed acute overdose, but there is little place for the routine use of this drug in the custodial setting or where the nature of the drug that has been taken is unknown. Reversal of benzodiazepine intoxication with this agent will not reduce the effects of any non-benzodiazepine drugs, and may also induce an acute withdrawal syndrome with anxiety, signs of sympathetic over-activity and convulsions in addicted patients.

Tolerance and addiction are well known to occur with benzodiazepines. This may represent a problem in the addict who is taken into custody and the supply of drugs suddenly ceased. An acute withdrawal syndrome may be precipitated resulting in anxiety, dysphoria, tremors and occasionally more severe manifestations, including panic attacks, acute psychotic reactions and convulsions, with their associated morbidity. Acute benzodiazepine withdrawal is rarely a medical emergency, but practitioners should be aware of the potential for the condition and should avoid precipitating it. Treatment should consist of very gradually withdrawing the drugs, preferably after substituting a long-acting benzodiazepine such as diazepam if shorter-acting members of the group such as temazepam or oxazepam are being taken.

Although therapeutic ranges of blood levels for many of these drugs are quoted, they are best considered as a guideline to consumption in most cases. It is very difficult to prove a consistent relationship between blood levels and clinical effect for these drugs especially in the presence of tolerance. Despite this limitation, toxicological tests can be useful in determining whether a drug has been administered and as a rough guide to dosage or tolerance. In cases where there is no reason for a benzodiazepine to be present, a positive blood or urine test can be very important evidence. An example of such a case might be a rape victim who may have been administered a drug concealed in a drink. In other cases a very high level of a drug may indicate extensive abuse and addiction.

## CANNABIS

Cannabis is probably the most commonly used illicit drug likely to be encountered in clinical forensic practice. Despite this it is often very difficult to detect clinically for a number of reasons. The drug is relatively short acting and there will be an inevitable time delay between administration and medical assessment that often allows acute signs of impairment to dissipate. General observations may be non-specific – reddened conjunctivae, partial ptosis, tachycardia and the characteristic smell. The clinical effects may be masked by the effects of co-administered nicotine or other drugs, particularly alcohol. Cannabis alone does not produce pupillary changes or nystagmus on eye examination.

The Standardized Field Sobriety Test (SFST) may therefore reveal little in the way of hard clinical signs as a result. In the psychomotor testing part of the test, users may have difficulty understanding or remembering instructions and will perform poorly on tests of co-ordination and divided attention tasks. Users may experience toxic psychosis, which may develop into schizophrenia in susceptible patients.[22] While clinical forensic examinations of 'pure' cannabis users are often unrewarding, it is important to be aware of co-morbidities such as this.

Cannabis use is reported by a great number of persons examined by clinical forensic physicians, but it is unusual for this alone to be a reason for the examination. Use of cannabis alone is not associated with violence or agitated behaviour, and intoxication with it in the absence of other drugs is not a condition producing concern regarding custodial issues. Acute intoxication may render a subject unfit to be interviewed due to confusion, but this is best assessed on general lines and will in most cases be short lived. Although tolerance and a degree of dependence have been documented, this is rarely of clinical significance. Any cannabis withdrawal syndrome occurring in the custodial setting is usually of a minor degree.

Passive smoking of cannabis is occasionally put forward as an explanation for positive blood or urine tests for the drug. Significant levels of THC metabolite have been found in urine following passive smoking of the drug.[23] However, the association with acute intoxication remains unclear.[24]

The effect on cannabis on driving is variable and subject to some controversy[25,26] (see also Section 4). At low levels of intoxication there is a decrease in aggression and slower, apparently more careful driving, but with an increase in steering errors and lateral deviation from a straight path. The capacity to make sudden decisions in stressful circumstances may also be degraded. While laboratory testing using driving simulators has demonstrated impairment of driving skills with cannabis, epidemiological studies show variable results depending on the design of the study. In combination with alcohol, the detrimental effect of both drugs may be enhanced.

Controversy exists regarding the interpretation of toxicological test for cannabis. The THC metabolite, carboxy-THC, is commonly reported in blood test results. However, since this substance is inactive it is not possible to infer any clinical effect whatsoever from its presence. Its long lifetime in the body reduces the significance of a positive test to confirmation that the drug had been taken some time in the preceding weeks. Mathematical models have been proposed for the estimation of time of consumption of cannabis from analysis of THC and carboxy-THC levels.[27] Use of such models for forensic purposes needs to be validated in both acute and chronic use settings and to take into account technical issues of THC analysis.

Direct measurement of THC in blood samples is not performed in all jurisdictions for forensic purposes in acute cases involving driving or suspected intoxication. Because of the short lifetime of THC it is often not possible to obtain a timely blood sample and the interpretation is difficult. There are also technical concerns regarding degradation of THC in stored samples. Detectable levels of THC can usually be interpreted as evidence of recent use of the drug; however, no clear dose–response characteristic has been established that would allow correlation of observed behaviour or impairment with THC levels.

## OPIOIDS

Opioids constitute a very common group of drugs of abuse that may lead to problems with the law and hence clinical forensic involvement. Clinical forensic practitioners very commonly see detainees or suspects who are heroin users or on methadone maintenance programmes. Practitioners may also need to treat persons who have suffered acute overdoses of opioids usually heroin, or conversely assess withdrawal. Since there are many opioid addicts who depend on medical prescriptions for their supplies, it is important for medical practitioners to be able to recognize drug-seeking individuals.

## Common drug effects seen in clinical medicine

A small proportion of opioid addicts seen in clinical forensic practice will be those who are addicted to licit drugs (usually morphine, pethidine (meperidine), codeine, oxycodone or dextromoramide) as a result of medical treatment of chronically painful conditions such as back pain or migraine. These patients will often attend doctors' surgeries with convincing stories to attempt to obtain prescriptions. In most jurisdictions there is provision for doctors to obtain permits to treat certain patients with large quantities of opioid analgesics, usually for painful terminal diseases. These patients do not often come to the attention of clinical forensic practitioners except perhaps after death in cases where there is an enquiry by the coroner. By far the most common aspect of opioid use likely to come under forensic scrutiny is the illicit use of heroin.

The use of heroin has reached epidemic proportions in Western societies, and an enormous amount of criminal activity, morbidity and mortality is associated with it. Heroin users come under very frequent police attention both because of activities including driving while intoxicated and because of criminal activities they engage in to sustain their habit.

The lifestyle of many opioid addicts is dominated by drug-seeking behaviour, including manipulative interactions with doctors (even in the forensic or custodial setting) aimed at obtaining drugs. Doctor shopping to obtain prescription drugs is common in societies where the medical system allows this. There is a strong association with crime and prostitution. Because the quality and concentration of street supplies of heroin are variable, unintentional overdosing may occur, often in 'epidemics'. Intravenous drug addicts will sometimes take any available drug in addition to or as a substitute for his or her preferred opioid. This may result in the intravenous administration of other substances, including methadone syrup and virtually any injectable drug obtained from various sources. Forensic practitioners must always be aware of the possibility of multiple drugs being present when assessing drug users in custody.

Heroin is usually consumed by intravenous injection, but a significant number of users smoke the drug in order to avoid the dangers of parenteral administration.

The clinical features of opioid use are primarily those of sedation, ranging from a drowsy dream-like state to profound coma with life-threatening respiratory depression. A characteristic sedated state with droopy eyelids and the ability to be roused before nodding off again is known as being 'on the nod'. Opioid intoxication produces miosis (pinpoint pupils). Pethidine (meperidine), however, may produce either constricted or dilated pupils in overdose because of its anti-cholinergic properties.

In SFST examinations the clues that result from opioid intoxication include pinpoint pupils with no nystagmus, the characteristic sedated state with slow pulse and blood pressure, truncal sway and staggering.

In emergency overdose situations the effects of opioids may be reversed by the use of the drug naloxone (Narcan). When administered by injection this drug produces a very rapid reversal of opioid effect, but the effect is short lived. The reversal of opioid effects may unmask the effects of other drugs as well as precipitating acute withdrawal. Addicts are usually very unappreciative of being woken, even from a coma, and may be aggressive after being given the drug. Naloxone does not reverse the sedative effect of benzodiazepines. Because of the short duration of action of naloxone, it is unwise to rely on a single dose as adequate treatment for profound intoxication with opioids, especially if long-acting opioids such as methadone have been taken. Patients who have been revived in this way must be monitored carefully for signs of opioid effect after the naloxone has worn off. Such patients are in general not fit for interview and incarceration should be contemplated with caution.

There is a high incidence of blood-borne viral infections in chronic intravenous drug users including hepatitis B and C and HIV. Users are prone to embolic phenomena leading to gangrene of extremities if intra-arterial injection is practised either intentionally or accidentally. Bacterial infections associated with poor injecting practice include thrombophlebitis, bacterial endocarditis and osteomyelitis. Chronic heroin users are invariably constipated with a palpable colon. Other findings include venous track marks that may be in unusual places as accessible veins are progressively destroyed by thrombosis and infection. Hypoxic brain damage and aspiration pneumonia are associated with sub-lethal overdoses. The general state of health and hygiene of many intravenous drug addicts is extremely poor.

Assessment of opioid users in custody hinges on the issues of fitness for interview, fitness for custody and the management of withdrawal.[28] This is a complex subject where policies may vary widely in different jurisdictions. While a detailed discussion of issues surrounding the determination of fitness to be interviewed is beyond the scope of this book, it is important to note the aspects of drug use and opioid use in particular that are important. The central question of whether the detainee is able to adequately represent his or herself in an interview may be influenced by intoxication on the one hand and the presence of withdrawal symptoms on the other. In some cases it can be argued that there is a 'window' of fitness between these two states, but assessment of this condition requires skill and experience. Although it is never possible for a medical assessment of this type to determine whether an interviewee will be truthful, it is possible to recognize factors that will affect comprehension and cerebration, as well as influences on motivation such as the presence of withdrawal symptoms.

The presence of acute intoxication with any sedative drug such as an opioid is a contraindication to incarceration in a non-monitored facility such as a police cell. In cases where the nature of drug use is unknown, and especially where there may be interactions between several drugs, it is essential that patients be transferred to a hospital or other monitored situation. The risks of death in custody are very high in these situations.

The characteristic withdrawal syndrome, while unpleasant, does not have the same serious medical potential as withdrawal from alcohol. The syndrome becomes evident at a variable time following the last dose, depending on the degree of tolerance and the dose interval to which the patient is accustomed. The syndrome begins with anxiety and a craving for the drug. It progresses to yawning, nasal congestion, mydriasis, piloerection myalgia, abdominal cramps, muscle spasms and gastrointestinal symptoms including diarrhoea. The syndrome abates after a few days leaving the subject drained and depressed. Although rarely serious or fatal, the onset of withdrawal is dreaded by most addicts. When addicts are taken into custody, it may be possible in some jurisdictions to continue methadone programmes. However, because of problems in obtaining details of a person's dosage, there may be a period of delay where withdrawal symptoms become apparent. In these circumstances, or where there is no provision for methadone, a considerate practitioner may institute treatment for the few days it takes for physical withdrawal to occur. Treatment is based on symptom alleviation and may include simple analgesics or NSAIDs, antispasmodics such as quinine, anti-diarrhoeals such as diphenoxylate/atropine and minor tranquillizers. Clonidine in small doses has a beneficial effect on the symptoms of withdrawal but may cause postural hypotension.

When asked to interpret drug levels found on blood or urine testing, it is important to bear in mind the known pharmacokinetics of the opioids (see also Section 5). The most commonly abused opioid, heroin, has a very short lifetime in the blood and is rapidly converted to 6-acetyl morphine (6-AM), which also has a very short lifetime. For this reason these substances are not often seen in blood test results taken from living persons in the forensic setting. Once excreted in the urine, however, metabolism of these substances ceases and the presence of 6-AM in urine tests is commonly used to detect illicit heroin use. 6-AM is in turn converted to morphine, which also has a comparatively short half-life of 4–6 h. Blood concentrations may have fallen to quite low levels by the time blood is taken even though the clinical effect has not yet diminished. Because of the phenomenon of tolerance in chronic opioid users, the specific blood level of morphine may be of little help in determining a degree of intoxication although it is generally good evidence of recent consumption.

Methadone is a long-acting semi-synthetic opioid that is used for maintenance treatment of heroin addicts.[29] It is usually dispensed in liquid form for immediate consumption under supervision, but under some circumstances it is prone to diversion and overdose. Because of its long half-life, methadone may accumulate over several days, even with once-daily dosing, and result in toxic levels, especially in combination with other drugs or if taken by a less tolerant patient. For this reason, there is a heightened danger of inadvertent overdose when first commencing treatment if dose levels are increased too soon. It is especially important for practitioners called upon to prescribe methadone to a previously unknown patient to obtain independent verification of the dose.

## ALCOHOL

Alcohol is the most common drug likely to be encountered in the forensic setting. Issues include fitness for interview, fitness for custody, effects of driving ability, disinhibition in relation to sexual activity, dealing with acute intoxicated states including violence, and management of withdrawal.

As with other drugs, histories may often be misleading. However, one positive feature is the ability to easily measure the blood alcohol concentration (BAC) by means of a breath test. This is often very helpful, as assessment of degree of intoxication by clinical means alone is notoriously unreliable, even with experienced examiners.[30] This is because of the wide range of tolerance that occurs to alcohol. Some experienced drinkers may appear superficially unaffected even at extremely high blood alcohol concentrations of the order of 0.3–0.4 g/100 mL. However this relative insensitivity of gross motor performance to alcohol does not extend to other skills such as judgement, concentration, coordination and the ability to perform divided attention tasks.

Clinical signs of alcohol effect include the smell of alcohol on breath, mood changes (raised or lowered), garrulousness, altered perception, ataxia and incoordination, slurred speech, peripheral vasodilatation and nystagmus. Pupillary changes may take the form of slight dilation, but this is not a consistent sign. Violence and aggression may present a major problem in management.

Intoxication may also be accompanied by signs of acute alcohol toxicity, including liver failure (acute alcoholic hepatitis) and depressed conscious state. Respiratory depression and reduced conscious state are important issues in determining fitness for custody where the risks of dying from aspiration of vomitus and alcohol toxicity are increased. A very significant risk is present in situations where consideration of other conditions is discounted by obvious signs of alcohol consumption.[31]

Alcohol intoxication alone is not usually determined in the field by SFST type examinations owing to the ease with which breath tests are conducted. There are very few subjects among the driving population who are not capable of providing an adequate breath sample.[32] Alcohol intoxication is commonly used in experiments with volunteers as a convenient and legal model of intoxication with which to train health professionals and police. The general effects of alcohol intoxication are very well known and the effects on a systematic procedure such as the SFST are a useful model of CNS depressant drug action.

Some controversy exists regarding the effect of alcohol on a subject's fitness to be interviewed. Because it is relatively easy to perform a breath test in most cases, information is usually available regarding the subject's BAC. Because of the wide variation in effect of alcohol, there may be a significant effect on a person's capacity to be interviewed even at low BACs. A reasonable course may be to judge a person unfit for interview if they are above the local legal limit for driving. On the other hand, alcohol withdrawal is a serious condition (see below) that would render a person not only unfit to be interviewed but in many cases unfit for custody as well. The decision is essentially a clinical one based on consideration of the person's drinking history and observations of signs of intoxication and/or withdrawal.

An enormous amount of material is available regarding the effects of alcohol on driving. It is well recognized that alcohol has a detrimental effect on driving skills and most jurisdictions have enacted legal limits on blood alcohol concentration for driving. It is extremely common for questions regarding all aspects of measuring and interpreting alcohol levels in drivers to be raised in legal proceedings. Although legal limits are defined based on scientific evidence regarding impairment, the levels chosen do not necessarily mean that all drivers will be significantly impaired at that BAC. Psychomotor impairment can be detected under laboratory conditions at the lowest measurable BACs. However, the statistical risk for driving impairment may not become significant until much higher levels are achieved. In many cases the legal limit is purposefully set at a level below that where the majority of drivers are impaired with the intention of preventing people from driving at dangerous levels of BAC.

In chronic alcohol abuse a number of physical signs may become evident as a result of the multi-system damage that occurs. These include the signs of chronic liver disease, endocrine changes, cardiomyopathy and bone marrow toxicity. Signs of peripheral neuropathy, Wernicke's encephalopathy (horizontal and vertical nystagmus, ataxia, confusion) and Korsakoff's psychosis (loss of short-term memory, confabulation and progressive dementia) may be evident. These signs are often accompanied by evidence of poor hygiene, neglect, malnutrition and injury, which are essential in assessing detainees in the forensic setting. Chronic ingestion of alcohol leads to a state of tolerance, physical dependence and addiction where the subject sustains elevated BAC on a virtually constant basis. Withdrawal from this state, often precipitated by being taken into custody, may precipitate a severe withdrawal syndrome that constitutes a medical emergency. In some cases where the patient is habituated to a sustained high BAC, signs of withdrawal can begin and may require treatment before the BAC has fallen to zero.

The alcohol withdrawal syndrome is a combination of nausea and vomiting, sweats, tremulousness, hyperreflexia, which may lead to seizures, and an acute psychosis. This may be accompanied by vivid and alarming visual hallucinations that are difficult for the patient to distinguish from reality. The symptoms usually peak within 24–36 h and dissipate after 48 h. Staging schemes have been developed to determine the degree of medical intervention that may be necessary. Mild cases may be treated outside a hospital with minor tranquillizers and supportive care under circumstances where there are no other serious medical complications and frequent review is possible.[33] In severe cases the syndrome progresses to hyperthermia, seizures and cardio-respiratory collapse. It is vital that forensic practitioners are able to recognize this condition in detainees as it requires urgent hospital treatment with thiamine and sedative drugs such as diazepam.[34]

The theory of alcohol absorption and metabolism has been presented elsewhere in this book. The elimination of alcohol can be modelled mathematically in a piecewise linear fashion by the use of the Widmark equation or variations of it and on this basis it is possible to estimate a blood alcohol level at some time prior to the time of a measurement of BAC (known as a read-back calculation). These methods assume a linear constant elimination rate between 0.01% and 0.02% per hour once the absorption peak level has been achieved. This is a reasonable assumption for most people and produces a realistic result as long as it can be assumed that absorption is complete. Since the exact elimination rate for any individual will not be known, such calculations can at best yield a range of possible values, which will diverge with the time between the test and the calculation. Another source of uncertainty is knowing when the peak occurs as there is a wide variation in absorption times quoted in the literature. Absorption may be influenced by factors such as food in the stomach, the presence of shock and traumatic injury or drugs which affect gastric emptying or extra hepatic metabolism. A commonly accepted range of absorption times is from 30 to 120 min, with most individuals probably falling into the lower end of this range.[35] BAC estimates may be made by simple interpolation during the absorption phase if it assumed that absorption is essentially constant during this period. This may not be a realistic assumption depending on the drinking scenario.

The Widmark theory is also used to determine the relationship between alcohol consumption and BAC (see Chapter 6.2). For most forensic purposes this usually takes the form of a single calculation of the BAC that could result from a given dose of alcohol, or the amount of alcohol in the body corresponding to a given BAC.[36] Attempts have been made to simulate alcohol absorption and metabolism by means of computer programs, which attempt to predict BAC from a forward analysis of alcohol consumption.[37] These have varying degrees of accuracy depending on the accuracy of the drinking history used to generate the data. In most law enforcement situations, the fixed points of driving times and the result of an objective measurement of BAC are known to have greater reliability than the drinking history given by the subject (see Case Report 6.2, p. 310).

359

# 8.6 Case reports

## CASE REPORT 8.1 FITNESS FOR INTERVIEW

A forensic physician was called to a police station at 2.55 p.m. in order to determine whether a 30-year-old man was fit to be interviewed. Attending police informed the doctor that the man had been arrested at approximately 11.30 that morning but had gradually become drowsy once he had been brought to the police station.

On examination he was a very drowsy man who appeared to be 'on the nod'. He was rouseable but rapidly slipped back into a stupor. The history was obtained with some difficulty. The man said that he had consumed approximately 20 Panadeine Forte tablets (each containing 30 mg of codeine and 500 mg of paracetamol (acetaminophen)) that morning together with 10 Valium tablets and 1 g of amphetamine intravenously. He also said that he had been taking heroin recently but he was unsure of when the last dose had been, but he thought it was the day before. He also said that when the police arrived that morning he swallowed four capsules of heroin in order to prevent the police from finding it. During his few lucid moments he said that he needed to eat and sleep as he had not slept for several days. A limited mental state examination was performed with some difficulty. This revealed the subject knew where he was and knew the month and the day of the week and the year. However, he was not able to answer more specific questions during the mental state examination.

Physical examination revealed a normal pulse and blood pressure. His pupils were not pinpoint. He was able to stand unsupported for a short period and his gait was extremely unsteady. The doctor assessed that he was severely impaired by the actions of various drugs and therefore unfit to be interviewed. He was taken by ambulance to a hospital.

*Discussion.* It was not safe for this man to remain in the police station because of his obviously intoxicated state and the possibility of further deterioration due to absorption of heroin. The lack of pinpoint pupils raised some doubt as to whether heroin or some other drug was responsible for his clinical state of intoxication. While drug ingestion histories are notoriously unreliable, in this case the possibility that 10 g of paracetamol (acetaminophen) had been taken also gave rise to concerns of potential developing hepatic toxicity.

## CASE REPORT 8.2 DRUG-AFFECTED DRIVING AND DOCTOR SHOPPING

Mr B was the driver of a car involved in a fatal collision. A blood sample taken at the hospital yielded the following results:

Amphetamine detected at a level of 0.05 mg/L.
Methylamphetamine detected at a level of 0.32 mg/L.

Pseudoephedrine detected.
Diazepam detected at a level of 2.07 mg/L.
Nordiazepam detected at a level of 2.36 mg/L.
Temazepam detected at a level of 0.60 mg/L.
Oxazepam detected at a level of 0.36 mg/L.
Nitrazepam detected at a level of less than 0.10 mg/L.
Morphine detected at a level of 0.02 mg/L.
Codeine detected at a level of 0.10 mg/L.

Mr B's medical and pharmaceutical history indicated that he was in the habit of visiting many doctors and received many prescriptions for psychoactive drugs in the period immediately prior to the accident.

*Descriptions of behaviour.* The only medical descriptions of Mr B's behaviour immediately after the crash were found in the notes from the hospital. At 2115 h (1 h following the collision) Dr M described him as 'drowsy' and having no memory of the accident. The doctor obtained a history of Mr B being on nitrazepam and the methadone maintenance programme as well as having obtained a prescription for 50 diazepam tablets 2 days previously, of which half were left in the pack. Dr C, a surgical registrar, described him at 2350 h as 'alert, orientated to time, place and person, appears compis mentis [sic]'. The emergency nursing notes described him as 'drowsy, orientated'. Mr B discharged himself against medical advice at 0315 h the next morning.

Sergeant T interviewed Mr B at 0200 h, nearly 6 h following the collision and described him as '... eyes were very droopy ... "far away stare" ... lapse into sleep and then recover within a second then lapse back into near sleep ... speech sometimes soft and slurred then he would give clear answers ...' While this is a good description of a person under the influence of a sedative drug, this must be considered in the setting of the time of the interview and recent stressful events.

*Analysis of blood and urine tests.* The urine drug screen taken from Mr B at 2310 h at the hospital revealed a very high level of benzodiazepines and a level of morphine so high as to overload the analysis instrument. There was also evidence of 6-AM and amphetamines. None of these drugs were given to Mr B in hospital or by the ambulance officers.

The blood sample taken from Mr B at the hospital contained several substances known to impair driving skills, either alone or in combination with other drugs. These include amphetamine and methamphetamine, which are not available as legal prescription items. Pseudoephedrine is a drug present in commercial over-the-counter cold and flu preparations, which is also used in the chemical synthesis of illegal amphetamines. Diazepam, nordiazepam, temazepam, oxazepam and nitrazepam are all benzodiazepine drugs or metabolic products of them and are consistent with consumption of the huge quantities of these drugs prescribed for Mr B by the various doctors he was visiting.

As part of his participation in the methadone programme, Mr B was required to submit random urine tests for drug screening. Although there was no urine test taken on the day of the crash, analysis of his medical records showed that every urine test within a few weeks of the crash showed 6-AM present as evidence of heroin consumption. The prescribing doctor did not seem to have taken any action on the basis of this information, and continued to prescribe methadone as well as large quantities of benzodiazepine drugs.

*Drug consumption.* In the 60 days prior to the collision, Mr B was issued with 22 prescriptions from several doctors. The majority of these prescriptions were for benzodiazepines, of which diazepam was the main drug. Assuming he took all the tablets, his average consumption of diazepam alone over the 60 days would have been 55 mg per day, equivalent to 11 tablets, each of 5 mg. This would have been in addition to several other benzodiazepines, as well as heroin and amphetamine.

It was obvious that Mr B was a severe chronic drug addict who was obtaining prescriptions for sedative drugs from several doctors as well as consuming illegal drugs such as heroin and amphetamines. 'Doctor-shopping' is a well-known and dangerous behaviour, and may be very easy under some primary care systems. It is usually difficult, if not impossible, for doctors to ascertain whether their patient has obtained prescriptions from other doctors. In addition, because doctor-shopping drug addicts rarely give accurate medical information to doctors, drugs may be prescribed inappropriately although with the best of intentions. The various medical notes contained many observations of Mr B being under the influence of drugs at the time he visited doctors as well as notes of occasions when he was refused prescriptions because of obvious intoxication and drug-seeking behaviour.

*Discussion.* Mr B had several drugs in his blood at the time of the collision, which were capable of causing impairment of driving skills. These included products of heroin metabolism as well as benzodiazepines and amphetamines. Hospital observations of him as being drowsy with no memory of the accident were consistent with the use of these drugs. The court accepted that his driving skills were adversely affected by the use of these drugs and he was convicted of culpable driving, an offence of equal significance to involuntary manslaughter.

## CASE REPORT 8.3 BENZODIAZEPINE OVERDOSE

A forensic opinion was sought regarding a 37-year-old female with a history of depression, multiple drug overdoses, and benzodiazepine dependency. She had attended several medical practitioners for prescriptions and developed negative relationships with several of them. She was on treatment consisting of nitrazepam and alprazolam tablets together with an antidepressant.

On the evening of 21 April she consumed 23 1-mg alprazolam tablets. Later she was picked up at 0400 h by a friend who described her as being very drowsy and sleeping for most of the day. In the evening she was described as '… very much under the influence of tranquillizers and staggering around the house …'

The following day she took a further overdose of multiple tablets as follows:

*0600*: Noted to be '… still very sedated …'
*0820*: Consumed eight nitrazepam tablets.

*0900*: Obtained 50 1-mg alprazolam tablets from a pharmacy. The pharmacist described her as '… in no way distressed …' and did not comment on drowsiness. She consumed 44 of these within 15 min.

*0930 (approximately)*: She engaged in sexual intercourse with a man in circumstances where her capacity to recollect the circumstances, give consent or resist was under question. She described feeling '… dopey and rather docile due to the tablets … in automatic mode'. He described her as driving and parking her car normally prior to the incident, verbalizing normally and without impairment of her co-ordination skills. He claims that she instigated sexual activity, actively enticed him to have sexual intercourse and that there was no evidence of passive resistance. Immediately after this she took a further eight alprazolam tablets.

*0953*: A policeman described her as having '… trouble keeping her eyes open … very groggy … speaking slowly and deliberately …' He supported her as she walked into the hospital and describes her as needing assistance to get into the bed.

*1000*: The woman was admitted to hospital and noted to be ' … ambulant, staggering with very slurred speech … needing support …' She was also described as '… vocal and agitated …' by the nurse in the A&E department, and was abusive to doctors.

*1115*: '… remained very drowsy … rouseable and responding to verbal stimuli …'

*1645*: Discharged herself from hospital. Described as '… ambulating slowly …'

*Discussion*. This woman tolerated significant overdoses of benzodiazepines and was still able to exhibit aggressive behaviour and be rouseable in the hours immediately after taking the overdose. She was able to discharge herself from hospital after 7 h. This indicated that she was tolerant of high doses, consistent with being addicted to benzodiazepines. A non-tolerant person consuming 40 mg of nitrazepam and 50 mg of alprazolam would be expected to be deeply unconscious or comatose for many hours.

Although the man described her as driving her car and parking normally before the incident, this would have been about 1 h after taking 40 mg of nitrazepam. The subject's ability to drive would be expected to have been severely impaired under these circumstances.

The drugs consumed by the subject immediately before having intercourse would not have reached their peak effect by 0930. Their blood levels would have been rising and her conscious state would have been deteriorating rapidly. It is very unlikely that she was fully conscious at the time of the incident. It is also possible however that she was disinhibited by the effects of the overdose and could have appeared transiently as the man described her. Her re-collection of events would be poor. She was considered to be incapable of being able to give valid consent for sexual intercourse thus satisfying one of the requirements for the charge of rape.

## CASE REPORT 8.4 METHADONE TOXICITY

An 18-year-old man died as a result of a suspected drug overdose. He was not subjected to full autopsy but an external inspection of the body resulted in the cause of death being given as 'unascertained'. Postmortem toxicology studies revealed the presence of methadone at a blood concentration of 0.3 mg/L, diazepam at ~0.1 mg/L and nordiazepam at ~0.2 mg/L. Other opioids were not detected and there was a qualitative positive result for cannabinoids in the urine.

The man had a past history of heroin use and attended Dr A on day one in order to commence a methadone programme. The following day he was prescribed his initial dose of 25 mg per day. Three days later, the man attended another doctor, Dr W, and stated that the current 25 mg dose was insufficient for him. Dr W increased the dose to 40 mg. The man attended a pharmacy later that day and took his first dose at the increased amount of 40 mg of methadone. He re-attended the next day (day 5) and took another dose of 40 mg. He was found dead on day 6 having not yet taken his dose for that day. The deceased was known to have a history of asthma, but was otherwise well.

Methadone is usually prescribed for heroin addicts at a starting dose between 20 and 40 mg. The dose may be increased gradually until the patient achieves a maintenance dose. Because levels may take up to a week to stabilize, increases of dosage in the first week of treatment must be made very carefully. In the context of this case, a starting dose of 25 mg with a subsequent increase to 40 mg would not be considered unusual. However, the timing of the increase may have been too soon. There is no clear correlation between blood levels and the effect of methadone as there is with other drugs.

The lack of detailed information in this case made it very difficult to give an opinion as to the dosage level of methadone and its possible involvement in causing death. However, there are some aspects of the methadone regimen that may have contributed to the man's death, especially an increase in dosage by 60% possibly before the initial dose level had time to reach equilibrium.

## CASE REPORT 8.5 ALCOHOL INTOXICATION

A forensic physician attending a police station was asked incidentally to 'take a quick look' at an unwell detainee. The 56-year-old man had been arrested 2 h previously for being 'drunk and disorderly'.

On examination an unkempt man was lying prone on the floor of the cell, snoring loudly with puddles of saliva around his mouth and urine around his groin. The hair on his head was matted with blood that appeared to be coming from a small laceration on his scalp. There was a strong smell of alcohol in the air. Attempts at rousing him were unsuccessful and he remained unconscious.

The man was taken to hospital urgently by ambulance, where his blood alcohol concentration was found to be 0.43% and a chest X-ray showed bronchopneumonia. He was admitted to the intensive care unit where he remained for 2 days and subsequently made an uneventful recovery. No evidence of closed head injury was found.

# References for Section 8

1. Carrigan TD, Field H, Illingworth RN, Gaffney P, Hamer DW. Toxicological screening in trauma. *J Accid Emerg Med* 2000; 17: 33–7.
2. McLay WDS, ed. *Clinical forensic medicine*, 2nd edn. London: Greenwich Medical Media; 1996.
3. Fenwick P. Automatism, Medicine and the Law. In: *Psychological medicine*. Cambridge University Press; 1990.
4. US National Highway and Traffic Safety Authority. *Horizontal gaze nystagmus – the science and the law*. US National Highway and Traffic Safety Authority; 1999.
5. Tharp V, Burns M, Moskowitz H. *Development and field test of psychophysical tests for DWI arrest*. US National Highway Safety Authority; 1981. Report no. DOT HS-805 864.
6. Kosnoski EM, Yolton RL, Citek K, Hayes CE, Evans RB. The Drug Evaluation Classification Program: using ocular and other signs to detect drug intoxication. *J Am Optom Assoc* 1998; 69(4): 211–27.
7. Davidson SE, Gossop M. The management of opioid addicts in police custody. *Med Sci Law* 1999; 39(2): 153–60.
8. Carter GL, Dawson AH, Lopert R. Drug induced delirium – incidence, management and prevention. *Drug Safety* 1996; 15(4): 291–301.
9. Gall JA, Freckleton I. Fitness for interview: current trends, views and an approach to the assessment procedure. *J Clin Forens Med* 1999; 6(4): 213–23.
10. Karch SB, Stephens BG. Drug abusers who die during arrest or custody. *J Royal Soc Med* 1999; 92: 110–13.
11. Odell MS. Drug-induced anisocoria in two detainees. *J Clin Forens Med* 1998; 5: 10–12.
12. Sachdev P. Attention deficit hyperactivity disorder in adults. *Psychol Med* 1999; 29: 507–14.
13. Arimany J, Medallo J, Pujol A, Vingut A, Borondo JC, Valverde JL. Intentional overdose and death with 3,4-methylenedioxyethamphetamine (MDEA; 'Eve'): case report. *Am J Forens Med Path* 1998; 19(2): 148–51.
14. Lan KC, Lin YF, Yu FC, Lin CS, Chu P. Clinical manifestations and prognostic features of acute methamphetamine intoxication. *J Formos Med Assoc* 1998; 97(8): 528–33.
15. O'Halloran RL, Frank JG. Asphyxial death during prone restraint revisited – a report of 21 cases. *Am J Forens Med Path* 2000; 21(1): 39–52.
16. Mirchandani HG, Rorke LB, Sekula-Perlman A, Hood IC. Cocaine induced agitated delirium, forceful struggle and minor head injury – a further definition of sudden death during restraint. *Am J Forens Med Path* 1994; 15(2): 95–9.
17. Farnham FR, Kennedy HG. Acute excited states and sudden death. *Br Med J* 1997; 315: 1107–8.

18. Mendelson JH, Mello NK. Management of cocaine abuse and dependence. *NEJM* 1996; 334(15): 965–72.
19. Woods JH, Winger G. Abuse liability of flunitrazepam. *J Clin Psychopharmacol* 1997; 17(3 suppl. 2): 1S–57S.
20. Rickert VI, Wiemann CM, Berenson AB. Flunitrazepam – more than a date rape drug. *J Pediatric Adolesc Gynecol* 2000; 13: 37–42.
21. Stark MM, Wells D. Drug-mediated sexual assault. *J Clin Forens Med* 1999; 6(1): 53–5.
22. McKay DR, Tennant CC. Is the grass greener? The link between cannabis and psychosis. *Med J Austr* 2000; 172: 284–6.
23. Hayden JA. Passive inhalation of marijuana smoke: a critical review. *J Subs Abuse* 1991; 3: 85–90.
24. Bussutil A, Obafunwa JO, Bulgin S. Passive inhalation of cannabis smoke: a novel defence strategy? *J Clin Forens Med* 1996; 3: 99–104.
25. Drummer OH. Drugs in drivers killed in Australian road traffic accidents. Melbourne: Department of Forensic Medicine, Monash University; March 1994. Report no. 0594.
26. Robbe HWJ. *Influence of marijuana on driving*. Maastricht, the Netherlands. CIP-Data Koninklinik Bibliothek, The Hague; 1994.
27. Huestis MA, Henningfield JE, Cone EJ. Blood cannabinoids. II. Models for the prediction of time of marijuana exposure from plasma concentrations of delta 9-tetrahydrocannabinol (THC) and 11-nor-9-carboxy-delta 9-tetrahydrocannabinol (THCCOOH). *J Anal Toxicol* 1992; 16(5): 283–90.
28. Davidson SE, Gossop M. The management of opioid addicts in police custody. *Med Sci Law* 1999; 39(2): 153–60.
29. Proceedings of Expert Workshop on the Induction and Stabilisation of Patients onto Methadone. Canberra: National Drug Strategy; 2000. Monograph Series no. 39.
30. McKnight AJ, Langston EA, Marques PR, Tippetts AS. Estimating blood alcohol level from observable signs. *Accid Anal Prev* 1997; 29(2): 247–55.
31. Milovanovic AV, DiMaio VJ. Death due to concussion and alcohol. *Am J Forens Med Path* 1999; 20(1): 6–9.
32. Odell MS, McDonald CF, Farrar J, Natsis JS, Pretto JF. Breath testing in patients with respiratory disability. *J Clin Forens Med* 1998; 5: 45–8.
33. Prater CD, Miller KE, Zylstra RG. Outpatient detoxification of the addicted or alcoholic patient. *Am Fam Physician* 1999; 60(4): 1175–83.
34. Holbrook AM, Crowther R, Lotter A, Cheng C, King D. Diagnosis and management of acute alcohol withdrawal. *CMAJ* 1999; 160(5): 675–80.
35. Winek CL, Wahba WW, Dowdell JL. Determination of absorption time of ethanol in social drinkers. *Forens Sci Internat* 1995; 77: 169–77.
36. Gullberg RG, Jones AW. Guidelines for estimating the amount of alcohol consumed from a single measurement of blood alcohol concentration: re-evaluation of Widmark's equation. *Forens Sci Internat* 1994; 69: 119–30.
37. Rockerbie DW, Rockerbie RA. Computer simulation analysis of blood alcohol. *J Clin Forens Med* 1995; 2: 137–41.

# Appendix

# Monographs of selected drugs

| | |
|---|---|
| **Explanations to monographs** | 368 |
| **Stimulants** | 369 |
| **Benzodiazepines** | 382 |
| **Other sedatives and anxiolytics** | 406 |
| **Opioids and related drugs** | 413 |
| **Other monographs** | 435 |
| **References for Appendix** | 442 |

# Explanations to monographs

| | |
|---|---|
| Class of drug | Pharmacological listing in prescriber information and pharmacopoeias and most common uses |
| Availability and proprietary or code names | Selected commercial names as registered by pharmaceutical company, and selected common street names |
| Properties | Common physical properties including: |
| | Chemical Abstracts Number (CAS) for base, unless otherwise indicated |
| | Molecular weight (MW) of free form |
| | Logarithm of acid equilibrium constant (pKa) |
| | Volume of distribution ($V_D$) |
| | Clearance (Cl) |
| | Logarithm of partition co-efficient of solubility in octanol to water, or phosphate buffer, pH 7 ($\log_P$) |
| | Degree of binding to blood plasma proteins (%) |
| | Bioavailability (%) |
| Blood half-life | Terminal elimination half-life, in hours |
| Effect of age and disease | Known effect on half-life and clearance as a result of age, liver and kidney disease, etc. |
| Metabolism | Type of biotransformation parent drug is likely to undergo |
| Metabolites | Products resulting from biotransformation of parent drug |
| Active metabolites | Metabolites whose activity is significant |
| Excretion | Type and amount of drug or metabolite excreted into urine |
| Common doses | Recommended or common doses, or common abused dose for illicit drugs |
| Blood concentrations | Blood concentrations following doses shown above, or following a defined listed dose |
| Postmortem artefacts | Any artefacts occurring after death that may affect accuracy of blood concentrations |
| Toxicity and abuse potential | Abuse potential, and minimum blood concentration capable of causing death in absence of other drugs, natural disease and injuries |
| Reviews and papers | Published review or key paper on drug providing more detailed account of pharmacokinetic or toxicological properties of drug |

# Stimulants

## AMPHETAMINE

| | |
|---|---|
| Class of drug and uses | Amphetamine prototype, stimulant and decongestant, used in narcolepsy, hyperkinetic disorders; an abused drug |
| Availability and proprietary or code names | Dexamphetamine, also known as desoxynorephedrine and dex-amphetamine, major metabolite of methamphetamine and ethylamphetamine, various names including Benzadrine, Dexedrine, Biphetamine, Durophet |
| Chemical form and solubility | Amphetamine sulphate, very soluble in water; also as phosphate salt, d-isomer active |

Properties

| | |
|---|---|
| CAS | 300-62-9 |
| MW | 135.2 |
| pKa | 9.9 |
| $V_D$ | 3–5 L/kg |
| Cl | |
| $Log_P$ | 1.8 |
| Protein binding | 15–42% |
| Bioavailability | High |

| | |
|---|---|
| Blood half-life (principle blood-borne species) | Amphetamine 4–30 h (pH dependent) |
| Effect of age and disease | Clearance is likely to decrease with age and liver or kidney disease; however mostly pH dependent |
| Metabolism | Deamination, oxidation, hydroxylation, conjugation |
| Metabolites | Norephedrine, hippuric acid; also a metabolite of anti-parkinson drug selegiline, clobenorex, amfetaminil, phenylamine, fenproporex, fenetylline, mefenorex, and benzphetamine |
| Active metabolites | Norephedrine and other hydroxylated metabolites |
| Excretion | Amphetamine 3–60% (pH dependent) |
| Common doses | Up to 40 mg daily for therapeutic use, up to 2 g when abused |
| Blood concentrations | Under 0.1 µg/mL after therapeutic use |
| Postmortem artefacts | Small postmortem artefactual changes |

| | |
|---|---|
| Toxicity and abuse potential | Moderate to high abuse potential, fatal concentration in peripheral blood probably >2 mg/L when used alone |
| Published papers | Rowland, 1969;[1] Angrist et al., 1987;[2] Smith-Kielland et al., 1997[3] |

# CATHINONE

| | |
|---|---|
| Class of drug and uses | Weak amphetamine-like stimulant |
| Availability and proprietary or code names | Main active alkaloid of khat (*Catha edulis*), grows in Arabian Peninsula and horn of Africa |
| Chemical form and solubility | Normally chewed from leaves, can be isolated and methylated to methcathinone |

Properties

| | |
|---|---|
| CAS | 492-39-7 |
| MW | 149.2 |
| pKa | 9.4 (cathine) |
| $V_D$ | Like amphetamine |
| Cl | |
| $Log_P$ | |
| Protein binding | |
| Bioavailability | Like amphetamine |

| | |
|---|---|
| Blood half-life (principle blood-borne species) | Cathinone 2–5 h |
| Effect of age and disease | Similar to ephedrines |
| Metabolism | Oxidation on keto to hydroxy metabolites |
| Metabolites | Norpseudoephedrine (cathine), norephedrine |
| Active metabolites | Activity mainly in pseudoephedrine/norephedrine |
| Excretion | 40% excreted unchanged, balance as above metabolites |
| Common doses | ~20–60 mg daily |
| Blood concentrations | Range up to 0.2 mg/L (acute doses) |
| Postmortem artefacts | Similar to ephedrines |
| Toxicity and abuse potential | Low to moderate abuse potential and toxicity |
| Published papers | Widler et al., 1994;[4] Mathys and Brenneisen, 1992;[5] Kalix et al., 1991[6] |

# DIETHYLPROPION (AMFEPRAMONE)

| | |
|---|---|
| Class of drug and uses | Weak stimulant used as an appetite suppressant |
| Availability and proprietary or code names | Tenuate, Tenuate Dospan, Tepanil, Prefamone, Regibon, Apisate, Aliped, Regenon, Anorex, Dobesin, Exipid, Keramin, Magrene, Tylinal |
| Chemical form and solubility | Hydrochloride salt soluble in water |
| Properties | |
| CAS | 90-84-6 |
| | 134-805 (HCl) |
| MW | 205.3 |
| pKa | |
| $V_D$ | |
| Cl | |
| Log$_P$ | |
| Protein binding | |
| Bioavailability | |
| Blood half-life (principle blood-borne species) | Diethylpropion ~2–8 h |
| Effect of age and disease | Likely to reduce with advanced age, and liver and kidney disease, and affected by urine pH |
| Metabolism | N-Dealkylation, reduction, deamination, N-hydroxylation conjugation |
| Metabolites | Various forms known |
| Active metabolites | Hydroxylated metabolites possibly active |
| Excretion | Diethylpropion 2% |
| | Nordiethylpropion 26% |
| | N,N-Diethylnorephedrine 16% |
| | N-Ethylnorephedrine 14% |
| | Norephedrine 26% |
| Common doses | To 75 mg daily |
| Blood concentrations | Diethylpropion levels range up to ~0.01 mg/L Main species nordiethylpropion and dinordiethylpropion (to 0.2 mg/L) |
| Postmortem artefacts | Not known |
| Toxicity and abuse potential | Low to moderate toxicity and abuse potential, fatal concentration in peripheral blood probably >5 mg/L when used alone |
| Published papers | Testa and Beckett, 1973;[7] Mihailova et al., 1974;[8] Wright et al., 1975[9] |

# EPHEDRINE

| | |
|---|---|
| Class of drug and uses | Nasal decongestant and bronchodilator, weak stimulant |
| Availability and proprietary or code names | Asmapax, Ephedrine, Franol and many others, extracted from *Ephedra* spp. |
| Chemical form and solubility | Usually as anhydrous substance, hydrochloride or sulphate salts, soluble in water |

**Properties**

| | |
|---|---|
| CAS | 299-42-3 |
| MW | 165.2 |
| pKa | 9.6 |
| $V_D$ | 2–4 L/kg |
| Cl | |
| $Log_P$ | 1.0 |
| Protein binding | |
| Bioavailability | Moderate |

| | |
|---|---|
| Blood half-life (principle blood-borne species) | Ephedrine 3–15 (6) h |
| Effect of age and disease | Likely to be affected by kidney disease, dependent on urinary pH |
| Metabolism | Demethylation, and oxidative deamination, conjugation |
| Metabolites | Norephedrine (phenylpropanolamine) |
| Active metabolites | Activity mainly in pseudoephedrine |
| Excretion | Pseudoephedrine ~55–80% <br> Norephedrine ~4–20% <br> Acid metabolites ~4–13% |
| Common doses | Up to 60 mg daily in divided doses |
| Blood concentrations | Range up to 0.2 mg/L |
| Postmortem artefacts | Small postmortem artefactual changes |
| Toxicity and abuse potential | Low abuse potential, low to medium toxicity, fatal concentration in peripheral blood probably >5 mg/L when used alone |
| Published papers | Roxanas and Spaulding, 1977;[10] Wilkinson and Beckett, 1968[11] |

# Stimulants

## FENFLURAMINE

| | |
|---|---|
| Class of drug and uses | Weak stimulant used as an appetite suppressant |
| Availability and proprietary or code names | Adifax, Ponderal, Pondimin, Ponderax Redux and others, also available as dexfenfluramine; street name 'fen', combined with phentermine and known as 'fen-phen' |
| Chemical form and solubility | Hydrochloride salt soluble in water |

Properties

| | |
|---|---|
| CAS | 458-24-2 |
| MW | 231.3 |
| pKa | 9.1 |
| $V_D$ | 12–16 L/kg |
| Cl | |
| Log$_P$ | |
| Protein binding | ~30% |
| Bioavailability | 68% |

| | | |
|---|---|---|
| Blood half-life (principle blood-borne species) | Fenfluramine | 11–30 h |
| | Norfenfluramine | ~32 h |
| Effect of age and disease | Likely to reduce with advanced age, and liver and kidney disease, excretion dependent on urinary pH | |
| Metabolism | De-ethylation and oxidation with conjugation | |
| Metabolites | Norfenfluramine, carboxylic acid conjugates | |
| Active metabolite | Norfenfluramine | |
| Excretion | Fenfluramine | 7–23% |
| | Norfenfluramine | 3–19% |
| Common doses | Up to 160 mg daily | |
| Blood concentrations | Range up to ~0.3 mg/L | |
| Postmortem artefacts | Not known | |
| Toxicity and abuse potential | Low to medium toxicity, weak abuse potential, fatal concentration in peripheral blood probably >5 mg/L when used alone | |
| Published papers | Campbell, 1970;[12] Fleisher and Campbell, 1969;[13] Mark et al., 1997[14] | |

---

## METHYLENEDIOXYMETHAMPHETAMINE (MDMA)

| | |
|---|---|
| Class of drug and uses | Designer amphetamine and powerful stimulant and hallucinogen, no significant medical uses |
| Availability and proprietary or code names | Adam, ecstasy, E, M&M, MDM, XTC |
| Chemical form and solubility | Soluble in water, also available as hydrochloride salt |

## Monographs of selected drugs

Properties

| | |
|---|---|
| CAS | 42542-10-9 |
| MW | 193.2 |
| pKa | |
| $V_D$ | |
| Cl | |
| Log$_P$ | |
| Protein binding | |
| Bioavailability | |
| Blood half-life (principle blood-borne species) | MDMA 8 h |
| Effect of age and disease | Likely to reduce with advanced age, and liver and kidney disease |
| Metabolism | Demethylation, ring opening and conjugation |
| Metabolites | MDA* and hydroxy conjugates |
| Active metabolites | MDA* also a powerful stimulant |
| Excretion | MDMA 65% |
| | MDA* 7% |
| Abused doses | Often 100–150 mg |
| Blood concentrations | Range up to ~0.3 mg/L |
| Postmortem artefacts | Small postmortem artefactual changes |
| Toxicity and abuse potential | Highly toxic and high abuse potential, fatal concentration in peripheral blood probably >0.1 mg/L when used alone |
| Published papers | Cook et al., 1993;[15] Maurer 1996[16] |

* Methylenedioxyamphetamine; see monograph for MDA.

## METHYLENEDIOXYAMPHETAMINE (MDA)

| | |
|---|---|
| Class of drug and uses | Designer amphetamine and powerful stimulant and hallucinogen, no significant medical uses |
| Availability and proprietary or code names | MDA, love pill, speed |
| Chemical form and solubility | Soluble in water, also available as hydrochloride salt |

# Stimulants

Properties

| | |
|---|---|
| CAS | 4764-17-4 |
| MW | 179.2 |
| pKa | ~10 |
| $V_D$ | L/kg |
| Cl | mL/min/kg |
| Log$_P$ | |
| Protein binding | |
| Bioavailability | |

| | |
|---|---|
| Blood half-life (principle blood-borne species) | MDA 3–8 h |
| Effect of age and disease | Likely to reduce with advanced age, and liver and kidney disease, and affected by urine pH |
| Metabolism | Ring fission, conjugation and deamination likely |
| Metabolites | Conjugated 3,4-dihydroxy metabolites likely |
| Active metabolites | Unknown but possible |
| Excretion | Largely as unchanged drug |
| Abused doses | Common doses 50–250 mg |
| Blood concentrations | Range up to ~0.4 mg/L |
| Postmortem artefacts | Small postmortem artefactual changes |
| Toxicity and abuse potential | Highly toxic with high abuse potential, usually as metabolite of MDMA, no minimum fatal concentration assignable |
| Published papers | Kunsman et al., 1996;[17] Maurer 1996[16] |

## METHAMPHETAMINE

| | |
|---|---|
| Class of drug and uses | Amphetamine and strong stimulant, limited medical uses |
| Availability and proprietary or code names | Also known as methylamphetamine, desoxyephedrine; available as Desoxyn, Fefamine and others; street names speed, crystal, crank, go, ice |
| Chemical form and solubility | Available as hydrochloride salt, soluble in water, d-isomer active |

## Properties

| | |
|---|---|
| CAS | 537-46-2 |
| MW | 149.2 |
| pKa | 10 |
| $V_D$ | 3–4 L/kg |
| Cl | |
| $Log_P$ | |
| Protein binding | Low |
| Bioavailability | High |

| | | |
|---|---|---|
| Blood half-life (principle blood-borne species) | Methamphetamine | 10–30 h |
| | Amphetamine | 4–15 h |
| Effect of age and disease | Likely to reduce with advanced age, and liver and kidney disease, and affected by urine pH | |
| Metabolism | Demethylation and hydroxylation | |
| Metabolites | Amphetamine, p-hydroxymethamphetamine; also a metabolite of anti-parkinson drug selegiline, benzphetamine, and other stimulants | |
| Active metabolites | Amphetamine | |
| Excretion | Methamphetamine | 40–45% |
| | Amphetamine | 4–7% |
| | p-Hydroxymethamphetamine | 15% |
| Abused doses | Range up to 2000 mg | |
| Blood concentrations | Range up to ~0.1 mg/L | |
| Postmortem artefacts | Small postmortem artefactual changes | |
| Toxicity and abuse potential | Moderate to high toxicity and abuse potential, fatal concentration in peripheral blood probably up to 0.1 mg/L when used alone | |
| Published papers | Valentine et al., 1995;[18] Cook et al., 1993;[15] Smith-Kielland et al., 1997[3] | |

## METHYLPHENIDATE

| | |
|---|---|
| Class of drug and uses | Medium-strong stimulant, used in attention deficit syndrome, narcolepsy and depression |
| Availability and proprietary or code names | Ritalin 2–20 mg tablets |
| Chemical form and solubility | Available as hydrochloride salt, soluble in water |

## Stimulants

| Properties | | |
|---|---|---|
| CAS | 113-45-1 | |
| MW | 233.3 | |
| pKa | 8.8 | |
| $V_D$ | 11–33 L/kg | |
| Cl | 90 mL/min/kg | |
| Log$_P$ | | |
| Protein binding | 15% | |
| Bioavailability | | |

| | | |
|---|---|---|
| Blood half-life (principle blood-borne species) | Methylphenidate | 2–4 h |
| Effect of age and disease | Likely to reduce with advanced age, and liver and kidney disease, and affected by urine pH | |
| Metabolism | De-esterification and oxidation | |
| Metabolites | Ritalinic acid, p-hydroxymethylphenidate and 6-oxoritalinic acid | |
| Active metabolites | p-Hydroxymethylphenidate | |
| Excretion | Methylphenidate | <1% |
| | Ritalinic acid | 60–80% |
| | 6-Oxoritalinic acid | 5–12% |
| Prescribed doses | Up to 60 mg daily | |
| Blood concentrations | 20 mg dose produces $T_{max}$ of 0.01–0.06 ng/mL | |
| Postmortem artefacts | Not known | |
| Toxicity and abuse potential | Low to moderate toxicity and abuse potential, fatal concentration in peripheral blood probably >3 mg/L when used alone | |
| Published papers | Hungrund et al., 1979;[19] Levine et al., 1986[20] | |

## PARA-METHOXYAMPHETAMINE (PMA)

| | |
|---|---|
| Class of drug and uses | Designer amphetamine and powerful stimulant and hallucinogen, no medical uses |
| Availability and proprietary or code names | Ecstasy in Australia |
| Chemical form and solubility | Available as hydrochloride salt, soluble in water |

Properties

| | |
|---|---|
| CAS | 23239-32-9 |
| MW | 165.2 |
| pKa | |
| $V_D$ | Moderate |
| Cl | |
| $Log_P$ | |
| Protein binding | |
| Bioavailability | Moderate |
| Blood half-life (principle blood-borne species) | |
| PMA | Unknown |
| Effect of age and disease | Likely to reduce with advanced age, and liver and kidney disease, and affected by urine pH |
| Metabolism | O-Demethylation and hydroxylation, conjugation |
| Metabolites | p-Hydroxyamphetamine and p-hydroxynorephedrine |
| Active metabolites | Unknown but hydroxy metabolites may contribute |
| Excretion | p-Methoxyamphetamine 15% |
| | p-Hydroxyamphetamine 28% (free and conjugates) |
| | p-Hydroxynorephedrine 4% |
| Abused doses | Usual doses 50–100 mg |
| Blood concentrations | Range up to ~0.2 mg/L |
| Postmortem artefacts | Unknown |
| Toxicity and abuse potential | Highly toxic and high abuse potential, fatal concentration in peripheral blood probably up to 0.2 mg/L when used alone |
| Published paper | Felgate et al., 1998;[21] Byard et al., 1998[22] |

## PHENTERMINE

| | |
|---|---|
| Class of drug and uses | Weak stimulant used as an appetite suppressant |
| Availability and proprietary or code names | Adipex-P, Dapex, Duromine, Fastin, Ionamin, Linyl, Lipopill, Minobea Forte, Mirapront, Obe-nix, Obephen, Obermine, Obestin, Parmine, Phentrol, Tora, Unifast, Wilpowr, and others; Street name 'phen' and as 'fen-phen' with fenfluramine |

# Stimulants

| | |
|---|---|
| Chemical form and solubility | Available as hydrochloride salt, which is soluble in water, and as an ion-exchange resin complex to delay and sustain release |

Properties

| | |
|---|---|
| CAS | 122-09-8 |
| MW | 149.2 |
| pKa | 10.1 |
| $V_D$ | 3–4 L/kg |
| Cl | |
| Log$_P$ | |
| Protein binding | |
| Bioavailability | Moderate |
| Blood half-life (principle blood-borne species) | Phentermine 7–24 h |
| Effect of age and disease | Likely to reduce with advanced age, and liver and kidney disease, and affected by urine pH |
| Metabolism | Hydroxylation and oxidation with conjugation |
| Metabolites | N- and p-Hydroxyphentermine |
| Active metabolites | Hydroxylated metabolites possibly active |
| Excretion | Phentermine Up to 90% |
| | N-Hydroxyphentermine ~5% |
| | p-Hydroxyphentermine <1% |
| Common doses | 15–40 mg daily |
| Blood concentrations | Range up to ~0.3 mg/L |
| | 30 mg chronic dosing produces blood levels of 0.08–0.14 µg/mL |
| Postmortem artefacts | Not known |
| Toxicity and abuse potential | Low to moderate toxicity and abuse potential, fatal concentration in peripheral blood probably >5 mg/L when used alone |
| Published papers | Groenewoud et al., 1993;[23] Hinsvark et al., 1973[24] |

## PSEUDOEPHEDRINE

| | |
|---|---|
| Class of drug and uses | Nasal decongestant and bronchodilator, weak stimulant |
| Availability and proprietary or code names | Sudafed and numerous other formulations often in combination with analgesics and anti-histamines |
| Chemical form and solubility | Usually as hydrochloride or sulphate salts, soluble in water |

379

## Monographs of selected drugs

Properties

| | |
|---|---|
| CAS | 90-82-4 |
| MW | 165.2 |
| pKa | 9.7–9.8 |
| V_D | 2–4 L/kg |
| Cl | |
| Log_P | 1.0 |
| Protein binding | |
| Bioavailability | Moderate |

| | |
|---|---|
| Blood half-life (principle blood-borne species) | Pseudoephedrine 3–16 h |
| Effect of age and disease | Likely to be affected by kidney disease, dependent on urinary pH |
| Metabolism | Demethylation |
| Metabolites | Norpseudoephedrine |
| Active metabolites | Activity mainly in pseudoephedrine |
| Excretion | Pseudoephedrine ~90%<br>Norpseudoephedrine ~1% |
| Common doses | Up to 240 mg daily in divided doses |
| Blood concentrations | Range up to 1 mg/L |
| Postmortem artefacts | Small postmortem artefactual changes |
| Toxicity and abuse potential | Low abuse potential, low toxicity, fatal concentration in peripheral blood probably >19 mg/L when used alone |
| Published papers | Kuntzman et al., 1971;[25] Lin et al., 1977[26] |

## COCAINE

| | |
|---|---|
| Class of drug and uses | Powerful stimulant and local anaesthetic, minor medical uses as topical anaesthetic in ophthalmological and otolarynological procedures (50 or 100 mg/mL) |
| Availability and proprietary or code names | Known as coke, snow, gold dust, lady, crack (freebase) |
| Chemical form and solubility | Usually as hydrochloride salt or free base, soluble in water |

Properties

| | |
|---|---|
| CAS | 50-36-2 |
| MW | 303.4 |
| pKa | 8.6 |
| $V_D$ | 1–3 L/kg |
| Cl | 10–30 mL/min/kg |
| Log$_P$ | |
| Protein binding | |
| Bioavailability | Low |
| Blood half-life (principle blood-borne species) | Cocaine 40 min to 2 h (dose-dependent) |
| Effect of age and disease | Unlikely to be significantly affected |
| Metabolism | Hydrolysis and conjugation |
| Metabolites | Benzoylecgonine, ecgonine methyl ester, ecgonine; cocaethylene produced when alcohol is co-consumed; anhydroecgonine methyl ester is produced when smoked |
| Active metabolites | Cocaethylene |
| Excretion | Mainly as benzoylecgonine and ecgonine methyl ester |
| Common doses | 10–100 mg |
| Blood concentrations | Range up to 0.5 mg/L |
| Postmortem artefacts | Small postmortem artefactual changes |
| Toxicity and abuse potential | High abuse potential, highly toxic, all concentrations potentially fatal in right circumstance if abused |
| Published papers | Barnett et al., 1981;[27] Cone 1995;[28] Wilkinson et al., 1980;[29] Isenchmid et al., 1992[30] |

# Benzodiazepines

## ADINAZOLAM

| | |
|---|---|
| Class of drug and uses | Sedative and hypnotic, used to treat depression |
| Availability and proprietary or code names | Deracyn etc. |
| Chemical form and solubility | |
| Properties | |
| CAS | 37115-32-5 |
| MW | 351.8 |
| pKa | |
| Cl | 4.3 mL/min/kg (parent) |
| | 0.8 mL/min/kg (metabolite) |
| $V_D$ | 2.2 L/kg (parent) |
| | 0.8 L/kg (metabolite) |
| Log$_P$ | |
| Protein binding | |
| Bioavailability | 40% |
| Blood half-life (principle blood-borne species) | Adinazolam 1–3 h |
| | Desmethyl adinazolam 2–4 h |
| Effect of age and disease | Half-life increased with age by ~40% |
| Metabolism | N-Demethylation |
| Metabolites | N-Desmethyl adinazolam |
| Active metabolites | N-Desmethyl adinazolam |
| Urinary excretion | N-Desmethyl adinazolam 50% |
| Common doses | 15–60 mg in divided doses |
| Blood concentrations | 10 mg s.d. produces peak levels of adinazolam and desmethyl metabolite of 0.063 and 0.10 mg/L at 0.6 and 0.9 h, respectively |
| | 50 mg s.d. produces peak levels of adinazolam and desmethyl metabolite of 0.363 and 0.46 mg/L at 0.4 and 0.8 h, respectively |
| Postmortem artefacts | Not known |
| Toxicity | Not known |
| Published reviews and papers | Fleishaker et al., 1990;[31] 1992;[32] 1991[33] |

# ALPRAZOLAM

| | |
|---|---|
| Class of drug and uses | Short-acting minor tranquillizer, anxiety, panic disorder, antidepressant |
| Availability and proprietary or code names | Alplax, Constan, Dominium, Frontal, Kalma, Ralozam, Solanax, Tafil, Trankimazin, Valeans, Xanax, Xanor, Zotran, etc. |
| Chemical form and solubility | Free form, soluble in ethanol, insoluble in water |

Properties

| | |
|---|---|
| CAS | 28981-97-7 |
| MW | 308.8 |
| pKa | 2.4 |
| $V_D$ | 0.7–1.3 L/kg |
| Cl | 1.2 mL/min/kg |
| $Log_P$ | 1.3 |
| Protein binding | 67–83% |
| Bioavailability | 90% |

| | | |
|---|---|---|
| Blood half-life (principle blood-borne species) | Alprazolam | 13 (6–22) h |
| | α-Hydroxy alprazolam | 1–2 h |
| Effect of age and disease | Elimination decreased with age | |
| Metabolism | α-Hydroxylation, conjugation with glucuronic acid | |
| Metabolites | α-Hydroxy and 4-hydroxy alprazolam | |
| Active metabolites | Minor contribution by α-hydroxy and 4-hydroxy alprazolam | |
| Urinary excretion | Alprazolam (12–20%), 5-chlorobenzophenone (17%), α-hydroxy alprazolam (15–17%), 4-hydroxy alprazolam (0.3%) as conjugates | |
| Common doses | 0.5–4 mg per day, once or in divided doses up to 10 mg for depression and panic disorders | |
| Blood concentrations | 1 mg s.d. 0.021 (0.015–0.032) mg/L at 1.5 h Steady-state levels after 3 mg chronic 0.03 mg/L, 6 mg 0.06 mg/L and 9 mg 0.10 mg/L | |
| Postmortem artefacts | Not significantly elevated in heart and femoral blood | |
| Toxicity | Toxic > 0.1 mg/L | |
| Published reviews and papers | Greenblatt and Wright, 1993;[34] Garzone and Kroboth, 1989[35] | |

# BROMAZEPAM

| | |
|---|---|
| Class of drug and uses | Short-acting minor tranquillizer used in anxiety, and as a muscle relaxant |
| Availability and proprietary or code names | Akamon, Bromiden, Bropax, Brozam, Lexotan, Lectopam, etc. |
| Chemical form and solubility | Free form, soluble in ethanol, sparingly soluble in water |

Properties

| | |
|---|---|
| CAS | 1812-30-2 |
| MW | 316.2 |
| pKa | 2.9, 11.0 |
| $V_D$ | 0.9 L/kg |
| Cl | |
| $Log_P$ | 1.6 |
| Protein binding | 70% |
| Bioavailability | |

| | |
|---|---|
| Blood half-life (principle blood-borne species) | Bromazepam  8–19 (mean 12) h |
| Effect of age and disease | Age reduces clearance |
| Metabolism | Hydroxylation, conjugation with glucuronic acid |
| Metabolites | 3-Hydroxy bromazepam and glucuronide Benzophenone (ABBP) and glucuronide |
| Active metabolites | Parent drug, possibly also 3-hydroxy metabolite |
| Urinary excretion | Bromazepam 2% |
| | Benzophenone 0.4% |
| | 3-Hydroxy glucuronide 27% |
| | Hydroxylated conjugated benzophenone 40% |
| Common doses | 10–30 mg in divided doses, up to a maximum of 60 mg |
| Blood concentrations | 12 mg s.d. p.o. peak levels 0.11–0.17 (mean 0.13) mg/L at 1–4 h |
| | 9 mg chronic, steady state levels averaged 0.12 mg/L (range 0.08–0.15) |
| Postmortem artefacts | Unknown |
| Toxicity | Toxic > 5 mg/L |
| Published review | Greenblatt, 1991;[36] Baselt and Cravey, 1990[37] |

## BROTIZOLAM

| | |
|---|---|
| Class of drug and uses | Short-acting potent hypnotic with anticonvulsant, muscle relaxant and antianxiety activity of thienotriazolodiazepine class |
| Availability and proprietary or code names | |
| Chemical form and solubility | Free form, probably soluble in ethanol and sparingly soluble in water |

Properties

| | |
|---|---|
| CAS | 57801-81-7 |
| MW | 393.7 |
| pKa | |
| $V_D$ | 0.66 L/kg |
| Cl | 7.8–15 L/h |
| $Log_P$ | |
| Protein binding | 89–95% |
| Bioavailability | 70% |

| | |
|---|---|
| Blood half-life (principle blood-borne species) | Brotizolam    4–10 (mean 5) h |
| Effect of age and disease | 1. Half-life doubled in the elderly |
| | 2. Half-life doubled in liver cirrhosis and increased volume of distribution, protein binding lowered significantly |
| | 3. No substantial effect by renal failure |
| Metabolism | Hydroxylation and conjugation with glucuronic acid |
| Metabolites | α-Hydroxy brotizolam |
| | 4-Hydroxy brotizolam |
| | α,4-Dihydroxy brotizolam |
| Active metabolites | Some activity of hydroxylated metabolites but rapidly inactivated by conjugation |
| Urinary excretion | Brotizolam    <1% |
| | α-Hydroxy brotizolam   Major metabolite |
| Common doses | 0.125–0.5 mg as hypnotic |
| Blood concentrations | 0.25 mg s.d. produced a peak concentration of 4.3 ng/mL at 1.2 h |
| Postmortem artefacts | Unknown |
| Toxicity | No cases reported |
| Published review | Langley et al., 1988[38] |

# CHLORDIAZEPOXIDE

| | |
|---|---|
| Class of drug and uses | Long-acting minor tranquilliser, also used in treating alcohol withdrawal |
| Availability and proprietary or code names | Calmoden, Librium, Libritabs, Risolid, Librax (with clidinium), Limitol (with amitriptyline), etc. |
| Chemical form and solubility | Free form and hydrochloride<br>Free form soluble in ethanol, insoluble in water<br>HCl is soluble in water and ethanol |

Properties

| | | |
|---|---|---|
| CAS | 58-25-3 | |
| | 438-41-5 (HCl) | |
| MW | 299.8 | |
| | 336.2 (HCl) | |
| pKa | 4.6–4.8 | |
| $V_D$ | 0.3–0.4 L/kg | |
| Cl | 0.2–0.5 mL/min/kg | |
| $Log_P$ | 2.5 | |
| Protein binding | 90–97% | |
| Bioavailability | ~100% | |

| | |
|---|---|
| Blood half-life (principle blood-borne species) | Chlordiazepoxide 12 (5–30) h<br>Nordazepam 30–100 h |
| Effect of age and disease | 1. Elimination decreased with advanced age<br>2. Liver cirrhosis significantly reduces clearance and increases half-life |
| Metabolism | N-Demethylation, deamination, hydroxylation with conjugation |
| Metabolites | Desmethyl chlordiazepoxide, medazepam, nordazepam, oxazepam |
| Active metabolites | Desmethyl chlordiazepoxide, medazepam, nordazepam, oxazepam |
| Urinary excretion | Chlordiazepoxide <1%<br>Demoxazepam 6%<br>Oxazepam glucuronide majority |
| Common doses | Up to 100 mg daily orally, although 300 mg may be given in alcohol withdrawal |

| | |
|---|---|
| Blood concentrations | 25 mg s.d. peak levels 0.86 (0.48–1.2) mg/L at 0.5–2 h |
| | 55 mg chronic dosing produces steady-state levels of 2.3, 1.4 and 0.7 mg/L of parent drug, desmethyl metabolite and nordazepam, respectively |
| Postmortem artefacts | Not significantly elevated in heart and femoral blood, chemically unstable and likely to degrade |
| Toxicity | Toxic > 26 mg/L |
| Published reviews and papers | Greenblatt et al., 1978[39] |

## CLOBAZAM

| | |
|---|---|
| Class of drug and uses | Long-acting sedative, anxiety, panic attacks, anti-convulsant |
| Availability and proprietary or code names | Clarmyl, Clopax, Frisium, Noifren, Sederlona, Urbadan, Urbanol, Urbanyl, etc. |
| Chemical form and solubility | Free form, soluble in ethanol, insoluble in water |

Properties
| | |
|---|---|
| CAS | 22316-47-8 |
| MW | 300.7 |
| pKa | |
| $V_D$ | 0.9–1.8 L/kg |
| Cl | 0.5 mL/min/kg |
| $Log_P$ | 0.9 |
| Protein binding | 85–90% |
| Bioavailability | |

| | |
|---|---|
| Blood half-life (principle blood-borne species) | Clobazam 25 (10–49) h |
| | Desmethyl clobazam 2–3 days |
| Effect of age and disease | Elimination decreased with advanced age |
| Metabolism | Hydroxylation and dealkylation |
| Metabolites | 4'-Hydroxy clobazam |
| | N-Desmethyl clobazam (norclobazam) |
| | 4'-Hydroxy desmethyl clobazam |
| Active metabolites | Parent drug and desmethyl clobazam |
| Urinary excretion | No data |
| Common doses | 10–60 mg per day, single or divided doses |

| | |
|---|---|
| Plasma concentrations | 20 mg s.d. peak levels clobazam 0.22–0.71 (mean 0.46) mg/L at 1.7 h, norclobazam 0.06–0.15 (mean 0.09) mg/L at 45 h<br>40 mg s.d. mean peak level clobazam 0.73 mg/L<br>Steady-state levels on 20 mg daily are 0.33 mg/L for clobazam and 2.8 mg/L for norclobazam |
| Postmortem artefacts | Unknown |
| Toxicity | No deaths reported from use alone |
| Published review | Brogden et al., 1980[40] |

## CLONAZEPAM

| | |
|---|---|
| Class of drug and uses | Potent long-acting anticonvulsant with uses in some neurological movement disorders, and in acute mania, schizophrenic/schizoaffective disorders, and panic attacks and other disorders |
| Availability and proprietary or code names | Clonazil, Clonopin, Epilax, Iktorivil, Klonopin, Paxam, Rivotril, etc. |
| Chemical form and solubility | Free form, slightly soluble in ethanol, sparingly soluble in water |

Properties
| | |
|---|---|
| CAS | 1622-61-3 |
| MW | 315.7 |
| pKa | 1.5, 10.5 |
| $V_D$ | 2–4 L/kg |
| Cl | 1.4 mL/min |
| $Log_P$ | 2.4 |
| Protein binding | 47–85% |
| Bioavailability | 80% |

| | |
|---|---|
| Blood half-life (principle blood-borne species) | Clonazepam 20–80 h |
| Effect of age and disease | Probably similar to flunitrazepam and nitrazepam |
| Metabolism | Reduction, acetylation, hydroxylation and conjugation |
| Metabolites | 7-Amino clonazepam, 7-acetamido clonazepam, 3-hydroxy clonazepam plus conjugates |

| | |
|---|---|
| Active metabolites | Parent drug only active |
| Urinary excretion | Clonazepam 0.5% |
| | 7-Amino clonazepam Major |
| | 7-Acetamido clonazepam Major |
| | 3-Hydroxy clonazepam |
| Common doses | Up to 1–8 mg in divided doses |
| Blood concentrations | 2 mg s.d. maximum levels 0.007–0.024 mg/L at 1–4 h |
| | 6 mg chronic steady-state levels 0.03–0.08 mg/L for clonazepam and 0.02–0.14 mg/L for 7-amino metabolite |
| Postmortem artefacts | Not significantly elevated in heart and femoral blood but must measure 7-amino clonazepam since almost all converted to this form after death |
| Toxicity | No deaths reported with drug alone |
| Published reviews and papers | Greenblatt, 1987;[41] De Vane et al., 1991;[42] Hvidberg and Dam, 1991[43] |

## CLORAZEPATE

| | |
|---|---|
| Class of drug and uses | Long-acting minor tranquilliser related to diazepam |
| Availability and proprietary or code names | Azene, Moderane, Noctran, Tranex, Transene, Tranxene, etc. |
| Chemical form and solubility | As di-potassium salt |

Properties

| | |
|---|---|
| CAS | 23887-31-2 |
| | 57109-90-7 (diK) |
| | 5991-71-9 (K) |
| MW | 314.7 |
| pKa | 3.5, 12.5 |
| $V_D$ | 0.5–2.5 L/kg |
| $Log_P$ | |
| Protein binding | 97% |
| Bioavailability | |

| | |
|---|---|
| Blood half-life (principle blood-borne species) | Clorazepate 2 h |
| | Nordazepam 30–100 h |
| Effect of age and disease | Elimination decreased |

| | |
|---|---|
| Metabolism | Decarboxylation, oxidation, hydroxylation and conjugation |
| Metabolites | Nordazepam, oxazepam glucuronide |
| Active metabolites | Nordazepam |
| Urinary excretion | Clorazepate 2–6% |
| | Nordazepam 1% |
| | Oxazepam glucuronide Balance |
| Common doses | Daily doses up to 60 mg |
| Blood concentrations | 15 mg s.d. peak levels of nordazepam 0.16 mg/L at 2 h |
| | 22.5 mg chronic dosing gives steady-state levels of nordazepam of 0.6 mg/L |
| | 50 mg chronic dosing gives levels of 1.6 (range 1.2–2.6) mg/L |
| Postmortem artefacts | Likely to be similar to diazepam/nordazepam |
| Toxicity | Likely to be similar to diazepam/nordazepam |
| Published review | United Nations, 1997;[44] |
| | Baselt and Cravey, 1990[37] |

## DIAZEPAM

| | |
|---|---|
| Class of drug and uses | Minor tranquillizer, sedative, hypnotic, anticonvulsant, panic attacks and muscle relaxant |
| Availability and proprietary or code names | Antenex, Dizac, Diazemuls, Ducene, Pro-Pam, Stesolid, Valium, Valrelease, Zetran, etc. |
| Chemical form and solubility | Free form, sparingly soluble in ethanol, chloroform, ether, insoluble water |

Properties

| | |
|---|---|
| CAS | 439-14-5 |
| MW | 284.7 |
| pKa | 3.3–3.4 |
| $V_D$ | 0.5–2.6 L/kg |
| Cl | 0.5 mL/min/kg |
| $Log_P$ | 2.7 |
| Protein binding | 98–99% |
| Bioavailability | 100% |

Blood half-life (principle blood-borne species)

| | |
|---|---|
| Diazepam | 30 (20–50) h |
| Nordiazepam | 50 (40–99) h |

| | |
|---|---|
| Effect of age and disease | Elimination decreased with age and protein binding and volume of distribution increases with age |
| Metabolism | N-Demethylation, 3-hydroxylation, conjugation with glucuronic acid |
| Metabolites | Nordiazepam (desmethyl diazepam, nordazepam), oxazepam, temazepam, and glucuronides of oxazepam and temazepam |
| Active metabolites | All non-conjuguated metabolites |
| Urinary excretion | Diazepam   Trace<br>Nordiazepam   Trace<br>Oxazepam   ~33% (as conjugate)<br>Temazepam   As conjugate |
| Common doses | 5–40 mg per day, once or in divided doses |
| Blood concentrations | 10 mg s.d. 0.2–0.6 mg/L at 0.5–2 h<br>30 mg chronic steady-state levels of diazepam 0.7–1.5 mg/L; nordiazepam 0.35–0.53 mg/L |
| Postmortem artefacts | Not significantly elevated in heart and femoral blood |
| Toxicity | Toxic > 5 mg/L |
| Published reviews and papers | Kaplan et al., 1973;[45] Mandelli et al., 1978[46] |

## ESTAZOLAM

| | |
|---|---|
| Class of drug and uses | Short-acting hypnotic |
| Availability and proprietary or code names | Esilagan, Urodin, Nuctalon, ProSom, etc. |
| Chemical form and solubility | Free form |
| Properties | |
| CAS | 29975-16-4 |
| MW | 294.7 |
| pKa | |
| $V_D$ | |
| Log$_P$ | |
| | 93% |
| Blood half-life (principle blood-borne species) | Estazolam   8–24 h |
| Effect of age and disease | Clearance reduced in elderly |
| Metabolism | Hydroxylation |

| | |
|---|---|
| Metabolites | 4-Hydroxy estazolam |
| | 1-Oxo estazolam |
| Active metabolites | Parent drug only |
| Urinary excretion | Trace parent |
| Common doses | 1–4 mg per day |
| Blood concentrations | 1 mg s.d. peak plasma level 0.04–0.07 (mean 0.05) mg/L by 2 h |
| | 2 mg s.d. peak plasma level 0.075–0.14 (mean 0.1 mg/L) |
| Postmortem artefacts | Not known |
| Toxicity | No data |
| Published reference | United Nations booklet, 1997[44] |

## ETIZOLAM

| | |
|---|---|
| Class of drug and uses | Anxiolytic used in panic attacks and as an anti-convulsant and muscle relaxant |
| Availability and proprietary or code names | Depas, Pasaden, Y-7131 |
| Chemical form and solubility | Possibly free form, soluble in alcohol |

Properties

| | | |
|---|---|---|
| CAS | 40054-69-1 | |
| MW | 342.9 | |
| pKa | | |
| $V_D$ | ~1.0 L/kg | |
| Cl | 3.1 mL/min/kg | |
| Log$_P$ | | |
| Protein binding | | |

| | | |
|---|---|---|
| Blood half-life (principle blood-borne species) | Etizolam | 3 h |
| | α-Hydroxy etizolam | 8 h |
| Effect of age and disease | Not known but likely to be affected | |
| Metabolism | Hydroxylation and conjugation | |
| Metabolites | α-Hydroxy etizolam and others | |
| Active metabolites | α-Hydroxy etizolam has similar activity to parent | |
| Urinary excretion | Etizolam <0.3% | |
| Common doses | 0.25–3 mg daily | |

| | |
|---|---|
| Blood concentrations | 0.5 mg s.d. gave peak levels of etizolam and α-hydroxy etizolam of 8.3 ng/mL at 0.9 h |
| | No significant accumulation with repeated dosing; concentration of metabolite is similar to parent drug |
| Postmortem artefacts | Unknown |
| Toxicity | Unknown |
| Published paper | Fracasso et al., 1991[47] |

## FLUNITRAZEPAM

| | |
|---|---|
| Class of drug and uses | Strong-short-acting hypnotic, used as a pre-operative anaesthestic |
| Availability and proprietary or code names | Darkene, Hypnodorm, Hypnor, Narcozep, Rohipnol, Rohypnol, Roipnol, Valsera, etc. |
| | Street names include Rhoies, Rophies, Ropies, Roofies, Ropes, Rohes, Rochas, Rochas Dos, Rophs, Ropers, Ribs, R-25, Roach-2s, Trip and Fall, Remember All, Mind Erasers, Forget Pills |
| Chemical form and solubility | Free form, slightly soluble in ethanol and ether, insoluble in water |

Properties

| | |
|---|---|
| CAS | 1622-62-4 |
| MW | 313.3 |
| pKa | 1.8 |
| $V_D$ | 3.4–5.5 L/kg |
| Cl | |
| Log$_P$ | 2.1 |
| Protein binding | 77–80% |
| Bioavailability | 70% |

| | | |
|---|---|---|
| Blood half-life | Flunitrazepam | 11–25 (mean 15 h) |
| | 7-Amino flunitrazepam | 10–16 h |
| | N-Desmethyl flunitrazepam | 23–33 h |
| Effect of age and disease | Elimination not affected significantly with advanced age | |
| Metabolism | Reduction, dealkylation, acetylation and hydroxylation | |

| | |
|---|---|
| Metabolites | 7-Amino flunitrazepam, 7-acetamido flunitrazepam, desmethyl flunitrazepam, 3-hydroxy flunitrazepam |
| Active metabolites | Flunitrazepam, minor contribution by 7-amino and desmethyl metabolites |
| Urinary excretion | Flunitrazepam <0.2%<br>7-Amino flunitrazepam 10%<br>7-Acetamido flunitrazepam 26%<br>3-Hydroxy flunitrazepam 3.5% |
| Common doses | 0.5–2 mg |
| Blood concentrations | 2 mg chronic gave steady-state levels of 0.010–0.020 mg/L |
| Postmortem artefacts | Not significantly elevated in heart and femoral blood but must measure 7-amino flunitrazepam since almost all converted to this form after death |
| Toxicity | Minimum fatal concentration 0.2 mg/L (total parent and 7-amino flunitrazepam) |
| Published review | Mattila and Larni, 1980;[48] Woods and Winger, 1997[49] |

## FLURAZEPAM

| | |
|---|---|
| Class of drug and uses | Long-acting hypnotic |
| Availability and proprietary or code names | Dalmane, Dalmadorm, Felison, Flunox, Irdal, Midorm A.R., Novoflupam, Paxane, Remdue, Somnol, Valdorm, etc. |
| Chemical form and solubility | Free form and HCl salt<br>Salt is soluble in ethanol and water |

Properties
CAS 17617-23-1
 36105-20-1 (HCl)
 1172-18-5 (diHCl)
MW 387.9
pKa 1.9, 8.2
$V_D$ 3.4–5.5 L/kg
Log$_P$ 2.3 (flurazepam)
 2.8 (desalkyl flurazepam)
Protein binding 83% (flurazepam)
 97% (desalkylflurazepam)
 65% (OH-ethylflurazepam)
Bioavailability

| | | |
|---|---|---|
| Blood half-life (principle blood-borne species) | Flurazepam | 1–3 h |
| | N-1-Desalkyl flurazepam | 80 (40–200) h |
| Effect of age and disease | Elimination decreased with age | |
| Metabolism | Dealkylation, oxidation and conjugation | |
| Metabolites | Flurazepam, N-1-desalkyl flurazepam, hydroxyethyl-flurazepam, flurazepam aldehyde and conjugated N-1-desalkyl-3-hydroxy flurazepam | |
| Active metabolites | Flurazepam, N-1-desalkyl flurazepam (14 times more active), hydroxyethyl flurazepam (1.2 times) and aldehyde metabolite (1.2 times) | |
| Urinary excretion | Flurazepam | Trace |
| | N-1'-Desalkyl flurazepam | 29–55% |
| | N-1-Desalkyl-3-hydroxy flurazepam | 1–2% conjugated |
| Common doses | 15–30 mg in divided doses | |
| Blood concentrations | 30 mg s.d. mean peak level flurazepam 0.002 mg/L at 1 h and 0.02 mg/L at 12 h for N-1-desalkyl flurazepam | |
| | 30 mg chronic steady-state N-1-desalkyl flurazepam levels are 0.03–0.11 mg/L | |
| Postmortem artefacts | Not known | |
| Toxicity | Toxic > 1.8 mg/L | |
| Published reviews and papers | Aderjan and Mattern, 1979;[50] Greenblatt, 1992;[51] Miller et al., 1988[52] | |

## LOPRAZOLAM

| | |
|---|---|
| Class of drug and uses | Short-acting hypnotic |
| Availability and proprietary or code names | Avlane, Dormonoct, Halvane, Havlane, etc. |
| Chemical form and solubility | Slightly soluble in water, ethanol |

Properties

| | |
|---|---|
| CAS | 61197-73-7 |
| MW | 464.9 |
| pKa | 6.2 |
| $V_D$ | 4 L/kg |
| Cl | 0.2 mL/min/kg |
| Log$_P$ | |
| Protein binding | 80% |
| Bioavailability | ~70% |

| | |
|---|---|
| Blood half-life (principle blood-borne species) | Loprazolam 3–22 (mean 8) h |
| Effect of age and disease | Clearance decreased with advanced age by 75%. |
| Metabolism | Hydrolysis, hydroxylation and conjugation |
| Metabolites | Piperazine N-oxide |
| Active metabolites | None |
| Urinary excretion | Loprazolam Trace |
| | Piperazine N-oxide 18% |
| | Polar metabolites 25% |
| | Hydroxy metabolite 3% |
| | Acetamido metabolite 4% |
| Common doses | 0.5–2 mg at night |
| Blood concentrations | 1 mg s.d. plasma levels 3–6 µg/L at 0.5–3 h |
| | Little accumulation with repeated administration |
| Postmortem artefacts | Unknown |
| Toxicity | Unknown |
| Published reviews and papers | Garzone and Kroboth, 1989;[35] Swift et al., 1985;[53] Clark et al., 1986[54] |

## LORAZEPAM

| | |
|---|---|
| Class of drug and uses | Hypnotic, anxiety, pre-operative medication |
| Availability and proprietary or code names | Ativan, Almazine, Control, Donix, Durazolam, Lorans, Loraz, Novolorazem, Orfidal, Pro Dorm, etc. |
| Chemical form and solubility | Free form, sparingly soluble in ethanol, soluble chloroform and acetone, insoluble in water |

Properties
CAS               846-49-1
MW                321.2
pKa               1.3, 11.5
$V_D$             0.8–1.6 L/kg
Cl                1.0 mL/min/kg
$Log_P$           1.0–2.4
Protein binding   90%
Bioavailability   90%

| | |
|---|---|
| Blood half-life (principle blood-borne species) | Lorazepam 13 (8–25) h |
| Effect of age and disease | Elimination not affected by advanced age |
| Metabolism | Glucuronidation, ring hydroxylation, quinazolines |
| Metabolites | Glucuronide and quinolone metabolite |
| Active metabolites | Parent drug only |
| Urinary excretion | Lorazepam glucuronide 75% |
| Common doses | 1–4 mg in divided doses up to 1–10 mg |
| Blood concentrations | 2 mg s.d. max. 0.018 mg/L at 2 h<br>10 mg m.d. steady state 0.181 mg/L (0.14–0.24 mg/L) |
| Postmortem artefacts | Not likely to be significantly elevated in heart and femoral blood |
| Toxicity | Toxic > 2.8 mg/L |
| Published review | Greenblatt, 1981[55] |

## MIDAZOLAM

| | |
|---|---|
| Class of drug and uses | Short-acting pre-operative, sedative, amnesic and hypnotic |
| Availability and proprietary or code names | Doricum, Dormicum, Hypnovel, Versed |
| Chemical form and solubility | Free, maleate and HCl forms, soluble in ethanol, insoluble in water |

Properties

| | |
|---|---|
| CAS | 59467-70-8 |
| | 59467-96-8 (HCl) |
| MW | 325.8 |
| pKa | 6.2 |
| $V_D$ | 0.5–2.5 L/kg |
| $Log_P$ | 3.2 |
| Protein binding | 97% |
| Bioavailability | |

| | |
|---|---|
| Blood half-life (principle blood-borne species) | Midazolam 2 (1.5–2.5) h<br>α-Hydroxy midazolam 1 h |
| Effect of age and disease | Variable effects with age, no clear pattern |
| Metabolism | Hydroxylation and conjugation |

## Monographs of selected drugs

| | |
|---|---|
| Metabolites | α-Hydroxy midazolam |
| | 4-Hydroxy midazolam |
| | α,4-Dihydroxy midazolam |
| Active metabolites | Parent and less active α-hydroxy metabolite (63%) |
| Urinary excretion | Midazolam &lt;1% |
| | α-Hydroxy midazolam glucuronide 60–80% |
| | 4-Hydroxy midazolam glucuronide 3% |
| | α,4-Dihydroxy midazolam 1% |
| Common doses | 0.07–0.08 mg/kg per hour i.m. (pre-operative sedation) |
| | 0.03–0.2 mg/kg per hour i.v. for anaesthesia |
| | 5–15 mg p.o. for induction of sleep |
| Blood concentrations | 10 mg s.d. p.o. peak level 0.06 mg/L at 1 h |
| Postmortem artefacts | Unknown |
| Toxicity | See Martindale for toxicity as pre-medication[56] |
| Published reviews and papers | Garzone and Kroboth, 1989;[35] Seppala et al., 1993[57] |

## NITRAZEPAM

| | |
|---|---|
| Class of drug and uses | Short-acting hypnotic and used to treat infantile spasms |
| Availability and proprietary or code names | Alodorm, Apodorm, Arem, Insoma, Mogadon, Paxadorm, Somnipar, etc. |
| Chemical form and solubility | Free form, soluble in ethanol and ether, but sparingly soluble in water |

Properties
| | |
|---|---|
| CAS | 146-22-5 |
| MW | 281.3 |
| pKa | 3.2, 10.8 |
| $V_D$ | 1.5–5 L/kg |
| Cl | 0.3–0.5 mL/min |
| $Log_P$ | 2.1 |
| Protein binding | 85–88% |
| Bioavailability | |

| | |
|---|---|
| Blood half-life (principle blood-borne species) | Nitrazepam 26 (16–48) h |

| | |
|---|---|
| Effect of age and disease | 1. Half-life and volume of distribution increased and protein binding reduced with advanced age<br>2. Liver cirrhosis has no significant effect on clearance and half-life<br>3. Mild to moderate renal insufficiency shows slight reduction in clearance only |
| Metabolism | Reduction, acetylation, ring cleavage and conjugation |
| Metabolites | 7-Amino nitrazepam, 7-acetamido nitrazepam, 3-hydroxy-2-amino-5-nitrobenzophenone plus conjugates |
| Active metabolites | Parent drug only |
| Urinary excretion | Nitrazepam 1%<br>7-Amino nitrazepam 31% plus conjugate<br>7-Acetamido nitrazepam 21% plus conjugate<br>Also 3-hydroxy-2-amino-5-nitrobenzophenone ~5% |
| Common doses | 5–10 mg at night, up to 20 mg for in-patients |
| Blood concentrations | 5 mg s.d. peak levels of 0.035 mg/L at 2 h<br>10 mg s.d. peak levels of 0.084 (0.068–0.11) mg/L<br>5 mg chronic steady-state levels of 0.04 mg/L |
| Postmortem artefacts | Not significantly elevated in heart and femoral blood but must measure 7-amino nitrazepam since almost all converted to this form after death |
| Toxicity | Toxic > 0.5 mg/L |
| Published reviews and papers | Kangas et al., 1979;[58] Jochemsen et al., 1983;[59] Oches et al., 1992[60] |

## NORDAZEPAM (NORDIAZEPAM)
## (PRAZEPAM, HALAZEPAM, KETAZOLAM, OXAZOLAM, PINAZEPAM)

| | |
|---|---|
| Class of drug and uses | Minor tranquillizer, sedative |
| Availability and proprietary or code names | Madar (nordazepam); Paxipam (halazepam); Centrax, Verstran, Demetrin, Lysanxia, Prazene and others (prazepam); Domar, Duna (pinazepam); Sedotime, Anxon, Loftran, Solatran, Centamex, Anseren (ketazolam); Tranquit, Serenal, Hializan (oxazolam), etc. |

## Monographs of selected drugs

| | | | |
|---|---|---|---|
| Chemical form and solubility | | Free form, soluble in ethanol, chloroform and ether, insoluble in water | |
| Properties | | | |
| CAS | 1088-11-5 | | |
| MW | 270.7 | | |
| pKa | 3.5, 12.0 | | |
| $V_D$ | 0.9–1.3 L/kg | | |
| Cl | | | |
| $Log_P$ | 1.7 | | |
| Protein binding | 97–98% | | |
| Bioavailability | | | |
| Blood half-life (principle blood-borne species) | | Nordazepam ~50–99 h | |
| Effect of age and disease | | Elimination decreased in elderly | |
| Metabolism | | 3-Hydroxylation, conjugation with glucuronic acid | |
| Metabolites | | Oxazepam and glucuronide of oxazepam | |
| Active metabolites | | Nordazepam, oxazepam | |
| Urinary excretion | | Primarily as conjugated 3-hydroxy metabolite Parent drug only excreted in trace quantities | |
| Common doses | | Nordazepam | 10 mg daily |
| | | Halazepam | 20–120 mg daily |
| | | Ketazolam | 15–60 mg daily |
| | | Oxazolam | 10–20 mg t.d.s. |
| | | Pinazepam | 5–20 mg daily |
| | | Prazepam | 20–60 mg daily |
| Blood concentrations | | 10 mg s.d. peak level 0.17 mg/L 20–30 mg chronic produces plasma levels of 0.6–1.8 mg/L (mean 1.1) at 10 h post-dose | |
| Postmortem artefacts | | Not significantly elevated in heart and femoral blood | |
| Toxicity | | See diazepam, no reported deaths with nordazepam or any of the pro-drugs | |
| Published reviews and papers | | Greenblatt et al., 1981;[61] Pacifici et al., 1983[62] | |

# Benzodiazepines

## OXAZEPAM

| | |
|---|---|
| Class of drug and uses | Short-acting hypnotic, sedative, alcohol withdrawal |
| Availability and proprietary or code names | Alepam, Anxiolit, Benzotran, Durazepam, Murelax, Oxapuren, Serax, Serepax, Serpax, Sobril, etc. |
| Chemical form and solubility | Free form, also occasionally as hemisuccinate, soluble in ethanol, ethyl acetate, chloroform, insoluble in water |

Properties

| | |
|---|---|
| CAS | 604-75-1 (free form) |
| MW | 286.7 |
| pKa | 1.7, 11.6 |
| Cl | 1.1 mL/min |
| $V_D$ | 0.5–2.0 L/kg |
| $Log_P$ | 2.2 |
| Protein binding | 95–98% |
| Bioavailability | 93% |

| | |
|---|---|
| Blood half-life | Oxazepam 8 (4–15) h |
| Effect of age and disease | Little effect on clearance with advanced age |
| Metabolism | Conjugation |
| Metabolites | Glucuronide |
| Active metabolites | Parent drug only |
| Urinary excretion | Oxazepam 70–80% as conjugate |
| Common doses | 15–60 mg per day, once or in divided doses |
| Blood concentrations | 15 mg s.d. peak level 0.31 mg/L at 1.5 h<br>45 mg s.d. peak level 1.1 (0.88–1.44) mg/L at 2 h<br>No accumulation during chronic dosing |
| Postmortem artefacts | Not significantly elevated in heart and femoral blood |
| Toxicity | Toxic >4.4 mg/L |
| Published papers and reviews | Greenblatt, 1981;[55] Sonne et al., 1988;[63] Ayd, 1990[64] |

## PRAZEPAM

| | |
|---|---|
| Class of drug and uses | Long-acting minor tranquilliser related to diazepam |
| Availability and proprietary or code names | Centrax, Demetrin, Lysanxia, mon-Demetrin, Prazene, Reapam, Trepidan, Verstran, etc. |
| Chemical form and solubility | Free form, soluble in ethanol, insoluble in water |

401

## Properties

| | |
|---|---|
| CAS | 2955-38-6 |
| MW | 324.8 |
| pKa | 2.7 |
| V_D | |
| Cl | mL/min/kg |
| Log_P | 3.7 |
| Protein binding | % |
| Bioavailability | % |

| | | |
|---|---|---|
| Blood half-life (principle blood-borne species) | Nordazepam | 29–192 h |
| Effect of age and disease | Elimination decreased | |
| Metabolism | N-Dealkylation, hydroxylation and conjugation | |
| Metabolites | Nordazepam, 3-hydroxy prazepam, oxazepam glucuronide | |
| Active metabolites | Nordazepam | |
| Urinary excretion | Nordazepam | Trace |
| | Oxazepam glucuronide | 60% |
| | 3-Hydroxy prazepam glucuronide | 3–35% |
| Common doses | Daily doses up to 60 mg | |
| Blood concentrations | 20 mg s.d. p.o. produces peak levels of nordazepam 0.07–0.17 (mean 0.14) mg/L at 2.5–72 h (mean 13) post-dose Parent drug not detected in blood | |
| Postmortem artefacts | Likely to be similar to diazepam/nordazepam | |
| Toxicity | Likely to be similar to diazepam/nordazepam | |
| Published paper | Allen, 1979[62a] | |

## QUAZEPAM

| | |
|---|---|
| Class of drug and uses | Selective hypnotic related to benzodiazepines |
| Availability and proprietary or code names | Oniria, Quazium, Selepam, Dorme, Doral, Quiedorm, etc. |
| Chemical form and solubility | Free form, soluble in ethanol, sparingly soluble in water |

Properties

| | |
|---|---|
| CAS | 36735-22-5 |
| MW | 386.8 |
| pKa | |
| V$_D$ | |
| Cl | mL/min/kg |
| Log$_P$ | 4.0 |
| Protein binding | >95% |
| Bioavailability | |

| | | |
|---|---|---|
| Blood half-life (principle blood-borne species) | Quazepam | 20–53 h |
| | 2-Oxoquazepam | 20–50 h |
| | Desalkyl flurazepam | 48–120 h |
| Effect of age and disease | Clearance reduced with age | |
| Metabolism | N-Dealkylation, oxidation, hydroxylation and conjugation | |
| Metabolites | 2-Oxoquazepam, N-desalkyl-2-oxoquazepam (desalkyl flurazepam) and conjugates | |
| Active metabolites | Parent, 2-oxoquazepam and desalkyl flurazepam | |
| Urinary excretion | Quazepam trace | |
| Common doses | 7.5–15 mg | |
| Blood concentrations | 25 mg s.d. p.o. peak levels of quazepam 0.15 mg/L at 1.5 h | |
| | 15 mg chronic produces steady-state plasma levels 0.011 mg/L | |
| | Plasma levels of 2-oxo and N-desalkyl-2-oxo metabolites are significant relative to parent drug | |
| Postmortem artefacts | Unknown | |
| Toxicity | Unknown | |
| Published papers and reviews | Ankier and Goa, 1988;[65] Kales, 1990[66] | |

## TEMAZEPAM

| | |
|---|---|
| Class of drug and uses | Short-acting hypnotic and pre-operative |
| Availability and proprietary or code names | Euhypnos, Nocturne, Nomapam, Normison, Temaze, Temtabs, Levanxol, Maeva, Planum, Remestan, Restoril, Temaz, Tenso, Z-Pam, etc. |
| Chemical form and solubility | Free form, soluble in ethanol and chloroform, insoluble in water |

# Monographs of selected drugs

Properties

| | |
|---|---|
| CAS | 846-50-4 |
| MW | 300.7 |
| pKa | 1.6 |
| $V_D$ | 0.8–1.4 L/kg |
| Cl | 1.2 mL/min/kg |
| $Log_P$ | 1.8 |
| Protein binding | 96–97% |
| Bioavailability | >80% |

| | | |
|---|---|---|
| Blood half-life (principle blood-borne species) | Temazepam | 10 (5–15) h |
| | Oxazepam | 7 (4–15) h |
| Effect of age and disease | Little change in clearance with age | |
| Metabolism | N-Demethylation, conjugation with glucuronic acid | |
| Metabolites | Oxazepam, and glucuronides of oxazepam and temazepam | |
| Active metabolites | All non-conjugated metabolites | |
| Urinary excretion | Temazepam | 1% in free form |
| | Temazepam | 73% as conjugate |
| | Oxazepam | 6% as conjugate |
| Active metabolites | All non-conjugated metabolites | |
| Common doses | 15–60 mg per day, once or in divided doses | |
| Blood concentrations | 10 mg s.d. peak levels 0.30 (0.20–0.43) mg/L at 15–90 min | |
| | 20 mg s.d. peak levels 0.67 (0.36–0.86) mg/L at 15–75 min | |
| | 30 mg s.d. peak level 0.87 (0.5–1.1) mg/L at 1.4 h | |
| Postmortem artefacts | Not significantly elevated in heart and femoral blood | |
| Toxicity | Toxic >3.8 mg/L | |
| Published review | Heel et al., 1981[67] | |

## TRIAZOLAM

| | |
|---|---|
| Class of drug and uses | Short-acting potent hypnotic |
| Availability and proprietary or code names | Apo-Triazo, Dumozolam, Halcion, Novodorm, Novo-triazolam, Nu-Triazo, Songar, Triazolam, etc. |

# Benzodiazepines

| | | |
|---|---|---|
| Chemical form and solubility | | Free form, also occasionally as hemisuccinate, soluble in ethanol, chloroform, insoluble in water |
| Properties | | |
| CAS | 28911-01-5 | |
| MW | 343.2 | |
| pKa | 1.5 | |
| $V_D$ | 1.1–2.7 L/kg | |
| Cl | 3.7–8.8 mL/min/kg | |
| $Log_P$ | 2.2 | |
| Protein binding | 78–90% | |
| Bioavailability | 44% | |
| Blood half-life | | Triazolam 3 (1.5–5.5) h |
| | | α-Hydroxy triazolam 4 h |
| Effect of age and disease | | Elimination decreased with age |
| Metabolism | | Hydroxylation and conjugation |
| Metabolites | | α-Hydroxy triazolam (or 1-hydroxy triazolam) |
| | | 4-Hydroxy triazolam |
| | | α-Hydroxy-4-hydroxy triazolam |
| Active metabolites | | Parent drug and α-hydroxy triazolam (activity 50–100% of parent) |
| Urinary excretion | | Triazolam 2% |
| | | α-Hydroxy triazolam 60–80% |
| | | 4-Hydroxy triazolam 10% |
| | | α-Hydroxy-4-hydroxy triazolam 2% |
| | | Others 2% |
| Common doses | | 0.125–0.25 mg at night |
| Plasma concentrations | | 0.25 mg s.d. peak levels 2.3–3.7 (mean 3.0) ng/mL at 0.75–1.5 h |
| | | 0.5 mg s.d. peak levels 1.7–9.4 (mean 4.4) ng/mL at 0.5–4 h |
| | | 1.0 mg s.d. peak levels 8.6 ng/mL at 1–1.5 h |
| Postmortem artefacts | | Not significantly elevated in heart and femoral blood |
| Toxicity | | Toxic > 0.04 mg/L |
| Published papers and reviews | | Garzone and Kroboth, 1989;[35] Pakes et al., 1981[68] |

## Other sedatives and anxiolytics

### BUSPIRONE

| | |
|---|---|
| Class of drug and uses | Short-acting azaspirone anxiolytic |
| Availability and proprietary or code names | BuSpar etc. |
| Chemical form and solubility | As hydrochloride, water soluble |
| Properties | |
| CAS | 3605-84-7 |
| | 33386-08-2 (HCl) |
| MW | 422.0 (HCl) |
| pKa | |
| $V_D$ | 1.3–6.6 L/kg |
| $Log_P$ | |
| Protein binding | 95% |
| Bioavailability | |
| Blood half-life (principle blood-borne species) | Buspirone 1–7 h |
| Effect of age and disease | Clearance probably reduced with age |
| Metabolism | Hydroxylation and conjugation |
| Metabolites | 5-Hydroxy buspirone and glucuronide |
| | 1-Pyrimidinylpiperazine (1-PP) |
| Active metabolites | Buspirone and 1-PP (0.25 of parent) |
| Urinary excretion | Buspirone |
| | 1-PP |
| | 5-Hydroxy buspirone |
| Common doses | 15–60 mg per day, in divided doses |
| Blood concentrations | 20 mg s.d. p.o. peak levels 0.5–3.1 (mean 1.2) ng/mL at 0.5–1 h |
| Postmortem artefacts | Unknown |
| Toxicity | No fatal cases reported |
| Published papers and reviews | Dalhoff et al., 1987;[69] Goldberg et al., 1983;[70] Napoliello and Domantay, 1991[71] |

# Other sedatives and anxiolytics

## ZALEPLON

| | |
|---|---|
| Class of drug and uses | Short-acting selective ($\omega_1$) hypnotic |
| Availability and proprietary or code names | Sonata, CL 284,846 |
| Chemical form and solubility | Free base, soluble in ethanol |
| Properties | |
| CAS | 151319-34-5 |
| MW | 305 |
| pKa | |
| $V_D$ | 1.3 (ss) L/kg |
| Cl | 0.9 L/h/kg |
| Log$_P$ | |
| Protein binding | |
| Bioavailability | 30% |
| Blood half-life (principle blood-borne species) | Zaleplon  1 h |
| Effect of age and disease | |
| Metabolism | N-Demethylation, oxidation and hydroxylation |
| Metabolites | Desethyl zaleplon, 5-oxo-zaleplon, 5-oxo-desethyl zaleplon, plus conjugates |
| Active metabolites | None |
| Urinary excretion | <1% excreted as zaleplon |
| Common doses | 5–10 mg at night |
| Blood concentrations | 5 mg oral dose gives blood concentrations to 0.1 mg/L (mean 0.06) at 1 h |
| Postmortem artefacts | Unknown |
| Toxicity | Unknown |
| Published papers and reviews | Sanger DJ et al., 1994;[72] Rush CR et al., 1999;[73] Rosen AS et al., 1999[74] |

## ZOPICLONE

| | |
|---|---|
| Class of drug and uses | Short-acting hypnotic<br>Effects reversed by flumazenil |
| Availability and proprietary or code names | Imovane, Zimovane, Ximovan, Datalon, Limovan, Siaten, etc. |
| Chemical form and solubility | Free base |

# Monographs of selected drugs

| Properties | | |
|---|---|---|
| CAS | 43200-80-2 | |
| MW | 388.8 | |
| pKa | | |
| V$_D$ | 1.5 L/kg | |
| Cl | 3.3 mL/min/kg | |
| Log$_P$ | | |
| Protein binding | 45% | |
| Bioavailability | 80% | |

| | | |
|---|---|---|
| Blood half-life (principle blood-borne species) | Zopiclone 2–6.5 h | |
| Effect of age and disease | Dose halved in elderly | |
| Metabolism | N-Demethylation and oxidation by P450 enzymes | |
| Metabolites | N-Desmethyl zopiclone and N-oxide | |
| Active metabolites | N-Oxide (some activity) | |
| Urinary excretion | Zopiclone | 4–7% |
| | N-Desmethyl zopiclone | 11–26% |
| | Zopiclone N-oxide | 8–12% |
| Common doses | 7.5–15 mg at night before retiring | |
| Blood concentrations | 7.5 mg dose produced peak plasma concentrations of 0.06–0.09 mg/L at 0.5–2 h | |
| | No change in kinetics occurs with repeated dosing | |
| | Shows stereoselective metabolism | |
| Postmortem artefacts | Relatively stable postmortem, no significant redistribution observed | |
| Toxicity | Toxic >0.6 mg/L | |
| Published papers and reviews | Houghton et al., 1985;[75] Hempel and Blaschke, 1996;[76] Goa and Heel, 1986;[77] Wadworth and McTavish, 1993[78] | |

## ZOLPIDEM

| | |
|---|---|
| Class of drug and uses | Short-acting selective ($\omega_1$) hypnotic |
| Availability and proprietary or code names | Ivadal, Stilnox, Stilnoct, Bikalm, Niotal, Cedrol, Dalparan, Ambien, etc. |
| Chemical form and solubility | Tartrate slightly soluble in water (23 mg/mL at 20°C) |

## Other sedatives and anxiolytics

| Properties | | |
|---|---|---|
| CAS | 82626-48-0 | |
| | 99294-93-6 (tartrate) | |
| MW | 392.4 | |
| | 764.9 (tartrate) | |
| pKa | 6.16 | |
| $V_D$ | 0.5–0.7 L/kg | |
| Cl | 0.25 mL/min/kg | |
| $Log_P$ | 2.4 | |
| Protein binding | 92% | |
| Bioavailability | 70% | |
| Blood half-life (principle blood-borne species) | Zolpidem | ~1.5–4.5 h |
| Effect of age and disease | 1. Clearance halved in elderly<br>2. Clearance three times higher in children than adults<br>3. No significant difference between racial groups and between genders<br>4. Clearance decreases in renal failure (halved)<br>5. Clearance reduced by one-third in liver cirrhosis<br>6. No significant chane in kinetics in obesity | |
| Metabolism | Hydroxylation and oxidation | |
| Metabolites | Carboxy metabolite of 4'-methyl, carboxy metabolite of 6-methyl, and ring hydroxylated metabolite | |
| Active metabolites | None | |
| Urinary excretion | Zolpidem | ~1% |
| | Carboxy metabolite of 4'-methyl | 30–50% |
| | Carboxy metabolite of 6-methyl | 1–11% |
| | Ring hydroxylated metabolite | Trace–10% |
| Common doses | 10–20 mg at night | |
| Blood concentrations | 20 mg s.d. produces peak plasma concentrations of 0.19–0.32 µg/mL at 0.75–2.6 h | |
| Postmortem artefacts | Unknown | |
| Toxicity | Only with significant natural disease and/or CNS depressant drugs | |
| Published papers and reviews | Salva and Costa, 1995;[79] Langtry and Benfield, 1990[80] | |

# AMYLOBARBITAL

| | |
|---|---|
| Class of drug and uses | Barbiturate hypnotic and sedative |
| Availability and proprietary or code names | Neur-Amyl, Amal, Amylbarb, Amytal, Etamyl, Stadodorm; also known as amylobarbitone |
| Chemical form and solubility | Sparingly soluble in water as free acid, sodium salt soluble |

**Properties**

| | |
|---|---|
| CAS | 57-43-2 |
| MW | 226.3 |
| pKa | 7.9 (salt) |
| $V_D$ | 1 L/kg |
| Cl | 0.5 mL/min/kg |
| $Log_P$ | 1.6 |
| Protein binding | 40–60% |
| Bioavailability | 95% |

| | |
|---|---|
| Blood half-life | Amylobarbital 8–40 h |
| Effect of age and disease | Clearance likely to decrease with advanced age and liver impairment |
| Metabolism | Hydroxylation and conjugation |
| Metabolites | 3′-Hydroxy metabolite and glucuronide |
| Active metabolites | 3′-Hydroxy metabolite (one-third activity) |
| Urinary excretion | Amylobarbital 1% |
| | 3′-Hydroxy metabolite 30–50% |
| | 3′-Hydroxy glucuronide 30% |
| Common doses | 30–600 mg daily |
| Plasma concentrations | 2–12 mg/L (therapeutic) |
| Postmortem artefacts | Stable postmortem, little redistribution |
| Toxicity | Toxic >5 mg/L, depending on tolerance |
| Published papers and reviews | Breimer, 1977[81] |

# SECOBARBITAL

| | |
|---|---|
| Class of drug and uses | Barbiturate hypnotic and sedative |
| Availability and proprietary or code names | Also known as quinalbarbital, meballymal, secobarbitone, quinalbarbitone Immenox, Proquinal, Quinbar, Seconal, Secogen, Seral, Tuinal, etc. |
| Chemical form and solubility | Very slightly soluble in water as free acid, sodium salt soluble |

**Other sedatives and anxiolytics**

| Properties | | |
|---|---|---|
| CAS | 76-73-3 | |
| MW | 238.3 | |
| pKa | 7.9 | |
| $V_D$ | 1.5 L/kg | |
| Cl | 0.8 mL/min/kg | |
| $Log_P$ | ~2 | |
| Protein binding | 70% | |
| Bioavailability | 95% | |

| | |
|---|---|
| Blood half-life | Secobarbital 15–30 h |
| Effect of age and disease | Clearance likely to decrease with advanced age and liver impairment |
| Metabolism | Hydroxylation, oxidation and conjugation |
| Metabolites | 3′-Hydroxy- and 3′-keto-quinalbarbital, secodiol |
| Active metabolites | Possibly similar to amylobarbital |
| Urinary excretion | Secobarbital <5% |
| Common doses | 50–200 mg daily |
| Plasma concentrations | 2–10 mg/L (therapeutic) |
| | 200 mg single dose produces peak plasma levels of ~2 mg/L |
| Postmortem artefacts | Stable postmortem, little redistribution |
| Toxicity | Toxic >5 mg/L, depending on tolerance |
| Published paper | Robinson and McDowell, 1979[82] |

## PENTOBARBITAL

| | |
|---|---|
| Class of drug and uses | Barbiturate hynotic and sedative |
| Availability and proprietary or code names | Nembutal, Mebumal, etc., also known as pentobarbitone |
| Chemical form and solubility | Slightly soluble in water as free acid, sodium salt soluble |

| Properties | |
|---|---|
| CAS | 76-74-4 |
| MW | 226.3 |
| pKa | 8.0 (salt) |
| $V_D$ | 0.7–1 L/kg |
| Cl | 0.3–0.5 mL/min/kg |
| $Log_P$ | 1.9 |
| Protein binding | 65% |
| Bioavailability | 95% |

| | |
|---|---|
| Blood half-life | Pentobarbital 15–48 h |
| Effect of age and disease | Clearance likely to decrease with advanced age and liver impairment |
| Metabolism | Hydroxylation and oxidation |
| Metabolites | 3-Hydroxy metabolites, N-hydroxy, 3-carboxy |
| Active metabolites | 3-Hydroxy metabolites likely |
| Urinary excretion | Pentobarbital 1% <br> 3-Hydroxy metabolite 7% <br> 3'-Hydroxy metabolite 30% <br> N-Hydroxy metabolite 7–14% <br> 3'-Carboxy metabolite 10–15% |
| Common doses | 100–200 mg daily |
| Plasma concentrations | 1–10 mg/L (therapeutic) |
| Postmortem artefacts | Stable postmortem, little redistribution |
| Toxicity | Toxic >5 mg/L, depending on tolerance |
| Published papers and reviews | Breimer, 1977[81] |

# Opioids and related drugs

## ALFENTANIL

| | |
|---|---|
| Class of drug and uses | Potent short-acting narcotic used in surgery as an analgesic and anaesthetic and to supplement other anaesthetics |
| Availability and proprietary or code names | Solution for injection, Rapifen; Alfenta, Fanaxal, Limifen |
| Chemical form and solubility | Available as base and hydrochloride, salt readily soluble in water, ethanol and methanol |

Properties
| | |
|---|---|
| CAS | 71195-58-9 |
| MW | 416.5 |
| pKa | 6.5 |
| $V_D$ | 0.6–1.0 L/kg |
| Cl | 2–8 mL/min/kg |
| Log$_P$ | 2.1 (moderate) |
| Protein binding | 90% |
| Bioavailability | N/A |

| | |
|---|---|
| Blood half-life (principle blood-borne species) | Alfentanil 1–2 h |
| Effect of age and disease | Expect lower clearance in elderly and in patients with impaired liver function |
| Metabolism | N- and O-dealkylation |
| Metabolites | N- and O-dealkylated products |
| Active metabolites | None |
| Urinary excretion | 1% parent drug excreted unchanged in urine |
| Common doses | Initial intravenous dose up to 0.5 mg, followed by maintenance doses |
| Blood concentrations | Expect plasma concentrations to 1.0 ng/mL |
| Postmortem artefacts | Unknown, redistribution likely |
| Toxicity | As for other potent opioids |
| Selected papers | Mather 1983;[83] Rubio and Cox, 1991[84] |

## BUPRENORPHINE

| | |
|---|---|
| Class of drug and uses | Potent partial agonist narcotic for relief of serious pain and as an adjunct to anaesthesia, used in opioid substitution programmes |

| | | |
|---|---|---|
| Availability and proprietary or code names | | Temgesic, Buprenex, Buprex, Finibron, Prefin tablets for sublingual use, solution for injections, skin patches |
| Chemical form and solubility | | Available as hydrochloride salt, soluble in water |
| Properties | | |
| CAS | 52485-79-7 | |
| MW | 467.6 | |
| pKa | 8.4, 9.9 | |
| $V_D$ | 2.5 L/kg | |
| Cl | 18 mL/min/kg | |
| $Log_P$ | 3.4 | |
| Protein binding | 96% | |
| Bioavailability | 50% (sublingual) 16% (oral) | |
| Blood half-life (principle blood-borne species) | | Buprenorphine 2–6 h |
| Effect of age and disease | | Small decline with age and liver disease |
| Metabolism | | N-Dealkylation and conjugation |
| Metabolites | | Norbuprenorphine and glucuronides |
| Active metabolites | | Norbuprenorphine shows only weak intrinsic activity |
| Excretion | | Excreted largely unchanged in urine (27%) and faeces (68%); high levels in bile |
| Common doses | | Given parenterally at 0.3–0.6 mg, and sublingually up to 24 mg daily |
| Blood concentrations | | Concentrations range up to 0.05 mg/L |
| Postmortem artefacts | | Unknown |
| Toxicity and abuse potential | | As for other opioids, may have a lower potential for producing dependence, but toxic in combination with benzodiazepines[85,86] |
| Selected papers | | Bullingham et al., 1983;[87] 1982;[88] Strang, 1985[89] |

## BUTORPHANOL

| | |
|---|---|
| Class of drug and uses | Synthetic narcotic analgesic, kappa agonist with mu-antagonist activity with antitussive activity, used in pre-operative and pre-anaesthetic states and in labour pains |

| | | |
|---|---|---|
| Availability and proprietary or code names | Stadol, Verstadol and others | |
| Chemical form and solubility | Tartrate salt, sparingly soluble in water | |
| Properties | | |
| CAS | 42408-82-2 | |
| MW | 327.46 | |
| pKa | | |
| $V_D$ | 3–7 L/kg | |
| Cl | 5–150 L/h | |
| $Log_P$ | 2.2 | |
| Protein binding | 80% | |
| Bioavailability | 60–70% (nasal) | |
| | 5–17% (oral) | |
| Blood half-life (principle blood-borne species) | Butorphanol 2–9 h (mean 5 h) | |
| Effect of age and disease | Advanced age and renal dysfunction increases half-life | |
| Metabolism | Hydroxylation and dealkylation | |
| Metabolites | Hydroxybutorphanol and norbutorphanol | |
| Active metabolites | No significant activity | |
| Urinary excretion | Butorphanol | 5% |
| | Hydroxybutorphanol | 49% |
| | Norbutorphanol | <5% |
| Common doses | 1–2 mg intranasally every 3–4 h | |
| Blood concentrations | 1–2 ng/ml at 0.6–1.0 h 1 mg intranasally | |
| Postmortem artefacts | Unknown | |
| Toxicity and abuse potential | Moderate to high | |
| Selected papers | Vogelsang and Hayes, 1991;[90] Gillis et al., 1995[91] | |

## CODEINE

| | |
|---|---|
| Class of drug and uses | Weak analgesic used for mild to moderate pain, as an antitussive and to treat diarrhoea |
| Availability and proprietary or code names | Various preparations, 8 mg with paracetamol (acetaminophen) over-the-counter, and 30–50 mg usually by prescription, and numerous other proprietary preparations |
| Chemical form and solubility | Available as hydrochloride, sulphate and phosphate salts, soluble in water |

Properties

| | |
|---|---|
| CAS | 76-57-3 (anhydrous) |
| MW | 317.4 |
| pKa | 8.2 |
| $V_D$ | 3.5 L/kg |
| Cl | |
| Log$_P$ | 0.6 (low) |
| Protein binding | 7% |
| Bioavailability | Moderate |

| | | |
|---|---|---|
| Blood half-life (principle blood-borne species) | Codeine | 2–4 h |
| Effect of age and disease | Little effect | |
| Metabolism | O-Demethylation to morphine and conjugation | |
| Metabolites | Morphine and 3- and 6-glucuronides | |
| Active metabolites | Morphine | |
| Urinary excretion | Codeine | 5–17% |
| | Norcodeine | 0–5% |
| | Morphine | Trace |
| | Codeine glucuronides | 32–56% |
| | Morphine glucuronides | 5–13% |
| Common doses | 8–60 mg 3 or 4 times daily | |
| Blood concentrations | 50 mg s.d. produces $C_{max}$ codeine level of 0.30 (0.12–0.31) mg/L at 0.5–2 h, and total codeine $C_{max}$ 4.4 (2–6) mg/L at 0.7–2 h, conjugated metabolite approximately 5–20-fold higher; morphine $C_{max}$ 0.008 mg/L, total morphine $C_{max}$ 0.18 mg/L | |
| Postmortem artefacts | No significant change postmortem in femoral blood | |
| Toxicity and abuse potential | Fatal concentration >0.4 mg/L;[92] has low abuse potential | |
| Selected papers | Gerostamoulos et al., 1996;[92] Lafolie et al., 1996[93] | |

## DEXTROMORAMIDE

| | |
|---|---|
| Class of drug and uses | Potent narcotic analgesic, 5–25-times the potency of morphine |
| Availability and proprietary or code names | Palfium, Jetrium and others |
| Chemical form and solubility | As tartrate, soluble in water |

Properties
CAS            357-56-2
MW             392.5
pKa
V$_D$
Cl
Log$_P$
Protein binding
Bioavailability

Blood half-life                 Dextromoramide   1.5–4 h
(principle blood-borne species)

Effect of age and disease       Unknown
Metabolism                      N-Oxidation, hydroxylation, and hydrolysis
Metabolites
Active metabolites
Urinary excretion
Common doses                    5–20 mg
Blood concentrations            Plasma concentration at 10–80 ng/mL after 5 mg intravenously

Postmortem artefacts            Likely to be subject to redistribution
Toxicity and abuse potential    40 ng/mL toxic
Selected papers                 Kintz et al., 1989;[94] Pagani et al., 1989;[95] Ufkes et al., 1998[96]

## DEZOCINE

Class of drug and uses          Potent opioid mixed agonist/antagonist (mu and kappa); used in analgesia and equipotent to morphine

Availability and proprietary or code names   Dalgan injection

Chemical form and solubility    Free base

Properties
CAS            53648-55-8
MW             245.4
pKa
V$_D$          10 L/kg
Cl             47–58 mL/min/kg
Log$_P$        0.2
Protein binding
Bioavailability   100% (i.m./s.c.)

## Monographs of selected drugs

| | |
|---|---|
| Blood half-life (principle blood-borne species) | Dezocine 0.6–7 h (mean 2 h) |
| Effect of age and disease | No significant change in clearance with advanced age and hepatic disease |
| Metabolism | Conjugation |
| Metabolites | Glucuronide and possibly sulphate |
| Active metabolites | None likely |
| Urinary excretion | Dezocine <1% |
| | Dezocine glucuronide/sulphate Balance |
| Common doses | 5–20 mg i.v./i.m./s.c. |
| Blood concentrations | 10–30 ng/mL peak concentrations i.m. at 10–90 min |
| Postmortem artefacts | Unknown |
| Toxicity and abuse potential | Low to moderate abuse potential |
| Selected paper | O'Brien and Benfield, 1989[97] |

## DIHYDROCODEINE

| | |
|---|---|
| Class of drug and uses | Weak narcotic analgesic and antitussive |
| Availability and proprietary or code names | Codox, Paracodin, Rikodeine, Co-dydramol, DF 118, DHC, DHC plus combination capsule with paracetamol (acetaminophen) and caffeine, and many others |
| Chemical form and solubility | Bitartrate salt |

Properties
| | |
|---|---|
| CAS | 125-28-0 |
| MW | 301.37 |
| pKa | |
| $V_D$ | 1.0–1.3 L/kg |
| Cl | mL/min/kg |
| Log$_P$ | |
| Protein binding | |
| Bioavailability | 20% |

| | |
|---|---|
| Blood half-life (principle blood-borne species) | Dihydrocodeine 3.5–4.5 h |
| Effect of age and disease | Similar to codeine |
| Metabolism | Demethylation and conjugation |
| Metabolites | Dihydromorphine and glucuronides |
| Active metabolites | Dihydromorphine |

| | |
|---|---|
| Urinary excretion | Likely to be similar to codeine with mainly glucuronides of dihydrocodeine and dihydromorphine |
| Common doses | 30–60 mg every 4–6 h |
| Blood concentrations | Peak concentration of 72 and 146 ng/mL after 30 and 60 mg, at 1.6–1.8 h |
| Postmortem artefacts | Probably similar to codeine |
| Toxicity and abuse potential | Low to moderate, fatal concentration >0.8 mg/L |
| Selected papers | Rowell et al., 1983;[98] Peat and Sengupta, 1977[99] |

## ETHYLMORPHINE

| | |
|---|---|
| Class of drug and uses | Narcotic analgesic and antitussive |
| Availability and proprietary or code names | Cosylan mixture and others |
| Chemical form and solubility | As hydrochloride salt; soluble in water |

Properties
CAS 76-58-4
MW 331.4
pKa
$V_D$
Cl
$Log_P$
Protein binding
Bioavailability

| | |
|---|---|
| Blood half-life (principle blood-borne species) | Ethylmorphine 2–3 h |
| Effect of age and disease | Similar to codeine, known poor metabolizers to ethylmorphine as for codeine |
| Metabolism | De-ethylation, glucuronidation |
| Metabolites | Morphine, morphine-3-glucuronide, morphine-6-glucuronide, ethylmorphine-6-glucuronide and others |
| Active metabolites | Morphine, morphine-6-glucuronide |
| Urinary excretion | Ethylmorphine 2–5% (median 4) Ethylmorphine-6-glucuronide 28–53% (median 41) Morphine 0.4–1.4% (median 0.8) |

## Monographs of selected drugs

|   |   |
|---|---|
| | Morphine-3-glucuronide 5–16% (median 12) |
| | Morphine-6-glucuronide 1.5–5% (median 3) |
| Common doses | 50 mg |
| Blood concentrations | Peak 0.1–0.3 mg/L at 45 min (60 mg) |
| Postmortem artefacts | Unknown, but likely to be similar to codeine |
| Toxicity and abuse potential | Low to moderate |
| Selected paper | Aasmundstad et al., 1995[100] |

## HEROIN (DIACETYLMORPHINE)

| | |
|---|---|
| Class of drug and uses | Potent short-acting narcotic analgesic for pain and pulmonary oedema and to control breathing in neonates |
| Availability and proprietary or code names | Illicit drug with some therapeutic uses; also known as diamorphine, diacetylmorphine, acetomorphine |
| Chemical form and solubility | Heroin is available as free base and hydrochloride salt; salt most water soluble; purity on the street varies typically from 3% to 70% |

Properties
| | | |
|---|---|---|
| CAS | 561-27-3 | |
| MW | 369.4 | |
| pKa | 7.6 | |
| $V_D$ | See morphine | |
| Cl | See morphine | |
| Log$_P$ | 0.2 | |
| Protein binding | See morphine | |
| Bioavailability | Very low | |

| | | |
|---|---|---|
| Blood half-life (i.v.) (principle blood-borne species) | Heroin | 2–7 min |
| | 6-Acetylmorphine | 3–25 min |
| Effect of age and disease | No studies, but likely to be similar to morphine | |
| Metabolism | Deacetylation and conjugation | |
| Metabolites | 6-Acetylmorphine, morphine, glucuronides | |
| Active metabolites | 6-Acetylmorphine, morphine | |
| Urinary excretion (i.v.) | Heroin | 0% |
| | 6-Acetylmorphine | 0.5% |
| | Morphine | 5% |
| | Morphine glucuronides | 55% |

| | |
|---|---|
| Usual doses | 5–10 mg up in adults |
| | 50–200 µg/kg loading dose in infants |
| Blood concentrations (20 mg i.v.) | Heroin and morphine concentrations 400 and 50 ng/mL at 2 min; heroin and morphine concentrations 0 and 20 ng/mL at 60 min |
| Postmortem artefacts | Postmortem metabolism to morphine |
| Toxicity and abuse potential | Highly toxic with high abuse potential, all morphine concentrations potentially fatal |
| Selected papers | Cone et al., 1991;[101] Boerner 1975[102] |

## FENTANYL

| | |
|---|---|
| Class of drug and uses | Potent short-acting narcotic analgesic used in surgery as an analgesic and anaesthetic and to supplement other anaesthetics |
| Availability and proprietary or code names | Fentanyl; Sublimaze solutions for injection, Duragesic, Fentanest, Leptanal, Tanyl, and other preparations |
| Chemical form and solubility | Available as citrate salt, soluble in water |

Properties
| | |
|---|---|
| CAS | 437-38-7 |
| MW | 336.5 |
| pKa | 8.4 |
| $V_D$ | 3–8 L/kg |
| Cl | 2–8 mL/min/kg |
| $Log_P$ | 2.3 (moderate) |
| Protein binding | 84% |
| Bioavailability | N/A |

| | |
|---|---|
| Blood half-life (principle blood-borne species) | Fentanyl 1–6 h |
| Effect of age and disease | Reduced clearance in elderly and in liver disease |
| Metabolism | Dealkylation, hydroxylation and deacylation |
| Metabolites | Norfentanyl and despropionylfentanyl |
| Active metabolites | None |
| Urinary excretion | Fentanyl 10–20% |
| Common doses | 50–200 µg intravenously |
| Blood concentrations | Usually less than 10 ng/mL |
| Postmortem artefacts | Unknown |

421

| | |
|---|---|
| Toxicity and abuse potential | Toxic, minimum lethal dose ~1–2 mg, fatal blood concentrations >0.2 ng/mL |
| Selected papers | Mather, 1983;[83] Bentley et al., 1982;[103] Henderson, 1991[104] |

# HYDROCODONE

| | |
|---|---|
| Class of drug and uses | Narcotic analgesic and antitussive |
| Availability and proprietary or code names | Vicodin combination tablet with paracetamol (acetaminophen), Hydrocet, Hycodan, Lorat, Lorcet, Lortab, Robidone, Tussionex, Vicoprofen, Zydone and others |
| Chemical form and solubility | Hydrated bitartrate salt, slightly soluble in water |

Properties
| | | |
|---|---|---|
| CAS | 125-29-1 | |
| MW | 299.4 | |
| pKa | | |
| $V_D$ | 3.3–4.7 /kg | |
| Cl | | |
| Log$_P$ | | |
| Protein binding | 25% | |
| Bioavailability | | |

| | |
|---|---|
| Blood half-life (principle blood-borne species) | Hydrocodone 3–9 h |
| Effect of age and disease | Likely small change with age and impaired liver function |
| Metabolism | O-Demethylation, N-demethylation and 6-keto reduction |
| Metabolites | Hydromorphone and others, including glucuronides |
| Active metabolites | Hydromorphone |
| Urinary excretion | Probably largely as glucuronides of demethylated and keto-reduced forms |
| Common doses | 5–10 mg every 4–6 h |
| Blood concentrations | Peak concentration 20–30 ng/mL after 10 mg, at 1.3 h |
| Postmortem artefacts | Likely to show small increase in blood concentration after death |
| Toxicity and abuse potential | Moderate to high, fatal blood concentrations >0.2 mg/L |
| Selected papers | Morrow and Faris, 1987;[105] Park et al., 1982[106] |

# LEVOMETHADYL ACETATE (LAAM)

| | |
|---|---|
| Class of drug and uses | Long-acting narcotic analgesic used in treatment of opioid dependence |
| Availability and proprietary or code names | Orlaam solution and others*, also known as acetylmethadol, LAAM, LAM |
| Chemical form and solubility | Hydrochloride salt, soluble in water acetyl derivative of a metabolite of methadone (methadol) |

Properties
| | |
|---|---|
| CAS | 1477-40-3 |
| MW | 353.5 |
| pKa | |
| $V_D$ | 20 L/kg |
| Cl | 3.7 mL/min/kg |
| Log$_P$ | 2.6 |
| Protein binding | |
| Bioavailability | |

| | | |
|---|---|---|
| Blood half-life (principle blood-borne species) | Levomethadyl acetate (LAAM) | 2–3 days |
| | NorLAAM | 2 days |
| | DinorLAAM | 4 days |
| Effect of age and disease | Unknown | |
| Metabolism | Demethylation (mono and di) | |
| Metabolites | NorLAAM, dinorLAAM | |
| Active metabolites | Both norLAAM and dinorLAAM more active | |
| Urinary excretion | | |
| Common doses | 60–100 mg 3 times weekly | |
| Blood concentrations | Peak concentration 0.02–0.15 (mean 0.06) mg/L at 4 h (50 mg), peak norLAAM concentration 0.06–0.19 mg/L, peak dinorLAAM concentration 0.06–0.12 mg/L | |
| Postmortem artefacts | Unknown, likely to be similar to methadone | |
| Toxicity and abuse potential | 20–40 mg toxic when first used, as for methadone | |
| Selected papers | Kaiko and Inturrisi, 1975;[107] Henderson et al., 1976[108] | |

---

* In some formulations naloxone is added to block the effects of the drug when given intravenously, in order to prevent abuse of LAAM. Oral consumption inactivates naloxone.

# Monographs of selected drugs

## LEVORPHANOL

| | | |
|---|---|---|
| Class of drug and uses | | Potent narcotic analgesic |
| Availability and proprietary or code names | | Levo-Dromoran injection and others |
| Chemical form and solubility | | As hydrated tartrate salt, soluble in water |

Properties
| | | |
|---|---|---|
| CAS | 77-07-6 | |
| MW | 257.4 | |
| pKa | 8.2 | |
| $V_D$ | 10–13 L/kg | |
| Cl | 13–18 mL/min/kg | |
| $Log_P$ | 1.1 | |
| Protein binding | 40% | |
| Bioavailability | Unknown | |

| | |
|---|---|
| Blood half-life (principle blood-borne species) | Levorphanol ~13 h |
| Effect of age and disease | Not likely to be affected greatly by advanced age, liver or kidney disease |
| Metabolism | 3-Glucuronidation |
| Metabolites | 3-Glucuronide |
| Active metabolites | None |
| Urinary excretion | Largely as 3-glucuronide |
| Common doses | 1 mg intravenously as slow infusion |
| Blood concentrations | 2 mg dose produces 5–10 ng/mL |
| | 20–50 mg dose produces 50–100 ng/mL |
| Postmortem artefacts | Unknown |
| Toxicity and abuse potential | High abuse potential, all doses toxic in opioid-naïve persons |

Selected papers

---

## METHADONE

| | |
|---|---|
| Class of drug and uses | Potent long-acting and orally active narcotic analgesic used for severe pain and for the treatment of opioid-dependent persons |
| Availability and proprietary or code names | Physeptone, Dolophine, Eptadone, Mephenon, Metasedin, Symoron, and other proprietary formulations |
| Chemical form and solubility | Available as hydrochloride salt, as tablets and as oral solution |

| Properties | | |
|---|---|---|
| CAS | 76-99-3 | |
| MW | 309.5 | |
| pKa | 8.6 | |
| $V_D$ | 3–5 L/kg | |
| Cl | 2 mL/min/kg | |
| Log$_P$ | 2.1 (moderate) | |
| Protein binding | 71–87% | |
| Bioavailability | 50% | |

$$CH_3CH_2-CO-\overset{\phantom{|}}{\underset{\phantom{|}}{|}}-CH_2CH(CH_3)N(CH_3)_2$$

| | | |
|---|---|---|
| Blood half-life (principle blood-borne species) | Methadone 15–72 h | |
| Effect of age and disease | Clearance reduced with age and with urine pH above 6 | |
| Metabolism | Demethylation and cyclization | |
| Metabolites | EDDP and EMDP (cyclized products), methadol | |
| Active metabolites | None with significant activity | |
| Urinary excretion | Methadone 5–50%  EDDP 3–25% | |
| Common doses | Range 10–120 mg daily, single dose | |
| Blood concentrations | Usual concentrations range to ~0.8 mg/L | |
| Postmortem artefacts | Moderately elevated in postmortem femoral blood | |
| Toxicity and abuse potential | Highly toxic in opioid-naïve persons, 20 mg can be fatal, fatal blood concentrations >0.1 mg/L; delayed onset of respiratory depression, high abuse potential | |
| Selected papers | Sawe, 1986;[109] Drummer et al., 1992;[110] Caplehorn and Drummer, 1999[111] | |

## MORPHINE

| | |
|---|---|
| Class of drug and uses | Potent narcotic analgesic used for relief of moderate to severe pain and associated anxiety, treatment of diarrhoea and dyspnoea associated with left ventricular failure and as an adjunct anaesthetic to surgery |
| Availability and proprietary or code names | Anamorph, Kapanol, Morphalgin, MS Contin, Ordine tablets and sustained release preparations and solutions for injection, Astramorph, Duramorph, Infumorph, Kadian, MSIR, Oramorph, RMS, Roxanol, and other proprietary products |

## Monographs of selected drugs

| | | |
|---|---|---|
| Chemical form and solubility | | Morphine is available as sulphate and hydrochloride salts, which are water soluble |

Properties
CAS         57-27-2 (anhydrous)
MW          303.4
pKa         7.95
$V_D$       1–6 L/kg
Cl          21 mL/min/kg
$Log_P$     Low
Protein binding 35%
Bioavailability 15–64%

| | | |
|---|---|---|
| Blood half-life (principle blood-borne species) | | Morphine 1–8 h |
| Effect of age and disease | | Clearance reduced with age, renal and liver disease |
| Metabolism | | Conjugation, demethylation |
| Metabolites | | N-Desmethyl, glucuronides at 3- and 6-positions |
| Active metabolites | | Normorphine and morphine-6-glucuronide |
| Urinary excretion | | Morphine 2–10%<br>M3G and M6G* 50–60% |
| Common doses | | Depends widely on need, 5–3000 mg daily |
| Blood concentrations | | Large range depending on dose, to 1000 ng/mL |
| Postmortem artefacts | | No significant change after death |
| Toxicity and abuse potential | | Highly toxic, fatal concentrations range from 0.01 mg/L; high abuse potential |
| Selected papers | | Glare and Walsh, 1991;[112] Osborne et al., 1990;[113] McQuay et al., 1990[114] |

* Morphine-3-glucuronide and 6-glucuronide.

## PETHIDINE (MEPERIDINE)

| | |
|---|---|
| Class of drug and uses | Potent short-acting narcotic analgesic used for the treatment of moderate to severe pain including labour pains and as an adjunct to anaesthesia |
| Availability and proprietary or code names | Pethidine 50 mg tablets and injection, Centraline, Demerol, Dolantin, Dolantina, Dolosal, Merpergan and others |
| Chemical form and solubility | Available as hydrochloride, soluble in water |

| Properties | | |
|---|---|---|
| CAS | 57-42-1 | |
| MW | 247.3 | |
| pKa | 8.6 | |
| $V_D$ | 3.7 L/kg | |
| Cl | 0.3 mL/min/kg | |
| $Log_P$ | 1.6 (moderate) | |
| Protein binding | 70% | |
| Bioavailability | 50% | |

| | | |
|---|---|---|
| Blood half-life (principle blood-borne species) | Pethidine | 2–6 h |
| | Norpethidine | 15–30 h |
| Effect of age and disease | Clearance halved in liver disease and acute viral hepatitis and in elderly, and reduced with basic urine | |
| Metabolism | N-Dealkylation and de-esterification | |
| Metabolites | Norpethidine and merperidinic acid | |
| Active metabolites | Norpethidine (acts also as a convulsive stimulant) | |
| Urinary excretion | Pethidine | 5–25% |
| | Norpethidine | 15–25% |
| | Meperidinic acid glucuronide | 40% |
| | Normeperidinic acid glucuronide | 20% |
| Common doses | 50 mg and higher, depending on need | |
| Blood concentrations | 100 mg s.d. oral dose produced $C_{max}$ of 0.17 mg/L at 1.3 h; 100 mg i.m. injection produced $C_{max}$ of 0.3 mg/L at 1 h, therapeutic to ~0.7 mg/L | |
| Postmortem artefacts | Possible slight elevation postmortem in femoral blood | |
| Toxicity and abuse potential | Toxic, particularly at blood concentrations >1.0 mg/L; norpethidine more toxic than parent; high abuse potential; designer analogues MPPP and MEPAP | |
| Selected papers | Edwards et al., 1982;[115] Clark et al., 1995[116] | |

## PROPOXYPHENE (DEXTROPROPOXYPHENE)

| | |
|---|---|
| Class of drug and uses | Weak orally active narcotic analgesic |
| Availability and proprietary or code names | Capadex, Digesic, Doloxene, Paradex tablets alone and with other drugs, Darvon, Dolene, Doxaphene, Wygesic and others |

# Monographs of selected drugs

| | |
|---|---|
| Chemical form and solubility | As hydrochloride and napsylate salt and is usually found in combination with paracetamol, (acetaminophen), aspirin and other drugs, soluble in water |

Properties
| | |
|---|---|
| CAS | 469-62-5 |
| MW | 339.5 |
| pKa | 6.3 |
| $V_D$ | 12–26 L/kg |
| Cl | 8–16 mL/min/kg |
| $Log_P$ | High |
| Protein binding | 78% |
| Bioavailability | 30–70% |

$$CH_3CH_2COO-C(CH_3)CH_2N(CH_3)_2$$

| | | |
|---|---|---|
| Blood half-life (principle blood-borne species) | Propoxyphene | 4–24 h |
| | Norpropoxyphene | 24–34 h |
| Effect of age and disease | Clearance reduced in elderly and in liver impairment | |
| Metabolism | N-Demethylation, de-esterification, hydroxylation and conjugation | |
| Metabolites | Norpropoxyphene and others | |
| Active metabolites | Norpropoxyphene (0.25–0.5 of parent) | |
| Urinary excretion | Propoxyphene | 1% |
| | Norpropoxyphene | 13% |
| Common doses | 128–390 mg as hydrochloride | |
| Blood concentrations | 130 mg s.d. produces $C_{max}$ 0.2 mg/L at 2 h; norpropoxyphene metabolite has $C_{max}$ of 0.3 mg/L at 4 h, chronic dosing produces accumulation of norpropoxyphene, steady-state levels 0.4 and 1.5 mg/L after ~200 mg daily | |
| Postmortem artefacts | Substantially increased postmortem, avoid central blood, smaller increases in femoral blood | |
| Toxicity and abuse potential | Highly toxic if abused, can be toxic at peripheral blood concentration >1.0 mg/L; medium abuse potential | |
| Selected papers | Young, 1983;[117] Pearson, 1984[118] | |

## OXYCODONE

| | |
|---|---|
| Class of drug and uses | Potent orally active narcotic analgesic used for treatment of moderate to severe pain |
| Availability and proprietary or code names | Endone, Proladone, Eubine, Eukodal, Oxycontin, OxyIR, Percodan, Percocet, Roxicodone, Supeudol, Tylox and others – tablets and suppositories |

| | |
|---|---|
| Chemical form and solubility | Available as hydrochloride, pectinate and terephthalate salts, soluble in water |

Properties
| | |
|---|---|
| CAS | 76-42-6 |
| MW | 315.4 |
| pKa | 8.9 |
| $V_D$ | 3 L/kg |
| Cl | 10 mL/min/kg |
| Log$_P$ | |
| Protein binding | 45% |
| Bioavailability | 60% (rectal) |
| | 80% (oral) |

| | |
|---|---|
| Blood half-life (principle blood-borne species) | Oxycodone 2–8 h |
| Effect of age and disease | Clearance reduced in renal disease and with advanced age |
| Metabolism | N- and O-demethylation and conjugation |
| Metabolites | Noroxycodone, oxymorphone |
| Active metabolites | Oxymorphone |
| Urinary excretion | Oxycodone and glucuronides 8–14% |
| Common doses | 30 mg suppositories 3 or 4 times daily; 5 mg tablet 4 times daily |
| Blood concentrations | 5 mg s.d. orally produces $C_{max}$ 0.02 (0.0089–0.037) mg/L at 1 h; 5 mg q.i.d. orally 4 days $C_{max}$ 0.016 mg/L |
| Postmortem artefacts | Possible slight elevation postmortem in femoral blood |
| Toxicity and abuse potential | Toxic at femoral blood concentrations > 0.2 mg/L; moderate abuse potential |
| Selected papers | Poyhia et al., 1991;[119] Leow et al., 1995[120] |

## OXYMORPHONE

| | |
|---|---|
| Class of drug and uses | Narcotic used as potent analgesic and to treat dyspnoea associated with left ventricular failure and pulmonary oedema |
| Availability and proprietary or code names | Numorphan |
| Chemical form and solubility | Hydrochloride salt, soluble in water |

## Monographs of selected drugs

| Properties | | |
|---|---|---|
| CAS | 76-41-5 | |
| MW | 301.3 | |
| pKa | 8.5, 9.3 | |
| $V_D$ | 2–3 L/kg | |
| Cl | | |
| Log$_P$ | Very low | |
| Protein binding | | |
| Bioavailability | | |
| Blood half-life (principle blood-borne species) | Oxymorphone | N/A |
| Effect of age and disease | N/A | |
| Metabolism | Conjugation and keto-reduction | |
| Metabolites | Glucuronides | |
| Active metabolites | Possibly 6-hydroxy oxymorphone | |
| Urinary excretion | Parent drug | <10% |
| | Oxymorphine glucuronide | 13–82% |
| | 6-Hydroxy metabolite | 0.1–3% |
| Common doses | 1–1.5 mg every 4–6 h intramuscularly or subcutaneously, or 5 mg rectally | |
| Blood concentrations | | |
| Postmortem artefacts | Unknown, but likely to be small | |
| Toxicity and abuse potential | High, potency 10-fold of morphine, lethal dose 50 mg | |
| Selected paper | Cone et al., 1983;[121] Hussain and Aungst, 1997[122] | |

## PENTAZOCINE

| | |
|---|---|
| Class of drug and uses | Narcotic analgesic with mixed agonist and antagonist activity, used as analgesic |
| Availability and proprietary or code names | Fortal, Fortral, Liticon, Fortalgesic, Pentafen, Talacen, Talwin, Sosenol and others |
| Chemical form and solubility | Hydrochloride salt soluble in water |

| Properties | |
|---|---|
| CAS | 359-83-1 |
| MW | 285.4 |
| pKa | 8.5, 10.0 |
| $V_D$ | 5.6 L/kg |
| Cl | 18 mL/min/kg |

| | |
|---|---|
| Log$_P$ | 2.0 |
| Protein binding | 60–70% |
| Bioavailability | 18% |
| Blood half-life (principle blood-borne species) | Pentazocine  1.5–10 h (mean 2.6 h) |
| Effect of age and disease | |
| Metabolism | Oxidation and conjugation |
| Metabolites | Carboxy metabolite of side chain, glucuronides |
| Active metabolites | Probably none |
| Urinary excretion | Pentazocine ~0.5–20% <br> Hydroxylated metabolite conjugates 10–30% |
| Common doses | 25 mg every 4 h, often combined with paracetamol (acetaminophen) or aspirin, up to 600 mg daily |
| Blood concentrations | 0.05–0.20 mg/L at 1 h (peak) |
| Postmortem artefacts | Unknown |
| Toxicity and abuse potential | Moderate abuse potential, minimum lethal dose ~300 mg, previously combined with tripelennamine (T's and Blues*), toxic at blood concentrations >0.2 mg/L |
| Selected papers | Bullingham et al., 1983;[87] Ehrnebo et al., 1977;[123] Polklis and Mackell, 1982;[124] Monforte et al., 1983[125] |

* In some formulations naloxone is added to block the effects of the drug when given intravenously, in order to prevent abuse. Oral consumption inactivates naloxone.

## REMIFENTANIL

| | |
|---|---|
| Class of drug and uses | Potent short-acting mu-opioid agonist used in surgery as an analgesic and anaesthetic and to supplement other anaesthetics |
| Availability and proprietary or code names | Ultra injection |
| Chemical form and solubility | Hydrochloride salt |

Properties

| | |
|---|---|
| CAS | 132875-61-7 |
| MW | 376.4 (base) |
| pKa | 7.07 |
| V$_D$ | 0.35 L/kg |
| Cl | 40 mL/min/kg |
| Log$_P$ | 1.2 |
| Protein binding | 70% |
| Bioavailability | N/A |

| | |
|---|---|
| Blood half-life (principle blood-borne species) | Remifentanil 10–20 min<br>Biological half-life 3–10 min |
| Effect of age and disease | Potency increases with advanced age, and liver dysfunction |
| Metabolism | Hydrolysis to carboxy form |
| Metabolites | Carboxy metabolite |
| Active metabolites | None known |
| Urinary excretion | Mainly as carboxy metabolite |
| Common doses | Initially 0.5–1.0 µg/kg/min, for 0.5–1 min, then reduced |
| Blood concentrations | Typically 1–3 ng/mL, following standard doses |
| Postmortem artefacts | Unknown |
| Toxicity and abuse potential | As for fentanyl |
| Selected papers | Servin, 1997;[126] Michelsen and Hug, 1996;[127] Patel and Spencer, 1996[128] |

## SULFENTANIL

| | |
|---|---|
| Class of drug and uses | Potent short-acting narcotic analgesic used in surgery as an analgesic and anaesthetic, and to supplement other anaesthetics |
| Availability and proprietary or code names | Available as parenteral solutions for injection; Sulfenta |
| Chemical form and solubility | Available as citrate salt |

Properties
CAS       56030-54-7
MW        396.7
pKa       8.0
$V_D$     2 L/kg
Cl        10 mL/min/kg
$Log_P$   3.2
Protein binding   92%
Bioavailability   N/A

| | |
|---|---|
| Blood half-life (principle blood-borne species) | Sulfentanil 2 h |
| Effect of age and disease | Clearance likely to decline with advancing age and liver dysfunction |
| Metabolism | N- and O-dealkylation |
| Metabolites | N-Desalkyl and O-desmethyl sulfentanil |

| | |
|---|---|
| Active metabolites | None with significant activity |
| Urinary excretion | 2% excreted unchanged in urine |
| Common doses | Variable doses depending on need, start at ~50 μg |
| Blood concentrations | Injection of 10 mg/kg dose gave a plasma concentration of 1 ng/mL at 60 min |
| Postmortem artefacts | Unknown, but likely to exhibit redistribution |
| Toxicity and abuse potential | Toxicity as for other opioids, therapeutic and toxic concentration overlap; high abuse potential |
| Selected papers | Mather, 1983;[83] Monk et al., 1988[129] |

## TRAMADOL

| | |
|---|---|
| Class of drug and uses | Central analgesic with low affinity for opioid receptors, used in treatment of moderate to severe pain |
| Availability and proprietary or code names | Tramal, Ultram |
| Chemical form and solubility | As hydrochloride, soluble in water |

Properties
CAS
MW 299.8 (HCl)
pKa 9.41
$V_D$ 2.6–2.9 L/kg
Cl
Log$_P$ 0.13
Protein binding 20%
Bioavailability 75%

| | |
|---|---|
| Blood half-life (principle blood-borne species) | Tramadol 5–7 h<br>M-1 metabolite 7 h |
| Effect of age and disease | Half-life increased with advanced age and loss of kidney and liver function |
| Metabolism | N- and O-demethylation, glucuronidation, sulphation |
| Metabolites | M-1 (O-desmethyl metabolite) |
| Active metabolites | M-1 metabolite |
| Urinary excretion | 30% excreted as unchanged drug |
| Common doses | 50–100 mg, up to 400 mg per day |
| Blood concentrations | Therapeutic to ~0.6 mg/L |
| Postmortem artefacts | Possibly small increases after death |

## Monographs of selected drugs

| | |
|---|---|
| Toxicity and abuse potential | Lower risk of respiratory depression to opioids, users do develop withdrawal symptoms on cessation, seizures are possible on misuse; minimum fatal dose uncertain |
| Selected papers | Lee et al., 1993;[130] Dayer et al., 1994[131] |

# Other monographs

## Δ⁹-TETRAHYDROCANNABINOL (THC)

| | |
|---|---|
| Class of drug and uses | Potent psychoactive component of cannabis used as an antiemetic |
| Availability and proprietary or code names | Dronabinol as Marinol (USA, available as oil-filled capsules, 2.5, 5.0 and 10 mg), also active component of cannabis |
| | Weed, grass, hemp, hashish, marijuana, marihuana, dagga |
| Chemical form and solubility | As Δ⁹-tetrahydrocannabinol in an oil base, insoluble in water, soluble in methanol and ethanol |

Properties
| | |
|---|---|
| CAS | 1972-08-3 |
| MW | 314.5 |
| pKa | Not ionized |
| $V_D$ | 9–11 L/kg |
| Cl | 14 mL/min/kg |
| $Log_P$ | High |
| Protein binding | 97–99% |
| Bioavailability | ~6% |

| | |
|---|---|
| Blood half-life (principle blood-borne species) | Δ⁹-Tetrahydrocannabinol  19–96 h (half-life shorter in regular users, average ~28 h) |
| Effect of age and disease | Unknown, likely to decrease with age and liver disease |
| Metabolism | Hydroxylation and oxidation with conjugation |
| Metabolites | 11-OH and 9-carboxy metabolites, 20 known metabolites |
| Active metabolites | 11-OH-Δ⁹-Tetrahydrocannabinol |
| Excretion | 30% in urine, 40% in faeces over several days |
| Common doses | 5–7.5 mg/m² every 3–4 h to 15 mg/m² |
| Blood concentrations | Range up to ~100 ng/mL |
| Postmortem artefacts | THC is likely to be redistributed |
| Toxicity and abuse potential | Low abuse potential, not regarded as capable of causing death, but can cause significant psychomotor and cognitive impairment, particularly with blood THC >2 ng/mL |
| Published reviews or papers on pharmacokinetics | Hunt and Jones, 1980;[132] Mason and McBay, 1985;[133] Nahas and Latour, 1992[134] |

# Monographs of selected drugs

## NABILONE

| | |
|---|---|
| Class of drug and uses | Synthetic cannabinoid used as an antiemetic, with anxiolytic activity |
| Availability and proprietary names | Cesamet (available as 1 mg capsules) |
| Chemical form and solubility | As $\Delta^9$-tetrahydrocannabinol in an oil base, insoluble in water, soluble in methanol and ethanol |

Properties
| | |
|---|---|
| CAS | 51022-71-0 |
| MW | 372.5 |
| pKa | Not ionized |
| $V_D$ | n/a |
| Cl | n/a |
| Log$_P$ | High |
| Protein binding | n/a |
| Bioavailability | n/a |

| | |
|---|---|
| Blood half-life (principle blood-borne species) | Nabilone 2 h |
| Effect of age and disease | Unknown, likely to decrease with age and liver disease |
| Metabolism | Probably oxidation with conjugation |
| Metabolites | Extensively metabolized |
| Active metabolites | Most likely |
| Excretion | Mainly through bile (70%) |
| Common doses | 1–2 mg every 6–12 h |
| Blood concentrations | Rapidly drop to below 1 ng/mL within 2 h |
| Postmortem artefacts | Unknown |
| Toxicity and abuse potential | Unknown |
| Published reviews or papers on pharmacokinetics | Rubin et al., 1977[135] |

## ETHANOL

| | |
|---|---|
| Class of drug and uses | Social drug with CNS depressant activity, and industrial and domestic solvent |
| Availability and common names | Widely available in alcoholic beverages, and as solvent in pharmaceuticals and many domestic products; alcohol, ethyl alcohol, grog, liquor, beers, spirits, wines and fortified wines |

# Other monographs

| | | |
|---|---|---|
| Chemical form and solubility | | Neutral molecule, liquid at room temperature, soluble in water in all proportions |
| Properties | | |
| CAS | 64-17-5 | |
| MW | 46.07 | |
| b.p. | 78.4°C | |
| pKa | None | |
| $V_D$ | 0.43 L/kg | |
| Cl | Concentration dependent | $CH_3CH_2OH$ |
| $Log_P$ | Distributed only to water compartment | |
| Protein binding | None | |
| Bioavailability | ~80% | |
| Blood elimination | | 0.012%/h in low alcohol consumers |
| | | 0.015%/h in medium consumers |
| | | 0.030%/h in alcoholics (heavy drinkers) |
| Effect of age and disease | | No significant effect on elimination, but body weight has appreciable effect for women and the elderly |
| Metabolism | | Oxidation and glucuronidation |
| Metabolites | | Metabolized to acetaldehyde, ethylglucuronide and carbon dioxide |
| Active metabolites | | None, but acetaldehyde toxic |
| Excretion | | Breath 0.7% |
| | | Urine 0.3% |
| | | Sweat 0.1% |
| Important doses | | Light drinkers <40 g ethanol per day |
| | | Medium drinkers From 40 to 80 g per day |
| | | Heavy drinkers >80 g ethanol per day |
| Blood concentrations | | 40 g ethanol peaks at 0.05% at ~60 min (men) |
| | | 30 g ethanol peaks at 0.05% at ~60 min (women) |
| Breath:blood ratios | | Expired air to blood ratio usually 2000–2800 : 1 |
| Postmortem artefacts | | Postmortem putrefaction capable of producing BAC levels greater than 0.2%, volatile chemical and therefore likely to dissipate |
| Toxicity and abuse potential | | Moderate to high abuse potential |
| Published reviews or papers on pharmacokinetics | | Holford, 1987;[136] Baselt, 1996;[137] Wilkinson, 1980[138] |

437

# LYSERGIC ACID DIETHYLAMIDE (LSD)

| | |
|---|---|
| Class of drug and uses | Hallucinogen, no current medical uses |
| Availability and proprietary or code names | Street drug sold as tabs, or tickets as paper impregnated with drug, soft-gel capsules, etc. Street names include acid, trip, mellow, tabs, blotters, dots, tickets, microdots, etc.; also known as lysergide |
| Chemical form and solubility | Soluble in water |

Properties
| | |
|---|---|
| CAS | 50-37-3 |
| MW | 323.4 |
| pKa | 7.5 |
| $V_D$ | 0.3 L/kg |
| Cl | |
| $Log_P$ | 3.0 |
| Protein binding | 90% |
| Bioavailability | Moderate to high |

| | |
|---|---|
| Blood half-life (principle blood-borne species) | LSD 2–6 h |
| Effect of age and disease | Unknown but likely to be affected |
| Metabolism | N-Dealkylation, oxidation, hydroxylation and glucuronidation |
| Metabolites | N-Desmethyl, desethyl, 2-oxo-3-hydroxy metabolites |
| Active metabolites | None |
| Urinary excretion | <1% excreted as unchanged drug |
| Common doses | 25–300 µg |
| Blood concentrations | Usually much less than 10 ng/mL |
| Postmortem artefacts | Unknown, but likely to undergo redistribution |
| Toxicity and abuse potential | Potent hallucinogen, low to moderate abuse potential |
| Selected papers | Aghajanian and Bing, 1964;[139] Upsall and Wailling, 1972;[140] Wagner et al., 1968;[141] Paul and Smith, 1999[142] |

# PHENCYCLIDINE

| | |
|---|---|
| Class of drug and uses | Hallucinogen, illicit drug |
| Availability and proprietary or code names | Not available readily in most jurisdictions, known as PCP; street names include angel dust, busy bee, cadillac, CJ, crystal, elephant tranquillizer, hog, peace, snorts, T, etc. |

## Other monographs

| | |
|---|---|
| Chemical form and solubility | Often as hydrochloride, soluble in water |
| Properties | |
| CAS | 77-10-1 |
| | 956-90-1 (HCl) |
| MW | 243.4 |
| pKa | 8.5 |
| $V_D$ | 5–8 L/kg |
| Cl | 0.14–0.77 L/min |
| Log$_P$ | |
| Protein binding | 60–80% |
| Bioavailability | 72% |
| Blood half-life (principle blood-borne species) | PCP  7–46 h |
| Effect of age and disease | Affected by pH of urine |
| Metabolism | Hydroxylation and glucuronidation |
| Metabolites | 4-Hydroxypiperidine and 4-cyclohexanol metabolites |
| Active metabolites | None |
| Urinary excretion | 4–19% as PCP, remainder largely as conjugates, affected by dose and acidity of urine |
| Common doses | 1–10 mg |
| Blood concentrations | Range to ~0.2 mg/L in active users |
| Postmortem artefacts | Not known |
| Toxicity and abuse potential | Highly toxic, levels greater than ~0.3 mg/L may cause death |
| Selected papers | Cook et al., 1982;[143] Cook et al., 1982;[144] Burns and Lerner, 1978[145] |

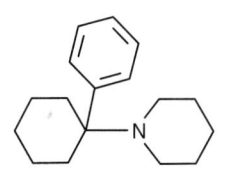

## KETAMINE

| | |
|---|---|
| Class of drug and uses | Induction agent for anaesthesia, and occasionally used recreationally |
| Availability and proprietary or code names | Ketaject, Ketalar, etc. as solution for injection Street names for ketamine include Special K, KitKat, vitamin K, K and ket |
| Chemical form and solubility | As hydrochloride salt, ketamine is also commonly cut with cocaine, amphetamine, LSD and heroin |

439

# Monographs of selected drugs

| Properties | | |
|---|---|---|
| CAS | 6740-88-1 | |
| | 1867-66-9 (HCl) | |
| MW | 237.7 | |
| pKa | 7.5 | |
| $V_D$ | 3–5 L/kg | |
| Cl | 17 mL/min/kg | |
| $Log_P$ | High | |
| Protein binding | 20–50% | |
| Bioavailability | Reasonable | |
| Blood half-life (principle blood-borne species) | | Ketamine 2–4 h |
| Effect of age and disease | | Likely to be similar to other amines |
| Metabolism | | Dealkylation, hydroxylation, conjugation |
| Metabolites | | Norketamine, hydroxyl metabolites and glucuronides |
| Active metabolites | | Norketamine weakly active |
| Urinary excretion | | 2% excreted unchanged |
| | | 2% norketamine |
| | | 16% dehydronorketamine |
| | | 80% conjugates |
| Common doses | | 1–4.5 mg/kg i.v. or 6.5–13 mg/kg i.m. |
| Blood concentrations | | May reach 6 mg/L in anaesthetic doses; plasma concentrations 1 h after 2 and 6 mg/kg doses are about 0.5 and 1.4 mg/L[146] |
| Postmortem artefacts | | Unknown |
| Toxicity and abuse potential | | Low to moderate toxicity, fatalities from 7 mg/L in absence of other factors |
| Selected papers | | Licata et al., 1994;[147] Moore et al., 1997;[148] Dalgarno and Shewan, 1996;[149] White et al., 1982[150] |

## GAMMA-HYDROXYBUTYRATE (GHB)

| | |
|---|---|
| Class of drug and uses | Illicit drug used in date rape; also limited clinical use for narcolepsy and to treat alcohol withdrawal syndrome |
| Availability and proprietary or code names | As liquid, powder or capsules |
| | Street names include easy lay, fantasy, georgia home boy, G, grievous bodily harm or GBH, G-Riffick, liquid ecstasy, liquid X, nature's quaalude and scoop |

| | |
|---|---|
| | Can be produced from 1,4-butanediol (Thunder nectar, FX), tetramethylene glycol (NRG3), and γ-butyrolactone (GBL) |
| Chemical form and solubility | Soluble in water |
| Properties | |
| CAS | 502-85-2 (Na salt) |
| MW | 104.12 |
| pKa | |
| $V_D$ | |
| Cl | |
| $Log_P$ | |
| Protein binding | |
| Bioavailability | |
| Blood half-life (principle blood-borne species) | GHB  <1 h |
| Effect of age and disease | Unknown |
| Metabolism | Oxidation, and metabolism through Krebs cycle |
| Metabolites | Succinic semi-aldehyde and succinic acid |
| Active metabolites | None |
| Urinary excretion | Rapidly excreted as unchanged drug, <5% unchanged |
| Common doses | 200 mg to 2 g |
| Blood concentrations | Usually <150 mg/L |
| Postmortem artefacts | GHB produced postmortem in blood up to ~50 mg/L, but not in urine |
| Toxicity and abuse potential | Low to moderate toxicity |
| Selected paper | Logan and Couper, 2000[151] |

# References for Appendix

1. Rowland M. Amphetamine blood and urine levels in man. *J Pharmaceut Sci* 1969; 58: 508–9.
2. Angrist B, Corwin J, Bartlik B, Cooper T. Early pharmacokinetics and clinical effects of oral d-amphetamine in normal subjects. *Biol Psychiat* 1987; 22(11): 1357–68.
3. Smith-Kielland A, Skuterud B, Mørland J. Urinary excretion of amphetamine after termination of drug abuse. *J Anal Toxicol* 1997; 21: 325–9.
4. Widler P, Mathys K, Brenneisen R, et al. Pharmacodynamics and pharmacokinetics of khat: a controlled study. *Clin Pharmacol Therapeut* 1994; 55(5): 556–62.
5. Mathys K, Brenneisen R. Determination of (S)-(−)cathinone and its metabolites (RS)-(−)norephedrine and (R,R)-(−)norpseudoephedrine in urine by high-performance liquid chromatography with photodiode array detection. *J Chromatogr* 1992; 593: 1–2.
6. Kalix P, Geisshusler S, Brenneisen R, Koelbing U, Fisch HU. Cathinone, a phenylpropylamine alkaolid from khat leaves that has amphetamine effects in humans. *NIDA Res Monogr* 1991; 105: 289–90.
7. Testa B, Beckett AH. Metabolism and excretion of diethylpropion in man under acidic conditions. *J Pharm Pharmacol* 1973; 25: 119–24.
8. Mihailova M, Rosen A, Testa B, Beckett AH. A pharmacokinetic investigation of the distribution and elimination of diethylpropion and its metabolites in man. *J Pharm Pharmacol* 1974; 26: 711–21.
9. Wright GJ, Lang JF, Lemieux RE, Goodfriend MJJ. The objective and timing of drug disposition studies, appendix III. Diethylpropion and its metabolites in the blood plasma of the human after subcutaneous and oral administration. *Drug Metab Rev* 1975; 4: 267–76.
10. Roxanas MG, Spaulding J. Ephedrine abuse psychosis. *Med J Austr* 1977; 2: 639–40.
11. Wilkinson GR, Beckett AH. Absorption, metabolism and excretion of ephedrine in man. I. *J Pharm Exp Ther* 1968; 162: 139–47.
12. Campbell DB. Gas chromatographic measurement of levels of fenfluramine and norfenfluramine in human plasma, red cells and urine following therapeutic doses. *J Chromatogr B* 1970; 49: 442–7.
13. Fleisher MR, Campbell DB. Fenfluramine overdosage. *Lancet* 1969: 1306–7.
14. Mark EJ, Patalas ED, Chang HT, Evans RJ, Kessler SC. Fatal pulmonary hypertension associated with short-term use of fenfluramine and phentermine. *N Engl J Med* 1997; 337(9): 602–6.
15. Cook CE, Jeffcoat AR, Hill JM, Pugh DE, Patetta PK, Sadler BM, et al. Pharmacokinetics of methamphetamine self-administered to human subjects by smoking S-(+)-methamphetamine hydrochloride. *Drug Metab Dispos* 1993; 21(4): 717–23.

# References

16. Maurer HH. On the metabolism and the toxicological analysis of methylenedioxyphenylalkylamine designer drugs by gas chromatography-mass spectrometry. *Therapeut Drug Monit* 1996; 18: 465–70.
17. Kunsman GW, Levine B, Kuhlman JJ, Jones RL, Hughes RO, Fujiyama CI, et al. MDA–MDMA concentrations in urine specimens. *J Anal Toxicol* 1996; 20(7): 517–21.
18. Valentine JL, Kearns GL, Sparks C, Letzig LG, Valentine CR, Shappell SA, et al. GC-MS determination of amphetamine and methamphetamine in human urine for 12 hours following oral administration of dextro-methamphetamine: lack of evidence supporting the established forensic guidelines for methamphetamine confirmation. *J Anal Toxicol* 1995; 19(7): 581–90.
19. Hungrund BL, Perel JM, Hurvic MJ, et al. Pharmacokinetics of methylphenidate in hyperkinetic children. *Br J Clin Pharmacol* 1979; 8: 571–6.
20. Levine B, Caplan YH, Kauffman G. Fatality resulting from methylphenidate overdose. *J Anal Toxicol* 1986; 10: 209–10.
21. Felgate HE, Felgate PD, James RA, Sims DN, Vozzo DC. Recent paramethoxyamphetamine deaths. *J Anal Toxicol* 1998; 22: 169–72.
22. Byard RW, Gilbert J, James R, Lokan RJ. Amphetamine derivative fatalities in South Australia – is 'Ecstasy' the culprit? *Am J Forens Med Pathol* 1998; 19(3): 261–5.
23. Groenewoud G, Schall R, Hundt HKL, Muller FO, van Dyk M. Steady-state pharmacokinetics of phentermine extended-release capsules. *Internat J Clin Pharmacol Ther Toxicol* 1993; 31: 368–72.
24. Hinsvark ON, Truant AP, Jenden DJ, Steinborn JA. The oral bioavailability and pharmacokinetics of soluble and resin-bound forms of amphetamine and phentermine in man. *J Pharmacokinet Biopharm* 1973; 1: 319–28.
25. Kuntzman RG, Tsai I, Brand L, Mark LC. The influence of urinary pH on the half-life of pseudoephedrine in man and dog and a sensitive assay for its determination in human plasma. *Clin Pharmacol Therapeut* 1971; 12: 62–7.
26. Lin ET, Brater DC, Benet LZ. Gas–liquid determination of pseudoephedrine and norpseudoephedrine in human plasma and urine. *J Chromatogr B* 1977; 140: 275–9.
27. Barnett G, Hawks R, Resnick R. Cocaine pharmacokinetics in humans. *J Ethnopharmacol* 1981; 3: 353–66.
28. Cone EJ. Pharmacokinetics and pharmacodynamics of cocaine. *J Anal Toxicol* 1995; 19(6): 459–78.
29. Wilkinson P, van Dyke C, Jatlow P, Barash P, Byck R. Intranasal and oral cocaine kinetics. *Clin Pharmacol Therapeut* 1980; 27: 386–94.
30. Isenschmid DS, Fischman MW, Foltin RW, Caplan YH. Concentration of cocaine and metabolites in plasma of humans following intravenous administration and smoking of cocaine. *J Anal Toxicol* 1992; 16: 311–14.
31. Fleishaker JC, Friedman H, Pollock SR, Smith TC. Clinical pharmacology of adinazolam and N-desmethyladinazolam mesylate after single oral doses of each compound in healthy volunteers. *CPT* 1990; 48: 652–64.
32. Fleishaker JC, Hulst LK, Ekernas S-A, Grahen A. Pharmacokinetics and pharmacodynamics of adinazolam and N-desmethyladinazolam after oral and intravenous dosing

in healthy, young and elederly volunteers. *J Clin Psychopharmacol* 1992; 12(6): 403–14.
33. Fleishaker JC, Smith TC, Friedman H, Phillips JP. N-desmethyladinazolam pharmacokinetics and behavioral effects following administration of 10–50 mg oral doses in healthy volunteers. *Psychopharmacology* 1991; 105: 181–5.
34. Greenblatt DG, Wright CE. Clinical pharmacokinetics of alprazolam. *Clin Pharmacokinet* 1993; 24(6): 453–71.
35. Garzone PD, Kroboth PD. Pharmacokinetics of the newer benzodiazepines. *Clin Pharmacokinet* 1989; 16: 337–64.
36. Greenblatt DJ. Benzodiazepine hypnotics: sorting the pharmacokinetic facts. *J Clin Psychiat* 1991; 52(9, suppl.): 4–10.
37. Baselt RC, Cravey RH. *Disposition of toxic drugs and chemicals in man*, 3rd edn. Foster City, CA: Year Book Medical Publishers; 1990.
38. Langley MS, Clissold SP. Brotizolam. A review of its pharmacodynamic and pharmacokinetic properties, and therapeutic efficacy as an hypnotic. *Drugs* 1988; 35(2): 104–22.
39. Greenblatt DJ, Shader RI, MacLeod SM, Sellers EM. Clinical pharmacokinetics of chlordiazepoxide. *Clin Pharmacokinet* 1978; 3(5): 381–94.
40. Brogden RN, Heel RC, Speight TM, Avery GS. *Drugs* 1980; 20: 161–78.
41. Greenblatt DJ, Miller LG, Shader RI. Clonazepam pharmacokinetics, brain uptake, and receptor interactions. *J Clin Psychiat* 1987; 48: 4–11.
42. De Vane CL, Ware MR, Lydiard RB. Pharmacokinetics, pharmacodynamics, and treatment issues of benzodiazepines: alprazolam, adinazolam, and clonazepam. *Psychopharmacol Bull* 1991; 27(4): 463–73.
43. Hvidberg EF, Dam M. Clinical pharmacokinetics of anticonvulsants. *Clin Pharmacokinet* 1976; 1(3): 161–88.
44. United Nations. Recommended methods for the detection and assay of barbiturates and benzodizepines in biological specimens. New York: United Nations; 1997.
45. Kaplan SA, Jack ML, Alexander K, Weinfeld RE. Pharmacokinetic profile of diazepam in man following single intravenous and oral and chronic oral administrations. *J Pharmaceut Sci* 1973; 62(11): 1789–96.
46. Mandelli M, Tognoni G, Garattini S. *Clin Pharmacokinet* 1978; 3: 72–91.
47. Fracasso C, Confalonieri S, Garaatini S, Caccia S. Single and multiple dose pharmacokinetics of etizolam in healthy subjects. *Eur J Clin Pharmacol* 1991; 40: 181–5.
48. Mattila MA, Larni HM. Flunitrazepam: a review of its pharmacological properties and therapeutic use. *Drugs* 1980; 20(5): 353–74.
49. Woods JH, Winger G. Abuse liability of flunitrazepam. *J Clin Psychopharmacol* 1997; 17(3, suppl. 2): 1S–57S.
50. Aderjan R, Mattern R. Eine toedlich verlaufene monointoxikation mit Flurazepam (Dalmadorm). *Arch Toxicol* 1979; 43: 69–75.
51. Greenblatt DJ. Pharmacology of benzodiazepine hypnotics. *J Clin Psychiat* 1992; 53 (6, suppl.): 7–13.

52. Miller LG, Greenblatt DJ, Abernathy DR, Friedman H, Luu MD, Paul SM, et al. Kinetics, brain uptake, and receptor binding characteristics of flurazepam and its metabolites. *Psychopharmacology* 1988; 94: 386–91.
53. Swift CG, Swift MR, Ankier SI, Pidgen A, Robinson J. Single dose pharmacokinetics and pharmacodynamics of oral loprazolam in the elderly. *Br J Clin Pharmacol* 1985; 20(2): 119–28.
54. Clark BG, Jue SG, Dawson GW, Ward A. Loprazolam: a review of its pharmacodynamic and pharmacokinetic properties and therapeutic efficacy in insomnia. *Drugs* 1986; 31: 500–16.
55. Greenblatt DJ. Clinical pharmacokinetics of oxazepam and lorazepam. *Clin Pharmacokinet* 1981; 6: 89–105.
56. Martindale W. *Martindale's: the complete drug reference*, 32nd edn. London: Pharmaceutical Press; 1999.
57. Seppala M, Alihanka J, Himberg JJ, Kanto J, Rajala T, Sourander L. Midazolam and flunitrazepam: pharmacokinetics and effects on night time respiration and body movements in the elderly. *Internat J Clin Pharmacol Ther Toxicol* 1993; 31(4): 170–6.
58. Kangas L, Iisalo E, Kanto J, Lehtinen V, Pynnonen S, Ruikka I, et al. Human pharmacokinetics of nitrazepam: effect of age and diseases. *Eur J Clin Pharmacol* 1979; 15(3): 163–70.
59. Jochemsen R, Van Beusekom BR, Spoelstra P, Janssens AR, Breimer DD. Effect of age and liver cirrhosis on the pharmacokinetics of nitrazepam. *Br J Clin Pharmacol* 1983; 15(3): 295–302.
60. Ochs HR, Oberem U, Greenblatt DJ. Nitrazepam clearance unimpaired in patients with renal insufficiency. *J Clin Psychopharmacol* 1992; 12(3): 183–5.
61. Greenblatt DJ, Shader RI, Divoll M, Harmatz JS. *Br J Clin Pharmacol* 1981; 11: 11S–16S.
62. Pacifici GM, Placidi GF, Fornaro P, Gomeni R. Pharmacokinetics of pinazepam in healthy volunteers. *Internat J Clin Pharmacol Res* 1983; 3(5): 331–7.
62a. Allen MD, Greenblatt DJ, Harmatz JS, Shader RI. Single-dose kinetics of prazepam, a precursor of desmethyldiazepam. *J Clin Pharmacol* 1979; 19: 445–50.
63. Sonne J, Loft S, Dossing M, Vollmer-Larsen A, Olesen KL, Victor M, et al. Bioavailability and pharmacokinetics of oxazepam. *Eur J Clin Pharmacol* 1988; 35: 385–9.
64. Ayd FJ, Jr. Oxazepam: update 1989. *Internat Clin Psychopharmacol* 1990; 5(1): 1–15.
65. Ankier SI, Goa KL. Quazepam. *Drugs* 1988; 35: 42–62.
66. Kales A. Quazepam: hypnotic efficacy and side effects. *Pharmacotherapy* 1990; 10(1): 1–12.
67. Heel RC, Brogden RN, Speight TM, Avery GS. *Drugs* 1981; 21: 321–40.
68. Pakes GE, Brogden RN, Heel RC, Speight TM, Avery GS. Triazolam: a review of its pharmacological properties and therapeutic efficacy in patients with insomnia. *Drugs* 1981; 22(2): 81–110.
69. Dalhoff K, Poulsen HE, Garred P, Placchi M, Gammans RE, Mayol RF, et al. Buspirone pharmacokinetics in patients with cirrhosis. *Br J Clin Pharmacol* 1987; 24: 547–50.
70. Goldberg ME, Salama AI, Patel JB, Malick JB. Novel non-benzodiazepine anxiolytics. *Neuropharmacology* 1983; 22(12B): 1499–504.

71. Napoliello MJ, Domantay AG. Buspirone: a worldwide update. *Br J Psychiat.* 1991; 12(suppl.): 40–4.
72. Sanger DJ, Benavides J, Perrault G, Morel E, Cohen C, Joly D, et al. Recent developments in the behavioural pharmacology of benzodiazepine (w) receptors: evidence for the functional significance of receptor subtypes. *Neurosci Biohav Rev* 1994; 18(3): 355–72.
73. Rush CR, Frey JM, Griffiths RR. Zaleplon and triazolam in humans: acute behavioral effects and abuse potential. *Psychopharmacology* 1999; 145(1): 39–51.
74. Rosen AS, Fournie P, Darwish M, Danjou P, Troy SM. Zaleplon pharmacokinetics and absolute bioavailability. *Biopharm Drug Dispos* 1999; 20(3): 171–5.
75. Houghton GW, Dennis MJ, Templeton R, Martin BK. A repeated dose pharmacokinetic study of a new hypnotic agent, zopiclone (Imovane). *J Clin Pharmacol Ther Toxicol* 1985; 23(2): 97–100.
76. Hempel G, Blaschke G. Enantioselective determination of zopiclone and its metabolites in urine by capillary electrophoresis. *J Chromatogr B Biomed Appl* 1996; 675(1): 139–46.
77. Goa KL, Heel RC. Zopiclone. A review of its pharmacodynamic and pharmacokinetic properties and therapeutic efficacy as an hypnotic. *Drugs* 1986; 32: 48–65.
78. Wadworth AN, McTavish D. Zopiclone. A review of its pharmacological properties and therapeutic efficacy as an hypnotic. *Drugs Aging* 1993; 3(5): 441–59. [Published erratum appears in *Drugs Aging* 1994; 4(1): 62.]
79. Salva P, Costa J. Clinical pharmacokinetics and pharmacodynamics of zolpidem. Therapeutic implications. *Clin Pharmacokinet* 1995; 29(3): 142–53.
80. Langtry HD, Benfield P. Zolpidem. A review of its pharmacodynamic and pharmacokinetic properties and therapeutic potential. *Drugs* 1990; 40(2): 291–313.
81. Breimer DD. Clinical pharmacology of hypnotics. *Clin Pharmacokinet* 1977; 2: 93–109.
82. Robinson AE, McDowell RD. The distribution of amylobarbitone, butobarbitone, pentobarbitone, and quinalbarbitone and the hydroxylated metbaolites in man. *J Pharm Pharmacol* 1979; 31: 357–65.
83. Mather LE. Clinical pharmacokinetics of fentanyl and its derivatives. *Clin Pharmacokinet* 1983; 8: 422–46.
84. Rubio A, Cox C. Sex, age and alfentanil pharmacokinetics. *Clin Pharmacokinet* 1991; 21: 81.
85. Reynaud M, Petit G, Potard D, Couty P. Six deaths linked to concomitant use of buprenorphine and benzodiazepines. *Addiction* 1998; 93(9): 1385–92.
86. Tracqui A, Ludes B. Buprenorphine-related deaths among drug addicts in France: a report on 20 fatalities. *J Anal Toxicol* 1998; 22: 430–4.
87. Bullingham RE, McQuay HJ, Moore RA. Clinical pharmacokinetics of narcotic agonist–antagonist drugs. *Clin Pharmacokinet* 1983; 8: 332–43.
88. Bullingham RE, McQuay HJ, Porter EJ, Allen MC, Moore RA. Sublingual buprenorphine used postoperatively: ten hour plasma drug concentration analysis. *Br J Clin Pharmacol* 1982; 13: 665–73.
89. Strang J. Abuse of buprenorphine. *Lancet* 1985; ii: 725.

90. Vogelsang J, Hayes SR. Butorphanol tartrate (stadol): a review. *J Post Anesth Nurs* 1991; 6(2): 129–35.
91. Gillis JC, Benfield P, Goa KL. Transnasal butorphanol. A review of its pharmacodynamic and pharmacokinetic properties, and therapeutic potential in acute pain management. *Drugs* 1995; 50(1): 157–75.
92. Gerostamoulos J, Burke MP, Drummer OH. Involvement of codeine in drug-related deaths. *Am J Forens Med Pathol* 1996; 17(4): 327–35.
93. Lafolie P, Beck O, Lin Z, Albertioni F, Boreus L. Urine and plasma pharmacokinetics of codeine in healthy volunteers: implications for drugs-of-abuse testing. *J Anal Toxicol* 1996; 20: 541–6.
94. Kintz P, Tracqui A, Mangin P, Lugnier AA, Chaumont AJ. Fatal intoxication by dextromoramide: a report on two cases. *J Anal Toxicol* 1989; 13(4): 238–9.
95. Pagani I, Barzaghi N, Crema F, Perucca E, Ego D, Rovei V. Pharmacokonetics of dextromoramide in surgical patients. *Fundam Clin Pharmacol* 1989; 3(1): 27–35.
96. Ufkes JG, de Vos JW, van Brussel GH. Determination and pharmacokinetics of dextromoramide in methadone maintenance therapy. *Pharm World Sci* 1998; 20(2): 83–7.
97. O'Brien JJ, Benfield P. Dezocine. *Drugs* 1989; 38(2): 226–8.
98. Rowell FJ, Seymour RA, Rawlins MD. Pharmacokinetics of intravenous and oral dihydrocodeine and its acid metabolites. *Eur J Clin Pharmacol* 1983; 25: 419–24.
99. Peat MA, Sengupta A. Toxicological investigations of cases of death involving codeine and dihydrocodeine. *Forens Sci Internat* 1977; 9: 21–32.
100. Aasmundstad TA, Xu BQ, Johannson I, Ripel A, Bjørneboe A, Christophersen AS, et al. Biotransformation and pharmacokinetics of ethylmorphine after a single oral dose. *Br J Clin Pharmacol* 1995; 39: 611–20.
101. Cone EJ, Welch P, Mitchell JM, Paul BD. Forensic drug testing for opiates: I. Detection of 6-acetylmorphine in urine as an indicator of recent heroin exposure; drug and assay considerations and detection times. *J Anal Toxicol* 1991; 15(1): 1–7.
102. Boerner U. The metabolism of morphine and heroin in man. *Drug Metab Rev* 1975; 4: 39–73.
103. Bentley JB, Borel JD, Nenand REJ, Gillespie TJ. Age and fentanyl pharmacokinetics. *Anaesthet Analges* 1982; 61: 968–71.
104. Henderson G. Fentanyl-related deaths: demographics, circumstances, and toxicology of 112 cases. *J Forens Sci* 1991; 236: 422–33.
105. Morrow PL, Faris EC. Death associated with inadvertant hydrocodone overdose in a child with a respiratory tract infection. *Am J Forens Med Pathol* 1987; 8(1): 60–3.
106. Park JI, Nakamura GR, Griesemer EC, Noguchi TT. Hydromorphone detected in bile following hydrocodone ingestion. *J Forens Sci* 1982; 27(1): 223–4.
107. Kaiko RF, Inturrisi CE. Disposition of acetylmethadol in relation to pharmacologic action. *Clin Pharmacol Therapeut* 1975; 18(1): 96–103.
108. Henderson GL, Wilson K, Lau DHM. Plasma l-a-acetylmethadol (LAAM) after acute and chronic administration. *Clin Pharmacol Therapeut* 1976; 21(1): 16–25.
109. Sawe J. High-dose morphine and methadone in cancer patients: clinical pharmacokinetic considerations of oral treatment. *Clin Pharmacokinet* 1986; 11: 87–106.

110. Drummer OH, Opeskin K, Syrjanen M, Cordner SM. Methadone toxicity causing death in ten subjects starting on a methadone maintenance program. *Am J Forens Med Pathol* 1992; 13(4): 346–50.
111. Caplehorn J, Drummer OH. Mortality associated with the NSW methadone program: lives lost and saved. *Med J Australia* 1999; 170: 104–9.
112. Glare PA, Walsh TD. Clinical pharmacokinetics of morphine: a review. *Therapeut Drug Monit* 1991; 13: 1–23.
113. Osborne R, Joel S, Trew D, Slevin M. Morphine and metabolite behaviour after different routes of administration: demonstration of the importance of the active metabolite morphine 6-glucuronide. *Clin Pharmacol Therapeut* 1990; 47: 12–19.
114. McQuay HJ, Carroll D, Faura CC, Cavaghan DJ, Hand CW. Oral morphine in cancer pain: influences on morphine and metabolite concentration. *Clin Pharmacol Therapeut* 1990; 48: 236–44.
115. Edwards DJ, Svensson CK, Visco JP, Lalka D. Clinical pharmacokinetics of pethidine: 1982. *Clin Pharmacokinet* 1982; 7: 421–33.
116. Clark RF, Wei EM, Anderson PO. Merperidine: therapeutic use and toxicity. *J Emerg Med* 1995; 13: 797–802.
117. Young RJ. Dextropropoxyphene overdosage. Pharmacological considerations and clinical management. *Drugs* 1983; 26: 70–9.
118. Pearson RM. Pharmacokinetics of propoxyphene. *Hum Toxicol* 1984; 3(suppl.): 37S–40S.
119. Poyhia R, Olkkola KT, Seppala T, Kalso E. The pharmacokinetics of oxycodone after intravenous injection in adults. *Br J Clin Pharmacol* 1991; 32: 516–18.
120. Leow KP, Cramond T, Smith MT. Pharmacokinetics and pharmacodynamics of oxycodone when given intravenously and rectally to adult patients with cancer pain. *Anaesthet Analges* 1995; 80: 296–302.
121. Cone EJ, Darwin WD, Buchwald WF, Gorodetzky CW. Oxymorphone metabolism and urinary excretion in human, rat, guinea pig, rabbit, and dog. *Drug Metab Dispos* 1983; 11(5): 446–50.
122. Hussain MA, Aungst BJ. Intranasal absorption of oxymorphone. *J Pharm Sci* 1997; 86(8): 975–6.
123. Ehrnebo M, Boreus LO, Loenroth U. Bioavailability and first pass metabolism of oral pentazocine in man. *Clin Pharmacol Therapeut* 1977; 22(6): 888–92.
124. Polklis A, Mackell MA. Pentazocine and tripelennamine (T's and Blues) abuse: toxicological findings in 39 cases. *J Anal Toxicol* 1982; 6: 109–14.
125. Monforte JR, Gault R, Smialek J, Goodin T. Toxicological and pathological findings in fatalities involving pentazocine and tripelennamine. *J Forens Sci* 1983; 28(1): 90–101.
126. Servin F. Remifentanil: when and how to use it. *Eur J Anaesthesiol* suppl. 1997; 15: 41–4.
127. Michelsen LG, Hug CC, Jr. The pharmacokinetics of remifentanil. *J Clin Anesth* 1996; 8(8): 679–82.
128. Patel SS, Spencer CM. Remifentanil. *Drugs* 1996; 52(3): 417–27; discussion 428.
129. Monk JP, Beresford R, Ward A. Sufentanil: a review of its pharmacological properties and therapeutic use. *Drugs* 1988; 36: 286–313.

130. Lee CR, McTavish D, Sorkin EM. Tramadol. A preliminary review of its pharmacodynamic and pharmacokinetic properties, and therapeutic potential in acute and chronic pain states. *Drugs* 1993; 46(2): 313–40.
131. Dayer P, Collart L, Desmeules J. The pharmacology of tramadol. *Drugs* 1994; 47(suppl.) 1: 3–7.
132. Hunt CA, Jones RT. Tolerance and disposition of tetrahydrocannabinol in man. *J Pharmacol Exp Therapeut* 1980; 215: 35–44.
133. Mason AP, McBay AJ. Cannabis: pharmacology and interpretation of effects. *J Forens Sci* 1985; 30(3): 615–31.
134. Nahas G, Latour C. The human toxicity of marijuana. *Med J Australia* 1992; 156: 495–7.
135. Rubin A, Lemberger L, Warrick P, Crabtree RE, Sullivan H, Rowe H, *et al*. Physiologic disposition of nabilone, a synthetic cannabinol derivative, in man. *Clin Pharmacol Therapeut* 1977; 22: 85–91.
136. Holford NH. Clinical pharmacokinetics of ethanol. *Clin Pharmacokinet* 1987; 13(5): 273–92.
137. Baselt RC. Disposition of alcohol in man. In: Garriott JC, ed. *Medicolegal aspects of alcohol*, 3rd edn. Tucson, Arizona: Lawyers and Judges Publishing; 1996. pp. 65–84.
138. Wilkinson PK. Pharmacokinetics of ethanol: a review. *Alcohol Clin Exp Res* 1980; 4(1): 6–21.
139. Aghajanian GK, Bing OHL. Persistance of lysergic acid diethylamide in the plasma of human subjects. *Clin Pharm Ther* 1964; 5: 611–14.
140. Upsall DG, Wailling DG. The determination of LSD in human plasma following oral administration. *Clin Chim Acta* 1972; 36: 67–73.
141. Wagner JG, Aghajanian GK, Bing OHL. Correlation of performance test scores with 'tissue concentration' of lysergic acid diethylamide in human subjects. *Clin Pharmacol Ther* 1968; 9: 635–8.
142. Paul BD, Smith ML. LSD – an overview on drug action and detection. *Forens Sci Rev* 1999; 11: 157–74.
143. Cook CE, Brine DR, Jeffcoat AR, Hill JM, Wall ME. Phencyclidine disposition after intravenous and oral doses. *Clin Pharmacol Ther* 1982; 31: 625–34.
144. Cook CE, Brine DR, Quin GD, Perez-Reyes M, DiGuiseppi SR. Phencyclidine and phenylcyclohexene disposition after smoking phencyclidine. *Clin Pharmacol Ther* 1982; 31: 635–41.
145. Burns RS, Lerner SE. Causes of phencyclidine-related deaths. *Clin Toxicol* 1978; 12: 463–81.
146. Grant IS, Nimmo WS, McNicol LR, Clements JA. Ketamine disposition in children and adults. *Br J Anaesth* 1983; 55(11): 1107–11.
146. Licata M, Pierini G, Popoli G. A fatal ketamine poisoning. *J Forens Sci* 1994; 39(5): 1314–20.
148. Moore KA, Kilbane EM, Jones R, Kunsman GW, Levine B, Smith M. Tissue distribution of ketamine in a mixed drug fatality. *J Forens Sci* 1997; 42(6): 1183–5.

149. Dalgarno PJ, Shewan D. Illicit use of ketamine in Scotland. *J Psychoactive Drugs* 1996; 28: 191–9.
150. White PF, Way WL, Trevor AJ. Ketamine – its pharmacology and therapeutic uses. *Anesthesiology* 1982; 56(2): 119–36.
151. Logan BK, Couper FJ. Determination of gamma-hydroxybutyrate (GHB) in biological specimens by gas chromatography-mass spectrometry. *J Anal Toxicol* 2000; 24: 1–7.

# Index

Entries are arranged in letter-by-letter alphabetical order. Page numbers in *italic* refer to figures and tables, those in **bold** indicate main discussion. *m* denotes a monograph.

absorption 22–3
   *see also under specific drugs/drug groups*
abstinence *see* withdrawal symptoms
abuse potential
   alcohol 297
   stimulants 79
6-acetylmorphine (6-AM) *228, 229*, 232, 233, 234, 251–2, 357
'ack ack' *see* smoking, heroin
ADD *see* attention deficit disorder
adenylate cyclase 197, 238
ADH *see* alcohol dehydrogenase
adinazolam *108*, 125, 126, 382*m*
adrenaline 52, 53
adrenoceptors 71, 74
adverse reactions 37
   *see also under specific drugs/drug groups*
AEME *see* anhydroecgonine methyl ester
agonists
   LSD 324
   opioid **222**, *223*, 238
agoraphobia 135, 143–4
AIDS chemotherapy 201
alcohol *see* ethanol/alcohol
alcohol dehydrogenase (ADH) 281, *282*, 295
   methanol metabolism 334
   nutritional status 285
   racial variations 283–4
aldehyde dehydrogenase 281, 283, 284
   inhibition 285
alfentanil *223*, 235, 242, 413*m*
alpidem *113*, 131
   *see also* imidazopyridines
alprazolam *108*, 109, 143–4, 145, 383*m*
   deaths 157
   in elderly 126
   in hair 159–60
   therapeutic uses 135
6-AM *see* 6-acetylmorphine
American Psychiatric Association 203
amfepramone *see* diethylpropion
'amotivational syndrome' 200

amphetamine 'binge' cycle 80
amphetamines 7, 50, **369–70***m*
   and alcohol 306
   case reports 93, 94, 95
   cut-off values 18
   effects
      cardiovascular 74
      CNS 75
      smooth muscle 74–5
   excretion 68–9
   half-life 67–8
   history 52–3
   mechanism of action 71
   oral absorption 63, 64
   production 4, 52, 56–7
   routes of adminstration 65
   street names 57
   structure and sources 55–7
   toxicology and pathology 84–8
   urine detection times 68–9
   urinary pH 67–8
amylobarbital 111, *112*, 410*m*
anaesthesia
   barbiturates 132
      thiopentone 111
   benzodiazepines 110, 142, 143
   cocaine 76
   ketamine 326, 327
   opioids 235, **242**, 255
      fentanyl 242, 247–8
analgesia
   cannabis 201–2
   opioid 231, 232, 238–9, **241**
anandamide 181, 197
anhydroecgonine methyl ester (AEME) 62
Antabuse 285, 307
antagonists
   LSD 324
   opioid **222**, *223*, 247
antibacterials 125, 285, 286, 307
antidiabetics 285, 307
antifungals 125, 285

**451**

# Index

antihistamines 7, 114
anxiety, treatment of 134–5
anxiolytics *see* benzodiazepines;
    sedatives/hypnotics
apnoea 142
appetite reduction *see* slimming tablets
arachidonic acid derivatives 181, 197
2-arachidonyl glycerol 181, 197
assays 17–18
ataxia 151–2
*Atropa belladonna* 53, 243
attention deficit disorder (ADD) 50, 77
azapirones (piperidinyl-piperazines) 111
  mechanism of action 132–3
  therapeutic uses 136–7
  *see also* buspirone

BAC *see* blood concentrations, alcohol
back calculation 26
  alcohol 359
  case reports
    alcohol 309–10
    cannabis (THC) 209–10
bacterial degradation of blood specimens
    10, 38–9
barbiturates 7
  and benzodiazepines 149
  deaths 157, *161*
  dependence 149
  half-life *119*
  mechanisms of action 132
  metabolism 120–1, *122*, 125–6
  pharmacokinetics in elderly 127
  side effects 146
  structure 111, *112*
  toxic reactions 157
  in treatment of insomnia 135–6
BD *see* 1,4-butanediol
behavioural aggression
  benzodiazepines 143–5
    case reports 164
  opioids 244
  *see also* violence
behavioural changes
  as adverse reactions 37
  alcohol 292
  cannabis 198–9
benzodiazepines 6–7, **104–75**
  absorption 116–17
  bioavailability 116–17
  case reports 163–5, 362–3
  chemical instability 38
  classification 110–11
  in clinical forensic settings 351–3
  cut-off values 18
  dependence 147–9
  driving skills *see* motor vehicle drivers

drug interactions 31–2, 124–6, 147, 247–8
  alcohol 289, **305–6**
  opioids 244
duration of action 123–4
effects
  behavioural aggression 143–5
  cardiovascular system 143, 152
  memory and cognitive functions 142
  nervous system 141
  respiration 142–3
  sexual behaviour 145–6
excretion 121–3
half-life 110–11, 117, *118*
intravenous administration 151, 157
lipid solubility 30, **123–4**
mechanism of action 130–2
medical uses **134–6**, 351
metabolism 119, *120*
  enzyme systems 121
non-medical use 138
overdose 152, 362–3
pharmacokinetics 126–8
postmortem changes 38–9
production 4
protein binding 30, 127, 128
routes of administration 116–17
structural features 105–10
therapeutic concentrations 138–9
tissue distribution 159–61
tolerance 147–9
toxic reactions to 151–7
benzoylecgonine 62, 66, 69, 90, 91
  alcohol effects 306
bile specimens 13
biliary excretion 28–9
  alcohol 303
  benzodiazepines 121, 159
  opioid metabolites 229–30
    morphine concentrations 11, 252
  PCP 328
bioavailability 22–3
  *see also under specific drugs/drug groups*
biochemical abnormalites, alcohol-induced
    294–5
bioconversion *see* metabolism
blood bourne infections 356
  AIDS chemotherapy 201
blood concentrations 29
  alcohol (BAC) 278–80, **302–3**, 357
    back calculation 279–80, 359
    CNS effects 292–3, 295
    elimination rates 282
    fatal 305, 306–7
    in forensic cases 300, 301
    ratios
      solid tissue 305
      synovial fluid 304

# Index

urine 304
    vitreous humour 304
    tolerance 298
benzodiazepines 138–9, 353
cannabis see under $\Delta^9$-tetrahydrocannabinol (THC)
LSD 323
normal and impaired clearance 32
opioids 357
    postmortem methadone 255–6
    postmortem propoxyphene 257
    toxic 258
oral administration 22
PCP 327, 328
postmortem changes 38–9
postmortem redistribution 39–41, 42
stimulants 62–5
blood loss and blood replacement effects 34–5, 302–3
blood specimens 9–10
'body packers' 342
bone marrow, alcohol concentrations 303
brain damage, chronic alcohol abuse 293, 298
brain haemorrhage, cocaine abuse 90
breastmilk 121–3, 236
breath analysis, alcohol **303**, 357, 358
bretazenil *108*, 131
bromazepam 111, 384*m*
brotizolam 385*m*
buprenorphine 224, 227, **254**, 413–14*m*
buspirone 7, 104, 113, 121, 406*m*
    dependence 149
    in elderly 146
    see also azapirones (piperidinyl-piperazines)
butane 333, 334
1,4-butanediol (BD) 329, 330
butorphanol 224, 414–15*m*

cancer
    alcohol-associated 295
    cannabis-associated 200
    opioid pharmacokinetics in sufferers 231
cannabinoids
    alternative sources 194–5
    endogeneous 178, 197
    synthetic 195
cannabis 6, **178–217**, 435–6*m*
    absorption 183–6
    active constituents and structure 180–1
    acute behavioural changes 198–9
    acute physiological effects 198
    -associated deaths 205–7
    bioavailability 183–6
    case reports 209–11
    chronic and adverse health effects 200–1
    in clinical forensic settings 353–4
    dependence 203–4

driving skills see motor vehicle accidents; motor vehicle drivers
    duration of action 189–94
    excretion 188–9
    historical aspects 179
    mechanisms of action 197
    medical uses 201–2
    metabolism and biological activity of metabolites 186–8
    prediction of time of ingestion 186
    production 4
    products 181
    species 179–80
    structures *180*
    synonyms 179
    tolerance 203
*Cannabis sativa* 179, 180–1, 194
carbohydrate deficient transferrin (CDT) 287
cardiac lesions, stimulant users 74, 86, 90
cardiovascular system
    alcohol 291, **293**, 294
    benzodiazepines 143, 152
    cannabis 198, 201
    opioids 243
    SFST observations 347
    stimulants
        amphetamine 74
        cocaine 76, 90
        non-amphetamine 89
*Catha edulis* 57
cathinone (khat) 57–8, 62, 65, 370*m*
CDT see carbohydrate deficient transferrin
central nervous system (CNS)
    alcohol
        effects 292–3
        mechanism of action 290–1
    amphetamines 75
    barbiturates 146
    benzodiazepines 141, 151–2
    cannabis 199, 207
    cocaine 76
    depressants 5
    opioids 243–4
    stimulants 5
cerebrospinal fluid 303
'chasing the dragon' see smoking, heroin
chemical instability 38
children
    attention deficit disorder (ADD) 50, 77
    clobazam and behavioural change 144
    pharmacokinetics in 34
        benzodiazepines 127
        opioids 230
    volatile substance abuse 334
chloral hydrate 7, *113*
chlordiazepoxide 386–7*m*

# Index

chronic interstitial pneumonia 90
cimetidine 124–5, 229, 286
*Claviceps purpurea* 323
clearance 25
clobazam 110, 141, 144, 387–8*m*
clonazepam 145, 146, 148, 388–9*m*
clorazepate 389–90*m*
CNS *see* central nervous system
*Coca erythroxylon* 7, 53, 58
cocaethylene 62, 91, 289, 306
cocaine 7, 50, 52, 380–1*m*
   and alcohol 62, 91, 289, **306**
   effects
      cardiovascular system 76
      CNS 76
      smooth muscle 76
   excretion 69
   half-life 68
   history 53–4, 82
   local anaesthetic activity 76
   mechanism of action 72
   metabolism 62
   postmortem redistribution 91
   routes of administration 66–7
      oral 62–3, 65
   structure and production 58
   toxicology and pathology 89–91
      case report 94–5
   urine detection times 69
codeine **235–6**, 242, 415–16*m*
   toxicity 254
cognitive function
   alcohol 292–3, 298
   benzodiazepines 142
   cannabis 199, 200
   hynotics/anxiolytics 146
   opioids 243, 244
coma 152, 330
   GHB, case report 332
commercial products
   alcohol content 277
   hemp 194–5
confirmation tests 17–18
   cut-off levels in urine 19
contamination of specimens
   blood 10, 38–9
   hair 14
   saliva 16
cough reflex, suppression of 242
'crack' 58
crime, drug-related 355
   *see also* violence
critically ill persons, pharmacokinetics in 33
   benzodiazepines 128
cross-tolerance
   barbiturates and benzodiazepines 149
   cannabis and alcohol 203

opioids 246
cut-off levels 17–18, *19*
cyclopyrrolones 112
   mechanism of action 132
   therapeutic uses 136
   *see also* zopiclone
CYP2D6 229, 235
CYP2E1 281
CYP3A 121
   inhibitors 125
   sedative substrates for *123*

date-rape 327, 329, 352
*Datura stramonium* 53, 243
dealkylation, opioids 227–9, 248
deaths
   alcohol 300–1, 305, 306–7
      and other drugs 305–6, *307*
   barbiturates 157, *161*
   benzodiazepines 104, **152–7**, *160*
   cannabis 205–7
   case reports
      cocaine 94–5
      flunitrazepam 165
   opioids 244, 253–8
      case reports 261–4
      *see also* heroin, deaths
   PCP 328
      case report 331
   risk of, in police custody 356
   sedatives *158*
   stimulants 83, 84–6
      cocaine 89–91
      non-amphetamine 88, 89
   sudden 2–3
dependence 36–7
   *see also under specific drugs/drug groups*
designer amphetamines 55–7, 60, 76
   MBDB 55, 56, 68–9
   MDA 64, 374–5*m*
   MDE 55–6, 91
   PMA 87, 91, 377–8*m*
   toxicology and pathology 84–7
   *see also* methylenedioxymethamphetamine (MDMA)
designer opioids 222, 255
dextromoramide **254**, 416–17*m*
dextropropoxyphene *see* propoxyphene
dezocine 417–18*m*
diabetic ketoacidosis 294, 298
diarrhoea 242
diazepam 390–1*m*
   bioavailability 116
   and cimetidine 125
   cognitive impairment 142
   deaths 157
   in hair 159–60

metabolism 119, 126
structure 106–7
tolerance 148
diethylpropion 7, 50, 55, 65, 371m
dihydrocodeine 255, 418–19m
disease states, pharmacokinetics in 33
see also under kidney disease; liver disease
disinhibition
  alcohol 292
  benzodiazepines 143, 144
    case report 164–5
    reversal 144–5
    sexual 145–6, 164
disulfiram (Antabuse) 285, 307
doctor shopping 355
  case report 360–2
dopamine
  amphetamine 71, 82
  cocaine 72, 82
  GHB 330
dose–response relationship 30, 348, 351, 354
driving under the influence see motor vehicle accidents; motor vehicle drivers
drug interactions 31–2
  cannabis 206
  opioids 229, 247–8
  see also under benzodiazepines; ethanol/alcohol
duration of action 29–31
  see also under specific drugs/drug groups
dysphoria 198–9

ecgonine methyl ester (EME) 62–3, 69, 91
ecstasy 56
  case report 94
  see also methylenedioxymethamphetamine (MDMA); p-methoxyamphetamine (PMA)
elderly
  pharmacokinetics in 32
    barbiturates 127
    benzodiazepines 126, 137
    opioids 230
    sedatives 126–7
  side effects of benzodiazepines 142, 144
embalming fluids 287
EME see ecgonine methyl ester
endocrine abnormalities, alcohol-induced 294–5
endogenous cannabinoids 178, 197
endogenous opioids 238, 244
endogogenous gamma-hydroxy butrate (GHB) 330
entero-hepatic recirculation 229–30
enzyme induction 32, 125–6, 286, 298
enzyme inhibition 197
  therapeutic drugs 31–2, 125, 229, 248, 285
enzyme systems
  alcohol 281, 298

benzodiazepines 121
opioids 229, 248
see also P450 enzymes
ephedrine 7, 54–5, 372m
  excretion 69
  and methcathinone 58
  oral absorption 64
epinephrine see adrenaline
ergot alkaloids 323
estazolam 391–2m
ethanol/alcohol 5–6, 274–320, 436–8m
  absorption 278–81
  abuse potential 297
  adverse reactions 297
  bioavailability 279
  cardiovascular effects 291, **293**, 294
  case reports 309–12, 364
  in clinical forensic settings 357–9
    case report 364
    prevalence 300–1
  clinical signs of intoxication 357–8
  CNS
    effects 292–3
    mechanisms 290–1
  collection artefacts 301
  content of beverages 276–7
  dependence 298
  drug interactions 285–6, 305–6, 307
    benzodiazepines 145, 147
    cannabis 203, 206
    cocaine 62, 91, 289, **306**
    opioids 244
  and drug pharmacokinetics 287–9
  duration of action 287
  excretion 281–2, 283
    and detection times 284–5
  gastrointestinal effects 293–4
  historical aspects and sources 276
  liver effects 293–4
  markers of consumption 286–7
  mechanisms of action 290–1
    peripheral nerves 291
  metabolism 281–4
    effect of age and gender 283
    effect of race 283–4
  pharmacological effects 292–5
  physical properties 275–6
  postmortem fermentation 301
  postmortem redistribution and diffusion 301–2
  structures 275
  therapeutic uses 295
  tissue concentrations 302–5
  tolerance 298
  toxicology and pathology 305–7
    acute 357–8
    chronic 358–9
  withdrawal symptoms 298, 359

# Index

ethyl glucuronide 281, **286**
ethylmorphine 223, 419–20*m*
etizolam 392–3*m*
euphoria 75, 198, 292
  medical use of opioids 241
excretion 28–9
  *see also under specific drugs/drug groups*
eye signs
  amphetamines 350
  benzodiazepines 352
  opioids 355
  PCP 327
  SFST observations 347

faecal excretion 28, 121, 188, 195
FAS *see* fetal alcohol syndrome
fatigue, case report 94
'fatty liver' 293–4
fenfluramine 7, 55, 67, 373*m*
  'fen-phen' 89
fentanyl 227, **235**, 421–2*m*
  anaesthesia 242, 247–8
  derivatives 222, 235
  drug interactions 247–8
  toxicity 255
fetal alcohol syndrome (FAS) 295
first-pass metabolism 22
flashbacks
  amphetamine 75
  cannabis 199
  LSD 324–5
flumazenil 108, 136
  as antidote to poisoning 144, 145, **152**, 352–3
flunitrazepam 138, 147–8, 151, 393–4*m*
  deaths 157, 306
    case report 165
  in forensic settings 351, 352
  in hair 159–60
flurazepam 157, 394–5*m*
flush reaction to alcohol 284, 293
food
  and alcohol effects 280
  hemp products in 194, 195
  ingestion of poppy seeds 259
  and opioid effects 244
  sources of alcohol 276
forensic practitioners
  interpretation of data 41–2
  opinions **348**, 351
  roles 340, 344, 354
  *see also* medical assessment
formalin 41
freebase
  cocaine 53
  heroin 233
Freud, S. 53–4, 80, 82
fructose 285

gamma-aminobutyric acid (GABA)
  barbiturates 132
  benzodiazepines 104, 130–1
  ethanol 290
  GHB 330
  sedatives 104, 132
gamma-glutamyl transferases (GGT) 287
gamma-hydroxy butrate (GHB) 4, **329–30**, 440–1*m*
  adverse reactions 329–30
  case reports 331–2
  excretion 329
  mechanism of action 330
  medical uses 329
  metabolism 329
  pharmacological actions 329–30
  street names 329
  tissue concentrations 329
  toxicity 330
gastric contents 11
gastrointestinal tract
  alcohol 293–4
  opioids 243
gender
  alcohol 283
  benzodiazepines 128
genetic differences and metabolism of opioids 229
genito-urinary system, opioid effects 243
GGT *see* gamma-glutamyl transferases (GGT)
GHB *see* gamma-hydroxy butrate (GHB)
glaucoma 201
glucuronidation 27
glucuronides 27
  alcohol 281, **286**
  cannabis (THC) 188
  opioid 229–32, 252
UPD-glucuronyl transferase 27, 281
glue sniffing 333, 334
G-protein coupling inhibition 197, 238

hair specimens 13–14
  benzodiazepines 159–60
half-life 25–7
  and duration of action 29–30
  *see also under specific drugs/drug groups*
hallucinogens 323–8
  production 4
  receptors 239
hashish 181
hash oil 181
health status **344**
hemp products 194–5
heroin 420–1*m*
  addicts in clinical forensic practice 355–7
  and benzodiazepine use 104
  and cannabis use 205
  chemical instability 38, 39

# Index

deaths 250–2
   case reports 261–3
   mechanisms 253
   urine specimens 10
pharmacokinetics 232–4
   intramuscular 234
   intravenous 232
   smoked 233–4
   snorted 234
production 221
street names 221
toxicology 249–53
history-taking 344, **345**
homicides, alcohol, case report 311
hospital admissions
   blood specimens 10
   see also medical emergencies
5-HT see 5-hydroxy tryptophan receptors;
   serotonin
hydrocodone 255, 422m
5-hydroxy tryptophan (5-HT) receptors 324
   5-HT$_{1A}$ 111, 132–3
   5-HT$_3$ 290
hyperthermia 76, 86, 87, 328
hypnotics see sedatives

imidazopyridines 112
   mechanism of action 132
   therapeutic uses 137
   see also zolipdem
insomnia, treatment of 135–6
International Narcotics Control Board (INCB) 3–4
intramuscular injection 23
   benzodiazepines 116–17
   heroin 234
intravenous injection 23
   benzodiazepines 151, 157, 351–2
   cocaine 67
   heroin **232**, *233*, 355
   methadone 236
   social and medical problems 344
isopropanol 275, 276, 301, 302

ketamine 326, 327, 439–40m
khat see cathinone
kidney
   alcohol effects 294
   cocaine effects 90
kidney disease
   pharmacokinetics in 33
      benzodiazepines 127–8
      opioids 230–1
   and rhabdomyolysis 75, 90

learning impairment see cognitive function;
   memory
levomethadyl acetate (LAAM) 423m

levorphanol 424m
lipid solubility 23, 25, 29–30
   benzodiazepines 30, **123–4**
   and obesity 33, 128
liver disease
   alcohol 286, 291, **293–4**
   pharmacokinetics in 33
      benzodiazepines 127
      opioids 230
liver specimens 11–13
*Lophophora williamsii* 57
loprazolam 108, 126, 395–6m
lorazepam 117, 143, 396–7m
   in hair 159–60
   pharmacokinetics 127–8
   in elderly 126
lung disease 200
   acute pulmonary oedema 241
lysergic acid diethylamide (LSD) **323–5**, 438m
   adverse reactions 325
   excretion 323–4
   mechanism of action 324–5
   metabolism 323–5
   pharmacological actions 324
   sources 323
   street names 323
   structures 323, *324*
   tissue concentrations 323–4
   toxicity 325

M6G see morphine 6-glucuronide
marijuana 181
   see also cannabis
maternal alcohol consumption 295
maternal drug use
   benzodiazepines 121–3
   cannabis 200
   methadone 236
   methamphetamine 87
MBDB 55, 56, 68–9
MDA see methylenedioxyamphetamine
MDE 55–6, 91
MDMA see methylenedioxymethamphetamine
medical assessment
   drug-affected drivers 341
   examination 345–7
      reasons for 341–3
   fitness for police interview 342, 352, 356
      case report 360
   health status 344
   history-taking 344, **345**
medical emergencies
   alcohol withdrawal 359
   overdose 342–3
      benzodiazepine 152, 362–3
      opioids 249–50, 355–6
      stimulants 351

# Index

medical treatment
  benzodiazepine withdrawal  353
  in custodial settings  342
  opioid withdrawal  356–7
medical uses
  benzodiazepines  **134–6**, 351
  cannabis  201–2
  GHB  329
  opioids  241–2
  stimulants  77, 349
memory
  alcohol  293
  benzodiazepines  142
  cannabis  200
  hypnotics/anxiolytics  146
MEOS *see* microsomal oxidizing system
meperidine *see* pethidine
mescaline  56, 57
metabolic interactions *see* drug interactions
metabolism
  first-pass  22
  phase 1 27, 28
  phase 2 27, 29
methadone  **236**, 424–5*m*
  half-life  227
  metabolism  228, 229
  postmortem redistribution  40
  tolerance  246
  toxicity  255–6
    case reports  263–4, 363–4
  treatment in custody  356, 357
methadone maintenance programmes (MMPs)  255–6
methamphetamine  50, 64, 375–6*m*
  excretion  68
  neurotoxicity  71
  oxblood  57
  -related deaths  87, 306
  routes of adminstration  65
  smoking  65, 74
methanol  **286–7**, 334
methcathinone  58
4-methylaminorex  58
methylecgonidine  62
methylenedioxyamphetamine (MDA)  64, 374–5*m*
  *see also* designer amphetamines
methylenedioxymethamphetamine (MDMA)  63, 64, 349, 373–4*m*
  excretion  68
  neurotoxicity  71
  pathology  87
  postmortem redistribution  91
  postmortem tissue concentrations  91
  *see also* designer amphetamines
methylphenidate  65, 77, 376–7*m*
metronidazole  285, 307

Michaelis–Menten kinetics  282
microsomal oxidizing system (MEOS)  281, 298
midazolam  108, 109, 397–8*m*
  cardiovascular effects  143
  in children  127
  cognitive function  142
  disinhibition  144, 145
  drug interactions  125, 247–8
  half-life  111, 128
  in obesity  128
  routes of administration  116–17
miosis *see* pupillary constriction
MMPs *see* methadone maintenance programmes
morphine  425–6*m*
  half-life  227
  metabolism  228
  pharmacokinetics  231–2
  postmortem blood concentrations  250–1
  postmortem urine concentrations  251–2
  production  4, 221
  *see also* opioids
morphine 6-glucuronide (M6G)  227, 228, 231, 232, 251–2
motor vehicle accidents
  alcohol  292–3
  cannabis  206–7
  case report  360–2
motor vehicle drivers
  assessment
    breath analysis  303, 357, 358
    *see also* Standardized Field Sobriety Test (SFST)
  benzodiazepines  141, 142, **146–7**, 352
    case report  163–4
  cannabis  199, 354
    case reports  209–11
  GHB, case report  331
  stimulants  80, 350
movement disorders  75
multiple-drug abuse  90, 250, 253
  case reports  261–3, 360–2
  hospital admissions  152
  intravenous drug addicts  351–2, 355

nabilone  **195**, 436*m*
NAD *see* nicotinamide adenine dinucleotide
naloxone  247, 249–50, 355–6
  and pentazocine  257
naltrexone  **236–7**, 244, 247
nasal decongestants  7, 77
nasal insufflation
  cocaine  23, 66, 67
  damage caused by  76
  heroin  227, 234
nausea and vomiting, opioids  242
neonates
  methamphetamine-related deaths  87

# Index

opioids
    medical use 241
    pharmacokinetics 230
neuroadaptation 36, 37
neuroleptic drugs 248, 325
neuropsychiatric diseases, chronic alcohol abuse 293
nicotinamide adenine dinucleotide (NAD) 281, 282, 285, 294–5
nitrazepam 126, 157, 398–9*m*
noradrenaline 52, 53
    amphetamines 71
    cocaine 72
nordazepam 159–60, 399–400*m*
norepinephrine *see* noradrenaline
nutritional status, alcohol 285, 293
nystagmus *see* eye signs

obesity, pharmacokinetics in 33–4
    benzodiazepines 128
one leg stand test 347
'on the nod' 355, 360
opioids 6, **220–71**
    absorption 225–7
    agonists **222**, 223
    agonists/antagonists, partial **222**, 224
    antagonists **222**, 223, 247
    bioavailability 225–7
    in clinical forensic settings 354–7
    dependence 246
    drug interactions 229, 247–8
        alcohol 306
        cannabis 201–2
    duration of action 227
    excretion 229–30
        ingestion of poppy seeds 259
    half-life 227
    mechanisms of action 238–40
    medical uses 241–2
    metabolism 227–9
        genetic differences 229
    non-medical uses 244
    overdose
        in custody 355–6
        hospital admission 249–50
    pharmacokinetics 230–1
        profiles 231–7
    receptors **238–9**, 241, 246, 258
    routes of adminstration 225–7
    side effects 242–4
    sources 221
    structural features 222–4
    therapeutic concentrations 244–5
    tolerance 246
    toxic concentrations 258
    toxicology and pathology 249–58
    urine profile, distinguishing sources from 258–9
    withdrawal symptoms 246–7
        treatment 356–7
oral absorption 22, *24*
overdose *see under* medical emergencies
oxazepam *106*, 119, 141, 157, 401*m*
    in hair 159–60
    in liver disease 127
    low dependence-producing liability 148
oxycodone 428–9*m*
oxymorphone 429–30*m*

P450 enzymes 27, *31*, 121, 281
    inhibitors and GHB 329
    opioids 229, 230
panic attacks 135, 143–4
*Papaver somniferum* 221
paranoia *see* psychoses
passive smoking, cannabis 194, 354
PCP *see* phencyclidine (PCP)
pentazocine 224, **257**, 430–1*m*
pentobarbital 111, *112*, 120–1, 411–12*m*
pethidine 230, 243, 355, 426–7*m*
    metabolism 228
peyote cactus 57
pharmacokinetics
    in children 34
    definition 22
    in disease states 33
    in elderly 32
    in obesity 33–4
    *see also under specific drugs/drug groups*
phencyclidine (PCP) **326–8**, 439*m*
    adverse reactions 327
    excretion 327
    mechanism of action 326–7
    metabolism 327
    pharmacological actions 327
    street names 326
    tissue concentrations 327
    toxicity 328
phentermine 7, 50, 55, 378–9*m*
    blood concentrations 63, 65, 67
    'fen-phen' 89
piperidinyl-piperazines *see* azapirones
p-methoxyamphetamine (PMA) 87, 91, 377–8*m*
    *see also* designer amphetamines
police 341, 344, 345
    fitness for interview with *see under* medical assessment
    risk of death in custody 356
poppy seeds 259
postmortem
    blood specimens 9–10

# Index

postmortem (*continued*)
  fermentation  301
  gastric contents  11
  interpretation of data  42
  metabolic changes  38–9
  putrefaction, case report  311–12
  redistribution  39–41, *42*
    stimulants  91
prazepam  401–2*m*
prevalence
  drug abuse in community  2, 3
  forensic cases
    alcohol  300–1
    cannabis (THC)  205
    stimulants  83
  sudden death  2–3
pro-drugs  22
  benzodiazepines  *106*, 109
  instability  38, 39
propoxyphene  257, 427–8*m*
protein binding  30
  benzodiazepines  124, 127, 128
pseudoephedrine  7, 54–5, 379–80*m*
  and methcathinone  58
  oral absorption  64
psychiatric assessment  351
psychiatric morbidity  344
psychoactive drugs
  classification  5
  manufacture and production  3–4
psychoses
  cannabis  199, **200–1**
  cocaine, case report  94–5
  ecstacy, case report  94
  PCP  327
  stimulants  79–80, 82
  *see also* flashbacks; violence
pulmonary hypertension  89
pulmonary oedema  241
pupillary constriction  **243**, 244, 355
  *see also* eye signs
putrefaction, case report  311–12
pyrazolopyrimidines  112

qat *see* cathinone (khat)
quality assurance  21
quazepam  124, 402–3*m*

race, alcohol metabolism  283–4
ranitidine  229, 286
rebound phenomenon
  benzodiazepines  148
  stimulants  82
receptors
  adrenoceptors  71, 74
  cannabanoid  178, 197
  opioid  **238–9**, 241, 246, 258
  *see also* dopamine; gamma-aminobutyric acid (GABA); 5-hydroxy tryptophan (5-HT) receptors
rectal administration  23
  benzodiazepines  117
  morphine  226
remifentanil  431–2*m*
reproductive system, cannabis  201
respiratory depression
  alcohol  293
  benzodiazepines  142–3
  opioids  **242**, 243–4, 253
  PCP  328
respiratory distress, neonatal  241
rhabdomyolysis  75, 76, 90, 328
rhinorrhoea  76, 246–7
Rohypnol *see* flunitrazepam
routes of administration  22–3
  *see also* smoking; *specific drug groups*

saliva specimens  15–16
  heroin  233–4
schizophrenia  200–1
screening tests  17–18
  occupational, case report  261
secobarbital  111, *112*, 410–11*m*
sedatives/hypnotics  6–7, 111–14, 136–7
  deaths  *158*, *160*, *161*
  half-life  *119*
  insomnia treatment  135
  mechanism of action  131
  metabolism  121, *122*
  pharmacokinetics in elderly  126–7
  *see also* benzodiazepines
serotonergic syndrome  137
serotonin (5-HT)
  alcohol  290
  azapirones (piperidinyl-piperazines)  111
  benzodiazepines  131–2
  cocaine  72
  LSD flashbacks  325
serotonin reuptake inhibitor antidepressants  41, 125, 293
  and azapirones (piperidinyl-piperazines)  137
  and LSD  325
  and methadone  236
sexual disinhibition, benzodiazepines  145–6
  case report  164–5
sexual fantasies, case report  164
SFST *see* Standardized Field Sobriety Test
side effects  37
sinsemilla  179, 181
slimming tablets  7, 52, 55, 75
smoking
  cannabis  183–6, 188
    passive  194, 354
    respiratory disease  200

460

# Index

cocaine 62, 66, 67
heroin 227, **233–4**
methamphetamine 65, 74
PCP 327
smooth muscle effects, stimulants 74–5, 76
'snorting' *see* nasal insufflation
solid organ specimens 11–13
  alcohol 305
solvents *see* volatile substances (VSA)
specimens 9–16
'speedball' 58
spinal cord, opioid receptors 238, 239, 242
Standardized Field Sobriety Test (SFST) 341, 346, *347*
  alcohol 358
  benzodiazepines 352
  cannabis 353
  opioids 355
  stimulants 350
stereoisomerism 54
stimulants **50–102**
  absorption 62–7
  abstinence 81–2
  abuse potential 79
  adverse reactions 79–80
  bioavailability 62–7
  case reports 93–5
  in clinical forensic settings 349–51
  dependence 81–2
  excretion 68–9
  half-life 67–8
  historical aspects 52–4
  legal 54–5
  mechanisms of action 71–3
  medical uses 77
  metabolism 60–2
  pharmacological actions 74–6
  postmortem redistribution 91
  postmortem tissue concentrations 91
  prevalence in forensic cases 83
  routes of administration 65–7
  structures and sources 54–8
  tolerance 80–1
  toxicology and pathology 84–91
  urine detection times 68–9
street names 344
  amphetamines 57
  cannabis 179
  GHB 329
  heroin 221
  LSD 323
  PCP 326
sulfentanil 235, 242, 432–3*m*
swallowed drugs 343
  'body packers' 342
sweat specimens 14–15
synovial fluid 304

temazepam 119, 126, 403–4*m*
  deaths 157
  in hair 159–60
  intravenous administration 151, 157
$\Delta^9$-tetrahydrocannabinol (THC) 6, 179–81, 435–6*m*
  blood concentrations 183–6, *190–1*, 203
  and duration of action 189, 198, *199*
  interpretation of data 207, 354
  case reports
    back calculation 209–10
    proof of cannabis use 209
  metabolites **186–8**
    carboxy-THC **184–5**, 186, 188, 189, *192–3*, 206–7, 354
    11-hydroxy-THC **185–6**, 189, 194
    urine detection times 188, 189, *192–3*, 194–5
  oral consumption 183, 189, 194, 195
  prevalence in forensic cases 205
  substances with THC-like activity 181
  *see also* cannabis
thienyldiazepines 109–10
thiopentone 120–1
tolerance 37
  *see also* cross-tolerance; *specific drugs/ drug groups*
toxicology **38–42**
tramadol 258, 433–4*m*
triazolam *108*, 111, 116, 404–5*m*
  drug interactions 125
tricyclic antidepressants 40, 137

ultrasonicating blender 12
uncertainty 19–21
urine analysis
  alcohol 304
  cannabis (THC metabolites) 186
  cut-off levels *18*, *19*
  opioids 229
    case report 261
    distinguishing sources 258–9
    heroin 357
    methadone 236
urine detection times
  alcohol 284–5
  cannabis (THC metabolites) 188, 189, *192–3*, 194–5
  codeine 235–6
  heroin 232
  LSD 323–4
  stimulants 68–9
  urinary pH 67–8
urine specimens 10

validation 18–21
violence
  alcohol 300–1

461

violence (*continued*)
    PCP, case report  331
    stimulants  80, 83, 350
        case reports  93
    *see also* behavioural aggression
vitreous humour  13
    alcohol  304
volatile substances (VSA)  **333–5**
    adverse reactions  334–5
    excretion  334
    mechanism and frequency of use  334
    metabolism  334
    pharmacological actions  334–5
    tissue concentration  334
    types  333–4
volume of distribution ($V_D$)  23–5
    and blood loss  35
    and postmortem redistribution  41
vomiting *see* nausea and vomiting

walk and turn test  346–7
water consumption
    with alcohol  294
    excessive  86
Widmark formula  279–80, 359
withdrawal symptoms  37
    alcohol  298, 359

benzodiazepines  148–9, 353
cannabis  204
GHB, case report  331–2
opioids  246–7
    treatment  356–7
stimulants  81–2
workplace, case reports  95, 261

zaleplon  7, 112, *113*, 146, 407*m*
    medical uses  137
    metabolism  121
    receptor affinity  104, 131
zolpidem  7, *113*, 146, 408–9*m*
    dependence  149
    in elderly  126–7
    in kidney disease  128
    metabolism  121
    receptor affinity  104, 131
    toxic reactions  157–9
    *see also* imidazopyridines
zopiclone  7, 104, *113*, 146, 407–8*m*
    and alcohol  147
    dependence  149
    metabolism  121, 125
    toxic reactions  159
    *see also* cyclopyrrlones